Sourcebook of Interactive Practice Exercises in Mental Health

Luciano L'Abate

Sourcebook of Interactive Practice Exercises in Mental Health

Springer

Luciano L'Abate
Georgia State University
Atlanta, GA 30345-3917
USA
llabate3@bellsouth.net

ISBN 978-1-4419-1353-1 e-ISBN 978-1-4419-1354-8
DOI 10.1007/978-1-4419-1354-8
Springer New York Dordrecht Heidelberg London

Printed on acid-free paper

Springer is part of Springer Science+Business Media (www.springer.com)

Dedication

To mental health professionals who want to practice in the twenty-first century.

Foreword

In olden days, when people were troubled they sought out a wise elder for counsel. Just talking about particular troublesome thoughts always seemed to help, regardless of the usefulness of the advice given. There has always seemed to be something magical about the simple relating and discussing of troublesome thoughts; perhaps it was just the reinforcement of "you are not alone" that provided the succor. And there was always the probability that the person listening would supply a new and different healing perspective or action. The various quests that people went on contained implied solutions to whatever their troublesome thoughts were. That expectation of finding answers was generally fulfilled.

Much later in our evolution, when writing materials became inexpensive and easily obtainable, the writing of personal thoughts and troublesome thoughts in diaries became a substitute mechanism for confronting troublesome thoughts and troubles. Again, the simple act of writing out these internal thoughts both concretized and externalized them. Those thoughts and feelings were no longer isolated within you. Somehow, when they were out there in that diary, they were more tractable and there was some surcease of the inner pain and turmoil. This was a personal sharing with a private and secret confidant.

Since Freud's time, face-to-face talk therapy has replaced wise elders and writing – in the age of experts, people needed to consult professional listeners. In a stroke of genius, Pennebaker found that simply writing for about 20 minutes/day about emotional troublesome thoughts had a significant beneficial effect. His discovery has led to the profusion of practice exercises, distance writing, and structured writing that has the potential of helping people with their troublesome thoughts via their own words. The designer of the practice exercise structures it to lead the writer through a well-thought-out series of questions and exercises, generally about a specific Troublesome thought. (Note that it is my bias to use the word *Troublesome thought* rather than the word *problem.*)

In this sourcebook, Professor L'Abate has provided a large number of well-thought-out practice exercises designed for both specific and general troublesome thoughts. In the first section the practice exercises are tied to specific diagnoses, such as those in the *Diagnostic and Statistical Manual of Mental Disorders* (DSM). The other sections include practice exercises for other areas, for dysfunctional and functional individuals, couples, and families. One of L'Abate's troublesome thoughts has always been to link therapeutic work to research, and his practice exercises provide a means of testing their usefulness to evaluate this link. By bringing together in one sourcebook all these practice exercises, he has made a major contribution to the field. This sourcebook will be a reference and an inspiration for further research. Perhaps the best way of proving this to yourself would be to pick a relevant practice exercise and just do it!

Rubin Battino, MS in Mental Health Counseling
Licensed Professional Clinical Counselor (Ohio)
Adjunct Professor of Human Services (Counseling)
Professor Emeritus of Chemistry
Wright State University

Acknowledgments

The Practice Exercises contained in this Sourcebook were produced from a variety of sources that constitute the basic building blocks for their contents. I am indebted to the sources listed below for providing, in some way, materials (lists of behaviors, items, factor analyses, symptoms, and syndromes) that compose these Practice Exercises. Every attempt was made to contact authors and publishers of the various sources used to produce these Practice Exercises. Their permissions were needed to publish Practice Exercises based on their materials (L'Abate, 2002). In spite of these attempts, some publishers forbid outright the use of their materials for Practice Exercises (obviously not produced here or anywhere else). Other responses ranged from absolutely no response, on one hand, to outrageous demands for what this author considered excessive payments well beyond his financial resources, on the other hand. Furthermore, some Practice Exercises are based on more than one source, requiring to request permission from them all, an impossible task because there was no way to allocate percentages of contribution to separate sources.

Consequently, once this initial attempt failed, I fell back on "fair use" laws (Elias, 1997; Stevens, 1997) to justify the uniform use of materials for a larger good, and that is, the expansion of inherently inert materials (tests, lists, etc.) to dynamic and interactive Practice Exercises. These Practice Exercises have the potential to intervene with populations that might not improve with talk but that could improve using programmed writing, as in Practice Exercises. These Practice Exercises expand the use of programmed distance writing past and expensive mental health services based mostly on talk interventions, requiring personal face-to-face talk-based contacts with a professional helper. The medium of programmed writing, through computers and the Internet, does reach people in need who may not be helped by talk but who, in addition to or, as a alternative or adjunct to talk, could use a different medium to improve their behaviors in ways that could not be obtained by talk alone. Even people who might improve with talk could obtain more lasting results if an additional medium of communication, such as distance writing, assigned as homework PEs is added to talk-based interventions (Kazantzis, Deane, Ronan, & L'Abate, 2005; Kazantzis & L'Abate, 2007; L'Abate (2002). I would like to thank the Copyeditor David Kaplan, the Project Manager Ragavia Ramakrishnan and SPi Global for the excellent job done.

Here are the sources, arranged by section, from which the practice exercise have been dervied.

Section 1. Self-help Practice Exercises for Individuals with Psychiatric Classification

Disorders of Internalization

Children and Youth

Anxiety: This practice exercise is based on the scale by the same name developed by Newcomer, Barenbaum, and Bryant (1994).

Anxiety Condition: This practice exercise is based on the work by Chorpita, Albano, and Barlow (1998).

Depression Condition: This practice exercise is based on the work by Chorpita, Albano, and Barlow (1998).

Fear Condition: This practice exercise is based on the work by Chorpita, Albano, and Barlow (1998).

Asperger Disorder: The list of symptoms used for this practice exercise was taken from the Diagnostic Statistical Manual for Mental Disorders-IV (DSM-IV). Washington, DC: American Psychiatric Association.

Depression: This practice exercise is based on the scale by the same name developed by Newcomer, Barenbaum, and Bryant (1994).

Post-Traumatic Stress: This practice exercise is based on the work of Anthony, Lonigan, and Hecht (1999).

Separation Anxiety: This practice exercise is based on the list of symptoms found in the Diagnostic Statistical Manual for Mental Disorders-IV (DSM-IV). Washington, DC: American Psychiatric Association.

Adults

Anxiety: The list of symptoms used for this practice exercise was taken from the Diagnostic Statistical Manual for Mental Disorders-IV (DSM-IV). Washington, DC: American Psychiatric Association.

Depressive Personality: This practice exercise is based on the research by Hartlage, Arduino, and Alloy (1998) about depressive characteristics.

Loneliness: Although loneliness is not a psychiatric dimension or category, this condition effects a great many people who suffer also from other conditions. One could say that loneliness is a concomitant of many psychiatric and non-psychiatric conditions, especially in youth. These are the reasons for including this practice exercise in this Section. This practice exercise was developed from the work of Hurtug, Audy, and

Cohen (1998) and of Peplau and Perlman (1982). A questionnaire found in Peplau and Perlman could be administered before and after completion of this practice exercise.

Phobias: This practice exercise was developed from the combined work of Levinson (1986) and Henley (1987).

Post-Traumatic Stress Disorder: This practice exercise is based on the factor analysis of research performed by King, Leskin, King, and Weathers (1998) as well as by Taylor, Koch, Koch, Crockett, & Passey (1998).

Procrastination: This practice exercise was derived from the work of Ferrari, Johnson, and McCown (1995).

Signs of Depression: This practice exercise was based on a variety of clinical and research sources.

Disruptive Developmental Disorders

Anger: This practice exercise is based on the factor analysis of Lahey, Frick, Loeber, Tannenbaum et al. (1990) and the work of Feindler (1995).

Conduct Disorder: The list of symptoms used for this practice exercise was taken from the Diagnostic Statistical Manual for Mental Disorders-IV (DSM-IV). Washington, DC: American Psychiatric Association.

Hyperactive/Attention Deficit: The list of symptoms used for this practice exercise was taken from the Diagnostic Statistical Manual for Mental Disorders-IV (DSM-IV). Washington, DC: American Psychiatric Association.

Juvenile Troublemaking: This practice exercise is based on the Child Troublemaking Scale developed by Lynam (1997).

Oppositional Defiant: The list of symptoms used for this practice exercise was taken from the Diagnostic Statistical Manual for Mental Disorders-IV (DSM-IV). Washington, DC: American Psychiatric Association.

Disorders of Externalization in Adults

Addendum to Social Training: This practice exercise is an elaboration of the original practice exercise on Social Training (L'Abate, 1992).

Anger Condition: This practice exercise is based on the work by Eckhardt and Deffenbacher (1995) and by Spielberger, Reheiser, and Sydeman (1995).

Hostility: This practice exercise is based on the work by Eckhardt and Deffenbacher (1995) and by Spielberger, Reheiser, and Sydeman (1995).

Agression: This practice exercise is based on the work by Eckhardt and Deffenbacher (1995) and by Spielberger, Reheiser, and Sydeman (1995).

Troublemaking: This practice exercise is based on the research by Kosson, Steuerwald, Forth, and Kirkhart (1997).

Severe Disorders

Mood Swings: The list of symptoms used for this practice exercise was taken from the Diagnostic Statistical Manual for Mental Disorders-IV (DSM-IV). Washington, DC: American Psychiatric Association.

Over-dependency: This practice exercise is based on a model of codependency developed by L'Abate and Harrison (1992), which is part of a relational theory of personality socialization and psychopathology in intimate relationships (L'Abate, 1997, 2005; L'Abate & Cusinato, 2007).

Severe Troublesome thoughts: The list of symptoms used for this practice exercise was taken from the Diagnostic Statistical Manual for Mental Disorders-IV (DSM-IV). Washington, DC: American Psychiatric Association.

Sexual Abuse: The contents of this practice exercise were taken from the vast literature on sexual abuse, with no single source being primary over others.

Section 2. Relational Self-help Practice Exercises for Conflicting Couples and Families

Children and Families

Bing Eating: This practice exercise was developed in collaboration with Monique Gray and published with her kind permission.

Divorce Adjustment in Children: This practice exercise was developed by Karin B. Jordan, Ph.D., and published here with her kind permission

Domestic Violence: This practice exercise was developed in collaboration with Fran Greenfield and published here with her kind permission.

Lying: This practice exercise was developed in collaboration with Maureen O'Toole and published here with her kind permission.

Shyness: This practice exercise was developed in collaboration with Sue Matthews and published Here with her kind permission.

Stealing: This practice exercise was developed in collaboration with Ernestine Williams and published here with her kind permission.

Temper Tantrums: This practice exercise is a substantial revision of a previously published practice exercise (L'Abate, 1992).

Time Out: This practice exercise is based on my clinical experience and one of the first Practice Exercises developed for children and their families.

Verbal Abuse: This practice exercise was developed from clinical experiences and considered as part of the Abusice-Apathetic style in relational competence theory (L'Abate, 2005; L'Abate & Cusinato, 2007).

Couples

A practice exercise for a structured interview: This practice exercise is derived from a structured interview derived from the 16 models of relational competence theory (L'Abate, 2005, 20006; 2008a; L'Abate & Cusinato, 2007; L'Abate & De Giacomo, 2003).

Arguing or Fighting: This practice exercise was developed from clinical experience and is based on a model of paradoxical psychotherapy presented by Weeks and L'Abate (1982; L'Abate, 2002, pp.124–125).

Complaints: This practice exercise is based on the research by Coyne, Thompson, and Palmer (2003).

Depression: This practice exercise is based on relational model of depression developed by L'Abate (1986).

Difficulties: This practice exercise was developed jointly by Keith Stanford and Luciano L'Abate from Sanford's research (2004). The help of Dr. Sanford is gratefully acknowledged.

Sexuality: The contents of this practice exercise were taken from the vast literature on sexuality, with no primary source being more relevant than others.

Violence: This practice exercise is based on the research by Eckhardt, Barbour, and Davison (1998).

Families

Hurt Feelings: This practice exercise is based on a model developed 30 years after this construct was developed (L'Abate, 1977), evaluated (L'Abate, Frey, & Holly, 1979) and resurrected by the important research by Vangelisti and her students (Vangelisti, 2009; Vangelisti and Beck (2007) and a chapter in her handbook (2009b; L'Abate, 2009b).

Intimacy: This practice exercise is based on a relational model of intimacy developed by L'Abate (1986, 1997, 2005; L'Abate, Cusinato, Maino, Colesso, & Scilletta, 2010).

Negotiation: This practice exercise is based on a relational model of negotiation developed by L'Abate (1986, 1997, 2005).

When Parents Argue: From the Child's Eyes: This practice exercise was developed from the research by Weston, Boxer, and Heatherington (1998).

When Parents and Child Argue: From the Child's Eyes: This practice exercise was developed from the research by Weston, Boxer, and Heatherington (1998).

Section 3. Self-help Practice Exercises for Individual Life-long Learning

Character Strengths: This practice exercise is based on the work of Peterson and Seligman (2004).

Emotional Expression: This practice exercise is based on a list of feelings developed by Bonanno and Keltner (1997).

Development of Emotional Competence: The contents of this practice exercise were developed from a variety of sources (Averill, 1997; Bradley, 2000; Cacioppo & Gardner, 1999; Gottman, Faisilber, & Hooven. 1997; Kennedy-Moore & Watson, 1999; L'Abate, 2002, p. 116; Mascolo & Griffin, 1998).

Multiple Abilities: This practice exercise was developed from various theories of intelligence (Bodine & Crawford, 1999; Campbell, Campbell, & Dickinson, 1999; Fogarty & Bellanca, 1998; Gardner, 1999; Mayer & Salovey, 1995; Sternberg, 1996; Sternberg & Kaufman, 1998).

Normative Experiences: Form AB5C: This practice exercise is based on the work of Goldberg (1999) and published with his expressed permission.

Normative Experiences: Form IPIP: This practice exercise is based on the work of Goldberg (1999) and published with his expressed permission.

Normative Experiences: Form PSC: This practice exercise is based on the work of Goldberg (1999) and published with his expressed permission.

Priorities: This practice exercise is based on a relational model of priorities that is part of a contextual theory of personality socialization (L'Abate (1994, 1997, 2005, 2006; L'Abate & Cusinato, 2007; L'Abate & De Giacomo, 2003).

Self-awareness: This practice exercise is based on a model of relationships developed by Piero De Giacomo translated into English and expanded (L'Abate, 2002, pp. 117–118; L'Abate & De Giacomo, 2003)

Self- Others Importance: This practice exercise was developed from a Selfhood model that makes the attribution of importance to self and intimate others the cornerstone of intimate and non-intimate relationships (L'Abate, 1994, 1997, 2002, 2003, 2005, 2006; L'Abate & De Giacomo, 2003).

Social Skills: This practice exercise was developed from the Inventory by the same name developed by Lorr, Youniss, and Stefic (1991).

Speak UP For Yourself: This practice exercise is based on the need to help fearful or insecure partners express themselves assertively in their intimate relationships without anger or aggression.

Who Am I? Aspects of Identity Formation: This practice exercise is based on a relational model of identity-differentiation that is part of a contextual theory of personality socialization developed (L'Abate, 1994, 1997, 2002, 2003, 2005, 2006; L'Abate & Cusinato, 2007; L'Abate et al., 2010; L'Abate & De Giacomo, 2003).

Section 4. Relational Self-help Practice Exercises for Life-long Learning of Couples and Families

Couples

Premarital Preparation: This practice exercise was developed from clinical experience with couples, indicating the crucial importance of marital preparation for many to-be married or not yet married couples.

Relational Quality 1: This practice exercise was developed from the research by Hassebrauck and Fehr (2002).

Relational Quality 2: This practice exercise was developed from the research by Hassebrauck and Fehr (2002).

Relational Quality 3: This practice exercise was developed from the research by Hassebrauck and Fehr (2002).

Relational Styles: This practice exercise is based on the Elementary Pragmatic Model of relationships developed by De Giacomo (L'Abate & De Giacomo, 2003).

Sexual Motivation: This practice exercise was developed from the research by Schachner and Shaver (2004).

Families

Foster/Adoptive Care: This practice exercise was developed by Mario Cusinato after an extensive review of the literature on adoptive parenting and translated by L'Abate.

Planned Parenting: This practice exercise is based on a variety of models that compose a developmental, contextual theory of personality socialization and psychopathology (L'Abate (1994, 1997, 2002, 2003, 2005, 2006; L'Abate & Cusinato, 2007; L'Abate & De Giacomo, 2003).

Section 5. Self-help Practice Exercises from Lists and Single- and Multiple-score Tests

Children: Mixed Internalizing and Externalizing Disorders

School Conduct Problems: This practice exercise was developed from the work of Brown and Hammill (1978), Kelly (1990), Kelly and Vitali (1992), and more general sources Such as Hersen and Last (1990) and Mash and Barkley (1996).

School Social Skills: This practice exercise was developed from the work of Brown, Black, and Downs (1984).

Unusual or Troublesome Behavior: This practice exercise was developed from Aman and Singh's (undated) Checklist for Aberrant Behavior.

Adults

Butcher Treatment Planning: This practice exercise was developed from the scale developed by Butcher (1998; Perry & Butcher, 1999) to evaluate individuals who are resistant to psychotherapeutic interventions.

Single Score Tests

Axis II Cluster C Internalizing Disorders:

Beck Anxiety: This practice exercise was developed from research by Joiner, Steer, Beck, Schmidt, Rudd, and Catanzaro (1999).

Beck Depression: This practice exercise was developed from research by Dozois, Dobson, and Ahnberg (1998) and the review by Katz, Katz, and Shaw (1999).

Hamilton Anxiety: This practice exercise was developed from research of Moras, Di Nardo, and Barlow (1992).

Hamilton Depression: This practice exercise was developed from research of Moras, Di Nardo, and Barlow (1992).

Help-seeking (Dependent): This practice exercise is based on lists of attributes for personality disorders developed by Davis and Millon (1999, p. 517).

Self-suffering (Masochistic): This practice exercise is based on lists of attributes for personality disorders developed by Davis and Millon (1999, p. 517).

Serious (Depressed): This practice exercise is based on lists of attributes for personality disorders developed by Davis and Millon (1999, p. 517).

What Are My Troublesome thoughts?: This practice exercise was developed from Blatt's et al., (1982) two factor model of depression, dependency and self-criticism.

Axis II. Cluster B Selected Personality Disorders:

Anger Expression: This practice exercise was developed from the work of Forgays, Forgays, and Spielberger, (1997).

Compelling (Compulsive): This practice exercise is based on lists of attributes for personality disorders developed by Davis and Millon (1999, p. 517).

Distinct (Schizoid): This practice exercise is based on lists of attributes for personality disorders developed by Davis and Millon (1999, p. 517).

Exciting (Histrionic): This practice exercise is based on lists of attributes for personality disorders developed by Davis and Millon (1999, p. 517).

Non-conformist (Negativistic): This practice exercise is based on lists of attributes for personality disorders developed by Davis and Millon (1999, p. 517).

Private (Avoidant): This practice exercise is based on lists of attributes for personality disorders developed by Davis and Millon (1999, p. 517).

Self-interested (Narcissistic): This practice exercise is based on lists of attributes for personality disorders developed by Davis and Millon (1999, p. 517).

Unpopular (Antisocial): This practice exercise is based on lists of attributes for personality disorders developed by Davis and Millon (1999, p. 517).

Unusual (Sadistic): This practice exercise is based on lists of attributes for personality disorders developed by Davis and Millon (1999, p. 517).

Mixed Internalizing and Externalizing Disorders

Personality Disorders: Form 1989: This practice exercise was developed from research of Livesley, Jackson, and Schroeder (1989).

Personality Disorders: Form 1990: This practice exercise is derived from research of Clark (1990).

Personality Disorders: Form 1992: This practice exercise was developed from a factor analysis of Schroeder, Wormsworth, and Livesley (1992)

Multiple Score Tests

Personality Dimensions from the MMPI: This practice exercise was developed from the 15 Content Scales of the Minnesota Multiphasic Personality Inventory-2 (Greene & Anderson, 1999).

Personality Dimensions from Neuroticism Extraversion Openness Inventory: This practice exercise was developed from the work by McCrae (1994) and Costa (Costa & Widiger, 1994).

Personality Dimensions from Personality Assessment Inventory: This practice exercise was developed from the work of Morey (1999) and Morey and Henry (1994).

Couples

Improving Relationships: This practice exercise was developed by Brenda Whaley, Ph.D. (L'Abate, 2002, pp. 121–122) and published with her kind permission.

Relationship Conflict: This practice exercise was developed from Bodin's (1996) Relationship Conflict Inventory and is published with the kind permission of Dr. Bodin.

Couple Satisfaction: This practice exercise was developed from Snyder's Inventory by the same name (L'Abate, 2002, pp. 122–123; Snyder, 1981; Snyder & Aikman, 1999) and reprinted with the kind permission of Western Psychological Service.

Families

Profile Form: This practice exercise was developed from an instrument developed by L'Abate and Weinstein (1987) and validated by Kochalka and L'Abate (1997).

Functioning: This practice exercise was developed from the factor analysis of self-report measures by Bloom (1985).

Contents

1

Background: Recent Advances in Mental Health Interventions

The purpose of this sourcebook is to provide a widely encompassing set of written self-help practice exercises that cover a variety of individual and relational conditions. They can be used as alternative or additional resources in the promotion of mental health as well as in the prevention, psychotherapy, and rehabilitation of mental illness.

This chapter discusses the development of self-help mental health practice exercises within the wider context of evolutionary if not revolutionary advances in the field of mental health interventions. The field has expanded so rapidly during the last generation that its advances can no longer be ignored by mental health professionals. These interventions, therefore, represent the historical background for the use of self-help practice exercises within the field of mental health interventions.

Mental health interventions entail the following approaches: (1) health promotion and lifelong learning; (2) prevention of emotional and mental illness, usually through structured psychoeducational social skills training programs for people at risk of future breakdown; (3) unstructured face-to-face talk-based psychotherapy for people who have had a breakdown and need immediate and close professional help; and (4) rehabilitation of anyone who has had a breakdown and needs to be brought back up, so to speak, to functional levels of adjustment. These uses of interventions demonstrate how self-help practice exercises are embedded within an evolutionary historical background.

L. L'Abate, *Sourcebook of Interactive Practice Exercises in Mental Health*, DOI 10.1007/978-1-4419-1354-8_1,

Perhaps the major revolutionary step that is occurring in the mental health field right now because of these advances lies in helping needy and troubled people at a distance, that is, from a remote location, without ever seeing them face-to-face or even talking with them. For mental health professionals who doubt the validity of that conclusive statement, the following chapters will demonstrate how valid that conclusion may be.

Why, then, would these approaches be included here right at the beginning? This is a legitimate question that deserves a legitimate answer: "The reasons for including these approaches in this sourcebook are clear. Self-help practice exercises apply to and can be administered in all four approaches." Of course, this answer does not mean that a interactive practice exercise written for a severe disorder could or should be administered to a well-functioning individual, any more than a practice exercise written for such an individual should be administered to an individual with a serious psychiatric disturbance. The range of practice exercises in this sourcebook is such that, as the reader will see, it covers as many clinical and nonclinical conditions as is humanly possible, with inevitable overlaps with practice exercises produced elsewhere (L'Abate, 2004a).

Another way to present the evolutionary progress of practice exercises would enable us to perceive them as the natural hand-in-hand extension of these four approaches in mental health. Practice exercises did not develop in a practical vacuum. They are a natural development, a mental health technology, so to speak, to help troubled people with more effective and perhaps more efficacious ways than face-to-face talk. These practice exercises represent an additional and alternative way to address a wide range of mental health problems.

HEALTH PROMOTION AND LIFELONG LEARNING

This approach has been called also primary prevention in the sense that it is universal and would include the majority of well-functioning individuals, couples, and families. This approach is discussed at greater length in Chap. 5. Practice exercises related to more effective functioning and lifelong learning for individuals, couples, and families are contained in Sections III and IV (L'Abate & Goldstein, 2007). Conceivably, in addition to the control practice exercise in Appendix E, practice exercises in those two sections could also be used as controls for practice exercises administered in Sections I, II, and V.

PREVENTION OF EMOTIONAL AND MENTAL ILLNESS

This approach has been called also secondary prevention to the extent that it is directed toward at-risk, targeted, but not yet diagnosable populations, such as adult children of alcoholics. The literature about this approach is extensive; the interested reader can review this approach historically in L'Abate (1990, 2007b) and L'Abate (2008d), where a great many representative psychoeducational social skill training programs are included. Most practice exercises in Section I for individuals, Section II for couples and families, and Section V could be administered to targeted individuals, couples, and families who may not be diagnosable yet but who are still at risk for a possible breakdown.

PSYCHOTHERAPY

This approach has been called also tertiary prevention or crisis intervention, to the extent that is designed to help people with serious, critical, chronic, clinical, and diagnosable emotional and mental disturbances. The literature for this face-to-face talk-based approach is extensive. Practice exercises in Sections I, II, and V address participants who could use these practice exercises in addition to face-to-face talk-based psychotherapy and medication (L'Abate, 1986, 1990, 2001, 2002, 2004a, 2004b).

REHABILITATION

This approach is administered to people who need to recover after a breakdown and during and after hospitalization. The interested reader is referred elsewhere for up-to-date sources (Corrigan, Mueser, Bond, Drake, & Solomon, 2007; Corrigan, Wassel, & Rafacz, 2008). Mental health rehabilitation is a completely wide-open field for the administration of self-help mental health practice exercises in all five sections of this volume.

CONCLUSION

The recent advances in the four approaches considered in this chapter as composing mental health interventions are discussed in the following chapters.

2

Computers and the Internet

The use of the Internet implies an interactive involvement in the process of acquiring information. To retain such information and incorporate it in one's daily life, that information needs to be in writing, either in printed form for reception or in one's handwriting or typing for recording reactions and responses (Pulier, Mount, McMenamin, & Maheu, 2007). If the Internet is indeed the most revolutionary development in the last generation, the information it yields will need to be transferred to participant records and documentation. This approach has made it relatively easy to help people through distance writing (DW) without ever seeing them face-to-face or even talking with them.

Consequently, reliance on DW, as the next inevitable step in the evolution of mental health interventions from face-to-face talk-based, suggests possibly a completely different paradigm. Ultimately, in its extreme, this DW-based paradigm implies never seeing participants face-to-face or talking with them, as happens every day online. DW includes a variety of approaches discussed in great detail in Chap. 6.

The ever-increasing role of the Internet in providing information to help people in need of greater knowledge about their perceived troublesome conditions is a topic considered briefly by Norcross (2006). This topic is discussed in greater detail in Chap. 3. There are at least four self-help advances not considered by Norcross. These advances have significant implications for the evolutionary progress of mental health interventions

L. L'Abate, *Sourcebook of Interactive Practice Exercises in Mental Health*, DOI 10.1007/978-1-4419-1354-8_2,

because they are evidence-based rather than based on the subjective impressions or personal opinions of mental health professionals, let alone participants: (1) the advent of DW as an additional or alternative approach to traditional face-to-face talk-based interventions (see Chap. 6), (2) greater use of homework assignments to increase and widen the scope and effect of face-to-face talk-based interventions (see Chap. 4), (3) the meteoric growth of written self-help mental health practice exercises and source-books (see Chap. 7), and (4) the rise of low-cost approaches to promote physical and mental health (see Chap. 5).

All these approaches involve the use of writing, a skill that does cover the majority of the population including psychiatric participants who seem able to type on computers what they seem unable to express verbally (Bloom, 1992). For those who protest this limitation, that is, the exclusion of illiterate people from this approach, one needs to be reminded that most illiterates are also excluded from talk-based approaches. Furthermore, this population can be helped by taped recordings or by volunteers who translate the written instructions and transcribe the participant's responses.

CONCLUSION

The Internet will become one of the major avenues of service delivery in the mental health field. Thus, I developed a graduate curriculum for middle-level professionals to become experts in delivering structured self-help mental health practice exercises for individuals, couples, and families (L'Abate, 2008d).

3

The Self-Help Movement in Mental Health: From Passivity to Interactivity?

This chapter expands and updates Norcross's (2006) original proposal to integrate self-help within psychotherapy through reading self-help books and autobiographies, and viewing films. This relatively passive approach can be expanded with active and interactive mental health interventions (health promotion, prevention, psychotherapy, and rehabilitation) through (1) distance writing (DW) in its various approaches (see Chap. 6), (2) homework assignments (see Chap. 4), (3) low-cost approaches to promote physical and mental health (see Chap. 5), and (4) structured mental health practice exercises (see Chaps. 7 and 8). These new approaches suggest a paradigm shift in mental health from direct face-to-face talk-based interventions to DW approaches that may mean interacting with participants online without ever seeing them directly.

Norcross's (2006) excellent suggestions about integrating self-help into the psychotherapy process can and should be expanded to include also the other three specialties of mental health interventions already listed above (see Chap. 1): health promotion (see Chap. 5), prevention, psychotherapy, and rehabilitation (see Chaps. 7 and 8).

Even before the publication of Norcross's proposal, a great many evolutionary advances have occurred in the field of mental health that were not considered in his excellent article. Except for community interventions, health promotion, prevention, psychotherapy, and even rehabilitation have been traditionally based on the face-to-face talk-based paradigm of the last century. In this century, mental health interventions may be slowly

L. L'Abate, *Sourcebook of Interactive Practice Exercises in Mental Health*, DOI 10.1007/978-1-4419-1354-8_3,

but inevitably and inexorably changing into a DW paradigm in its many interactive forms (L'Abate, 2007d). This relatively new DW paradigm is based on the increasing use of the Internet, as Norcross notes in his proposal, and in recent advances in the use of homework assignments in prevention, psychotherapy, and rehabilitation, especially the growth of self-help sourcebooks or practice exercises, and low-cost approaches to promote physical and mental health, topics discussed in the chapters to follow.

THE PASSIVE-ACTIVE-INTERACTIVE DIMENSION IN SELF-HELP

In defining self-help, Norcross (2006) includes reading self-help books and autobiographies and viewing films related to a variety of clinical and nonclinical conditions. The lists he presents about these three approaches also include rankings by a large number of psychologists who use them in their professional practices. Norcross, however, did not report any evidence to support the ancillary use of these three approaches in psychotherapy. The failure to provide evidence for his proposal seems strangely contrary to the need to support professional practices with evidence rather than with just consensus or personal opinion. For instance, there were no baseline data to evaluate what kind of participants would benefit by which approach. Without such information it would be impossible to evaluate the outcome of such approaches.

Nonetheless, Norcross's 16 practical suggestions to integrate self-help into psychotherapy are right on target and should be heeded by mental health professionals who use or plan to use self-help information and materials in their clinical, community, and preventive practices. (The interested reader can refer to Norcross's original article to review his 16 suggestions.)

Consequently, we are in Norcross's debt for providing an ample and distinct background for this expansion and updating of self-help approaches. He provides a completely thorough review of the literature, with a full-scale rationale for the introduction of self-help approaches in mental health interventions.

Instead of conceiving of self-help as connected solely to psychotherapy, however, self-help could and should be conceived of as forming a tier of interventions with characteristics of its own, independent of traditional mental health interventions. These characteristics may run hand in hand along a continuum of community and prevention approaches consisting of universal primary, targeted secondary, and tertiary prevention (Harwood & L'Abate, 2010; Mrazek & Haggerty, 1994), and already introduced in Chap. 1.

Consequently, self-help interventions can stand alone, depending, for instance, on whether they are directed toward functional populations in health promotion or primary prevention, or toward at-risk semiclinical targeted populations, such as adult children of alcoholics in secondary prevention, or toward clinical populations in crisis in tertiary prevention or psychotherapy and rehabilitation.

The introduction of self-help approaches would produce and, it is hoped, obtain a synergistic outcome with combinations of these approaches. Self-help should be paired with traditional face-to-face talk-based mental health interventions. Nonetheless, self-help should be shown empirically to produce positive outcomes of its own, before coupling it with any mental health intervention, in community, primary, secondary, or tertiary prevention approaches and rehabilitation (Harwood & L'Abate, in press).

No matter how interesting and even absorbing the reading of self-help books and autobiographies and the viewing of films may be, they are all passive activities. They entail receptively experiencing input and processing throughput rather than the expressive output side of information processing. They do not demand an active or interactive involvement and investment on the part of readers and viewers. These activities perhaps may be valuable in the precontemplative and contemplative phases of any intervention, maybe encouraging potential participants to ask for professional help. During treatment, these passive activities may increase to an unknown degree participants' involvement in the process. However, this information about the outcome of these three assigned activities is missing in Norcross's proposal, a strange omission when the field of psychotherapy is totally immersed in the quest for evidence-based practices. As Norcross himself notes, there is no evidence that these activities perform a positive role in the outcome of psychotherapy, except for subjective therapist and perhaps participant satisfaction. However, no information or evidence for consumer satisfaction was given, let alone outcome. Satisfaction in and of itself does not account for the outcome of any intervention. It may be part of the process and may contribute to the variance of outcome, but it does not guarantee that participants' behavior has been changed significantly. Consequently, the evidence to support these three passive activities is either lacking or questionable. Can we do better?

The passive-receptive nature of reading self-help books, autobiographies, and viewing films, for instance, stands in stark contrast to the many studies about the level of active involvement required by therapists as well as by participants for change to occur. The level of activity on the part of therapists and of participants, for instance, predicts a more positive outcome. The greater the level of activity from both parties, the more positive will be the outcome (Bergin & Garfield, 1994; Hubble, Duncan, & Miller, 1999; Snyder & Ingram, 2000). One would suspect that the same outcome would be present in other types of mental health interventions not included in Norcross's review. Of course, it all depends on the type of activity we are talking about. Activity per se does not make for a positive outcome. It is important to specify the nature of the activity (positive-negative, frequency, duration, intensity, and satisfaction), how it is prescribed (face-to-face, talk-based, online, mail, fax, phone, etc.), how it is implemented and evaluated by both professionals and participants, and how it is received and used by participants.

Independently of the three approaches advocated by Norcross, which could be considered minimal and self-absorbing, there are some relatively new advances in the field of self-help that require the active and even interactive involvement of participants in mental health interventions.

Table 3.1 A classification of the self-help movement in mental health

I. New advances in mental health interventions
   A. Advent of the Internet and distance writing: working at a distance from participants (see Chap. 6)
   B. Advent of homework assignments in psychotherapy: increase in psychotherapeutic directiveness (see Chap. 4)
   C. Advent of low-cost approaches to promote physical and mental health (see Chap. 5)
   D. Conclusion: a new paradigm for psychotherapy?

II. Self-support approaches: initiated and maintained by participants
   A. Nutrition and diets
   B. Exercise
   C. Self-support face-to-face groups
   D. Self-support groups online
   E. Self-help books (popular psychology)

III. Self-help approaches: initiated, administered, guided, maintained, and monitored by professionals for participants
   A. Bibliotherapy
   B. Distance writing (see Chap. 6)
   C. Online therapy
   D. Manuals for practitioners (Muller, Rego, & Sanderson, 2008)
   E. Miscellaneous (movies, videos, popular psychology books)
   F. Self-help approaches for specific conditions: anxieties, depressions, eating disorders, addictions, personality disorders, severe psychopathology, medical conditions

Adapted from Harwood and L'Abate (2010)

As introduced in the previous chapters and discussed in greater detail in the following chapters, these advances were not considered in Norcross's otherwise interesting and important proposal. These advances require an interactive involvement by participants to become part of the process of change since they require participants to demonstrate their motivation to change with actions rather than solely with words (Bohart & Tallman, 1999). A list of most self-help approaches is included in Table 3.1. The major distinction made in this table involves whether these approaches are consumer-led or administered by professionals.

CONCLUSION

The self-help movement might allow a great many people to take control of their mental health in ways that were unconceivable a generation ago. This movement offers so many choices and opportunities for both consumers and professionals that it will be imperative to evaluate which self-help approach is more effective than other approaches. This is the reason why Harwood and L'Abate (in press) undertook to review the empirical evidence to support self-help practices with and without the presence and influence of mental health professionals.

4

Growth in the Use of the Between-Session Homework Assignments

The field of mental health technology is full of advertising from major publishing houses about handouts, sourcebooks, reproducible instructions, and materials that can be used by partcipants. These advertisements attest to the tremendous growth of between-session homework assignments in psychotherapy (Kazantzis, Deane, Ronan, & L'Abate, 2005; Kazantzis & L'Abate, 2007). The rationale for the use of these approaches is relatively simple. We need to make sure that whatever is learned in the professional's office transfers outside that setting into the home, school, or work. This process has been called "generalization." Consequently, any mental health intervention must fulfill two requirements: (1) generalization to the home/school/work settings, and (2) duration of positive changes above and beyond the immediacy of the help proffered.

A taxonomy of counseling goals and methods (Frey & Raming, 1979), based on content analyses and multivariate taxonomic procedures, for instance, produced seven goal clusters. The cluster most relevant to the advances in mental health interventions considered here was "transfer of therapy learning to outside situations." The other six clusters are still relevant to mental health interventions in general but not to this particular sourcebook. The primary goal of any mental health intervention, be it in the community, school, clinic, private office, or hospital, is to ensure that whatever positive behaviors or relationships are considered and discussed in those settings will generalize to home/school/work settings. In line with this goal, in the last few years the evidence in support of homework assignments to increase generalization from the office to the home has grown

L. L'Abate, *Sourcebook of Interactive Practice Exercises in Mental Health*, DOI 10.1007/978-1-4419-1354-8_4,

exponentially (Kazantzis et al., 2007). Administration of homework, for instance, may be minimal in nondirective and psychoanalytical psychotherapies, but it achieves much wider applications in most other psychotherapeutic approaches for a wide range of clinical conditions. The most relevant conclusion that can be made about homework assignments lies in their not yet having received systematic application. Many homework assignments seem to be administered helter-skelter, without clear plans or replicable prescriptive plans, as discussed below.

However, most homework assignments (Kazantzis et al., 2007; Kazantzis & L'Abate, 2007) rely in large part on written instructions, and in some cases require writing in practice exercises for partcipants. Thus far, homework assignments, in spite of their being used by many psychotherapeutic schools, as shown in Table 4.1, have not produced a model for their systematic administration, perhaps with the exception of Brown-Stanbridge's (1989) model that relies solely on verbal instructions rather than on writing. However, that model can be expanded by adding two modalities of intervention: writing and nonverbal (L'Abate, 2008d). Nonetheless, the potential for homework assignments in mental health interventions is immense and in need of being explored and exploited fully in research and practice (L'Abate, 2004b).

Table 4.1 Homework assignments in health promotion, prevention, psychotherapy, and rehabilitation

A. Schools of psychotherapy
1. Behavior approaches (Kazantzis et al., 2007)
2. Participant-centered
3. Cognitive
4. Emotion-focused
5. Interpersonal
6. Psychodynamic
7. Acceptance and commitment
8. Brief strategic family therapy
9. Personal constructs
B. Participant populations
1. Children and teenagers
2. Adults
3. Couples
4. Families
C. Specific problems
1. Borderline personality disorders
2. Chronic depression
3. Chronic pain
4. Eating disorders
5. Low self-esteem
6. Obsessions and compulsions
7. Psychosis
8. Sexual dysfunction
9. Substance abuse
10. Traumatic head injury

Adapted from Kazantzis & L'Abate, 2007

ISSUES IN THE ADMINISTRATION OF HOMEWORK ASSIGNMENTS

There are five issues that are relevant to the use of homework assignments, and even more relevant to the administration of written self-help practice exercises included in this sourcebook: (1) homework assigned ad hoc, (2) relationship to a theory or model, (3) verbally administered, or (4) administered in writing, and (5) resistance to homework assignments in the mental health professions (Kazantzis & L'Abate, 2007).

Ad-Hoc Assignments

These assignments are administered on the spurt of the moment and intuitively, by the whim and will of the professional. They may seem related to the problem at hand but are independent of theory or of any systematic therapeutic approach. This kind of assignments may be the most frequent in the practice of psychotherapy.

Relationship to a Theory or Model

Homework assignment can be independent of, related to, or derived from any theory or model. As shown in Table 4.1, most schools of psychotherapy do use homework assignments to one extent or another: none in nondirective therapy, some in psychodynamic therapy, and a great deal in cognitive-behavioral therapies. However, what is difficult to demonstrate in most cases is the relationship of these assignments to a theory or model. This relationship is even more difficult to demonstrate if assignments are administered and answered verbally. As will be discussed in greater detail in Chap. 7, and as was cited in the Acknowledgements, practice exercises can be classified according to their relationship with a model or a theory. Assignments can be completely independent of any theory or model, as in ad-hoc assignments, discussed above, that are based entirely on clinical experience and practice, as in the arguing and fighting in couples practice exercise (Section II). However, in the case of the practice exercises contained in this sourcebook, their written nature makes them automatically replicable from one professional to another and from one setting to another. In this way these practice exercises can be evaluated for their health promotional, preventive, psychotherapeutic, and rehabilitative impact.

Some practice exercises, on the other hand, are related to a model, as in the case of practice exercises derived from Blatt, Quinlan, Chevron, McDonald, and Zuroff, 1982), the two-factor model of depression, among others. Some practice exercises are directly derived from models composing relational competence theory (L'Abate, 2005, 2006; L'Abate & Cusinato, 2007; L'Abate & De Giacomo, 2003). In this latter fashion, then, practice exercises become direct instruments of validation for specific models of a theory, in a much more dynamic way to evaluate a theory than just through talking or through inert psychological tests. Examples of these practice exercises are a practice exercise from a structured interview (see Section II), intimacy and negotiation (see Section II), identity formation (see Section III), and planned parenting (see Section IV).

Verbally Administered Assignments

As can be readily seen from what has been written above, I do have a distinct bias toward talk-based interventions because they are so difficult to evaluate, as I have discussed in previous writings (L'Abate, 1991, 1992, 1999, 2001, 2002, 2004a, 2004b). Nevertheless, there is no question that many mental health professionals persist in this practice, perhaps because it might emphasize their importance, creativity, intuition, and autonomy. This is why the field of psychotherapy can be considered as a chaotic Tower of Babel, with each practitioner having his or her idiosyncratic way without regard to scientific or even professional standards (L'Abate, 2007d).

Assignments Administered in Writing

This is a preferred way to administer assignments because in this fashion it is possible to evaluate whether assignments were completed and, if completed, how well they were completed (L'Abate et al., 2005). Talk-based instructions can be forgotten, distorted, or produce conflicting memories in multirelational partcipants, such as couples, families, or groups. Hence, completion or noncompletion of written homework assignments becomes a much more direct way to evaluate motivation to change in partcipants rather than just talk.

Resistance to Administration of Homework Assignments in the Mental Health Profession

Just as completion or noncompletion of homework assignments is one way to evaluate motivation to change in partcipants, the same could be said of mental health professionals who avoid using DW and the administration of homework assignments. It is a question of whether those professionals want to update their practices to enter the twenty-first century or want remain in the past century (L'Abate, 1997a, 1997b, 1999). Whether these professionals like it or not, DW will be the preferred medium of communicating and healing in mental health interventions if not in the present very likely in the near future.

CONCLUSION

If the goal of mental health interventions is to ensure and increase the generalization of positive behaviors from professional offices to the partcipants' homes, schools, and work settings, then this outcome is maximized by DW, administration of homework assignments, written practice exercises from self-help sourcebooks, and low-cost approaches to promote physical and mental health. These recent advances perhaps suggest a possibly different paradigm most appropriate to the mental health troublesome thoughts and practices of this century, namely, helping partcipants at a distance without ever seeing them.

5

Low-Cost Approaches to Promote Physical and Mental health

Another advance relevant to the evolution of self-help in mental health interventions lies in low-cost approaches to promote physical and mental health. These approaches are based on the substantial evidence of positive outcomes in survival and mortality rates derived from (1) nutrition (diet, omega fatty acids, vitamins, and supplements); (2) nonverbal activities (relaxation, meditation, exercise, expressive movement such as dancing, and pleasant activities, such as gardening, playing cards, hobbies, etc.) (L'Abate, in press-b); (3) various types of writing (see Chap. 6); (4) close physical nonerotic contacts (massage, affection, hugging, holding, huddling, cuddling, etc.); and (5) relational bonds (friendships, social support, animal companions, prayer, spirituality, etc.) (L'Abate, 2007b).

The major implication of these approaches lies in their requiring identification of levels and types of functionality for the appropriate administration of homework to strengthen average or even superior functioning in mental health interventions. The large sizes of populations in both primary and secondary prevention make face-to-face talk-based interventions unrealistic or impossible to implement. Identification of functional and semifunctional populations on the basis of voluntary participation or self-report paper-and-pencil tests may be difficult. Most psychological tests are designed to measure psychopathology and dysfunctionality, with

L. L'Abate, *Sourcebook of Interactive Practice Exercises in Mental Health*, DOI 10.1007/978-1-4419-1354-8_5,

little attention to the evaluation and specification of average or superior functioning. It is important, therefore, to discriminate level and type of functionality from actual positive behavior rather than from indirectly evaluated personality inventories.

Consequently, in line with the approaches listed above and in L'Abate (2008b, 2008d), a rating list was developed to assess positive activities for individuals, couples, and families. The contents of this rating list are in line with the positive psychology movement that emphasizes the positive rather than the negative aspects of life. This list has not been validated as yet, but it was presented in a replicable form that should allow distinguishing among levels of functioning. Responses to items in this list would allow development of a plan for helping individuals, couples, and families in more cost-effective ways than we have available at present. For instance, participants scoring within the most functional range, without a presenting reason for referral, could be administered any of the self-help activities listed above or in any of the nonclinical practice exercises in Sections III and IV of this sourcebook. Participants scoring in the middle range and presenting a reason for referral, such as adult children of alcoholics, could be administered targeted sourcebooks directed toward a specific conflict area. Participants scoring in the low range with a clinical reason for referral and in clear distress could be seen for face-to-face talk-based crisis-intervention psychotherapy and medication, and can be assigned practice exercises directly related to psychiatric diagnosis and the reason for referral. A more detailed proposal for an arithmetical model to evaluate intimate relationships can be found in L'Abate et al., (2010).

CONCLUSION

Low-cost approaches to promote physical and mental health constitute an inexpensive tier of their own within the field of self-help interventions that could be paired with other types of interventions to maximize synergistic outcomes.

6

Distance Writing and Its Applications

The use of distance writing (DW) in health promotion, prevention, psychotherapy, and rehabilitation has come of age in many ways (Esterling, L'Abate, Murray, & Pennebaker, 1999; L'Abate, 2007a, 2007c, 2007d; Lepore & Smyth, 2002), including autobiographies (Demetrio & Borgonovi, 2007), journaling and diaries (Levine & Calvanio, 2006), expressive writing or the Pennebaker paradigm (Kacewicz, Slatcher, & Pennebaker, 2007), and self-help mental health practice exercises (L'Abate & Goldstein, 2007). Writing has become even more important with the increasing use of the Internet (Pulier, Mount, McMenamin, & Maheu, 2007) and homework assignments in psychotherapy (Kazantzis, Deane, Ronan, & L'Abate, 2005; Kazantzis & L'Abate, 2007).

Consequently, given the high costs of psychiatric and psychological treatments, DW, rather than talking, will become the most cost-effective, mass-oriented, versatile form and vehicle of health promotion, illness prevention, treatment, and rehabilitation of emotional and mental disorders in the immediate future (L'Abate, 1992, 2001, 2002, 2008a, 2008b). When talk in psychological treatments is paired with practice exercises for homework or online administration (Kazantis & L'Abate, 2007) perhaps their efficacy might be increased.

Distance writing is a progressive step in the evolution of mental health interventions. This statement is made in an emphatic style that leaves no doubt where my biases lie. I have discussed the advantages and disadvantages of DW at length in previous publications that are cited here.

L. L'Abate, *Sourcebook of Interactive Practice Exercises in Mental Health*, DOI 10.1007/978-1-4419-1354-8_6,

Table 6.1 Classification of distance writing and written homework practice exercises

A.	Automatic writing is of questionable usefulness and in need of more controlled research before considering its use (Sweeney, in press)
B.	Dictionary-based writing to produce changes regardless of age, gender, educational, socioeconomic background and level or type of dysfunctionality (see Chap. 8)
C.	Expressive writing, as in Pennebaker's paradigm, which entails writing about hurts and traumas heretofore not discussed with others for 15 minutes a day for four consecutive days (Esterling et al., 1999; Kacewicz et al., 2007; Lepore & Smyth, 2002)
D.	Focused writing, as in autobiographies (Demetrio & Borgonovi, 2007).
E.	Guided writing, as in answering written questions, as illustrated in various practice exercises of this sourcebook
F.	Programmed writing, as in practice exercises for targeted clinical participants (children and teenagers, single individuals, couples, and families) and for nontargeted conditions for lifelong learning in nonclinical participants (L'Abate, 1986, 1990, 1991, 1992, 2001, 2002, 2004a, 2004b; L'Abate & De Giacomo, 2003; L'Abate & Goldstein, 2007)
G.	Open-ended writing, as in personal information gathered through diaries or journals (Levine & Calvanio, 2007)

Adapted from L'Abate (2004a)

Consequently, I shall limit this chapter to a list of various types of distance writing (Table 6.1); each type has its advantages and disadvantages (see cited references).

Programmed writing consists of sourcebooks or practice exercises administered as in-between therapy sessions homework assignments distinct from the other types of DW listed in Table 6.1. This approach includes prevention for individuals not diagnosed with any syndrome, such as high school and college students, or individuals at risk for becoming diagnosable, such as adult children of alcoholics, or as an additional way to add to the effectiveness of face-to-face talk-based individual, couple, or family therapy writing (Kazantzis & L'Abate, 2005; L'Abate, 2007a, 2007b, 2007c, 2007d).

CONCLUSION

The various types of DW indicate how a great deal of the information that is usually gathered verbally by professionals from participants can be obtained just as well in writing. This process would allow professionals to focus their expertise on more specific issues and important troublesome thoughts. These types of DW allow immediate documentation and may spare a great deal of expensive professional time.

7

The Role of Self-Help Practice Exercises in Mental Health Interventions

A parallel advance in the field of mental health, in line within the advent of DW and homework assignments, has been the growth of self-help mental health sourcebooks or practice exercises. The practice exercises entail participants doing DW and receiving verbal or written feedback from professionals (L'Abate, 1991, 1992, 2001, 2002, 2004a, 2004b, 2007a, 2007b, 2007c; L'Abate & Goldstein, 2007). Many practice exercises for individuals are based on, and derived directly from, lists of symptoms found in the *Diagnostic and Statistical Manual of Mental Disorders*, fourth edition (DSM-IV), as indicated in the Acknowledgments. Here is where the dictionary procedures listed in Table 6.1 come into being, which are discussed at greater length in Chap. 8.

EVALUATION AND SELF-HELP PRACTICE EXERCISES

Practice exercises in this sourcebook are the outcome of more than 20 years of work. I began to use (L'Abate, 1992) programmed writing in my clinical practice and research (L'Abate, 2004b; L'Abate, Boyce, Fraizer, & Russ, 1992; L'Abate, L'Abate, & Maino, 2005; Smyth & L'Abate, 2001). Many of the practice exercises in this sourcebook match evaluation instruments that make it possible to link treatment with evaluation in much more specific and documentable ways than talk-based psychotherapy alone

L. L'Abate, *Sourcebook of Interactive Practice Exercises in Mental Health*, DOI 10.1007/978-1-4419-1354-8_7,

permits. Not only do some practice exercises match evaluation instruments, but also, as will be shown below and in Chap. 8, it is very easy to convert evaluative instruments into practice exercises themselves.

For instance, Ben-Porath (1997) reviewed the use of personality assessment instruments in empirically guided treatment planning, summarizing a variety of reasons for the need to construct an entirely new kind of assessment instrument in order to prescribe treatment more accurately. This viewpoint parallels similar arguments made about the use of programmed writing in health promotion, prevention, psychotherapy, and rehabilitation (L'Abate, 1990, 1991, 1992, 1997a, 1997b, 1999), that as long as psychological treatment is based solely on talk, it will be very expensive to validate what therapists do or say or what they think they did or said. One would have to tape-record what was said in the therapy session, transcribe it, and eventually code it for classification. This process, although relevant and important, is limited to a handful of researchers who have the tenacity and motivation, not to mention grant money, to verify the validity of the therapeutic process and link it to an assessment instrument.

To support these arguments in favor of using writing as a much more specific way to intervene and to link evaluation with treatment, a variety of practice exercises that are isomorphic with their corresponding assessment instruments were developed. In addition to practice exercises derived from assessment inventories, practice exercises based on some of the most frequent reasons for clinical referral have been developed; these reasons for referral include anxiety, anger, codependency, sexual abuse, loneliness, procrastination, moodiness, and phobias. All these practice exercises point to the need to construct a new class of assessment instruments that are constructed to encompass not only the old standby criteria of diagnosis and prediction but also a third criterion – prescription (L'Abate, 1990, 1997a, 1997b, 1997c, 1999).

One such instrument, for example, is the Problems in Relationships Scale and Practice exercise. The scale is composed of 240 items to cover 20 dimensions of couple relationships matched with 20 practice exercises derived from the very same dimensions (L'Abate, 1992). The discrepancy score between partners correlates negatively and significantly with Spanier's Dyadic Adjustment Scale, among other tests (McMahan & L'Abate, 2001). From the profile produced by this instrument, therefore, it is possible to identify which areas of conflict are present in a couple, and to administer the appropriate practice exercise. How to arrive at this process is detailed in Chaps. 8 and 9. One can take any assessment instrument and develop from its items, dimensions, or profile a matching programmed practice exercise that can direct treatment in more specific ways that through face-to-face talk-based contacts. These practice exercises demonstrate that given any evaluated and even nonevaluated dimension, it is possible to develop a practice exercise with matching practice exercises for any area or dimension of assessment covered by any instrument (Ben-Porah, 1997; Butcher, 1998; Perry & Butcher, 1999). In this way, in addition to the three criteria of understanding, predicting, and controlling, the latter criterion of control can be achieved in a much more specific way through prescriptive practice exercises (L'Abate, 1990).

It is hoped that the practice exercises in this sourcebook will help in contributing a new and different aspect to face-to-face talk.

RESEARCH ON MENTAL HEALTH PRACTICE EXERCISES

A consistent attempt has been made to evaluate the clinical usefulness of self-help practice exercises from the very beginning of their development (L'Abate, 1977a; L'Abate et al., 1992). Reworked statistical evidence for various studies performed in my laboratory more than 30 years ago can be found in L'Abate (2004b). For instance, a more recent meta-analysis of six sourcebooks for physical health and 12 for mental health yielded effect sizes of 0.25 and 0.44, respectively (Smyth & L'Abate, 2001). These low and medium effect sizes, although not very high, must be considered within the context of their administration. These sourcebooks were administered to individuals or couples at a distance, with little if any contact with professionals, thus reducing costs of professional time to a minimum. The results from these administrations (L'Abate, 2004a; & 2004b) demonstrated that we can indeed change behavior and relationships at a distance without ever seeing or talking with participants face-to-face. Research on the outcome of a practice exercise administrated to incarcerated inmates is reported by Reed, McMahan, and L'Abate (2001) and McMahan and Arias (2004).

Additional research to support the use of practice exercises as self-help in psychotherapy was performed by L'Abate et al. (2005). In over 25 years of part-time private practice, this research divided individuals, couples, and families into two groups. One group received face-to-face talk-based therapy without practice exercises. The other group received self-help practice exercises involving DW as homework assignments in addition to face-to-face talk-based psychotherapy. On the basis of my frequent claims of cost-effectiveness made for self-help practice exercises, it was expected that the second group of participants would have a lower number of psychotherapy sessions. Results demonstrated this expectation to be completely incorrect. The second group had a significantly greater number of therapy sessions than the first group. On the other hand, a problem-solving sourcebook administered to women hospitalized with personality disorders in Buenos Aires showed a significantly shorter length of hospitalizations and lower remission rates for participants who completed the sourcebook (L'Abate & Goldstein, 2007).

These contradictory results indicate that it is important to evaluate the outcome of any intervention with and without sourcebooks, and to evaluate the sole effect of sourcebook administration without any other interventions, as was already performed (L'Abate, 2004b) but is in dire need of replication. Future evaluations need to include the nature (structure, contents, topic, etc.) of sourcebooks themselves, the setting where this administration is occurring (school, community center, clinic, outparticipant, hospital, etc.), and the type of problem addressed by a particular sourcebook.

For clinical or research purposes, in addition to an interview, participants should ideally receive a battery of objective tests, before and after the administration of a practice exercise. The purpose of these tests is

(1) to establish a baseline about the level functioning of participants before the administration of practice exercises, (2) to confirm or disconfirm diagnostic labels assigned to a particular participant that should match the practice exercise administered, and (3) to evaluate whether there was an improvement in the level of functioning after completion of a practice exercise.

A control/comparison practice exercise (Appendix E) was created for administration to participants who did not receive a clinical practice exercise but who were given psychiatric diagnoses similar to those in the experimental group. However, this control/comparison group needs to have the same criteria as the experimental group. In addition to similar diagnoses and demographic information (age, gender, socioeconomic status, and education), control/comparison participants should be required to write for specific periods of time (a minimum of 20 minutes to a maximum of 60 minutes) for each practice exercise, as do participants in the experimental group.

This control/comparison practice exercise, therefore, would match practice exercises administered to an experimental group by using the same medium (writing) and requiring the same amount of time spent in writing. However, it is different from clinical practice exercises in terms of its supposedly neutral content. The content of this practice exercise requires writing about seemingly impersonal topics or common topics without the emotional valence of practice exercises containing signs or symptoms of a disorder. "Supposedly neutral" is said advisedly, because it means that the neutrality of the content cannot be determined beforehand. Seemingly neutral topics for one participant may provoke extremely intense emotional response for someone else. Therefore, an attempt was made to select neutral topics for this control/comparison practice exercise. However, the neutrality of its contents cannot be guaranteed at this time. It needs to be determined.

These practice exercises, therefore, add a different perspective by treating any clinical and nonclinical condition with a matching intervention, after an objective evaluation is completed, by a paper-and-pencil, self-report test, rating sheet, or questionnaire.

FUNCTIONS OF SELF-HELP PRACTICE EXERCISES IN MENTAL HEALTH

These practice exercises can be administered as systematic structured interviews in traditional face-to-face talk-based psychotherapy, or can be done in between session as handouts, worksheets or sourcebooks, or practice exercises (Kazantzis & L'Abate, 2007). Each specific psychiatric disorder has a matching practice exercise with a set of practice exercises directly written for each symptom or sign of that disorder. In some cases, such as depression, there is more than one practice exercise that deals with the condition (L'Abate, 2002). This approach follows medical practice that for each illness there is one or more specific medication to treat it. Of course, it might take more than one practice exercise to treat many psychiatric disorders, given their multidimensional and comorbid nature, as shown in case studies presented in Chap. 9.

ETHICAL AND PROFESSIONAL TROUBLESOME THOUGHTS

To avoid any possible ethical and professional issues provoked by using any practice exercise, participants, or in the case of children, their close relatives or caregivers, should be cognizant of the possible troublesome thoughts that may arise from the administration of a practice exercise (L'Abate, 2001, 2002). Participants and guardians should sign an informed consent form. A sample of this form is found in Appendix A.

Practice exercises in Section I are based on the reason for referral being a psychiatric diagnosis assigned to participants by a responsible mental health professional from a list of symptoms composing that diagnosis. Other practice exercises in Section V are based on single- or multiple-score tests for disorders where different sources – self-report, paper-and-pencil tests – are used to reach a psychiatric classification and diagnosis (L'Abate, 2002).

ADVANTAGES OF SELF-HELP PRACTICE EXERCISES

The advantages of programmed self-help practice exercises as homework assignments have been touted from the beginning of their applications in mental health interventions (L'Abate, 1986, 1990, 1992, 2001, 2002, 2004b, 2007c, 2008, 2008b , L'Abate & Sweeny (in press)). Here is a list of at least eight possible advantages:

1. ***Cost-effectiveness***: The jury on this alleged advantage is still out. As L'Abate et al. (2005) found with participants in a private practice setting, administration of self-help practice exercises increased rather than decreased, as predicted, the number of face-to-face talk-based psychotherapy sessions with individuals, couples, and families. On the other hand, Goldstein (L'Abate & Goldstein, 2007) found a significant decrease in the number of days in a charity hospital in Buenos Aires for women with Cluster B and C personality disorders. Clearly, this is a basic advantage that needs a great deal of further research.
2. ***Documentation***: Self-help, written practice exercises of any kind, programmed or otherwise, answered by participants, serve as an ideal source of documentation, above and beyond what professionals may have recorded in their notes. This practice is well served in the case studies reported in Chap. 9.
3. ***Explicitness***: Especially programmed writing, more than other types of distance writing, expands on a confusing, vague, and threatening diagnostic label or superficial reason for referral. Matching a diagnosis or reason for referral with a treatment plan is the clearest way to help participants make sense of how evaluation leads directly to treatment. The treatment is isomorphic with evaluation in ways that would be difficult if not impossible to achieve verbally.
4. ***Interactivity***: Practice exercises involve participants in ways that would be impossible to do only with face-to-face talk-based interventions, allowing participants to become involved and take responsibility for the process of treatment and its possible outcome. The increased

involvement of participants may explain why they stayed longer in psychotherapy (L'Abate et al., 2005).

5. ***Mass-orientation***: Practice exercises can be administered to single individuals (children, teenagers, adults), couples, families, and groups of various sizes, including even Internet administration.
6. ***Specificity***: How can it more specific than to match a diagnosis or reason for referral with treatment? This is a kind of specificity that is difficult to demonstrate using face-to-face talk-based interventions.
7. ***Versatility***: Practice exercises can be administered as preparatory for interventions, during and after interventions, as adjunct additions, or as alternatives to face-to-face talk-based interventions in clinics, hospitals, jails (as shown in Chap. 9), schools, and private practice offices, through the mail, Internet, and faxes.
8. ***Verifiability***: By their very nature of being written and therefore reproducible ad infinitum, practice exercises can be evaluated easily for their alleged advantages and usefulness. However, their advantages should not blind us to their potential and possible dangers and disadvantages.

DANGERS AND DISADVANTAGES OF SELF-HELP PRACTICE EXERCISES

Like any interventions in mental health, practice exercises are not free of dangers and disadvantages, especially when administered irresponsibly, insensitively, or unprofessionally. Consequently, practice exercises must be administered after a full explanation of their functions are explained fully, and an informed consent form has been signed by participants (Appendix A), with a structured or unstructured interview (see practice exercise for a Structured Interview in Section II, L'Abate, 2007a), and administration of a battery of self-report, paper-and-pencil psychological questionnaire or tests (L'Abate, 2008d, in press-a).

Discovery or Uncovering of Thus Far Avoided and Undisclosed (Denied, Repressed, or Suppressed) Experiences, Feelings, and Traumas

A participant may ask for professional help for his anxiety. After a review of the origin, frequency, duration, rate, and intensity of the symptom (without administration of a test to measure anxiety or other symptoms or a signed informed consent form), the participant is administered an anxiety-related practice exercise. The practice exercise is completed but the participant reports that this approach did not help at all, and in fact it made him worst because now he feels that the professional is in cahoots with the federal government and the FBI. This example may be exaggerated. However, mental health professionals practicing with a nontraditional approach such as distance programmed writing need to consider the worst possible scenario and prepare for it. This is why it is so important to evaluate the symptom or reason for referral, the participant, as well as the participant's intimate and social network.

Mismatch Among Diagnosis, Evaluation, and Reason for Referral Possibly Originating from a Cavalier Administration of Practice Exercises

The administration of a particular practice exercise should be based on multiple sources: (1) symptom or reason for referral, (2) results from psychological tests, and (3) the participant's opinion. For instance, given the wide availability of different practice exercises to deal with the same symptom, such as anxiety, depression, or acting out, some information should be given to participants about the various choices they have available, especially when dealing with couples and families.

Failure to Assure Participants of the Importance of Confidentiality on the Part of the Mental Health Professional

In case there is any doubt about the veracity of distance communications between the professional and the participant or about the confidentiality of whatever is disclosed and discussed, there are two ways to be sure: use of a password, and use of encryption. These fail-safe ways apply also when the professional needs to be reassured that the individual, couple, or family that is communicating is the real one, and not someone else. When DW is concerned, the handwriting can be the best source of reassurance that the same participant was completing all assignments (see Chap. 9).

Avoidance of Possible Cheating from Participants, such as Having Someone Else Answer and Complete Homework Assignments

If a interactive practice exercise is administered through correspondence and regular mail, as in the case of two participants reported in Chap. 9, handwriting is the major clue to observe whether there have being changes on the part of participants. When a practice exercise is administered through the Internet, passwords and encryption can be used to ensure that the same person is responding to the professional.

Poorly Written Practice Exercises with Hortatory, Exhortatory, Verbose Attempts to Influence the Thinking and Behavior of Participants

Every attempt has been made to ensure that practice exercises will not brainwash, indoctrinate, or influence participants to think according to whoever originated the practice exercise. In other words, the practice exercise should be neutral in wording and in specific biases. Whether that is the case in these practice exercises is left to professionals and participants to judge. However, as shown in most case studies in Chap. 9, explanation and interpretation of behavior needs to follow some systematic framework such as relational competence theory (L'Abate, 2005; L'Abate & Cusinato, L'Abate et al., 2010).

Bias and Resistance of Mental Health Professionals Who Are Threatened by This New Technology that They Might Perceive as Possibly Encroaching on Their face-to-face talk-based Practice

I have written already (L'Abate, 1997b, 1999) about the paradox that mental health professions, who claim to be dedicated to help people change for the better, are the very ones who rigidly adhere to past practices that may be ineffective and nonefficacious, such as face-to-face talk-based psychotherapy. Eventually, new practices will be adopted when the livelihood of those professionals is endangered by competing, more cost-effective and efficacious practices.

STRUCTURE

With few exceptions, practice exercises in this sourcebook follow the same structured format. The first practice exercise asks participants to define a list of terms (signs, symptoms) about specific behaviors. Here the use of a dictionary or equivalent online information is strongly recommended (see Chap. 8). Each participant must also give two examples of the behavior, or rate terms given for each specific disorder. After completing definitions and examples or ratings (nomothetic step), participants are asked to rank-order all the terms they have just defined or rated according to how these terms apply to them (idiographic step). This rank-order is then used to administer practice exercises according to a standard format (Appendix B) that covers historical origin, frequency, rate, meaning, and context of each behavioral term (sign or symptom). A final feedback practice exercise allows participants to express how they feel about the practice exercises they completed (Appendix C). Some practice exercises for children and teenagers with a few changes could be also administered to adults.

Essentially, this Sourcebook allows mental health professionals to add to and augment their therapeutic armamentarium by including programmed DW and practice exercises as an additional alternative or supplementary medium of treatment and intervention for psychiatric disorders or human conditions.

ADMINISTRATION OF PRACTICE EXERCISES

Administration of practice exercises should take place after a therapeutic alliance has been formed and an informed consent form (Appendix A) has been signed by participants, or by caregivers in the case of a minor. This signed form represents the formal contract between professional helpers and participants.

Practice exercises must be administered one at a time with feedback from the professional after each one is completed. No practice exercise should be given in its totality to any participant because it might present too much information that would be difficult if not impossible to process without systematic feedback. As already noted, administration of practice exercises can take place face-to-face, when each practice exercise becomes a structured interview, or as between-session homework, or administered though the mail, fax, and or Internet after professional and ethical issues about online administration are discussed.

After completing the initial practice exercise, in some practice exercises there is a standard format practice exercise (Appendix B) that can be administered with the behavior, sign, or symptom to be discussed according to its developmental origin, frequency, duration, and intensity. These practice exercises cover the behaviors that have been rank-ordered, and they are administered in the sequence given in that rank-order. They are numbered according to the sequence given in the first practice exercise. In this way, as already noted, each practice exercise can be geared idiographically to the particular, stated rank-order given by a participant. If a professional strongly disagrees with that rank-order, negotiation between the participant and the professional about the rank-order may be necessary.

For instance, if a participant complains of being depressed, and has been assigned a psychiatric diagnosis by a physician, it may be useful to administer the Hamilton Depression Inventory. If indeed the participant's score on this instrument is within the clinical range, then discussion about completing written homework concerning depression in between face-to-face talk-based sessions may produce a positive response. After signing an informed consent form, the participant would be given the first practice exercise of the Beck Depression Inventory that asks the participant to define its items using a dictionary, to give two concrete examples, and to rank-order the items based on how much they apply to him- or herself. This completed practice exercise would be returned during the second face-to-face talk-based session with the therapist, who, after discussing the first practice exercise and other issues pertaining to the participant's depression, gives the participant a standard practice exercise with the sign of depression that the participant rank-ordered as applying to his depression the most. The same sequence is followed in future sessions.

Some practice exercises have their own concluding feedback form, and some do not. Hence, a standard feedback form to use with practice exercises that do not have one is available in Appendix B. Another feedback form for separate practice exercises is available in Appendix. An example of a concluding feedback form for practice exercises is available in Appendix D.

The order of administration of the practice exercises can be arranged in three different ways. One way would follow the rank-order given by the participant in the first practice exercise, as stated. Another way would follow a test profile administered beforehand, either from the most elevated score to the least elevated one or, vice versa, from the least to the most elevated score, depending on the nature of the test and the specific condition of a participant. A third alternative, especially if there is a large discrepancy between the participant's subjective rank-orders and the objective profile, would be to discuss this discrepancy with the participant and arrive at a compromised, negotiated order of administration.

Table 7.1 Classification of self-help practice exercises in mental health[a]

Composition of participants: singles (adults, children, teenagers), couples, families, groups
Reason for referral: troublesome thoughts, diagnoses, single versus dual or multiple problems, symptoms
Level and type of functionality: DSM-IV or reason for referral
Functional: no diagnosis
Externalizations: Axis II. Cluster B
Internalizations: Axis II. Cluster C
Severe: Axis I
Administration for a specific symptom versus general condition or lifelong learning
Symptom-free versus symptom-related and diagnosis-linked
Theory-derived, theory-related, theory-independent
Format: fixed (nomothetic); flexible (idiographic); or mixed (nomothetic and idiographic)
Style: linear versus circular (paradoxical)
Derivation: single versus multiple score tests, e.g., Beck Depression Inventory vs. Minnesota Multiphasic Personality Inventory.
Content: clinical addictions, affective disorders, Axis I and Axis II, Clusters A, B, and C

[a]Adapted from L'Abate (2002, 2004b), L'Abate and De Giacomo (2003)

CONTENTS OF PRACTICE EXERCISES

As detailed in Table 7.1, one level of classification of practice exercises includes a classification of practice exercises according to their content, a process present in the practice exercises of this sourcebook. Section I practice exercises match or are isomorphic with many major, supposedly nonoverlapping psychiatric disorders. Some other practice exercises are derived from the DSM-IV. Section II practice exercises cover a variety of conditions about relational conflicts in couples and families. Section III includes a variety of practice exercises that could provide lifelong learning for individuals. Section IV includes a variety of practice exercises that could provide lifelong learning for couples and families. Section V includes practice exercises derived from research-based lists of attributes or behaviors from single or multiple self-report, paper-and-pencil tests. These practice exercises could be used to bolster any psychiatric condition or diagnosis considered in Section I.

SECTION I: INDIVIDUALS WITH A DIAGNOSED OR DIAGNOSABLE PSYCHIATRIC CONDITION

This section contains practice exercises that are aligned with major, comorbid DSM-IV disorders, such as (1) disorders of internalization in children, teenagers, and adults; (2) disruptive developmental disorders; and (3) disorders of externalization in adults.

Disorders of Internalization (Axis II, Cluster C of DSM-IV)

This subsection contains practice exercises dealing with intra-psychic, internalizing behaviors rather than externalizing behaviors. Cluster C contains internalizing personality disorders. Cluster B contains externalizing personality disorders. Here the disorder is not expressed externally unless the paticipant discusses it with significant others or with a professional helper; such disorders include anxieties, depressions, and fears.

Disruptive Developmental Disorders

These disorders include impulsive anger, prolonged hostility, and frequent aggression.

Disorders of Externalization (Axis II, Cluster B of DSM-IV)

This subsection contains practice exercises dealing with disorders where Discharge stands for explosive, acting out behaviors, such as aggression, temper tantrums, and violence with a minimum of forethought or planning about the future consequences of their actions. Responsibility for their actions are ascribed to external sources ("The devil made me do it").

SECTION II: RELATIONAL PRACTICE EXERCISES FOR CONFLICTUAL COUPLES AND FAMILIES

This section contains practice exercises for (1) distressed or troubled children and their families, (2) couples, and (3) families that might be helped by learning more effective ways of getting along. Except for the divorce practice exercise, all the other practice exercises for children and families follow the same format of description, explanation, and prescription (Weeks & L'Abate, 1982). In contrast to the previous section, which was devoted to individuals, using an overall diagnostic classification loosely based on the DSM-IV, there is no equivalent classification for children, couples, and families (L'Abate, 2005, 2006). Practice exercises contained in this section cover as many possibly dysfunctionalities as possible. They can be administered as structured interviews prior to face-to-face talk-based prevention, psychotherapy, and rehabilitation, or alongside any of those approaches as between-session homework practice exercises, or after those approaches are terminated as additional ways of helping, based on DW rather than on talking.

SECTION III: PRACTICE EXERCISES FOR INDIVIDUAL LIFELONG LEARNING

The practice exercises contained in this section are different from those contained in the two preceding Sections, which contained practice exercises for clinical or conflictual personal or relational conditions. The practice exercises in this section, on the other hand, are oriented toward functional or normal individuals who have not been diagnosed with a psychiatric or clinical condition. Conceivably, the practice exercises in this section can be self-administered for the promotion of mental health and lifelong learning (L'Abate & Goldstein, 2007), perhaps preventing mental illness. They could be used also after termination of psychotherapy or even medication to provide "booster-shots" that would reinforce whatever gains have been obtained through face-to-face talk-based processes or medications. Under certain conditions, this process could conceivably occur without face-to-face contact with a professional helper but through the mail, fax, computer, and the Internet. In some cases, due to their repetitive nature, the standard practice exercises are found only in Appendix B. Furthermore, for research purposes, given the possibly emotional nature of the control practice exercise (Appendix E), the presumably neutral nature of many practice exercises in this section could allow them to be used as controls for practice exercises in Section I.

The details, rationale, and background for some of the practice exercises contained in this section have been described elsewhere (L'Abate, 2002). However, others have been added since then, and their background is acknowledged in Section I (L'Abate & Goldstein, 2007).

SECTION IV: RELATIONAL PRACTICE EXERCISES FOR LIFELONG LEARNING OF COUPLES AND FAMILIES

The practice exercises in this section are designed to improve the level of functioning of couples and families without a clinical or diagnosable disorder. Couples and families that have undergone and terminated psychotherapy or some form of prolonged face-to-face talk-based intervention might profit from doing these practice exercises, which would serve as "booster-shots" to avoid and prevent possible relapses by strengthening their resources. Furthermore, for research purposes, the presumably neutral nature of the contents of many practice exercises in this section makes them ideal as controls for the clinical couples or families of Section II.

Partners in couples or parents in families should receive their own separate copies of practice exercises to be completed separately. After completing their practice exercises separately, the partners or parents should be told to make appointments with each other at least 24 h ahead to compare, contrast, and discuss their answers to the practice exercises. They should also take notes of their discussion for their records and possibly discuss their answers and notes with the professional who is administering these practice exercises.

SECTION V: SELF-HELP PRACTICE EXERCISES FROM LISTS AND TESTS

This section includes practice exercises derived from lists of behaviors and from single- and multiple-score tests. Many practice exercises in the previous sections were based solely on research-derived lists of behaviors and other factor-analyzed characteristics, but not on current and widely used psychological tests. Many practice exercises in this section are based on or derived from the basic dimensions of a test, as in the case of multiple-score tests, or from items in single-score tests or lists developed from factor analyses or other research.

The links of self-help practice exercises, psychological tests, and treatment through programmed DW enables matching treatment with evaluation in ways that would be difficult if not impossible to achieve by talk alone. Furthermore, by asking participants to define each dimension or item and to give two examples of each, the large semantic gap between professionals and participants is decreased considerably (see Chap. 8). Once a stigmatizing and threatening term such as *depression* or *anxiety* is used by professionals, they have to explain verbally what that term means. By reading and defining each term that makes up a specific clinical Troublesome thought, participants could achieve a much better understanding of their ascribed diagnosis. They can also use a dictionary or online information to define items or dimensions, as expanded on in Chap. 8. That understanding would be difficult if not impossible to achieve when face-to-face communication between professionals and participants is based on talk alone (L'Abate, 2004b).

In addition, by then asking participants to rank-order items or dimensions according to how they apply specifically and differently to them, it is possible to administer subsequent written practice exercises according to a systematically idiographic rather than a nomothetic order. That systematic order is also difficult if not impossible to obtain verbally.

In the case of lists or items from factor-analytic research as well as items or dimensions from well-documented tests, it is possible to replicable, standard operating evaluations and interventions, as in the laboratory method that would be difficult if not impossible to replicate verbally (L'Abate, 2008d). The simple, written application of definitions, examples, and individual rank-orderings of items in otherwise statically and passively inert factor analyses or even psychological tests opens new vistas on how evaluation can be linked directly to DW interventions and the Internet (L'Abate, 1990).

The large number of tests available in the psychological marketplace with few if any clinical applications except evaluation could open the way to a dynamically active and interactive expansion with administration of new and as-yet-untreated or even unreachable populations of potential participants in ways that were difficult if not impossible to reach through talk alone. The heretofore passive and inert psychological tests turned into self-help practice exercises could become active and interactive ways to help functional and dysfunctional people in ways that would be difficult if not impossible to obtain through talk. Reliance on the written rather than on the spoken word may also decrease costs of face-to-face contacts between professionals and participants, adding an alternative medium that in the long run may be more cost-effective than face-to-face talk.

CONCLUSION

Self-help mental health practice exercises expand the health promotional, preventive, psychotherapeutic, and rehabilitative horizons of existing professional practices. The future is completely open to research and practice with clinical and nonclinical populations.

8

The Use of the Dictionary in Mental Health Interventions

This chapter expands on the use of the dictionary in the various mental health approaches discussed in the previous chapters. Many practice exercises in this sourcebook require the use of a dictionary. Therefore, it is important to proffer a rationale for this requirement, which is not yet based on sufficiently supported empirical evidence. Unfortunately, I have no data to support it, except for my clinical experience. Essentially, this proposal was the outcome of years of clinical work using programmed DW with individuals, couples, and families (L'Abate, 1986, 2008a, 2008b).

The seemingly preposterous thesis of this chapter might inevitably produce perplexity, puzzlement, and wonder in many mental health professionals. How can a dictionary be a vehicle of change? The aim of this chapter is to answer that very question from conceptual, practical, and clinical perspectives. The outlandish aspect of this proposal does not lie only in its title and thesis, but also in its being based on complete speculation and not on any kind of evidence, except for my limited clinical experience. Furthermore, the entirely undocumented and unproven nature of this proposal is completely inconsistent with my emphasis on clinical psychology as a laboratory science (L'Abate, 2008d). I cannot prove the thesis of this proposal because I am retired from both clinical practice and teaching. Consequently, I do not have available participants to evaluate its validity. Nonetheless, this proposal is proffered for evaluation by mental health professionals to judge whether the procedures presented here work for most participants (children, teenagers, single adults, couples, and families).

L. L'Abate, *Sourcebook of Interactive Practice Exercises in Mental Health*, DOI 10.1007/978-1-4419-1354-8_8,

THE FUNCTIONS OF A DICTIONARY

A dictionary is inexpensive and it provides valuable information. If a participant does not own one, a selection of dictionaries can be easily found online or in public or university libraries. Consequently, dictionaries (or equivalent information) are freely available to anybody who can read. Also, they are very easy to read because they use short sentences. Another advantage is that they force readers to think. Just by looking up a word, readers become actively involved in taking responsibility for their vocabulary and perhaps their thinking. Furthermore, dictionaries are completely free of partisan theories or models, unless the terms to be defined are related to a theoretical model or to a practical framework.

If words are basic to thought (Pinker, 2007), and if thought is basic to living, could learning more appropriate words improve one's thinking? A large vocabulary, in and of itself, does not guarantee more appropriate or functional behavior. Appropriate thinking is basic to more functional behavior (Bearson & Zimiles, 1986; Grieger & Grieger, 1982; Vetter, 1970). Appropriateness certainly cannot be determined by a large vocabulary. Some psychopathic and criminal personalities, for instance, may have large vocabularies, but their words are used to manipulate others. Hence, if these premises are correct, any improvement in verbal skills obtained through the use of a dictionary might improve one's thinking, but with provisos. Words in and of themselves are not enough. They are only the beginning of a process. With more appropriate and expanded thought processes, perhaps there could be an improvement in one's behavior. Whether these premises and provisos are correct remains to be seen.

FILLING THE SEMANTIC GAP BETWEEN THERAPISTS AND PARTICIPANTS

Information in a dictionary can perhaps fill the semantic gap between participants and mental health professionals. The therapeutic value of information can be expanded through homework assignments, DW, and self-help mental health practice exercises contained in this sourcebook (Kazantzis & L'Abate, 2007; L'Abate, in press-b).

One could argue that processes in mental health interventions are based on an exchange of information between mental health professionals and participants. Participants disclose painful events and feelings in their lives. Professionals acknowledge the importance of the disclosure by reciprocating with emotional or cognitive information, such as a reflection of the participant's feelings, a positive reframing of events, an interpretation of dysfunctional patterns, and suggestions and recommendations for more positive choices, among other approaches. This information, it is hoped, will move participants toward more functional ways of thinking, behaving, and relating to others. How accurate, empathic, and helpful the information is depends on whether participants can use it to improve their attitudes, feelings, thoughts, and relationships.

The amount and type of information exchanged between therapists and participants is increased by assigning homework, using DW (Kazantzis & L'Abate, 2005). A homework assignment could include asking participants to use the dictionary to define words that are relevant to a participant's Troublesome thoughts.

Mental health professionals are linguistically articulate individuals. Even if they do not talk much and limit themselves to a few well-chosen words or sentences in their practices, mental health professionals possess a wide vocabulary that is further augmented by professional jargon and scientific terms. Participants who are bright and literate may also possess a wide vocabulary equivalent or, in some instances, superior to the therapist's. However, in most cases, they may be unaware of self-defeating, destructive patterns. Consequently, their awareness of painful or self-defeating areas in their lives for which they are seeking help may be limited (Beltman & Nair, 2004). How can one's restricted awareness be expanded above and beyond whatever information is exchanged in a professional's office? Could the use of a dictionary as an initial homework assignment lead to a participant's increased awareness and, perhaps, to improved behavior? Here the emphasis is on "initial" because, admittedly and clearly, solely enlarging one's vocabulary in and of itself is not sufficient to increase one's awareness or improve behavior. However, looking up words in a dictionary, specifically to uncover their meanings and their experiential, cognitive, and behavioral connotations and implications related to individuals, couples, or families, may lead to widening one's awareness and perhaps improving one's behavior.

Participants with a limited understanding of their condition may be confronted with frightening diagnostic labels and esoteric terms whose meanings may not be fully understood. Could the use of a dictionary with words whose meanings closely define their plight, Troublesome thought, or condition lead participants toward a more articulate understanding of their condition? Would this understanding lead to more constructive relationships between individuals, couples, and entire families? Again, this is possible, provided the meaning of words encompasses past and present experiences and relationships.

In addition, participants may react negatively to their being diagnosed with a seemingly disparaging or derogatory label, such as depression, anxiety, or personality disorder. Furthermore, they may deny being an alcoholic or a drug addict, let alone as an abuser or sexual predator. Participants may also lack an internal dialogue, preventing them from understanding in more nuanced terms what it means to be diagnosed and labeled with a clinical condition. This dialogue may be developed by providing participants with more appropriate words related to their underlying Troublesome thoughts or conditions. Consider, for instance, alexithymic individuals with a restricted vocabulary of emotion-related words, limiting their awareness of feelings and emotions (Sifneos, 1973). How would these individuals define emotion-related words? How would the behavior of relatively inarticulate, acting-out, impulsive youngsters who are not thinking about the negative consequences of their actions be improved? Can an expanded and enriched vocabulary describing the consequences of their acting out lead to changes in their feelings and thinking and, perhaps, move them toward a more appropriate behavior? How about distressed couples that are unaware of their own repetitively reactive patterns in their relationship? Is there a way of making partners more aware of such patterns (L'Abate, in press)?

HOW THE DICTIONARY MAY BEGIN TO ENLARGE AWARENESS AND PERHAPS IMPROVE BEHAVIOR

Two examples of how the dictionary can initially be used to possibly expand awareness and improve behavior are self-help practice exercises and DW for distressed couples. In addition to the approaches listed in Table 6.1, one DW step in the process of acquiring and expressing information interactively lies in the use of the dictionary. Instead of receiving and answering a test instrument, such as the Beck Depression Inventory, which implies a diagnosis of depression, why not ask participants as homework to follow progressively these three steps? First, define in writing items in the Beck Depression Inventory (or any single-item test) using a dictionary. Second, give two examples of how each item applies to the participant's personal experience. Third, rank-order the items according to how they apply to the participant's experience with depression, going from extremely applicable to not applicable. Instead of a totally undifferentiated global diagnosis, now the term *depression* becomes more specific and unique to the participant's personal and individual experience. The first two steps are nomothetic. The third step is idiographic. Now depression becomes a more specific condition that is experienced uniquely by individual participants and not shared with anyone else. The same approach can be used with nonclinical instruments for individuals, couples, and families (L'Abate, 2007b).

Participants now define, give two examples, specify, and rank-order which behaviors, signs, or symptoms apply directly to them and are more applicable to themselves than other behaviors, signs, or symptoms. Standard practice exercises consequently are assigned according to the rank-order of behaviors, signs, or symptoms endorsed initially by participants. In this fashion, through programmed DW, it is possible to link evaluation or diagnosis with mental health interventions in ways that are difficult to replicate by talk alone.

SEQUENTIAL STEPS IN PRACTICE EXERCISE ADMINISTRATION

The procedure for administering self-help practice exercises with or without the dictionary in health promotion, prevention, psychotherapy, and rehabilitation is relatively simple and straightforward. Participants first sign an informed consent form. Completion of homework assignments is one way to evaluate motivation for change in participants. Whether the professional helper will accept participants who have not completed homework is left to the therapist's own discretion (Omer, 1985).

Step 1. The participant signs an informed consent form after the therapist explains the functions of these homework assignments, either verbally or in writing. Explanation of what is requested of participants, such as making appointments with self or others at specific times and places and frequency of homework, should be specified beforehand.

Step 2. Administration of (a) a single-item questionnaire, such as the Beck Depression Inventory; (b) a list of symptoms, such as those found in the *Diagnostic and Statistical Manual of Mental Disorders* (DSM-IV); (c) a list of behaviors obtained from readily available factor analyses; or (d) a list of content scales from multiple-scale tests, such as the content scales of the Minnesota Multiphasic Personality Inventory (see Section V). This step establishes a baseline for functioning and an objective way to assess the context of the reason for referral.

Step 3. Administration of items from instruments that are different from those administered to set a baseline of functioning and to evaluate degree and type of symptomatology. For instance, if the Beck Depression Inventory was administered beforehand, administer another single-item scale measuring depression, such as the Hamilton Depression Scale.

Step 4. Either verbally or in writing instruct participants that for between-session homework assignment they will need a dictionary to define all the items in the practice exercises and give two specific examples to indicate how that term applies to them. This is essentially a nomothetic assignment that may take more than 1 week to complete. However, if the explanation and rationale for its administration is sufficiently clear, participants who are motivated will complete this task in due time.

Step 5. After completion of definitions and examples, an extra copy of the answers should be made for the therapist's files and use and for the records of participants. They will need their answers to rank-order items according to how they apply specifically to themselves, an idiographic task. In couples and families, an appointment may be set up for partners or family members to arrive at a multirelational consensus on how items apply to individuals as well as to couples or families.

Step 6. After this rank-order is completed, the therapist would have available a more specific treatment plan than would be available verbally. The first rank-ordered item would then become grist for the therapeutic mill. If the item is sufficiently covered and resolved, either verbally or through a standard practice exercise, the therapist can move on to the second-ranked items, and so on.

CONSTRUCTION OF SELF-HELP PRACTICE EXERCISES

Many self-help mental health practice exercises in this volume are based on lists of items found in most common assessment tests or on factor analyses of behaviors, signs, and symptoms. These lists include practice exercises developed from, among others, the DSM-IV.

To summarize what has been presented above and what needs repeating here, one can take any list of items from a myriad of psychological tests, such as items in the Beck Depression Inventory, and expand those items to fit a written practice exercise or sourcebook with concomitant practice exercises. This outcome is obtained with a very simple procedure. Participants are asked to (1) define each item in writing (using a dictionary or online information), and (2) give two examples for each item. By defining and giving examples participants are now becoming aware of what a professional means by the label *depression*. After completing this nomothetic task, participants rank-order items according to how closely the items apply to them. Rank-ordering is an idiographic task because results vary from one participant to another, forcing them to prioritize and to determine which items are more important than others. Supposedly, the processes of defining, exemplifying, and prioritizing should increase an internal and relational dialogue.

Once this practice exercise is completed, another standard exercise is administered, based on the rank-order of each item. Thus, each term, behavior, or symptom in a list becomes the title in a sequence of standard practice exercises or sourcebooks. Each term in the title can expand upon the original definition by answering questions about the title's historical/developmental background, its nature, frequency, rate, intensity, direction, and functionality. The same procedure is followed for practice exercises that include lists of items for children, teenagers, couples, and families. With this simple procedure, evaluation leads also to intervention in ways that would be difficult to obtain through talk alone.

DESTRUCTIVELY REACTIVE PATTERNS IN COUPLES THERAPY

A second therapeutic application of an initial dictionary approach could be used in couples therapy (L'Abate, in press). It pertains to a list of single words describing destructive relationship patterns derived from Gottman's (1994) empirical work and from L'Abate's (L'Abate, 2005; L'Abate & Cusinato, 2007) theoretical/clinical models. Prior to seeing the therapist face-to-face, couples seeking couples therapy could be asked to complete a questionnaire of positive individual and relational activities. After this task is completed, the couple would be asked to define each single-word pattern, with the help of a dictionary, and to provide one example of each pattern. After rating those patterns for frequency and severity, the partners rank-order them according to which patterns are more destructive to their relationship. Based on this rank-order, therapists can develop treatment plans at a distance, using standard forms for practice exercises. Plans can be administered in writing or verbally, face to face. Again, as in the case with written practice exercises, words in a dictionary become the building blocks for change. Partners may become aware of their own destructive patterns, first through their definitions and examples, and second through their ratings of frequency, severity, and rank-order. The whole process, therefore, starts with definitions of words and an understanding of their personal and interpersonal meanings.

A FINAL NOTE ON HURT FEELINGS IN MENTAL HEALTH

Years ago I recommended that therapists should help participants approach those very hurt feelings they were spending their energies to avoid (L'Abate, 1977b, 1986). For that purpose, I created an intimacy sourcebook with three of six practice exercises devoted to help participants recognize, express, and discuss with relevant intimates whatever trauma or abuse or negative event had been experienced in the past and that they had avoided discussing with most intimates (see Section II). This avoidance was usually based on years of being rejected and discounted. Eventually, to help participants who were unable to express these feelings in writing, I developed an face-to-face exercise that allowed participants to get in touch with those feelings and to discuss them with loved ones. The verbatim instructions for this approach are available in L'Abate and Cusinato (2007, p. 325).

Since then, however, I become aware of how often I was asking participants to rely on the dictionary to complete practice exercises. The dictionary, therefore, is a way to approach what has been avoided perhaps for many years: feared hurt feelings and the memory of painful events. This approach is in keeping with the empirical evidence about exposing participants to feared stimuli or to painful memories: approach what you have avoided (L'Abate, 1984). The literature about the evidence for exposure therapy is so large that only three selected and already outdated references are cited (Dobson & Craig, 1998; Nathan & Gorman, 1998; Roth & Fonagy, 1996). Consequently, the dictionary becomes another avenue of repeated exposure to access avoided hurt feelings and memories of painful events.

The dictionary, however, has another function recently suggested by Pennebaker and Chung (2008). They proposed that writing words helps put into a digital perspective whatever unclear and undefined analogic experiences have occurred. This process was called "going from A to D." If this model is valid, it serves as a simple conceptual tool to help participants use the dictionary to go from an amorphous mass of unclear analogic states (repressed or suppressed, unconscious, conscious, or preconscious feelings and memories) to a more specific digital verbal or written states (De Giacomo, L'Abate, Pennebaker, & Rumbaugh, 2010). As Pinker (2007, p. 162) commented on this issue, reinforcing the conclusion of these authors, "language is not an analogue medium but a digital one." If this is the case, then this model would serve as an empirically based rationale for the use of the dictionary. A more recent practice exercise based on a wider definition of hurt feelings is available in Section II.

CONCLUSION

Unfortunately, this proposal by its very nature cannot be supported by empirical evidence or even by clinical experience, since it is based on guesswork and speculation from a variety of sources in my past, and not vast, clinical experience. No empirical support is as yet available to document the usefulness of the dictionary in widening awareness and perhaps changing behavior for the better. Since I am retired from academic and clinical pursuits, I no longer have willing participants available except for the inmates presented in the next chapter and those I saw in my part-time private practice years ago. More empirically minded and able colleagues might be able to produce evidence to either support or not support this proposal.

ACKNOWLEDGMENT

A previous version of the chapter was published in L'Abate (2007a). It is reprinted here with revisions from the original article with the kind permission of Deborah Cox, editor of *The Family Psychologist.*

9

Selected Case Studies for Sourcebook Sections

The selected case studies in this chapter are taken from our files of years ago, when Bess L. L'Abate and I started to introduce programmed writing and self-help practice exercises in our part-time private practice (L'Abate et al., 2005). (The three individuals presented below for Section I gave written permission.) A complete practice exercise of social training, designed to decrease impulsivity with pretreatment and posttreatment evaluation in an imprisoned individual, was reported in L'Abate (1992). No permission was obtained from the participants at the time because publication was not contemplated; thus, many studies reported in this chapter are composites of cases for Sections II and V, to make sure that no identification is possible. Few case studies can be presented for Sections III and IV because we were not able to administer written homework assignments to functional or semifunctional participants. Furthermore, many of the practice exercise in this volume had not been created then.

Nonetheless, one diagnostically questionable case is presented for Section IV, strictly for illustrative purposes. These cases are presented to demonstrate the process of programmed distance writing and not as proof of its effectiveness. This issue was covered in Chap. 7, which briefly presented past research with practice exercises. For a more detailed presentation of research conducted with programmed distant writing in the Family Study Center of Georgia State University more than 30 years ago, the interested reader is referred to (L'Abate 1977a) and (L'Abate 2004b).

Three caveats are necessary at the outset. First, tests used over 20 years ago were mostly monadic and not dyadic or multirelational, as were not available at the time. However, some recent couple or family

L. L'Abate, *Sourcebook of Interactive Practice Exercises in Mental Health*, DOI 10.1007/978-1-4419-1354-8_9,

evaluation instruments have minimal or no connection to theoretical models or theories. Therefore, throughout the last decade my Italian collaborators and I developed and validated a battery of paper-and-pencil self-report tests or tasks derived from models of relational competence theory (L'Abate, 2005; L'Abate & Cusinato, 2007).

Hence, years ago, our evaluation for most referrals was unsystematic and incomplete. I was still wrestling with the development of relational, multipersonal paper-and-pencil self-report tests that would derive from models of relational competence theory. We relied mostly on the Minnesota Multiphasic Personality Inventory-2 (MMPI-2) for screening and baseline purposes in spite of its strictly monadic orientation. Furthermore, our failure to make retesting at termination part of the initial informed consent form did not permit evaluating outcomes except through the number of sessions (L'Abate et al., 2005).

Second, many of the practice exercises included in this Sourcebook were not yet developed 20 years ago. Consequently, the repertory of practice exercises available up to the time that Bess L. L'Abate and I retired from part-time practice in 1998 was quite limited; the Arguing and Fighting practice exercise, for instance, was the most frequently used with couples and in some cases with families.

Third, no examples of actual responses to practice exercises could be given in this chapter because it would have been difficult to decide which one would be most illustrative and because it would make the chapter too long. Furthermore, little information could be derived from isolated examples of practice exercises. The letters included in some cases explain what is happening in the process of practice exercise assignment and completion. Consequently, we usually summarize the process, except where it is important to illustrate it through letters in response to completed practice exercises. The letters were written voluntarily, as in the second and third cases in Section I. Most letters indicate what kind of practice exercise was assigned.

SECTION I: SELF-HELP PRACTICE EXERCISES FOR PSYCHIATRIC CLASSIFICATION

The first participant who volunteered to enroll in a programmed distance writing practice exercise-based program administered through the mail was charged \$480, with \$160 refundable if he completed the program. This fee was paid by the participant's father who referred him and his grandmother, who was involved in his welfare. The second and third participants were helped pro bono, given the experimental nature of this approach and given the reality of their being inmates in state prisons without income or resources.

Even though it was difficult to assign a reliable psychiatric diagnosis to all three cases, the nature of the alleged crime in the first two participants and the admission of guilt from the third participant would indicate personality disorders, the first and third as Axis II Cluster B antisocial personality disorders, and the second as possibly Axis II Cluster C obsessive–compulsive personality disorder. All three participants had no prior criminal records and were jailed for the first time.

The criterion of only one single criminal occurrence and no previous record of criminality is an important one to keep in mind when administering practice exercises to inmates. This criterion is recommended for selection of potential participants in a distance-writing program. This recommendation is based on many failed attempts to apply this program to individual participants with multiple-crime records. In those cases participants might be better candidates for different kinds of practice exercises than those administered to these three participants, including those dealing with psychopathic conditions (Sections I and V). Nonetheless, more experience and evidence will be necessary to reach a more definitive conclusion about what kind of inmates or participants will benefit from what kind of practice exercise (McMahan & Arias, 2004; Reed, McMahan, & L'Abate, 2001).

Caution should be taken in administering these practice exercises to groups of participants at the same time, especially those groups in punitive institutions or with Cluster B personality disorders. In instances of this type, where discharge and externalization is the major characteristic, inmates tend to discuss the process among themselves, which minimizes the value of the process and the value of the test instruments, practice exercises, and trainers, producing much worse MMPI-2 profiles completed at the end of the process than at the beginning.

This process is predictable from the selfhood model of relational competence theory (Cusinato et al., 2008; L'Abate, 2005; L'Abate & Cusinato, 2007) that makes attribution and bestowal of importance the most important resource exchanged in intimate and non-intimate relationships (L'Abate et al., 2010). Cluster B personality disorders tend to devalue the importance of others to elevate self-importance. Consequently, the process of programmed distance writing with Cluster B personality disorders should be conducted on a one-to-one basis to avoid discussion with other inmates, which could be detrimental to the whole process and outcome. This model is described in greater detail below.

Cluster C personality disorders, on the other hand, in which delay and internalization are the major characteristics, tend to devalue self and elevate the importance of others, according to the selfhood model (described below). Outparticipant group therapy with Cluster C participants, where each participant receives a different practice exercise based on the diagnosis or referral reason, also may produce unsatisfactory results. Issues of confidentiality, among others, might get in the way, and a chaotic process would occur because each participant responds to a different practice exercise. It would be preferable if everybody in the group were to be administered the same practice exercise, as determined by the nature of the group, such as a group dedicated to dealing with anxiety, depression, past physical or sexual abuse, posttraumatic stress disorder, or other clinical or nonclinical conditions. In all instances, the informed consent form (Appendix A) should specify the reason for referral and how the practice exercise will be used.

An Impulsive Armed Robber

Tom, a 20-year-old inmate, was referred by both his father, who had participated in a previous face-to-face therapy program that included written homework practice exercises, and his uncle, who had participated with his wife and son in face-to-face psychotherapy combined with a distance writing program. Tom had been sentenced to 4 years in jail for armed robbery, accepting stolen property, and resisting arrest. The nature of this therapy program was explained to him in a letter. He was told that he would have to complete a test (MMPI-2) before the program was started and after the program was finished, and again some time after termination of the program. The program consisted of his completing written homework practice exercises through the mail. He would receive written feedback about each completed practice exercise.

Tom agreed (in writing) to these terms, and he took the first MMPI-2. As shown in Fig. 9.1, his score on the Psychopathic Deviate (Pd) scale reached the 90th percentile with above-average scores on the Schizophrenia (Sc) and Mania (Ma) scales. It took 1 year of discussion among his father, his mother (who was divorced from his father), and his paternal grandmother to clarify the nature of this program.

Letter 9.1

January 28, 1989

Social Training
Atlanta, Georgia 30345

Dear Tom,

I am sorry it took such a long time to get back to you to start the social training program. I was forced to wait until we squared away a few details with your folks. Your father paid $480 for this program. If and when you finish (including testing right after completion and 3 months after completion), he will be refunded one third of this fee, namely $160. If you do not finish he will not be refunded anything. OK?

Now we can start and I look forward to working with you on this program. I am enclosing the Agreement form and the first lesson of the program.

Please answer all the questions and return to me ASAP. From now on, I will answer you within 48 h of receipt, giving you feedback on each lesson and, if your answers are satisfactory, I will send you the next lesson. OK? Of course, you are welcome to add whatever you want to each lesson, as you see fit. Do not be shy in adding whatever is important to you. You are also welcome to ask any questions you want answered. I cannot guarantee I can answer all your questions, because I may not know the answer!

I am delighted to be working with you and I look forward from hearing from your soon.

Sincerely yours.

Luciano L'Abate, Ph.D.

[Note: At the time I was using the term "lesson" to denote what are now called practice exercises.]

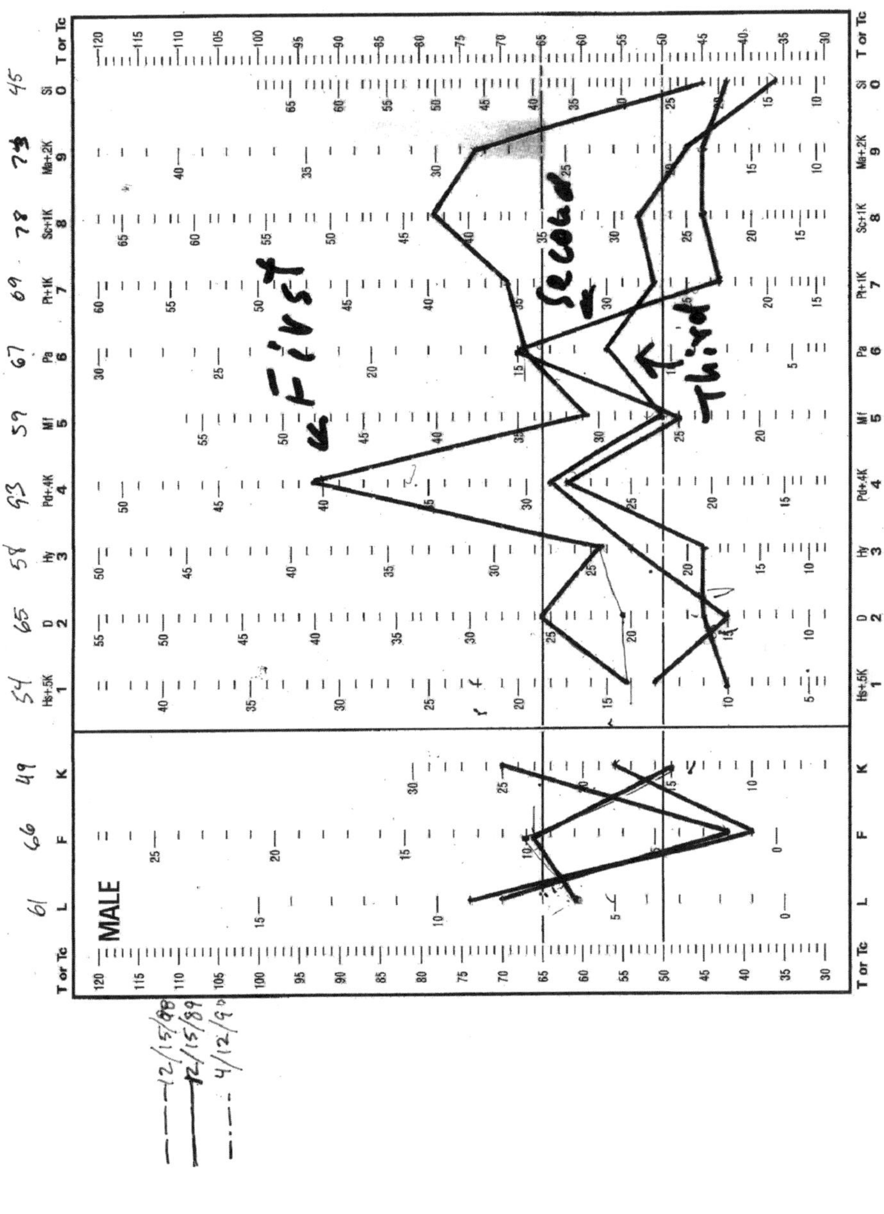

Fig. 9.1 Pre-post-and follow-up MMPI Profiles of a Personality Disorder administered interactive Practice Exercises over a period of time.

Tom was sent the first practice exercise of the anger practice exercise. From previous cases [and from theory (L'Abate, 2005)], I had learned that before starting a distance-writing program with impulsive individuals, it was more useful to deal with anger from the outset, before administering other practice exercises. As part of this practice exercise, Tom was to record examples of when and how he became angry and what the outcome was.

As a result of completing the first practice exercise, Tom was told that if he wanted to learn to control his anger he would have to schedule it for a certain time, detailing beforehand how, if, and when he would become angry (L'Abate, 1984; Weeks & L'Abate, 1982). He would have to record in writing all these instances. In another letter, Tom admitted taking responsibility for losing a paying job in jail, but he would be allowed to have a home visit for Easter on a short pass.

Tom was then started on the Social Training Program, the first practice exercise produced to deal with impulsivity (L'Abate, 1992) and with goals and wants as the first practice exercise, which he completed quite well. He ranked as his No. 1 and No. 2 goals to improve his behavior and to become a better person. The next practice exercise dealt with reactivity, which is an important part of impulsivity. Over the next 3 months, he completed practice exercises about mistakes, control, the law, humility, responsibility, and self. In a letter sent with the practice exercise about love, he admitted having a problem with "showing and sharing" love, following this letter with completion of a practice exercise about care and caring. A feedback letter complimented him on his progress and commented about his answers to some of the practice exercises and mailed the "Seeing the Good in Self and Others" exercise. I gave him some feedback about the practice exercises he completed thus far. In another letter he wrote that he had decided to become an actor, including plans on how to pay for tuition. He then completed the practice exercise about respect for parents as part of the original Social Training practice exercise. A second reactivity practice exercise was administered to reinforce establishment of controls over himself. Tom then wrote another and completed the forgiveness practice exercise [which is part of an intimacy practice exercise (L'Abate, 1986) that appeared in print long before forgiveness had become an acceptable factor in psychological and psychotherapeutic circles (L'Abate, 1986; Root & McCullough, 2007)], in which he related forgiving himself for what he had done during the robbery and receiving forgiveness from his family. A practice exercise about conflictful situations was unremarkable, raising questions about its usefulness and its vague and nonspecific nature. The same can be said about the practice exercise on actions and decisions.

Given the cognitive aspects of the program thus far and seeing the necessity to approach feelings and emotions, the next practice exercise was on that topic. However, since he did not complete this practice exercise, the unfinished portion was sent back to Tom to complete, underlying how important it was to feel first, think second, and think before acting third. He completed the unfinished part as well as a practice exercise about thinking. In his accompanying letter, Tom wrote:

> I feel like my thinking and judgment is [sic] the most things I need to work on. I always have to catch myself and watch myself because I'll react quick if I'm not thinking and I believe that is my biggest problem. It always has been in the past ... After taking all these tests I can say I am a better thinker because of taking the test themselves and having to think about myself ... I have to love myself before I can love someone else.

Tom complete the follow-up practice exercise, titled "Putting it All Together," and wrote two consecutive letters. In one, he wrote:

> Over the last ten months I have been taking these test lesions [sic] and all I feel I have learned a few things about myself... it really hit hard about my not thinking before I act. I feel like that is my biggest problem and that scares me. I feel like I can say 100% sure I am not going to get in any trouble with the law again... I sure don't want to fail at something just because I didn't think before I acted. I have really been watching myself the past couple of days just to see my actions and I noticed there are little things I do that I need to watch. I guess maybe I did con people in my past just to get them off my back but now I am realizing that I have grown up and I have to start taking care of myself and become a productive person. I guess that is why I would make a good actor since I've been acting most of my life. I have noticed one major change in me since I have been taking these test [sic] and that is, is b'n able to communicate better with my family. I used to argue with my dad but now I don't anymore... I respect people more... Some of your lessons were easy going for me some were real hard because I had to really look at myself and I feel like I really need to continue to look at myself to keep old habits from coming back, because that scares me the most... I would be lying if I said I have changed to a totally straight up person with no problems... I have saved every piece [sic] of paper, letters etc. you have sent me and I can go back and read things that remind me of areas to grown in and watch.

In my feedback letter, I asked Tom whether he felt he was part of a deadly triangle between his father and his uncle's wife who did not get along (L'Abate, in press). He admitted feeling like the victim, persecutor, and rescuer, but he was giving up these roles because he wanted to understand his family better than he did in the past without getting involved in triangles set up by family members.

Tom next wrote to discuss his feelings about the jail's assistant warden's suicide and how that event affected him. He also completed the second administration of the MMPI-2, which showed a significant decrease in the Pd scale but a significant increase in the paranoia scale (Pa; Fig. 9.1). I congratulated him about the decrease, but questioned him about issues of trust and seeing authority figures as threatening and punitive. At Tom's request, I mailed him a practice exercise about fears, which prompted a two-page letter and completion of that homework, informing me of his involvement with a 30-year-old woman with a child. In confessing his fears, he also said he thought that fear controlled his father "for a long time."

In another letter he informed me about his plan to attend school in the morning and to work afternoons with his uncle in the family business. He also mentioned "negative thinking," attributed to depression, which he agreed to work on. He then completed the first practice exercise about depression, defining it as not having self-worth. He completed a second practice exercise about negative thinking and a practice exercise about characteristics of negative thoughts. He had been promoted to trustee, and was given a more interesting job. He then completed the practice exercise about typical errors in negative thinking.

However, in completing the next practice exercise on correcting negative thoughts, he reported a "bad attitude" because his passes for home visits have been canceled over his reacting to a very controlling guard. Tom completed two final practice exercises about correcting self-downing thoughts and practicing rational thinking. A third retest of the MMPI-2 showed a continued decrease in the whole profile with a peak on the Histrionic scale (Fig. 9.1), well in keeping with his goal of becoming an actor. As a result of his completing the program, the $160 from the initial charge was refunded. An unexpected letter asked me to write a letter on his behalf to his uncle's friend for a possible job when released from jail, which I did.

Toward the end of the program, I received a phone call from Tom's grandmother expressing her pleasure about how much Tom had changed. A couple of years later, his cousin informed us that Tom had continued to work after he had been released from jail and doing "real well."

As far as I know, this is the first case of someone treated completely through programmed distance writing (DW) without any face-to-face talk-based (talk-based) contacts, suggesting among other evidence my collaborators and I collected over 30 years ago (L'Abate, 1977), that DW can be used as an alternative or adjunct to the verbal medium to help people improve their behavior.

An Allegedly Innocent Child Molester

Bill was first seen at Cross Keys Counseling Center, in Forest Park, Georgia. This was a church-affiliated clinic where I had been a consultant for years. He was middle-aged and in the process of being divorced from his second wife, who accused him of molesting her 9-year-old daughter from her previous marriage. He acknowledged being seriously depressed by the accusation and by his wife's threat "to take me to the cleaners." As a result of this accusation, being arrested and having to go to court to defend himself, he had lost his job and was at the end of his emotional and financial resources. The only contact he admitted about the accusation consisted of holding his step-daughter on his lap while showing her how to work on a computer. However, he denied ever touching her in any way except lovingly. According to him, his wife exaggerated his holding the step-daughter on his lap as a sexual position that according to her was "completely unnecessary."

After the first session, at his own request, Bill took the MMPI-2 to evaluate whether his profile would be similar to profiles of sex offenders. The score on the Depression scale demonstrated the depression that was the original reason for referral. There was no indication that his profile was similar to those of sex offenders. In my limited experience with sex offenders, I had not seen any who would volunteer for professional help; if forced by court order to undergo it, sex offenders would be extremely resistant to any therapeutic intervention.

During the few months I saw him face to face, Bill returned to a city where he had previously lived to find out why his wife had divorced her first husband, the father of her child. He discovered in the court proceedings that his wife had accused the child's father of sexual molestation, while acknowledging also that she had been molested by her father at about the same age (6–9 years). He showed me a copy of the proceedings, but the copy he gave to his lawyer disappeared mysteriously. The lawyer "lost" it and therefore could not bring it up in court in the participant's defense. I saw Bill for a few sessions before he had to go on trial to face his wife's accusation. He was found guilty, and according to state law, sentenced to 10 years in the penitentiary. The prosecuting attorney was a relative of his ex-wife and apparently politically useful to the defendant's own lawyer. Readers may draw their own conclusions.

After being incarcerated for 4 years, Bill contacted Cross Keys Counseling Center to ask me asking for help with his anger, an emotion he considered unacceptable given his Christian religion. I had already retired from clinical practice, so Bill's counseling was supervised and monitored by a licensed clinical psychologist, Doris Hewitt, Ph.D., who was the clinical director at Cross Keys Counseling Center. Here is a copy of the agreement between Sourcebooks for Better Living LLC and Cross Keys Counseling Center:

The above letter was written after Bill wrote to let me know how eager he was to work in a distance-writing program but how worried he was about whatever we wrote being under the scrutiny of the prison personnel. There was nothing I could do but reassure him from my part. However, I could not control what the prison personnel would do except to make sure that the correspondence would occur without interference.

Evaluation and Informed Consent Form

After completing a battery of self-report paper-and-pencil tests, and receiving and signing an informed consent form (Appendix A), Bill was administered the following:

1. Self-Information Form (L'Abate, 1992) a structured 85-item questionnaire that covers most possible situations in a person's life. A major characteristic of this test is the use of weights to evaluate answers according to levels of functionality. Bill reported being a college graduate, employed for the last 2 years, attending church regularly, and being active in half a dozen social clubs and fraternities, but having very few friends. He did not smoke and did not drink, denying having anything to do with drugs. His sleep was very irregular and he did not get enough. Bill followed a regular schedule of exercise and played volleyball at least twice a week. He had two children from his first marriage, a girl and a boy. He saw himself as a very good provider. He reported that his mother drank heavily until he was 10 years old. He was more dissatisfied by his mother than his father, but viewed both as being very authoritarian and restrictive. Bill had four other siblings, all middle-aged. Consequently, a great deal of very relevant information, not included here, could be gathered from this type of structured interview. However, more information about his family, and especially his parents was freely offered throughout the course of this program.

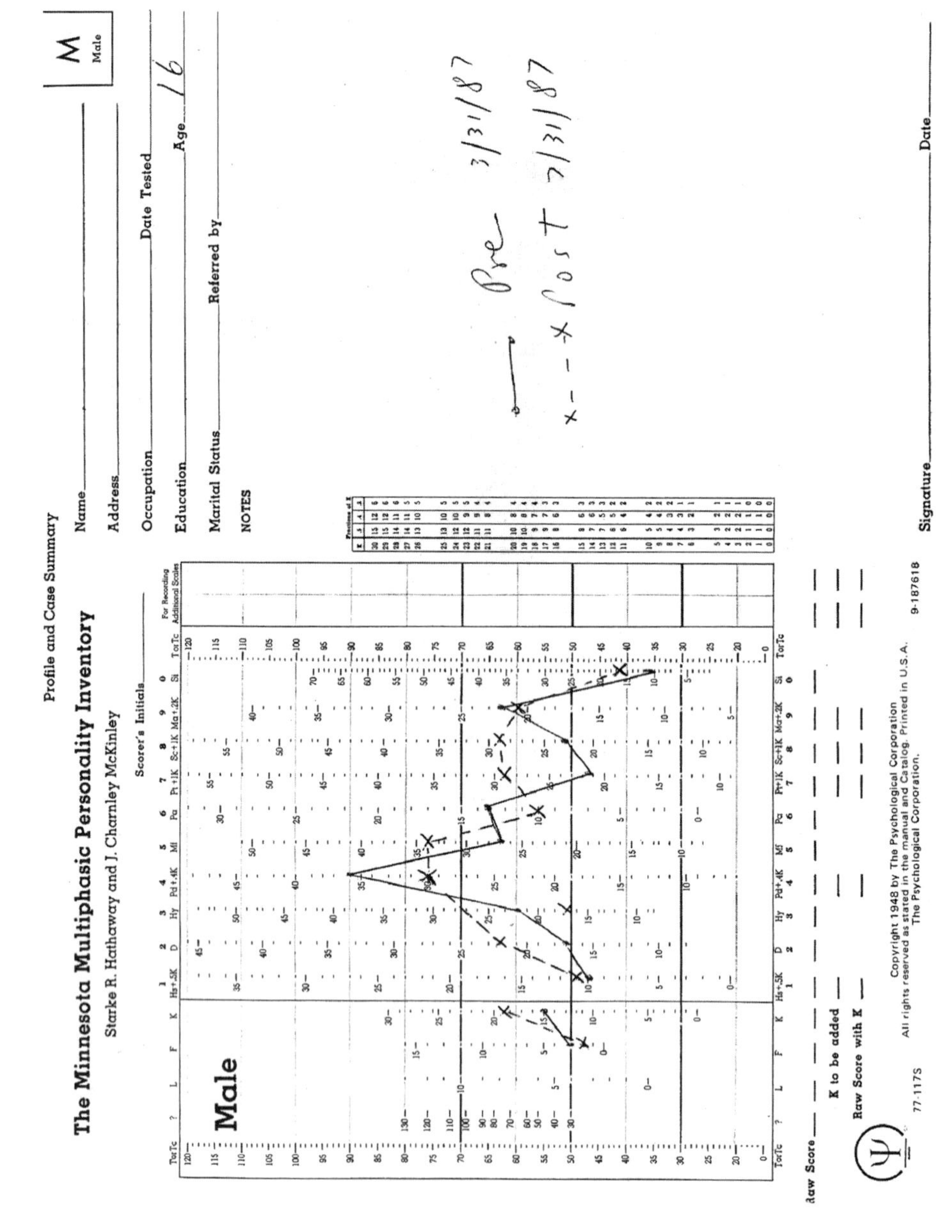

Fig. 9.2 The Minnesota multiphasic personality inventory.

2. *Evaluation of Troublesome thoughts*: This 20-item rating sheet was developed from Blatt et al.'s (1982) distinction of two different types of depression – self-criticism and dependency – rated on a three-point scale of often, sometimes, and never. On this scale, Bill scored above average for depression.

Process of Programmed Writing Through the Mail

Letter 9.2

June 27, 2002

Dear ______:

Thank you for completing the first assignment from the Anger Expression sourcebook. Your answers were very complete and very thoughtful. It is also clear that many of your reactions are related to your past relationship with your ex-wife and the present, oftentimes arbitrary and unfair, correctional practices. Is there anyone you can petition to receive permission to see your grandson? Can your present lawyer do anything about it? I can see how a great deal of your anger and angry reactions come from the deep hurts, disappointment, and betrayals you have received from people who you loved and you thought loved you (prison personnel not included!).

On the basis of your answers, I am enclosing the second assignment about "hate," which you ranked as being your No. 1 problem. You are going to decide whether hate is going to control you or whether you are going to be in control of your hate.

I look forward to seeing the completion of the enclosed assignment and finding out whether these assignments are useful to you or not.

Cordially yours,

Luciano L'Abate

Letter 9.3

October 12, 2002

Dear ________:

Thank you for completing the first assignment of the Addendum to Anger Sourcebook. As usual your answers are complete and full. I am enclosing an assignment about anger as the smoke for hurts, that, as you indicated, is the major source of your anger (L'Abate, in press-a).

I appreciate also your sharing with me all the many sources of frustration that arise from living where you are now. I am sorry because I can only answer with just one response and some suggestions and I cannot do anything else.

In the first place, only late in my life did I realize that fairness is not present in this world, and to expect it from imperfect human beings, especially correction officers, is unrealistic and impossible. Jails and penitentiaries, after all, are settings that continue the abuse that has been perpetuated by the very same persons who have been lodged there.

I am sorry that you have been put into the same settings, even though you do not deserve it. In addition, your good works, and your behavior, which is a complete denial of why you were condemned, must rankle some correction officers, because you really do not belong there, you do not fit the mold, and unfortunately, they think they are above and beyond the law. However, there is something you can do about it.

In the second place, I suggest you record in detail:

1. The time of day
2. Date
3. Exact place of occurrence
4. Officer's or officers' name(s)
5. A specific description of the behavior, with a minimum of interpretation, just what took place. If there were other witnesses you can rely on who were present, include their names

Once you have a list of about ten or 12 such incidents, I suggest you send this list to your wife with the name of your lawyer as the address on the top of the letter. However, before you include the list of incidents, introduce this list along with a list of your many accomplishments since you have been in jail.

Once copies of this letter are made, send one copy to your lawyer, and one copy to the head of the Georgia Department of Corrections, not your warden, but the chief honcho of the state. If your lawyer is willing to send this letter, so much the better. By all means, have your wife keep a copy of the letter. You are welcome to send me a copy if you like.

I am enclosing a copy of the second assignment. I hope you find helpful. If not, we have many other options. I look forward hearing from you.

Sincerely yours,

Luciano L'Abate, Ph.D.

Letter 9.4

November 14, 2002

Dear ___________:

I am in receipt of your last assignment about distinguishing anger from other feelings. After reading your answers and reviewing your previous answers to past assignments, I have concluded that your anger is circumscribed and focused mostly on your ex-wife, rather than on anybody else.

Consequently, if this conclusion is valid, and I would appreciate your letting me know if it is or isn't, I have changed the direction of your assignments, focusing more on feelings and emotions in general rather than only and strictly on anger. However, if you disagree with me or have other ideas on how these assignments could be of help to you, please let me know. I am open to suggestions and corrections.

On this basis, I am enclosing the first assignment of a sourcebook that deals strictly with feelings and emotions in general. I hope that these assignments might help you get rid of your ex-wife in your mind. You are spending a great deal of good energy on her, giving her the power to control your life even though she is physically out of your life. She is still in your mind.

It would be much more helpful to you if anytime you think about your ex-wife you would (1) stop yourself, and (2) direct your thinking toward a more positive direction, be it (3) completing a homework assignment, (4) reading parts of the Bible that appeal to you, (5) starting a positive activity that will enhance you, or (6) writing letters to your loved ones.

Even more importantly, you could also write a goodbye letter to her (without sending it to her, of course) in which you express all the feelings that you have felt about her. Write that letter and send it to me (not her). This might be another way to wash her completely out of your system. The goodbye is for your benefit not hers. OK?

I look forward to receiving your goodbye letter to your ex-wife and your answers to the enclosed assignment.

Sincerely yours,

Luciano L'Abate

Letter 9.5

November 19, 2002

Dear _________:

I just received your letter concerning the need and importance of a psychological evaluation to obtain a parole from the State Board. I agree completely with your attorney, that even though she is an extremely competent and highly valued professional and dear friend, Dr. Hewitt indeed is not an expert in the field of pedophilia, and for that matter, neither am I.

You would need to tell me the name of the specialist you have found, and I certainly can scout around to find another one who might perform the same service for less money. To be sure, you or your attorney can call the Georgia Psychological Association and find who, in Atlanta, specializes in that field. I do have a couple of friends who might be able to help me in case you need another name or, whether they would be willing to help. However, I do not think they consider themselves specialists in that field. It would only take me a couple of phone calls, if you need another name.

Of course, I will be more than delighted to write a letter on your behalf to the Parole Board, anytime you need one.

I hope this information is helpful to you. Just let me know.

Cordially,

Luciano L'Abate

Letter 9.6

December 21, 2002

Dear ____________:

Thank you for writing to me about your troubles in writing a letter to your ex-wife. Please keep in mind that that letter is not to be sent to her. On the contrary, that letter is to be written for your benefit and not hers. It would not do any good to write to her and I am sure she would use it to make things harder for you. It would serve the function of getting out all the negative feelings you accumulated over the years. Hence, I hope you will reconsider writing it for yourself only and absolutely not for her.

As far as the evaluation from an expert goes, I agree with your lawyer. It would be absolutely disastrous to your case to have someone testify who is not fully prepared and qualified. After asking some trusted colleagues (without, of course, disclosing my reason for asking), I came up with exactly the same two names you came up with.

Can your lawyer receive permission to have you come to Atlanta to be evaluated by either one of these two experts? You are not dangerous to anyone. You are not going to leave and fly away. The costs of the experts coming down there may seem outrageous but not out of line, considering that it would take 1 day to come down there and examine you and even one more day to examine the results and report on them.

If you think about surgeons charging ten or 20 times more for a few hours, you can see how professional time is expensive. That is why I am using writing to decrease the costs of psychological interventions and make them more available to more people than would be the cost of talk and face-to-face contact between professionals and participants. As you can understand, many professionals are not very keen on this approach.

I look forward to receiving your next assignment, and I am very sorry that you will not be able to spend Xmas with your loved ones. Just think that all of them, will be thinking of you and wishing the best for you.

Sincerely yours,

Luciano L'Abate, Ph.D.

Letter 9.7

March 2, 2003

Dear _________:

Thank you for explaining to me the abusive role that your parents, and especially your mother, played in your upbringing. Growing up in the horrendous circumstances you describe took a look of grit and courage. I am also happy to see that you have forgiven them, not an easy thing to do in light of their behavior. You made something of yourself in spite of them and the hurtful circumstances. Even now, where you are, it shows that you have been able to rise above what life has given you. Congratulations! You are one of the few resilient souls who go above and beyond adversities.

I appreciate the fact that you did not mail your letter to your former wife. She could and would have made things worse for you. I just hope you are able to let go of the past and work for the present and the future.

I look forward to hearing what your counselor says in response to the suggestion of using self-help sourcebooks to help men who do want to better themselves while in jail. If she could get in touch with me, I would be glad to see what we can do to help and to use you as an intermediary in the process.

There are a couple of pieces of unfinished business that I need to take up with you. One is the role of your siblings in your growing up. You commented on your not being close to them. I wonder why? I think it would complete the picture of your background to know more about them.

The second piece of unfinished business has to do with depression. When I evaluated you years ago, your profile showed a relatively high depression score. I am enclosing a short checklist (questionnaire) to be answered IN THE PRESENT, not as you felt years ago, but how you feel now, to see whether you still suffer from that condition.

I understand from how you answer about your siblings and from your answers to the enclosed checklist. I look forward hearing from you.

Sincerely yours.

Luciano L'Abate, Ph.D.
Enclosure: "Signs of Depression" questionnaire

Letter 9.8

October 15, 2003

Dear _________:

I am glad to know that you are keeping very busy with very positive endeavors. I am very proud of you and of all the work you are doing to improve yourself spiritually and mentally.

Surely God has a plan for you, to use your God-given skills and abilities for the betterment of people who did not have a chance to learn how to behave, except in hurtful ways. I am absolutely sure that you will find your niche once you have the opportunity to shine through. Of course, I will continue to send assignments that are relevant to your needs, whatever they may be. I think we have finished all we can do with depression, unless you still feel you want to work on this topic. I have plenty of sourcebooks in this area. What other areas would like to work on?

I am delighted you have chosen to help someone else through the help of sourcebooks. Tell Mr. _______ to write to me directly to let me know what areas of his life he wants to work on and why.

I will send to you the papers and assignments for him to answer because, since I still do not know him as yet, I want to make sure he answers and completes them in front of you, unless you trust him not to show or discuss these papers with anyone else and to answer all the questions himself.

I know I can trust you, but I want to be doubly sure that all questions are answered by him and no one else. I hope you understand.

Cordially yours,

Luciano L'Abate, Ph.D.

Letter 9.9

January 5, 2004

Dear _____________:

Thank you for writing to me after a long lapse of time. I was beginning to worry about you since my letter of October 15, 2003. I am glad you are feeling all right and sounding like you are pleased and proud of yourself as you should be.

No, I do not have a copy of your latest assignment. It could have been lost in the process of changing my mailing address (Please note the change!). Consequently, as for your request, I am enclosing that assignment.

I appreciate a lot what you are saying about all that you have learned. But, if anything was learned and you changed the way you feel and think, that is due solely to you, your positive attitude, and your winning spirit, and energy. I am very proud of you and I hope you will continue to go forward according to God's and your plan.

I look forward to hearing from you again soon. I wish you and your wife a healthy and constructive new year.

Cordially,

Luciano L'Abate
Enclosure: Standard Assignment

Letter 9.10

January 19, 2004

Georgia Pardon and Parole Board
Atlanta, Georgia

Dear Honorable Members of the Pardon and Parole Board:

I am writing this letter to possibly correct a serious miscarriage of justice in the sentence assigned to Mr. ________. I hope this miscarriage can be corrected by the leniency that this man deserves.

I first met him face to face in 1995, while I was a consultant to the Cross Keys Counseling Center in Conley, GA. I saw him for about 1 year on an outparticipant basis and resumed the relationship in 2002, after he wrote to me asking for my professional help at a distance, since he was incarcerated. Therefore, my relationship during this period consisted of his completing written homework assignments based on sourcebooks I have produced dealing with his anger and his depression, among many other sourcebooks I have produced about many other conditions. I have spent the last 20 years of my life based on the conviction that talk is too expensive and too inefficient to deal with and possibly heal the myriad of human problems facing our society.

On the basis of psychological tests I administered to him in 1995 throughout my prolonged face-to-face talks with him and again in 2002, plus what he wrote during the last 2 years, I have come to the following conclusion: Mr. ________ is not in any way, shape, or form a sexual deviate or predator. He is in no way a danger to children and to society. His sentence and subsequent incarceration are due to factors that I hope will be explained by his lawyer.

I have arrived at my conclusion on the basis of 42 years of clinical practice, but more substantially, on the basis of the following evidence:

1. His test patterns in no way conform to those of sexual deviates or predators. He did not lie and he answered all the test items in an extremely consistent and reliable fashion. This is not a pattern found usually in sexual deviates or inmates who want to con a professional.
2. His asking for therapy and professional support goes against anything I know about sexual deviates. They avoid professional mental health contacts like the plague. When forced to use such contacts, they resist them as a form of denial and avoidance of personal, internal conflict.
3. During his completion of written homework assignments (a cost-effective approach that I made available at no charge years ago to the Georgia DOC, without even the courtesy of a reply!), Mr. ________ was exemplary in the honesty and thoroughness of his replies. I have used this approach with many inmates and I think I know what I am talking about. His digging into himself, and looking at himself as directly and honesty as he has done, remains

unequaled in comparison to individuals who are notoriously resistant to this process.

Can I have been conned by Mr. ________? Of course, I can and I am completely aware of that possibility, personally and professionally. However, considering all the evidence I have gathered during 3 years of professional contacts with Mr. _______, I would conclude that that possibility is extremely remote. I stake my reputation on this conclusion. In 42 years of practice, I have never gone out on a limb to defend and support a man like Mr. _____. He amply deserves your leniency.

Please let me know what else I can do and how I can be of further help to Mr. ____ and to members of this board.

Respectfully yours,

Luciano L'Abate, Ph.D.
Diplomate and former Examiner
American Board of Examiners in Professional Psychology
Enclosure: Brief CV

I never received any reply to any letter I wrote to the Prison and Parole Board. The chair of that board, as a political appointee, was a funeral director with a high school education.

Afterwards, it seemed possible to see whether the level of intimacy between Bill and the wife he married before going to jail could be increased. Therefore, with her permission and signed informed consent form, it was agreed to pursue this line of intervention, which leads to the reciprocal discussion of hurts (Section II). The process of helping participants deal with their hurt feelings is an important one, because many participants, especially those with personality disorders, have difficulty expressing these feelings (L'Abate, in press).

Letter 9.11

May 22, 2004

Dear Bill and Peggy:

Thank you both for your excellent completion of the second assignment in the Intimacy sourcebook. I hope you both had a chance to compare, contrast, and discuss your answers for each assignment face to face or through regular correspondence. If you have not done so, I urge you to do it as soon as possible, because part of intimacy is sharing one's deepest feelings and thoughts with someone we love and who loves us.

If you have not retained copies of this assignment, I will be glad to send them back to you for discussion and sharing. Otherwise, without this sharing the major purpose of these assignments would be lost.

Bill, I would prefer it if you were to use the personal pronoun "I" rather than the impersonal pronoun "You." The use of "You" is too abstract by referring to a nonexistent person. Using "I" allows you to see the existence of a real person, you! You want Peggy to know about you, not about an abstract nonexistent person. OK?

Neither one of you completed the homework assigned at the end. Is there any particular reason why it was not completed? I appreciate your clarifying this point for me.

Cordially,

Luciano L'Abate, Ph.D.

Enclosure: two copies of Assignment No. 3 in the Intimacy sourcebook

---

Letter 9.12

June 8, 2004

Dear Bill:

I am responding to your letter concerning the latest assignment of the Intimacy sourcebook. I understand your difficulties in completing it and discussing it with your wife. If not now, eventually you will need to discuss the completed assignments in this sourcebook if you want to increase the closeness in your marriage.

I am glad to hear that you have become aware of how important it is to use the personal pronoun "I" rather than an impersonal, hypothetical "you."

In the spirit of sharing with Peggy, I am sending her a copy of this letter and from now on I will mail the assignments directly to her. OK?

I look forward to seeing your completed assignment and I hope that when you and Peggy get together you will be able to discuss, compare, and contrast your answers, because the next assignments in this sourcebook are going to be the most difficult ones.

Please let me know what else I can do to help.

Cordially,

Luciano L'Abate, Ph.D.

Bill was able to complete his practice exercises on the intimacy practical exercise but his wife was unable to complete it. I do not know why except to wonder whether she was afraid to express her hurt feelings. However, at the completion of that practice exercise, Bill raised the question about whether he was too passive and not strong enough to assert and stand up for himself. Consequently, a practice exercise about that topic was mailed to him (Section III).

Letter 9.13

January 4, 2005

Dear Bill:

I just received your completed assignment about standing up for yourself. I believe that this was a breakthrough assignment because after you completed it, you poured out things about yourself that you had only hinted about indirectly in the past.

With this outpouring I guess you were able to get in touch with all the hurts you received since childhood, where you were bullied and continued the role of becoming a victim marrying a woman who eventually betrayed you. I hope you will become aware of how much your life might have been a continuation of growing up as a poor victim of external circumstances, seemingly beyond your control.

I do not know whether this is going to be helpful, but being a victim is part of a deadly triangle made up of persecutor, savior, and victim roles. Perhaps you have become aware of having played the role of victim and less aware of how you also might have played the role of persecutor, as seen from Peggy's eyes. You saw her first as a savior and adored her as such, until she became your persecutor in spades! Please be aware of this deadly triangle! Become aware of its existence in your life and make sure not to be part of it as soon as you see its presence. You may think of it as the devil! To avoid at all costs.

I am enclosing another assignment in the Normalization sourcebook. I look forward to hearing from you.

Cordially,

Luciano L'Abate, Ph.D.

Enclosure: Remaining assignment of Normalization sourcebook

Here I raised the question about the presence of the deadly triangle that I raised with the previous participant, and whether this triangle is valid and present mainly in abusive relationships (L'Abate, in press) and whether in bringing it up I was brainwashing Bill or other participants, such as the preceding and the following ones. In writing these practice exercises, I tried as much as I could to avoid indoctrination and even worse brainwashing. However, that line can be crossed easily and I may be just as guilty of crossing it and perhaps seeing it even when it does not exist. However, in this case, the deadly triangle seemed to be very relevant when Bill revealed in his previous letter that in childhood he would take the place of his sister to protect her from the abusive physical punishment from their mother for whatever transgression his sister had done.

Letter 9.14

April 11, 2005

Dear Bill:

I am responding to the request in your latest letter in regard to more information about the deadly triangle in your life. I suspect that that triangle started when you started to protect/rescue your sister from your mother's whippings. By assuming the role of protector/rescuer you also assumed the role of victim, becoming the object of your mother's whippings that you really did not deserve. Keep in mind that all three roles, victim, rescuer, and persecutor, are intertwined with each other.

This theme of becoming the undeserving victim was repeated in your marriage to Peggy, whom you perceived initially as a savior/protector/rescuer, but who eventually, on the basis of that triangle being strong in her life, repeated it in her relationship with you. I do not remember the details of your first marriage, but I would not be surprised if that triangle was repeated there as well.

It might help if you start writing about all the possible past incidences where you played one of those three roles, to make sure you are not repeating it in your present relationships. Do you become involved with saviors who then become persecutors with you playing the victim role?

I wish you the best in your attempts at petitioning the Pardon and Parole Board. Let me know if there is anything I can do. I still cannot get over your finding what Peggy did in Jacksonville in her previous marriage all that crucial; important information getting lost. I wonder whether I made a copy of the transcript you showed me but I doubt it. I did when I saw you at Cross Keys Counseling Center years ago.

Let me hear from you at your earliest convenience.

As ever,

Luciano L'Abate, Ph.D.

By now, finding practice exercises and practice exercises that would be helpful to Bill became a problem, since he would find acceptable and complete practically any practice exercises I was mailing him. However, the next practice exercise seemed to be relevant to what he told me about his life in the previous practice exercises and correspondence.

Letter 9.15

August 3, 2005

Dear Bill:

It looks like our assignment on impulse control was right on the mark! Your finding emotional fulfillment in food rather than in intimate relationships tells me how deprived you feel, and indeed are, wanting warmth, acceptance, and love in reciprocity from those you love and who love you.

You awareness of how you are using food to fulfill your emotional needs is quite unique, and it indicates the level of personality development that you have reached.

On the basis of the above, I am enclosing another assignment on nurturance. Can we nurture ourselves before or while we also nurture those we love and who love us?

By now you should be able to understand that no relationships, intimate or otherwise can last without the law of reciprocity, which you might know as the Golden Rule.

I look forward to seeing your completion of the enclosed attachment.

As ever, cordially

Luciano L'Abate, Ph.D.
Enclosure: Nurturance assignment

The practice exercise about the Golden Rule can be found in the practice exercise devoted to negotiation (Section II).

Letter 9.16

February 25, 2006

Dear Bill:

I was happy to hear from you but very unhappy to learn what had been done to you. I am attaching a letter of protest to Mr. Nix. I leave it up to you whether you want to send it to him or not. I did not send it myself because I do not know whether it would help or hinder.

Under the present circumstances, I do not see how sending you any homework would help. I just hope that whatever you have learned in the past is going to bear fruits in the present, because now all your resources are being tested.

See whether keeping a daily journal will help, in which you write your deepest feelings and thoughts. Mail copies to me as your see fit.

Of course, I am very concerned about you and I will do whatever I can to help you.

Cordially, as ever,

Luciano L'Abate, Ph.D.
Attachments: Letter of protest to Mr. Nix

Bill continued to work on various practice exercises on a once-a-month basis but inclusion of all the correspondence during this period would lengthen this chapter unduly.

Letter 9.17

September 4, 2005

The Honorable Mr. Milton E. Nix, Chairman
State Board of Pardons and Paroles
Atlanta, Georgia

Dear Mr. Nix:

I am writing this letter to support Mr. _______'s request for a reduction in his sentence of 10 years for child molestation. I have known Mr. _____ professionally since he sought my help on an outparticipant basis in 1995, when I was a consultant to the Cross Keys Counseling Center in Conley, GA. I evaluated him through objective psychological tests then and saw him for about ten counseling sessions to deal with depression related to his ex-wife's accusation of child molestation.

Once in custody, Mr. _____ sought my help again about 3 years ago. Since then he has worked with me on completing written self-help mental-health sourcebooks I devised to help lower impulsivity and other troubling conditions in criminals and mentally ill persons. I do not believe that talk therapy works well with this type of individual. I prefer to rely on the written word.

On the basis of all the tests I have administered to him plus all the completed written homework assignments, I can testify unequivocally that Mr. ______ fails to show any signs of being a sexual predator or pedophile. I do believe, and I am ready to put my scientific and professional reputation on the line, that Mr. _____ is of no danger to society in any way, shape, or form. Indeed, I believe him to be an outstanding citizen who has paid his debt to society. Nothing would be gained by retaining him in custody any longer.

FYI, I am attaching a brief copy of my CV. Please let me know if I can be of further service to you and to the P&P Board.

Respectfully yours.

Luciano L'Abate, Ph.D.
Diplomate and Former Examiner

American Board of Examiners in Professional Psychology

Letter 9.18

October 15, 2005

Dear Bill:

Thank you for completing the nurturance assignment in the usual completeness and depth that you have used throughout our correspondence. Thank you also for enclosing a copy of the GDOC Group Contract. I admire your decision. However, I am afraid that it may not help you in the long run. Let me know what happens.

As far as loving your wife more than yourself, please read Matthew 23, where Jesus in reply to a question answered: "Love your God with all your might, and love your neighbor as yourself." If we do not nurture ourselves, how can we nurture others? However, our self-nurturance must not take place at the expense of others.

I am attaching a blank assignment form for you to choose which area of your life we have not covered. Feel free to name that area and then complete the form accordingly. I look forward to seeing what area you chose.

As ever, cordially

Luciano L'Abate, Ph.D.

As this point in the process Bill was moved to another jail that was set up by the state to treat pedophiles provided they admit their guilt, which produced a conflict in Bill: How could he admit something he had not done? He did not see himself as a pedophile, yet in order to receive treatment and therefore very likely shorten his time in prison, he would have to lie in order to be treated! He was given the choice either to confess and lie or to be true to himself. He wrote extensively to me about this conflict, which I acknowledged, reassuring him that whatever choice he made would not change his relationship with me but I could not make this choice for him. He chose to refuse admission of guilt and, therefore, was moved to the worst prison in the state system.

Consequently, I wrote the following letter to the chairperson of the system.

Letter 9.19

February 25, 2006

The Honorable Mr. Milton E Nix, Chairman
State Board of Pardons and Paroles
Atlanta, Georgia
RE: Mr. ________
Dear Mr. Nix:

I am writing to you to protest in the strongest possible way the punitive and unnecessary changes to the prison conditions of Mr. ________.

As I wrote you in my previous letter of September 4, I put my national and international reputation on the line in declaring Mr. _________ not to be a sexual predator or pedophile. He has maintained his innocence throughout the period he has been imprisoned. His record throughout these years of incarceration has been impeccable. He has not received any negative note or punishment; he has earned many achievements throughout these years and has shown excellent behavior.

To be punished for maintaining his innocence is abusive, punitive, and unnecessary. To try to break this man through punishment and retribution is inhumane and uncalled for.

I hope you can correct what I consider an inhuman and abusive attempt to break this man into declaring what he is not. He is not a pedophile or a sexual predator, in spite of what the court has determined.

My professional opinion, of course, may not count. However, the consequences of a negative, punitive action toward Mr. ______ will count, especially when that action is not needed.

Respectfully yours,

Luciano L'Abate, Ph.D.
Diplomate and former Examiner
American Board of Examiners in Professional Psychology
President, Sourcebooks for Better Living

At this point, running out of relevant practice exercises but knowing Bill's religious conviction, I asked whether he would be willing to work on a spirituality practice exercise not contained in this book. In this practice exercise I attempted to separate the church as a concrete institution from religion as a set of special beliefs and practice, and from spirituality, which is a much more abstract and often indefinable state of mind.

Letter 9.20

April 23, 2006

Dear Bill:

I am glad that you liked the first assignment of the Spirituality Sourcebook. I am enclosing it with the second assignment because you will need to use the ratings from the first assignment to complete the second.

I am absolutely delighted to know that you will be taking a computer course, since I do not believe one can survive in today's world without computer literacy. That knowledge will allow you to expand your work to unlimited heights, besides getting a job after your leave the "system."

I look forward to continuing working with you on the spirituality sourcebook that I developed with the folks at the Church of God Theological Seminary in Cleveland, TN, where I lectured months ago.

I hope you will be able to give me some corrective feedback about it because I have another spirituality sourcebook based on sentences rather than words that need to be improved.

Cordially,

Luciano L'Abate, Ph.D.

Enclosures: Second Assignment of Words Spirituality Sourcebook

Bill was coming close to the time of discharge, and at this time he expressed his anxieties and fears about facing the real world after 10 years in a completely different world. I tried to allay his fears the best I could. His transition to real life was made easier by the presence of his wife and by the welcome of his family and friends who knew and supported him. He reported to the parole officer regularly and attended a post-imprisonment program required of all released felons. Fortunately, after a negative experience with a representative of one such program, he was able to meet and relate well with a representative of another program who had been a past collaborator and colleague of mine years earlier. Bill obtained a job driving a truck, but he was waiting for a much better job in another state offered to him by another friend. He still keeps me informed about whatever relevant information is going on in his life.

Termination

In terminating the process of distance writing while he was still imprisoned, Bill asked me whether I would be willing to help another inmate who was aware of his work with me and asked whether I would help him with his depression. I agreed to become involved, provided this friend would abide by the same conditions set up in the informed consent form and complete a battery of self-report paper-and-pencil tests before and after completion of the writing program.

Bill reassured me that his friend would abide by these requirements. Consequently, below is a representative sample of this case.

A Depressed Murderer Recruited by the Previous Participant

Bob was in his middle forties and imprisoned for killing a man to defend his then girlfriend (more of this in the following correspondence). He was administered the Self-Other Profile Chart produced to evaluate the selfhood model alluded to before, in which the propensity for the attribution of importance to self and others is measured (L'Abate et al., 2010; L'Abate,

2005; L'Abate & Cusinato, 2007). His ratings indicated a positive view of himself and an even higher positive view of his family, a tendency that is in the opposite direction for externalizing personality disorders in Cluster B, as indicated earlier in this chapter.

Letter 9.21

December 1, 2004

Dear Bob:

Thank you so much for leveling with me about your being accused of manslaughter when you tried to defend yourself. I am sorry that the jury did not give you the benefit of the doubt. But I hope that your case will be reviewed in your favor. Gook luck! I am pulling for you!

You completed the assignments I sent you admirably! Congratulations! You did well. I would recommend, however, that you try to complete each assignment at a preset time by making an appointment with yourself beforehand rather than doing it at any time. In this fashion, you learn to control your depression rather than the depression controlling you.

I am enclosing the assignment that you ranked ordered as third in your first assignment. I look forward to seeing it completed.

Cordially yours,

Luciano L'Abate

Enclosure: Assignment on losing interest in hobbies and pleasurable activities

---

Letter 9.22

January 29, 2005

Dear Bob:

Thank you for completing the assignment on losing interest in pleasurable activities and hobbies. I understand from what you write that you cannot concentrate and that your mind wanders from one thing to another. Consequently, you have trouble completing things. Nonetheless, you did complete this and previous assignments well. That means that you can complete a task if you are motivated enough to do it.

Instead of enclosing the next assignment of your sourcebook, we need to change our plan somewhat by concentrating on the reasons for your depression. Consequently, I suggest that you start writing your autobiography starting from the earliest times you can remember. Write by concentrating only on your earliest memories, and when you come to a point when you feel like wanting to stop, do stop and mail me what you have written up to that point.

After you mail me that first part, you can go on to write about your elementary- and middle-school years. Write as much in detail as you can, because once you have written about those years, we are not going back to them unless we have reasons to do it.

One thing that I do not understand thus far is your idealization of your family. Given your idealizing them so much, why did you divorce your wife? Who divorced whom? You said you "smothered" them. What do you mean by that and what did you do to "smother" them? I would like some answers to these questions, if and when you can or want to.

Once we find the reasons for your depression (in addition to being in jail) and not being able to enjoy life (I do not expect you to enjoy yourself where you are now!), we will go back to the assignments in your sourcebook.

I hope this slight change of direction meets with your approval. If not, let me know and we can continue with the assignments in the depression sourcebook.

Cordially yours.

Luciano L'Abate

Bob explained his divorce as something that surprised him and found him unprepared to deal with it, but his then wife insisted on it and Bob felt he had no choice but to go along with it. However, he continued his relationship with his daughters. His ex remarried and was apparently happy with her second marriage according to reports he received from his daughters, who came to visit him in jail.

Letter 9.23

March 2, 2005

Dear Bob:

I have received a very satisfactory explanation of the reason for the divorce (dominance at one level and fear at another level?). What were you afraid of? Losing them? Have you have thought about the reasons for that control and dominance? From at least the first part of your autobiography, it seems clear that your grandfather was extremely dominant and controlling. Hence, this characteristic may have been handed down from one generation to another.

I would like to have your thoughts about these issues.

As far as the first part of your autobiography is concerned, you did an excellent job. However, do not be afraid of writing as much as you want.

The more detailed your writing, the better. We want to get out as much as we can from your past to understand the present. You will need to fill the gap from the time you graduated from high school to when you married and your marriage years.

From what you tell me thus far, it seems that you were raised in an abusive family atmosphere, at least by today standards. Whipping would be considered abuse and your mother would lose custody of the children. With this abuse there must have been a great deal of emphasis on doing rather than on being close. Doing and performing might have been more important than being together, as apparently is taking place now. You report being close to your siblings. However, the role of savior of your sister and accepting the role of victim to be punished by your "persecuting" mother, raise the question whether this deadly triangle (victim, rescuer/savior, and persecutor) was existing in your family of origin and whether it was present in your family of procreation. I would like to know what you think about this triangle.

Part of what I glimpse from your report is the inability to discuss hurts and feelings of hurt. Even your writing does not convey the presence of "soft" feelings, only the macho, "grin-and-bear-it" facade of a pseudo-man who does not cry, does not express any feelings, but goes into action without thinking about the consequences of his actions. Is that what happened when you were involved in the death that put you in jail? I would like to know what you think this. Does it make any sense? Do you agree with what I said? Feel free to disagree with whatever I say. It is not cast in stone. I value your explanation and understanding rather than mine!

I look forward to hearing from you at your convenience.

Cordially yours.

Luciano L'Abate

Letter 9.24

April, 2005

Dear Bob:

You do not owe me an apology. You are a grown man who can be and is responsible for his own actions. I do not expect anything from you except answers to my questions, a task that you have accomplished fully and well. How fast you respond is up to you. I am not in a hurry. The only thing I am concerned with is to be of help to you in the best way I know how, and that is through writing.

I appreciated your sharing with me your love for your daughters and their sharing with you issues and problems in their lives, in spite of your being in jail. That is quite an achievement I hope you are very proud of having accomplished such a result in spite of your present position. Congratulations on achieving something many men would like to achieve in much better conditions than yours.

Your motivation to achieve, in part due to being (feeling) short in stature, I hope is by now gone. Perhaps God had a plan for you in putting you in a condition where you have to reflect and introspect about your past life and possible mistakes. If you can learn from such introspection, perhaps all the years you are spending where you are now will not be lost.

There are still empty places in your autobiography that need filling, such as what happened to you since you graduated from high school. Can you do that? It would help if you could put dates or at least years to your recollections. You were a man of (impulsive or driven?) action with little time for reflection. I hope now you can decrease your action and increase your thinking before acting.

As noted above, there are no deadlines to complete these assignments. You work at your own speed, as you think through and reflect on your past. I will be there for you as you go, no matter what.

Cordially yours.

Luciano L'Abate, Ph.D.

Earlier, in a previous letter (March 2, 2005), I mentioned another model of my relational competence theory called the triangle of living (Cusinato et al, 2008; L'Abate, 2005; L'Abate & Cusinato, 2007). This triangle was adopted from resource exchange theory (Foa & Foa, 1974) that includes six resources continually exchanged among intimates and nonintimates: status, love, information, services, possessions, and money. I renamed "status" as "importance" and "love" as "intimacy," but kept the other four resources unchanged. Combining importance with intimacy produces a modality of being present and available emotionally and instrumentally to oneself and intimates. Combining information with services produces a modality of doing or performance. Combining possessions with money produces a modality of having or production. Functionality occurs when being is at the base of this triangle, with doing and having sharing in equal proportions in the triangle. Dysfunctionality occurs when the base of the triangle, "being present," is missing, forcing increments in doing and having. Here Bob showed very clearly how emphasis on doing and performing occurred at the expense of his being available to himself and loved ones.

From resource exchange theory, "status" was changed to "importance" and expanded into the selfhood model, where importance can be exchanged according to four propensities: self-fulness, when importance is exchanged reciprocally between self and intimate others; selfishness, when self-importance is achieved at the expense of others, as in Cluster B, where basic narcissism produces an uneven exchange in favor of the self and by putting down others; selflessness, when the self is put down and others are put up; no-self, when neither self or others are viewed as important (L'Abate, 2010). Models such as the triangle of living, selfhood, the drama triangle, and sharing of joys as well as hurt feelings feature prominently in my explaining relationships to participants in ways that seem to make sense to them. Recently, to reduce seemingly abstract models into concrete, specific, easy to understand ways, a theory-derived structured interview was created (L'Abate, 2008a).

At this point, I asked Bob to start writing his autobiography to learn more about him and his family background (Demetrio & Borgonovi, 2007).

Letter 9.25

April 28, 2005

Dear Bob:

Thank you for your letter and for your autobiography. Now that I have all the information I need, I am ready to discuss with you what I have learned thus far about you. Of course, I do not know whether what I concluded is correct or not. It will be up to you to judge.

Most of your life, and in most of your drive to achieve, your energy and troublesome thoughts have been directed toward performing (doing) and producing (having). What seems to be missing in your life is the third most important part of a triangle, the very basis of a triangle, and that is presence, or being emotionally available to yourself and to your loved ones – feeling important regardless of your achievements.

For instance, are you happy or feel satisfied if you do nothing? Are you important even if you do not achieve anything? Do you need to produce and perform to feel important? As long as your sense of importance comes from your production and your performance, I doubt whether you will ever feel satisfied because you are missing your feeling of importance regardless of what you achieve, produce, or perform. Can you accept that you are important because you are a human being, created in the image of God? What would happen to your sense of importance if or when you were no longer able to perform or to produce?

Please try to answer the questions asked above, and if my conclusion is halfway correct, we can then work on increasing your presence, since you already know how to perform and how to produce.

I look forward to hearing from you.

Cordially yours,

Luciano L'Abate, Ph.D.

Letter 9.26

May 11, 2005

Dear Bob:

Thank you for your honest and complete answers to my questions. Even though you claim to be important even if you do not perform, you make quite a few contradictory statements. I am enclosing a copy of your page to let you check out how consistent or inconsistent you may have been in your answers.

The major issue relates to what you report about your wife. You loved her a lot but were unable to express your love for her. Why? There are three possible answers to that question. I may be incorrect on all three counts. Consequently, correct me if I am way off.

In the first place, you were raised in a family where love was demonstrated by doing and not by saying. How could you express words of love if you did not have models about how to do it as you were growing up? Please comment on this possible answer.

In the second place, apparently you were so driven that it was impossible for you to express what you may have felt but for which you did not have words. Your priority to achieve seemed to have been stronger than to love and to be loved by the woman you loved.

In the third place, there is your perfectionism, which is one of the worst drawbacks in your background. Even though you profess to be a Christian, you seem to forget that God sent His Son because of our imperfect, incomplete nature. We were told to be "perfect as my Father who is in Heaven." You forget that we are still on earth, and, therefore, perfectionism can be obtained only when we go to Heaven.

All of the above tends to support the conclusion that you are still in need of becoming more aware of your feelings and emotions, learning a new language that has nothing to do with doing or having. If that is the case, and you agree, at least in part, we can then start working on a sourcebook on feelings and emotions, to prepare and enlarge the part of you, your presence, that has been weakened by your stress on performance and production.

Let me know what you think about the above. I do not have a stake in being correct. I do have a stake in being helpful. Let me know if I am.

Cordially yours,

Luciano L'Abate, Ph.D.

Letter 9.27

July 20, 2005

Dear Bob:

Thank you so much for all the information you shared in the latest assignment on seeing the good. I see that you have been able to reflect on a great many issues relating to your former wife. Your information seems to support the possibility that you stressed doing (performance) and having (money, possessions) by trying to buy her love through gifts rather than through emotional availability (being present). It seems that you have been able to appreciate the importance of emotional availability over doing or having. If we cannot be available emotionally to ourselves, how can we be available to those we love and who love us?

However, I am not still convinced that you are able to let go of your stress on performance (to the point of exhaustion?). The test for this conviction lies in your being able to DO NOTHING and still feel good about yourself. Try to do absolutely nothing for 10 minutes by the clock and see how you feel during and after those 10 minutes. I am very interested in your trying this test and seeing what happens.

I am enclosing the third assignment of the Intimacy sourcebook. I think you have made enormous strides in this area.

As ever, cordially yours,

Luciano L'Abate, Ph.D.

Enclosure: Third assignment of Intimacy sourcebook

The second practice exercise above, about seeing the good in self and others, is part of the intimacy practice exercise (Section II) that leads to three of the six practice exercises focusing on discussing hurt feelings, as shown in the next letter.

Letter 9.28

August 23, 2005

Dear Bob:

I have received your completed assignments No. 3 on love-forgiveness from the Intimacy sourcebook as well as your added letter. As usual you completed it very well and I congratulate you for a job well done, at least verbally. How words will translate into actions remains to be seen.

The important issue brought into focus by your letter relates to the 10 minutes of doing nothing exercise that deals with your being able to do nothing and still love yourself. Again, while you were doing nothing, you wanted to accomplish something, but the very issue is whether you can still love yourself if you do not accomplish anything! Even in doing nothing you "kept on thinking" about what you needed to do. It looks like you are so hooked on performance that it seems impossible to give it up. Can you understand what I am saying?

Apparently, if you perform and perform well you might reach some kind of perfection, or approval, or even love. What will happen when you will not be able to perform because of age or sickness? Life is not about being perfect but about developing skills to manage imperfection! We are back to the whole issue of intimacy: can you share your hurts with yourself first and with those you love and who love you?

I hope that the next assignment will get you onto a more balanced track. I hope it helps you think about what is important in life – performance and production (gifts, money, things, possessions), or presence, being available to yourself and loved ones when you or they hurt.

I look forward to seeing your completion of the enclosed assignment and your reactions to it and to what I have said in this letter.

As ever, cordially,

Luciano L'Abate, Ph.D.
Enclosure: Fourth assignment of Intimacy sourcebook

Letter 9.29

August 24, 2005

Dear Bob:

I have received in record time your completed assignment No. 4 of the Intimacy sourcebook. I am glad that you finally understood what I mean by presence versus doing or having, that is, being available emotionally not only to ourselves but particularly to our loved ones, in order to discuss our hurts reciprocally.

How good are these feelings if we cannot express them reciprocally with those who care for us? Allowing the feelings to fester inside us will only increase our blood pressure and push us into acting out against others without thinking, acting only on impulse, without reflection about the consequences of our actions. Becoming aware of our feelings is the first step. Expressing them verbally rather than in actions (performance) is the second step.

Your attribution of not being able to discuss your inner feelings to "machismo" is partially correct. I believe also that the way you were raised may have a great deal to do with your inability to discuss your inner feelings. From what you have told me, in growing up you might have been caught in between two contrasting and extreme models of emotionality. Your mother was a model of anger coupled with abuse. Your father was a model of stoic, silent suffering without any expression of feelings, keeping them inside and keeping himself isolated from others. Perhaps you may want to reflect on this possibility and let me know what you think about it.

I am enclosing the fifth assignment of the Intimacy sourcebook. Please let a little more time elapse between assignments to allow more time to reflect on what is being asked and what you answer.

As ever, cordially,

Luciano L'Abate, Ph.D.
Enclosure: Fourth assignment of Intimacy sourcebook

Letter 9.30

September 22, 2005

Dear Bob:

I have received your completed fifth assignment on love and intimacy. I see that you understand how important it is to discuss our deepest emotions, hurts, with those who love us, provided this sharing takes place reciprocally. If there is no reciprocity, asked for, expected or requested, and received, there is little chance of a deep relationship being present. If and when we ask for reciprocity and we do not receive it, then the chances of the relationship being meaningful and lasting are very slim.

I understand perfectly your seeing that today's abuse was yesterday's correctedness, especially within the context of your family. Your father was the model of bottling up feelings, of a "grin-and-bear-it" approach. You seem to have learned from him quite well, at least until now.

I just hope that what you write so well has really sunk in. You have done very, very well.

I am enclosing the sixth and last assignment of the Intimacy sourcebook and I look forward to your reply.

As ever, cordially,

Luciano L'Abate, Ph.D.
Enclosure: Sixth assignment of Intimacy sourcebook.

Letter 9.31

October, 2005

Dear Bob:

I received your completed last assignment for the Intimacy sourcebook. I am delighted by your answers and I am glad to know you found this sourcebook useful. Nonetheless, to make it more formal, I am enclosing a feedback form to evaluate how useful was this sourcebook to you.

Since we have been dealing with hurts, one hurt that has been avoided and I do not know much about relates to another human being no longer alive because of your actions, whether in self-defense or otherwise. I cannot help wonder how you feel about that action. Given what you have learned thus far, how could you have avoided what happened then, and what would you do if that same situation were to happen again in your life?

You will need to decide whether you have completed what you wanted to work on and stop here, or whether you want to continue with another sourcebook of your choice. If you choose to stop working with me, I shall send you some forms that you completed at the beginning of this program.

Please understand that as much as I enjoyed working with you, either choice will be OK with me. I want you to feel completely free to make either choice without regrets.

Cordially,

Luciano L'Abate, Ph.D.
Enclosure: Seventh assignment of Intimacy sourcebook

Letter 9.32

November 13, 2005

Dear Bob:

Thank you for completing the feedback form well. I am glad to hear that finally you have come to terms with your depression and that it still controls you rather than you controlling it. Apparently, we failed to learn from the first sourcebook. On the other hand, God gave us depression to face so that we can deal with feelings. This is a gift that many of the people who are there with you cannot experience. They can experience anger, hostility, and aggression (which equals abuse), but not depression. Anger, hostility, and aggression together are smoke that hides the underlying feelings of hurt, and that is what you are reexperiencing now. Unfortunately, other people there cannot.

From what you told me, it seems clear to me that we need to deal with depression in a different way from the first time. Of course, I do not know whether this program will help or not. However, let's see how it works for you. I am sure you will let me know.

Make sure that you make appointments with yourself, for a specific, constant time and place when you are going to deal with your depression. If you do not do that, depression will become your enemy (attacking you when you least expect it), instead of your friend, that you invite in when it is convenient for you and when you are ready for it. OK?

I look forward to seeing how you complete this assignment.

Cordially,

Luciano L'Abate, Ph.D.
Enclosure: 1st assignment of Depression 1986 sourcebook

Letter 9.33

December 13, 2005

Dear Bob:

I received your completed homework assignment for the Depression sourcebook. Unfortunately, it was completed in a completely different way than is was meant to be.

The three parts of persecutor, victim, and rescuer are all negative parts, played within the family, in which each family member switches from one part to another, as in the case of you assuming the role of victim to rescue your sister (another victim) from the persecutor (mother).

Hence, you will have to dig into your past to see how you played these parts within the family first, and then later with a girlfriend who set you up by assuming the role of victim and making you her rescuer. Then, to defend her, you became a persecutor of her former boyfriend. As a victim of her double-dealing, you were involved in a very deadly triangle, weren't you? This triangle is still played by inmates who play these roles with each other and with the guards.

The examples you gave me do not include the rescuer role as defined in the deadly triangle. All the examples you cited were part of a job or responsibility assigned to you, requiring rational presence rather than emotionality. You helped but did not rescue the people you helped. With your daughter you played the role of a father, not a therapist. I do not mean to take away from your achievements in this area, but the examples you gave did not involve a triangle.

I am not sure you can see the negative and destructive aspects of this triangle. Therefore, I would suggest that you think about past occurrences of this triangle in your life. Another way to become aware of this deadly triangle is to see how your "neighbors" play these parts now in jail as well as in their past lives. You could ask some of them to recount to you whether and how and when this triangle was present in their lives.

You could transcribe these experiences, provided that you respect the privacy of these men and not give any information that would identify them.

Let me know how you feel about what I have said and suggested in this letter. I do not think we can go forward with this sourcebook until we have exorcised this triangle from your life.

I am sure that it will be hard to spend these holidays away from people you love and who love you. I just wish you the very best under the situation you are in. I look forward to hearing from you at your convenience.

Cordially, as ever,

Luciano L'Abate

Letter 9.34

December 31, 2005

Dear Bob:

Thank you so much for completing extremely well the first assignment of the Depression sourcebook. Keep in mind that whatever you do is not for me. It is for you!

I hope that by now you have been able to see how the deadly triangle works. In trying to rescue who you perceived as a victim, you became the persecutor of whom you perceived as a persecutor. In rescuing your sister, for instance, you assumed the role of victim. This triangle is beautifully illustrated in what happened with Christie, who was a professional victim, asking you to rescue her from alleged persecutors, while asking them to rescue her from you as a persecutor/abuser.

I hope you can see how deadly this triangle can be and I applaud you staying away from fights and other triangles that come up everyday in a situation like yours. I hope that by now you have become painfully aware how a triangle established in childhood persisted in adulthood. In making all the decisions for your family members you were trying to rescue them from making decisions. At least your ex-wife felt victimized and perceived you as a persecutor. Eventually, given your drivenness and lack of insight in what you were doing, the only choice she had was to get out of that triangle to avoid keeping the victim role with you playing the rescuer/persecutor role. If you are aware of how deadly this triangle is, perhaps you will be able to avoid getting into it in the future.

It would be relevant, if possible, without creating any antagonism among the other inmates, if you could explore the existence of this triangle in them. Doing it and getting more information from them may add to your awareness of this deadly triangle. After all, don't inmates feel victimized by the courts and the guards, and the "system" that put them there, such as an unfair judge, a bad lawyer, nasty/abusive guards, and so on?

I am enclosing the second assignment of the Depression sourcebook to see whether it will be as helpful to you as the first assignment was.

I wish you and yours the best possible year under the circumstances you are in.

As ever, cordially,

Luciano L'Abate
Enclosure: Second assignment of Depression sourcebook

Letter 9.35

February 5, 2006

Dear Bob:

Thank you for completing the third assignment of the Depression sourcebook. I hope that by now you have realized that you are a lucky one among a few in the place where you are. You are strong enough to admit being depressed. It takes a strong person to admit to being weak, equating erroneously being depressed with weakness, an extremely destructive equation (L'Abate, Hevict, & McMahan, 2007; Weeks & L'Abate, 1982). Many "weak" people cannot admit it. I am willing to bet that many of the other inmates would be unwilling to admit being depressed because they need to cling to a facade of the strong macho man who needs to assert being strong no matter what.

Being depressed allows us to be introspective and reflect, while many impulsive individuals, as you should well know by now, are unable or unwilling to be introspective and reflect about their past and present behavior. Count your blessings on being able to be and become depressed.

I am attaching the fourth assignment of the Depression sourcebook that I hope you will find useful, especially if you make appointments with yourself about 24 h before allowing yourself to become depressed. If you start it on a regular basis, you will acquire the strength to stop it, just like inviting a friend into your house. Enemies come in when you least expect them, ambushing you with hurts that are then difficult to sweep away. I hope that I am clear in what I am saying and require of you. I am sure that we will be able to see whether this approach works or not. The previous sourcebook did not seem to work because you were still depressed after you completed the sourcebook.

I look forward to seeing your completed assignments.

As ever, cordially,

Luciano L'Abate
Enclosure: Fourth assignment of Depression sourcebook

Letter 9.36

March 10, 2006

Dear Bob:

Thank you for answering completely and well the previous assignment. Please keep in mind that you are not writing these assignments for my satisfaction but rather for your satisfaction. It's you who must feel good, proud, and satisfied about the work you do, not me. I am completely satisfied by the help I am able to give you, hoping that it will be useful to you. I am only performing a service. Whether this service is useful remains in the minds and hands of those who participate. OK?

As far as your answers to the fifth assignment are concerned, it looks like you have been able to make friends with your depression rather than considering it an enemy, when in the past you allowed it to ambush you when you least expected it.

As far as your inability to cry is concerned, it is indeed a very relevant and valid Troublesome thought. Perhaps, under the right circumstances, yet unknown, you may be able to cry. However, I do believe that you have been crying silently for years. Perhaps you were too macho to express your tears and anguish to discuss it with those you loved and who loved you. Perhaps your major role models did not show their tears either. Perhaps you may think more about other possibilities for this inability, as they come to you in the future. If and when they do, make sure you write them down. I would be very interested to read what you come up with.

I hope you will find the next assignment, No. 6, useful. Keep in mind that I do not expect all assignments to be equally useful. I am aware that some are more useful than others.

I look forward to hearing from you.

Cordially,

Luciano L'Abate
Enclosure: Sixth assignment of Depression sourcebook

Letter 9.37

April 3, 2006

Dear Bob:

Thank you for your very thoughtful answers to questions in the sixth assignment of the Depression sourcebook. It looks like you are beginning to control and profit from your depression rather than being controlled and consumed by it.

In your answers I still detect the old tendency to perform and to spring into action, on one hand, while you are now beginning to think through your past behaviors, accepting them as they happened and accepting your responsibility (no blame please!) for them.

It is also very evident from this assignment that you have been able to mourn past losses of your family and of your self-esteem as a result. I am happy to know that you are satisfied by the process and progress made thus far. Of course, I hope you will let me know if you are not. My satisfaction comes from the process of helping you change for the better and demonstrating that behavior can be changed at a distance without ever meeting and talking with a participant face to face.

I hope you understand how important that process is because it means that perhaps many lives could be changed for the better without face-to-face talk therapy but just through programmed distance writing. You and Bill helped to demonstrate that it is possible to do it. Am I correct?

Cordially,

Luciano L'Abate
Enclosure: Seventh assignment of Depression sourcebook

Here is what I received from Bob to answer the question asked in the last paragraph of the letter above:

> I feel as though I was helped *more* this way. I felt more comfortable. I feel that I thought my answers through more thoroughly, and I feel my answers came more from my heart this way. I'm sure we could have discussed things more in depth face to face, but I don't feel that my answers would have been as honest, would not have been thought out as deeply, and I would not have felt as comfortable with the worry of what you think of my answers or with the thought of my time running out.

Letter 9.38

April 21, 2006

Dear Bob:

Thank you so much for completing the seventh assignment on depression and answering my request for validation of my work. I really appreciated what you said and I hope you will let me use it (without of course ever mentioning your name).

I found your use of an imaginary respondent very creative and important. I think that the ability to discuss issues with someone else, even imaginary, is very important. It allows you to consider another perspective besides your own.

I am attaching the last assignment of the Depression sourcebook, which will be followed by a feedback form after I receive your completed form. After that you will have to decide whether to stop this correspondence altogether or to continue this correspondence; if you choose to continue, in what direction you would like to go? I am open to whatever choice you make.

If you choose to stop, I would ask you to take again the same questionnaires I gave you at the beginning. If you choose to continue, you need to think about what kind of further help you need from me about your depression, anxiety, or whatever area you want to explore that I can help you with. You do not need to make this choice now. Wait until you have completed the feedback form.

Cordially,

Luciano L'Abate
Enclosure: Eighth assignment of Depression sourcebook

Letter 9.39

May 2, 2006

Dear Bob:

I am in reception of your completed last assignment for depression. The major point in learning to control and use depression is to make sure to schedule appointments rather than giving in to depression any time it creeps up on you. For instance, if you feel a depressive or sad thought during the day, write yourself a note (if you can) about the thought and postpone it until your appointment time, perhaps in the evening when you are in the cell, to really spend time with that thought. Make sure that you write down whatever is coming up in your mind. By writing it down, you are getting that thought out of your mind, allowing room for other thoughts. OK?

Thank you for allowing me to use your experiences to help others. I guarantee complete and absolute anonymity. If you know of others who could be helped by this method, I will consider only one-crime-only inmates, like you and Bill. I have learned that inmates with multiple crimes do not profit by this approach, even though I am open to other possibilities.

I am attaching the follow-up questionnaire for the Depression sourcebook. I look forward to receiving it well completed, as usual. Let me know whether you want to continue working with me, and if you do, which sourcebook would be of interest to you. If you feel you have received enough from me, that will be OK too. No problem about ending this work.

Cordially,

Luciano L'Abate
Enclosure: Feedback questionnaire of Depression sourcebook

Administration of the same instruments given at the outset of the program showed a slight increase in self-importance on the self-other profile chart and a definite decrease in the level of depression. No further contact has occurred since the date of the last letter.

Disruptive Developmental Disorders

Some case studies of these disorders will be reported in Section II.

SECTION II: RELATIONAL SELF-HELP PRACTICE EXERCISES FOR COUPLES AND FAMILIES IN CONFLICT

The first case of sibling rivalry illustrates the process followed by all the practice exercises in this section, except for divorce. The first practice exercise asks for information, origin, frequency, rate, and intensity of the symptom. The second practice exercise reframes the symptom positively. The third practice exercise assigns the symptom at home according to specific instructions to be followed to the letter by parents, guardians, or caregivers. One case should sufficiently illustrate how this process occurs. The two cases of an acting-out adolescent and an adolescent who was involved in conflictful relationships with his family as well as with school and community are summarized here. In both cases, the outcome was measured with the MMPI-2.

Sibling Rivalry

Jackson was an 8-year-old boy who was bitterly involved in a power struggle with his 6-year-old sister, Betsy, for attention from the parents. Their parents, in their late 20s, had been referred by their pediatrician who did not know how to help them with this problem. They were college graduates, both working in middle-level management positions, and highly involved with their children. They completed independently the questions asked in the sibling rivalry practice exercise in Section II with a great deal of agreement about the nature of this rivalry. Jackson would initiate most battles by hitting Betsy, stealing her toys, making fun of her, and essentially doing his best to make her life miserable. The mother could only deal with them after she came back from work and waited for the husband to come home to punish the culprit, usually Jackson.

Otherwise, this rivalry was not evident in other settings outside the home. During the first face-to-face talk-based session, sibling rivalry was reframed positively as Jackson really caring a great deal for Betsy and Betsy really caring for Jackson a great deal since they spent a great deal of time together when they could have played with their own age peers instead. Predictably, Jackson expressed his marvel by demonstrating a picture of surprise and disbelief on his face, that is, the "paradoxical face."

After completing the diagnostic first practice exercise, the second practice exercise included a positive reframing of the symptom according to circular paradoxical instructions (L'Abate, 1984; Weeks & L'Abate, 1982), giving parents room to explore other positive reframings of the symptom and their own explanation. The third practice exercise gave detailed instructions on how to prescribe the symptom when both parents were present. As explained in previous work (L'Abate, 1984), having the parents achieve control over the symptom, and changing the direction of the symptom from the parents to the children, changes the context of the symptom, which helps to change the symptom.

The parents came back after completing the third practice exercise reporting that their children no longer were involved in the rivalry, were much more relaxed, making age-consistent choices of playmates, and making life pleasant for everybody. We expressed skepticism about this "sudden and unexpected" change and predicted that the change would not last long. Nonetheless, we gave the parents a fourth appointment to check whether this change was temporary or real. One week before the appointment, the parents called to cancel the appointment because they felt the change was real and lasting. They said they would call us if or when the need for help arose.

An Acting-Out Adolescent

The mother of Joshua, a 17-year-old, brought him to see us after he was suspended from school for rebellious behavior. This was the third high school he had attended. The father was busy with work commitments, raising questions about his possibly being a workaholic and being relatively distant from the wife and son.

The face-to-face approach, therefore, was conducted with his mother according to a paradoxical positive relational reframing of Joshua's acting-out behavior as protection for his mother's loneliness and middle-age depression. Consequently, we bet Joshua five dollars that he would continue acting out in school and home for the next 2 weeks. When they came back for the next session, Joshua announced proudly that he had won the bet and that we owed him five dollars. The money was given to him with skepticism that that improvement was temporary, and that it would not last very long. Therefore, the bet was renewed. The mother asked us to talk without Joshua being present, and a separate appointment with her alone was set up.

During this appointment she disclosed that when her husband was away, she would wake up at night to write about her "demons." She refused to divulge the nature of these demons and refused to let us look at her journals. We discussed how she was managing Joshua under these circumstances, and she admitted being very inconsistent with her parenting practices, ranging from being very lenient to being overly punitive with him. Nonetheless, she would be willing to let Joshua participate in a program of distance writing. Joshua came back after 2 weeks, reporting triumphantly that he had not received any teacher's reports and that he had lettered in tennis as the best in his high school team. Nonetheless, he did agreed to take the MMPI-2 and to participate in a distance-writing program through the mail since his family was moving to another town because of his father's work. Before his family's leaving town, we secured a final face-to-face appointment with both parents, where the father's overcommitment to his job was producing deleterious effects in his wife and his son. He agreed to become more involved with his wife and son, but we do not have any information whether this agreement was kept.

Joshua's MMPI-2 profile showed high scores (77th percentile) on the Pd and PA scales, with the Sc scale at the 70th percentile. From the start to the end of the program, Joshua completed 20 practice exercises from the social training practice exercise in addition to writing long letters accompanying his completed homework. On retest, his MMPI-2 showed a high score on the PA scale (85th percentile). Hence, in our closing report, we discussed the nature of his distrust of people and whether he would consider seeing a professional helper in his hometown. We were reassured that he would. No further information was received afterward.

Another Acting-Out Teenager

Acting out in this 16-year-old consisted of making sure he would be expelled from school for disciplinary rather than academic reasons. According to his parents, he succeeded in being expelled by the best private high schools in the metropolitan area in just a few weeks after attending each one. After helping his parents with being more consistent within and between themselves in dealing with their son's provocative behavior, he was given a choice of either going to a military high school or pursuing a programmed distance writing program through the mail. After his parents signed an informed consent form, he was administered the MMPI-2 and then, on the basis of the profile, the social training practice exercise was administered on a once-a-week basis through the mail. Figure 9.2 shows the results of this approach within the 4-month period it occurred. During and after completion of this approach, he was not expelled by the public high school he now was attending, where he completed the school year successfully with an increased involvement in basketball.

This profile shows an increase in the K scale with a subsequent decrease in the Pd, but a concomitant increase in the Mf, Pt and Sc scales. When his parents were contacted a year later, they expressed satisfaction with the outcome and reported that their son had continued to attend school without any troubles, finding success and even achievement in basketball.

SECTION III: SELF-HELP PRACTICE EXERCISES FOR INDIVIDUAL LIFELONG LEARNING

We have not administered any practice exercises in this section on any participants because our clientele was self-referred and clinical in the sense of showing definite symptoms or reasons for referral. Practice exercises were written to be used in health promotion and prevention with at-risk individuals without a psychiatric diagnosis or reason for referral. Nonetheless, we do have a record of a 20-year-old man who was referred by his mother. The social training practice exercise was initiated with the mother after she had been in about 10 years of on-and-off family therapy with a psychiatrist. She was divorced, and she brought various lovers to us after the divorce for our evaluation. Verbal therapy was discontinued when the results of her MMPI-2 showed how impulsive she was, with the Psychopathic Deviate (Pd) scale at the 95th percentile. Administration of the social training practice exercise was conduced at a distance with written feedback for a period of about 1 year.

After completing the social training practice exercise with a successful outcome, in that her Pd score had gone down to the 55th percentile, she wanted her children to undergo the same experience. Her teenage daughter came for an interview but was not interested in pursuing a distance-writing program or face-to-face therapy. On the other hand, her 20-year-old brother agreed to undertake such a program, and signed an informed consent form. He was pursuing this program to improve himself, please his mother, and see whether he should continue dating his present girlfriend, who was from a different religious and ethnic background and whom his mother did not approve of. His MMPI-2 profile showed a K scale score at the 68th percentile, while his Pd was at the 71st percentile, with Masculinity–Femininity and Paranoia both at the 68th percentile. Henry was administered through correspondence practice exercises from the social training practice exercise, which he answered fully and in ample detail, adding additional notes that he wrote at will to communicate in addition to the practice exercises he completed.

In a chance meeting with his mother a couple of years later, she informed us that she had married a professional man and that Henry had completed college and was doing quite well. No information was given about his relationship with the girl he was dating during the process of the DW program.

SECTION IV: RELATIONAL SELF-HELP PRACTICE EXERCISES FOR LIFELONG LEARNING OF COUPLES AND FAMILIES

We have not administered any of these Practice Exercises to participants. They were written to be used in health promotion and prevention, possibly with at-risk participants. Nonetheless, we are including one example of a couple that even though by coming to see us would be classified as being "clinical" and therefore relegated to Section II, they are placed her because of the mildness of their referral reason, that is, their reactivity toward each other. Their MMPI-2 profiles well within normal limits. They could not be assigned a formal psychiatric diagnosis, on one hand, but could not be dismissed from treatment, on the other hand. They were seen for six face-to-face talk-based sessions, with the husband completing three and the wife ten practice exercises. The husband received and answered the negative treatment indicators for participants who are resistant to or not interested in accepting professional help and, in this case, written homework assignments.

SECTION V: SELF-HELP PRACTICE EXERCISES FROM LISTS AND SINGLE- AND MULTIPLE-SCORE TESTS

Disorders of Internalization in Adults

A Very Disturbed Young Woman

This 24-year-old woman was seen in face-to-face talk therapy for 38 sessions. On the MMPI-2 she scored at the 80th percentile on the F scale (validity), at the 85th percentile on the Depression scale, at the 76th percentile on the Psychopathic Deviate scale, and at the 74th percentile on the Paranoia, Psychasthenia, and Schizophrenia scales. She completed 19 practice exercises on a one-a-week basis and wrote several letters. Most practice exercises dealt with depression but were inconsistently and incompletely answered. Verbally as well as in writing we labeled depression positively as a friend to welcome through appointments rather than trying to avoid it like an enemy (L'Abate, 1986; Weeks & L'Abate, 1982). Seeing, however, that our efforts did not produce any changes, we planned to support her by referring her to a psychiatric consultant for treatment with medication. At termination, her MMPI-2 profile was essentially a duplicate of the first profile but with even more extreme scores on the same scales.

We felt that essentially we failed to help her and realized that talk therapy should have been paired with medication from the very outset of treatment. On the basis of this experience and others, we changed our evaluation from one to three sessions, where evaluation occurred through an initial interview, administration of a battery of paper-and-pencil self-report tests, and offering an informed consent form to be discussed at home between the first and second interviews. The scoring of tests was returned at the second interview, and the test results discussed at the third interview.

We later received a card from her with the following message:

Dear Luciano & Bess:

Please accept the enclosed gift certificate as a token of appreciation for all you have done for me. I learned a great deal during our sessions and I will continue to use what you both taught me. I know now that it is alright to feel depressed, as long as I set up appointments with myself to sort out my feelings and not let them control me. Thank you again and all my love.

Who knows? Perhaps our efforts were not in vain?

Disruptive Developmental Disorders

A Troublesome Teenager

This family came to see us because of the inability of the parents to set clear and consistent guidelines with their teenage son, Dick, while their younger daughter was doing well and was not considered problematic by them. However, she also attended family sessions but had little to contribute except as a "tattle-tale" of her bother's misbehaviors in school. The father, with a high school education, was employed as a mechanic in a large industrial Troublesome thought, while the mother, also a high school graduate, worked as a school clerk. Both parents were in their late 30s. Even after helping the parents set clear and consistent guidelines, Dick continued to act out by getting traffic tickets for speeding and getting into car accidents. He also had fights in school, and had a poor academic record. Taking away the car from him would have penalized his sister, who needed Dick to drive her to school because the parents had to leave for work.

Since we felt that the parents were now working together, we gave Dick a choice of whether we should refer the family to Juvenile Court or whether he would like to cooperate on a distance-writing program, the social training practice exercise, that at the time had been completed by an inmate (L'Abate, 1992). He agreed to work on this program. He was administered the MMPI-2, which showed an F scale (validity) score at the 70th percentile, a 98 profile, with the Mania scale at the 86th percentile and the Schizophrenia scale at the 73rd percentile. Since at that time this was the only practice exercise available for impulsivity, he agreed to work on it on a once-a-week basis through the mail, since the family lived 40 miles from our office.

The program was initiated lasted a year and a half. During this period, Dick completed 14 practice exercises with written feedback on each one, with the exception of a couple of practice exercises that were sent back to him because they had not been answered satisfactorily. On the first practice exercise about goals and wants, Dick reported improving his behavior as his first goal followed by feeling better as a person and lowering the stress he was under. After a couple of practice exercises, it became evident that anger was still a problem, and a supplementary practice exercise on anger was mailed to him with an explanation of why this topic had to be addressed before going on with the practice exercise.

At the end of this practice exercise he announced that he really never got angry. As a result, he was told to try to get angry at least once a day and try to record what happened when he got angry – how, with whom, when, what, and why. Instead of once every 1 or 2 weeks, his completed homework slowed down to once a month.

At one point in the practice exercise he wrote us an unsolicited letter:

Lou:

I'm doing fine, I have a really best friend that I can trust and that won't screw me over like girls do. I am not turning gay or anything but I don't think I can handle girls right now. I heard some people at my school were supposed to tear up my yard and egg my house tonight. It's because I egged this guy's girlfriend's house. Well, I got a loaded 20 gauge that should do the trick. And I bet you anything that my house doesn't get messed up. I got a C in Spanish and English, a B in History and Algebra, and an F in Art. The art teacher grades harder. No joke! I'm really a good artist. Well, Gotta go.Your friend, Dick

In a follow-up addendum to his completed practice exercise, Dick added the following footnote:

It turned out I didn't get the opportunity to use the 20 gauge. I am trying to do well in all my subjects in school now. For real I even started using my head about fighting in school. I had the opportunity to but I didn't want to get suspended and fail and then not be able to play baseball. I got me a job at the Dwarf House in (a suburb south of Atlanta). I like it pretty much. The people there are nice and some of the girls there put Christy Brinkley to shame. I got the job to earn money for a new stereo for my Monte Carlo. I hope you have had a Merry Christmas. I am sure that I will.

Your friend, Dick

P.S. I've been getting drunk every weekend for 3 weeks now. Just kidding. SCARED YOU, DIDN'T I?!!?

Dick proceeded to complete the remainder of the social learning practice exercise at a much slower pace than at the beginning of the program, also because he became heavily involved with his baseball team. In fact, he invited me to attend some of his games. I replied that we could not attend his ballgames for reason of distance and our work schedule. However, we would attend an important game if he let us know 2 or 3 weeks in advance.

I did not hear from him for a while, and then received this note:

Sorry it has took so long to sent this back. I have been traveling a lot with my baseball team. We won the Georgia State Championship. I got the game-winning RBI and the game winning catch. I was also in the newspaper. We went to [a southern state] for the South-East Regional. We didn't do good but I was in the newspaper. That is why it took so long.Your friend, Dick

Dick did not complete the retest with the MMPI-2, but when I called his parents to ask about him, they answered that Dick had been doing extremely well. They were very pleased with the outcome and felt that Dick did not need to take another test.

CONCLUSION

These case studies illustrate how it is possible to obtain significant positive changes in participants willing to become involved in the process of change through the use of programmed DW. It will be left to other mental health professionals who are skeptical of this approach to evaluate whether this approach is useful and cost-effective.

ACKNOWLEDGMENT

I am greatly indebted to Phillip Webb of Georgia State University School of Art and Design for his help with this chapter.

10

Implications of Recent Advances in Mental Health Interventions

As summarized in the previous chapters, one admittedly extreme advance relevant to the conduct and delivery of mental health interventions in this century is the administration of homework assignments interspersed with rare, infrequent face-to-face talk-based sessions. The purpose of the sessions would be to check on the immediate outcome obtained by doing homework after completing each assignment or practice exercise, as in the technique developed, among others, by Lambert and Whipple (2008). This checking could be performed online, once the correct identity of participants is confirmed. Instead of face-to-face talk-based sessions interspersed with homework assignments, the valued and expensive presence and talk of a professional could become contingent on participants completing homework assignments (L'Abate, 2007d, 2008b; Omer, 1985). This is standard operating procedure in medical practice, and there is no rational or empirical reason why the same practice should not be pursued in mental health intervention, except for the guild interests of most mental health disciplines.

This implication might seem preposterous to many mental health professionals who value their personal presence and their words. However, it could be argued that because the presence and expertise of the professional are so important, these qualities should be used sparingly and selectively, not just on the basis of words, but on the basis of deeds, that is, how well participants complete the prescribed homework assignments. This is the best way to assess whether participants are interested in working

L. L'Abate, *Sourcebook of Interactive Practice Exercises in Mental Health*, DOI 10.1007/978-1-4419-1354-8_10,

for change or whether they want to depend on the therapist to shoulder the major responsibility.

A less extreme implication of these advances relevant to mental health interventions involves successive stages. First, after an informed consent form about homework and DW is signed by participants, assignments could consist of the most concrete, easy-to-complete behaviors, such as completing a questionnaire about positive individual, couple, and families activities. Second, assignments of activities that are the most frequently performed and enjoyed by participants could progress to more difficult and complex homework with sourcebooks specific to individual functioning of partners and family members. Face-to-face talk-based therapy, for instance, could occur at the same time as participants complete practice exercises and homework assignments specific to individual or relational conflicts or disorders.

CONCLUSION

The proposals presented here lead to a possibly new paradigm for mental health interventions: Plan A: self-help; Plan B: Written Interactive Practice Exercises: Plan C: face-to-face talk-based interventions: Plan D: medication. If Plan A does not work, apply Plan B. If Plan B does not work, apply Plan C. If plan C does not work, apply Plan D. If Plan D does not work, apply hospitalization or incarceration. If necessary all these plans can be applied all together synergistically in most severe cases.

Section 1
Interactive Practice Exercises for Psychiatric Classification

Disorders of Internalization

Children and Teenagers
Separation Anxiety
Anxiety Disorder
Depression
Fears
Posttraumatic Stress
Asperger's Disorder

Adults
Depressive Personality
Phobias
Procrastination
Anxiety
Depression
Posttraumatic Stress Disorder
Loneliness

Disorders of Externalization

Children and Teenagers
Disruptive Developmental Disorders
Hyperactive/Attention Deficit
Anger
Conduct Disorder
Oppositional Defiant
Troublemaking

Adults
Anger
Hostility
Aggression
Antisocial Behavior
Troublemaking

Other Disorders
Overdependency
Sexual Abuse
Psychological Problems
Mood Swings

Separation Anxiety*

Name ________________________________ Sex____Date_________

The purpose of this practice exercise is to learn more about the disorder that is affecting your child and your family. Please answer all questions or instructions fully.

---

*To be administered to child and/or major attachment figure(s) after they have signed the Informed Consent Form (Appendix A), Standard Format; they also should fill out the practice exercises (Appendix B) and the Concluding Feedback Form (Appendix C). If the wording is too advanced or complicated for a child, then the care-taker should be involved in explaining it to the child/youth.

L. L'Abate, *Sourcebook of Interactive Practice Exercises in Mental Health*, DOI 10.1007/978-1-4419-1354-8_11,

Instructions: Please rank-order the behaviors listed below according to how much they apply to your child, with No. 1 being the one that applies the most, No. 2 being the one that applies second, No. 3 being the one that applies third, and so on. If some behaviors do not apply at all, mark them N/A (not applicable).

Behaviors	*Rank-order*
a. Recurrent excessive distress when separated from home or from major attachment figure occurs or when separation is anticipated	_________
b. Persistent and excessive worry about losing major attachment figures, or about possible harm befalling them	_________
c. Persistent and excessive worry that an untoward event will lead to separation from a major attachment figure (e.g., getting lost or being kidnapped)	_________
d. Persistent reluctance or refusal to go to school or elsewhere because of fear of separation	_________
e. Persistent and excessive fear or reluctance to be alone or without major attachment figures at home or without significant adults in other settings	_________
f. Persistent reluctance or refusal to go to sleep without being near a major attachment figure or to sleep away from home	_________
g. Repeated nightmares involving the theme of separation	_________
h. Repeated complaints of physical symptoms (such as headaches, stomachaches, nausea, or vomiting) when separation from major attachment figures occurs or is anticipated	_________

Anxiety

The purpose of this practice exercise is to help you deal with anxious and fearful behaviors that make it hard for you to do well in school, outside of school, and, perhaps, at home. This beginning practice exercise tries to help you learn more about behaviors that are anxious and fearful to you.

Practice Exercise 1. Definitions and Meanings

Name______________________________Sex_____Date____________

1. Give the meaning of each behavior listed below as you understand it. Give two examples to make sure you understand each meaning. It might take you more than one sitting to write down all these meanings and their examples. Take your time.

Behaviors and Meanings	*Examples*
a. Feeling sad ______	Example 1 ______
______	______
______	Example 2 ______
______	______
b. Having bad dream ______	Example 1 ______
______	______
______	Example 2 ______
______	______
c. Feeling lonely ______	Example 1 ______
______	______
______	Example 2 ______
______	______
d. Feeling sick ______	Example 1 ______
______	______
______	Example 2 ______
______	______
e. Worry about dying ______	Example 1 ______
______	______
______	Example 2 ______
______	______
f. Worry about keeping my friends ______	Example 1 ______
______	______
______	Example 2 ______
______	______
g. Feeling frightened ______	Example 1 ______
______	______
______	Example 2 ______
______	______
h. Feeling like crying ______	Example 1 ______
______	______
______	Example 2 ______
______	______
i. Having trouble going to sleep ______	Example 1 ______
______	______
______	Example 2 ______
______	______

j. Not liking food ______________

Example 1 ______________

Example 2 ______________

k. Having nightmares ______________

Example 1 ______________

Example 2 ______________

l. Getting along with other children or teenagers my age ______________

Example 1 ______________

Example 2 ______________

m. Not enjoying school ______________

Example 1 ______________

Example 2 ______________

n. Not working hard in class ______________

Example 1 ______________

Example 2 ______________

o. Whining and complaining often ______________

Example 1 ______________

Example 2 ______________

p. Being moody ______________

Example 1 ______________

Example 2 ______________

q. Daydreaming often ______________

Example 1 ______________

Example 2 ______________

r. Not being able to sit still because of my nervousness ______________

Example 1 ______________

Example 2 ______________

s. Worrying about things often — Example 1 ______ Example 2 ______

t. Being easily frightened — Example 1 ______ Example 2 ______

u. Crying easily — Example 1 ______ Example 2 ______

v. Becoming upset easily — Example 1 ______ Example 2 ______

w. Having a chip on my shoulder — Example 1 ______ Example 2 ______

x. Sulking a lot — Example 1 ______ Example 2 ______

y. Being moody often — Example 1 ______ Example 2 ______

z. Complaining often — Example 1 ______ Example 2 ______

2. Rank-order the behaviors defined above according to how hurtful and painful they are to you. Rank-order as No. 1 the most hurtful and painful behavior, rank as No. 2 the next most hurtful behavior, and so on; if a behavior or behaviors are not hurtful or painful to you, mark them N/A.

Behaviors	*Rank-order*	*Behaviors*	*Rank-order*
a. Feeling sad	________	o. Whining often	________
b. Having bad dreams	________	p. Being moody	________
c. Feeling lonely	________	q. Daydreaming often	________
d. Feeling sick	________	r. Not being able to sit still because of my nervousness	________
e. Worry about dying	________	s. Worrying about things often	________
f. Worry about keeping my friends	________	t. Being easily frightened	________
g. Feeling frightened	________	u. Crying easily	________
h. Feeling like crying	________	v. Becoming upset easily	________
i. Having trouble going to sleep	________	w. Having a chip on my shoulder	________
j. Not liking food	________	x. Sulking a lot	________
k. Having nightmares	________	y. Being moody often	________
l. Getting along with other children or teenagers	________	z. Complaining often	________
m. Not enjoying school	________		
n. Not working hard in class	________		

3. Why did you rank-order these behaviors they way you did? Please explain.

____
____
____
____
____

Homework: During the coming week, think about these behaviors and how you rank-ordered them. Perhaps the more you approach these behaviors instead of avoiding them, the easier it will be for you to forget about them and for them to have an effect on your behavior, before going on with the next practice exercise, you need to answer these two questions in writing: (1) What will happen to you if you go on with the same anxious and fearful behaviors? (2) What would happen to you if you were to change these behaviors from anxious to relaxed and from fearful to secure?

____
____
____
____
____

Standard Practice Exercise for Anxiety

Standard Practice Exercise No.______________________

Title (name behavior)______________________________

Name____________________________Sex_____Date___________

The purpose of this practice exercise is to understand more about the behavior listed in the title above.

1. How does this behavior apply to you? Please explain in detail.

____
____
____
____
____

2. How often do you behave this way?

a.	Practically every day	______	d.	Once a month	______
b.	Once a week	______	e.	Once every 6 months	______
c.	A couple of times a month	______	f.	Once a year	______
			g.	Once every few years	______

Please explain further.

____
____
____
____
____

3. How did this behavior come about? Do you remember when it started? Check which answer fits best:

   a. When I was a child (younger than 5 years of age) ______
   b. When I was in elementary school ______
   c. When I was in middle school ______
   d. When I was in high school ______
   e. Any other time ______

Please explain further.

4. Is this behavior acceptable (OK) or unacceptable (not OK) to you? Why is this behavior acceptable (OK) to you? Why is it unacceptable (not OK) to you? Please explain.

5. Give three specific examples of how this behavior was hurtful and painful to you in the past.

Example 1

Example 2

Example 3

6. Give three specific examples of how this behavior is hurtful and painful to you now.

   Example 1

   Example 2

   Example 3

7. Give three specific examples of how this behavior will be hurtful and painful to you in the future.

   Example 1

   Example 2

Example 3

____
____
____
____

Homework: Next week pretend (make it up and put it in writing) to bring about or repeat this hurtful and painful behavior at preset times (for instance, at 8 a.m., 12 noon, 4 or 7 p.m.) on at least 3 days (Monday, Wednesday, and Friday, or Tuesday, Thursday, and Saturday). It may sound strange to you to be asked to repeat this behavior, especially when it is so hurtful and painful to you. However, keep in mind that *if you can start it, you can control it.* If you can learn to control it, you may be able to let it go. Otherwise, this behavior may come back when you least expect it. Each time you pretend to do (make up) this behavior, write down what you thought would happen in detail. Make sure to answer in writing the following four questions:

a. What behavior did you start?
b. How did you start it?
c. How did it end?
d. What did this behavior get you?

Time 1 (write the time you started__________)

a. ____
____
____

b. ____
____
____

c. ____
____
____

d. ____
____
____

Time 2 (write the time you started __________)

a. ____
____
____

b. ____
____
____

c. ____
____
____

d. ____
____
____

Time 3 (write the time you started__________)

a. ____
____
____

b. ____
____
____

c. ____
____
____

d. ____
____
____

Please check one of the following choices to show how you feel about this practice exercise:

a. Completely useless __________
b. Somewhat useless __________
c. So-so __________
d. Somewhat useful __________
e. Extremely useful __________

Explain in greater detail how you feel about this practice exercise and what you got out of it.

____
____
____
____
____

Concluding Follow-Up Form for Anxiety

Name______________________________Sex_____Date___________

The purpose of this form is to review whether this practice exercise was helpful to you or not.

____

____

____

____

1. Please select the answer that best fits how you feel about this practice exercise:

   a. I did not like working on this practice exercise at all. I wish I never saw it. _________
   b. I did not like this practice exercise at all, but I am glad I got to work on it. _________
   c. I am happy I got a chance to work on this practice exercise. _________
   d. I am not only delighted about working on this practice exercise, but I wish all children who suffer from the same painful experience had a chance to work on it. _________

2. How helpful was it to work on this practice exercise? Check the answer that applies to you:

   a. Not helpfull at all _________
   b. Somewhat helpful _________
   c. Helpful _________
   d. Very helpful _________

3. Which practice exercise did you *like best or was it most helpful to you*? Please rank-order the practice exercises; rank as No. 1 the one you liked best or was most helpful to you, rank as No. 2 the one you liked next best, and so on; if there is one you did not like at all or that did not apply to you, mark it N/A.

Behaviors	*Rank-order*	*Behaviors*	*Rank-order*
a. Feeling sad	_________	j. Not liking food	_________
b. Having bad dreams	_________	k. Having nightmares	_________
c. Feeling lonely	_________	l. Getting along with other children or teenagers	_________
d. Feeling sick	_________	m. Not enjoying school	_________
e. Worry about dying	_________	n. Not working hard in class	_________
f. Worry about keeping my friends	_________	o. Whining often	_________
g. Feeling frightened	_________	p. Being moody	_________
h. Feeling like crying	_________	q. Daydreaming often	_________
i. Having trouble going to sleep	_________		

Behaviors	*Rank-order*	*Behaviors*	*Rank-order*
r. Not being able to sit still because of my nervousness	________	v. Becoming upset easily	________
s. Worrying about things often	________	w. Having a chip on my shoulder	________
t. Being frightened easily	________	x. Sulking a lot	________
u. Crying easily	________	y. Being moody often	________
		z. Complaining often	________

4. Why did you rank-order the practice exercises the way you did? Please explain your reason(s) for your rank-order of the practice exercises.

____
____
____
____
____

5. Feel free to write any comments that might improve this practice exercise.

____
____
____
____
____

Anxiety

Practice Exercise 1. Definitions

Name______________________________Sex_____Date___________

The purpose of this practice exercise is to help you deal with emotions that may be handicapping your life, and to help you understand and cope with these feelings and emotions in better ways than you may have done in the past.

____
____
____
____
____

1. Below you will find a list of feelings that are related to each of three emotions: fear, anxiety, and depression. Write how you have experienced each feeling listed below; give two examples. If you have not experienced a particular feeling, give two reasons, instead of examples, of why you have not experienced that particular feeling.

a. General worries ____________ Example 1 ____________

Example 2 ____________

b. Fear of impulses ____________ Example 1 ____________

Example 2 ____________

c. Need to be perfect ____________ Example 1 ____________

Example 2 ____________

d. Feeling nervous or tense ____________ Example 1 ____________

Example 2 ____________

e. Feeling self-conscious ____________ Example 1 ____________

Example 2 ____________

f. Worries about being hurt ____________ Example 1 ____________

Example 2 ____________

g. Worries about the future ____________ Example 1 ____________

Example 2 ____________

h. Worries at bedtime ____________ Example 1 ____________

Example 2 ____________

i. Indecision ____________ Example 1 ____________

Example 2 ____________

j. Worries about my body ________ Example 1 ____________________
____________________ ____________________
____________________ Example 2 ____________________
____________________ ____________________

k. An anxious feeling not listed above; name it: ____________________ Example 1 ____________________
____________________ ____________________
____________________ Example 2 ____________________
____________________ ____________________

2. Now that you have written about these feelings, rank-order them from No. 1 for the feeling that is greatest and strongest in you to begin with to feelings that, although present, do not effect you as much (N/A). Rank as No. 1 the strongest feeling, rank as No. 2 the next strongest feeling, until the last feeling that you have experienced above. Do not rank-order feelings that you do not experience or that you do not think effect you at all.

Feelings and Emotions	*Rank order*	*Feelings and Emotions*	*Rank order*
a. General worries	________	g. Worries about the future	________
b. Fears of impulses	________	h. Worry at bedtime	________
c. Needs to be perfect	________	i. Indecision	________
d. Nervous, tense	________	j. Worries about the body	________
e. Self conscious	________	k. An axious feeling not listed above, name it	________
f. Worries about being hurt	________		

Homework: During the next few days think about what you have written in this practice exercise and how you have ranked your feelings. Would you want to rank-order your feelings in a different way than the way you just completed? If you do, let the professional who is working with you on this sourcebook know about it.

____
____
____
____

Depression

Practice Exercise 1. Definitions

Name________________________Sex______Date____________

The purpose of this practice exercise is to help you deal with emotions that may be handicapping your life, and to help you understand and cope with these feelings and emotions in better ways than you may have done in the past.

1. Below you will find a list of feelings that are related to each of three emotions: fear, anxiety, and depression. Write how you have experienced each feeling listed below; give two examples. If you have not experienced a particular feeling, give two reasons, instead of examples, of why you have not experienced that particular feeling.

a. Prefers to be alone ________________ Example 1 ________________

Example 2 ________________

b. Staring blankly ________________ Example 1 ________________

Example 2 ________________

c. Sulking ________________ Example 1 ________________

Example 2 ________________

d. Underactive ________________ Example 1 ________________

Example 2 ________________

e. Unhappy ________________ Example 1 ________________

Example 2 ________________

f. Withdrawn ________________ Example 1 ________________

Example 2 ________________

g. Dislike being with others ________________ Example 1 ________________

Example 2 ________________

h. Feeling alone ________________ Example 1 ________________

Example 2 ________________

i. Having no fun at school or at work ______________________________ Example 1 ______________________________ Example 2 ______________________________

j. Having no friends ______________________________ Example 1 ______________________________ Example 2 ______________________________

k. Must push myself to work ______________________________ Example 1 ______________________________ Example 2 ______________________________

l. Nothing is fun ______________________________ Example 1 ______________________________ Example 2 ______________________________

m. A depressive feeling not listed above; name it: ______________________________ Example 1 ______________________________ Example 2 ______________________________

2. Now that you have written about these feelings, rank-order them from No. 1 for the feeling that is greatest and strongest in you to begin with to feelings that, although present, do not effect you as much (N/A). Rank as No. 1 the strongest feeling, rank as No. 2 the next strongest feeling, until the last feeling that you have experienced above. Do not rank-order feelings that you do not experience or that you do not think effect you at all.

Feelings and Emotions	*Rank-order*	*Feelings and Emotions*	*Rank-order*
a. Prefers to be alone	________	h. Feeling alone	________
b. Staring blankly	________	i. No fun at school	________
c. Sulking	________	j. No friends	________
d. Underactive	________	k. Must push self to work	________
e. Unhappy	________	l. Nothing is fun	________
f. Withdrawn	________	m. A depressive feeling not listed above, name it:	________
g. Dislike of being with others	________		

Homework: During the next few days think about what you have written in this practice exercise and how you have ranked your feelings. Would you want to rank-order your feelings in a different way than the way you just completed? If you do, let the professional who is working with you on this sourcebook know about it.

Fears

Practice Exercise 1. Definitions

Name______________________________Sex_____Date___________

The purpose of this practice exercise is to help you deal with emotions that may be handicapping your life, and to help you understand and cope with these feelings and emotions in better ways than you may have done in the past.

1. Below you will find a list of feelings that are related to each of three emotions: fear, anxiety, and depression. Write how you have experienced each feeling listed below; give two examples. If you have not experienced a particular feeling, give two reasons, instead of examples, of why you have not experienced that particular feeling.

Emotion	*Your Experience and Examples*
a. Dizziness ______________________	Example 1 ______________________
______________________	______________________
______________________	Example 2 ______________________
______________________	______________________
b. Nausea ______________________	Example 1 ______________________
______________________	______________________
______________________	Example 2 ______________________
______________________	______________________
c. Stomachaches ______________________	Example 1 ______________________
______________________	______________________
______________________	Example 2 ______________________
______________________	______________________
d. Vomiting ______________________	Example 1 ______________________
______________________	______________________
______________________	Example 2 ______________________
______________________	______________________

e. Breathlessness ________________
____
____
____

Example 1 ________________________
____
Example 2 ________________________
____

f. Tiredness ________________
____
____
____

Example 1 ________________________
____
Example 2 ________________________
____

g. Becoming mad easily ____________
____
____
____

Example 1 ________________________
____
Example 2 ________________________
____

h. Sleeping poorly ________________
____
____
____

Example 1 ________________________
____
Example 2 ________________________
____

i. Wiggling in seat ________________
____
____
____

Example 1 ________________________
____
Example 2 ________________________
____

j. Stomach ache ________________
____
____
____

Example 1 ________________________
____
Example 2 ________________________
____

k. A fear not listed above; name it:
____
____
____

Example 1 ________________________
____
Example 2 ________________________
____

Feelings and Emotions	*Rank-order*
a. Dizziness	________
b. Nausea	________
c. Stomach aches	________
d. Vomiting	________
e. Breathlessness	________
f. Tired	________

Feelings and Emotions	*Rank-order*
g. Mad easily	________
h. Poor sleep	________
i. Wiggle in seat	________
j. Upset stomach	________
k. A fear not listed above, name it:	________

Homework: During the next few days think about what you have written in this practice exercise and how you have ranked your feelings. Would you want to rank-order your feelings in a different way than the way you just completed? If you do, let the professional who is working with you on this sourcebook know about it.

____
____
____
____
____

Standard Practice Exercises for Anxiety, Depression, and Fears

Practice Exercise No._____Title of Feeling:____________________

Name______________________________Sex_____Date____________

The purpose of this practice exercise is to learn more about the feeling listed in the title.

1. How does this feeling trouble you? Please explain in detail.

____
____
____
____
____

2. How often does this feeling trouble you? Check which answer applies to you:

a. Practically every day	_______	d. Once a month	_______
b. Once a week	_______	e. Once every 6 months	_______
c. A couple of times a month	_______	f. Once a year	_______
		g. Once every few years	_______

3. Please explain further.

____
____
____
____
____

4. How did this feeling come about? Do you remember when you started feeling it? Check which answer fits best:

a. When I was a child (younger than 5 years of age)	______
b. When I was in elementary school	______
c. When I was in middle school	______
d. When I was in high school	______
e. After high school	______
f. Any other time	______

5. Please explain further.

____
____
____
____
____

6. Give three specific examples of how this feeling troubles you.

Example 1

____
____
____
____
____

Example 2

____
____
____
____
____

Example 3

____
____
____
____
____

Homework: Next week, in order for you to learn to control this feeling ("Start it if you want to stop it!"), plan to repeat this feeling at preset times (for instance, at 8 a.m., 12 noon, 4 or 7 p.m.) on at least 3 days (Monday, Wednesday, and Friday, or Tuesday. Thursday, and Saturday). Write down what happened in detail. For each time, make sure to answer in writing the following four questions:

a. How did you start this feeling?
b. What followed after you felt this feeling?
c. How did this feeling end?
d. What did this feeling get you?

Time 1 (write the time you started __________)

a. ______________________________
____
____

b. ______________________________
____
____

c. ______________________________
____
____

d. ______________________________
____
____

Time 2 (write the time you started __________)

a. ______________________________
____
____

b. ______________________________
____
____

c. ______________________________
____
____

d. ______________________________
____
____

Time 3 (write the time you started__________)

a. ______________________________
____
____

b. ____
____
____

c. ____
____
____

d. ____
____
____

Please check which of the following shows what you got out of this practice exercise:

a. Completely useless _______
b. Somewhat useless _______
c. So-so _______
d. Somewhat useful _______
e. Extremely useful _______

Feel free to explain how you feel about the homework practice exercise and what you got out of it.

____
____
____
____
____

Concluding Feedback Form

Name______________________________Sex_____Date__________

The purpose of this last form is to find out how you feel about the practice exercises you completed in this practice exercise.

1. Please select the answer that best fits how you feel about this sourcebook:

   a. I did not like working on this sourcebook at all. I wish I never saw it. _________
   b. I did not like this sourcebook at all, but I am glad I got to work on it. _________
   c. I am delighted I got a chance to work on this sourcebook. _________
   d. I am not only delighted about this sourcebook but I wish all anxious, fearful, or depressed people had a chance to work on it. _________

2. How helpful was it to work on this sourcebook? Check the answer that applies to you:

a. Not helpful at all	_______	c. Helpful	_______
b. Somewhat helpful	_______	d. Very helpful	_______

3. Rank-order each practice exercise according to how much you liked it. Rank-order as No. 1 the practice exercise you liked the most. Rank as No. 2 the practice exercise that you liked second best, and so on, until you reach a practice exercise that did not apply to you (N/A).

Feelings and Emotions	*Rank-order*
I. Fear	_________
a. Dizziness	_________
b. Nausea	_________
c. Stomachaches	_________
d. Vomiting	_________
e. Breathlessness	_________
f. Tiredness	_________
g. Becoming mad easily	_________
h. Sleeping poorly	_________
i. Wiggling in seat	_________
j. Upset stomach	_________
k. A fear not listed above; name it:	_________
II. Anxiety	
a. General worries	_________
b. Fear of impulses	_________
c. Need to be perfect	_________
d. Feeling nervous or tense	_________
e. Feeling self-conscious	_________
f. Worries about being hurt	_________
g. Worries about the future	_________
h. Worries at bedtime	_________
i. Indecision	_________
j. Worries about my body	_________
k. An anxious feeling not listed above; name it: (___________)	_________
III. Depression	
a. Prefer to be alone	_________
b. Staring blankly	_________
c. Sulking	_________
d. Underactive	_________
e. Unhappy	_________
f. Withdrawn	_________
g. Dislike being with others	_________
h. Feeling alone	_________
i. Having no fun at school or work	_________
j. Having no friends	_________
k. Must push myself to work	_________
l. Nothing is fun	_________
m. A depressive feeling not listed above; name it: (___________)	_________

4. Why did you rank-order the practice exercises the way you did?

____

____

____

____

5. Which practice exercise was the most *helpful* to you? Sometimes what we like most is not necessarily the most helpful. Consequently, could you rank the practice exercises according to their helpfulness to you? Rank as No. 1 the most helpful, No. 2 the next most helpful, and so on until the least helpful practice exercise.

Feelings and Emotions	*Rank-order*
I. Fear	
a. Dizziness	________
b. Nausea	________
c. Stomachaches	________
d. Vomiting	________
e. Breathlessness	________
f. Tiredness	________
g. Becoming mad easily	________
h. Sleeping poorly	________
i. Wiggling in seat	________
j. Upset stomach	________
k. A fear not listed above; name it: (__________)	________
II. Anxiety	
a. General worries	________
b. Fear of impulses	________
c. Need to be perfect	________
d. Feeling nervous or tense	________
e. Feeling self-conscious	________
f. Worries about being hurt	________
g. Worries about the future	________
h. Worries at bedtime	________

Feelings and Emotions	*Rank-order*
i. Indecision	________
j. Worries about my body	________
k. An anxious feeling not listed above; name it: (__________)	________
III. Depression	
a. Prefer to be alone	________
b. Staring blankly	________
c. Sulking	________
d. Underactive	________
e. Unhappy	________
f. Withdrawn	________
g. Dislike being with others	________
h. Feeling alone	________
i. Having no fun at school	________
j. Having no friends	________
k. Must push myself to work	________
l. Nothing is fun	________
m. A depressive feeling not listed above; name it: (__________)	________

6. Why did you rank the practice exercises the way you did?

____
____
____
____
____

7. Feel free to write any comments that might improve this sourcebook.

____
____
____
____
____

Depression

The purpose of this practice exercise is to help you deal with sad and unhappy feelings, thoughts, and behaviors that are painful to you and make it hard for you to do well in school, outside of school, and, perhaps, at home. This beginning practice exercise tries to help you learn more about these behaviors that are sad and unhappy to you.

Practice Exercise 1. Definitions and Examples

Name______________________________Sex_____Date___________

The purpose of this practice exercise is to understand more fully what depression means to you.

1. Give the meaning of each behavior listed below as you understand it. Give two examples to make sure you understand each meaning. It might take you more than a day to write down all these meanings and their examples. Take your time.

Behaviors and Meanings	*Examples*
a. Feeling like I am a bad person	Example 1 ______________
b. Feeling dumb and stupid	Example 2 ______________
c. Thinking I am ugly	Example 1 ______________ Example 2 ______________
d. Thinking most other children or teenagers hate me	Example 1 ______________ Example 2 ______________

e. Wishing I could run away ____________________ Example 1 ____________________
____________________ Example 2 ____________________

f. Having trouble getting along with other children or teenagers ____________________ Example 1 ____________________
____________________ Example 2 ____________________

g. Feeling like killing myself ____________________ Example 1 ____________________
____________________ Example 2 ____________________

h. Hating myself ____________________ Example 1 ____________________
____________________ Example 2 ____________________

i. Feeling like things don't matter anymore ____________________ Example 1 ____________________
____________________ Example 2 ____________________

j. Causing troublesome thought for everybody ____________________ Example 1 ____________________
____________________ Example 2 ____________________

k. Feeling tired all the time ____________________ Example 1 ____________________
____________________ Example 2 ____________________

l. Feeling listless often ____________________ Example 1 ____________________
____________________ Example 2 ____________________

m. Feeling easily upset ____________________ Example 1 ____________________
____________________ Example 2 ____________________

n. Getting down on myself easily ______ Example 1 ______

Example 2 ______

o. Feeling nervous and edgy ______ Example 1 ______

Example 2 ______

p. Having few friends ______ Example 1 ______

Example 2 ______

q. Feeling unusually fearful ______ Example 1 ______

Example 2 ______

r. Seeming too serious-minded ______ Example 1 ______

Example 2 ______

s. Unable to enjoy life ______ Example 1 ______

Example 2 ______

t. Feeling sad very often ______ Example 1 ______

Example 2 ______

u. Feeling sullen often ______ Example 1 ______

Example 2 ______

v. Not knowing how to have a good time ______ Example 1 ______

Example 2 ______

w. Lacking in self-confidence ______ Example 1 ______ Example 2 ______

x. Depending too much on others ______ Example 1 ______ Example 2 ______

y. Lacking in sense of humor ______ Example 1 ______ Example 2 ______

z. Feeling sick often ______ Example 1 ______ Example 2 ______

aa. Not liking to go to school ______ Example 1 ______ Example 2 ______

bb. Feeling lonely ______ Example 1 ______ Example 2 ______

cc. Spending a lot of time sleeping or lying around ______ Example 1 ______ Example 2 ______

dd. Thinking of myself as a failure ______ Example 1 ______ Example 2 ______

2. Rank-order the behaviors defined above according to how hurtful and painful they are to you. Rank-order as No. 1 the most hurtful and painful behavior, rank as No. 2 the next most hurtful behavior, until you reach a behavior or behaviors that are not hurtful or painful to you (N/A).

Behaviors	*Rank-order*
a. Feeling like I am a bad person	______
b. Feeling dumb and stupid	______
c. Thinking I am ugly	______
d. Thinking most other children or teenagers hate me	______
e. Wishing I could run away	______
f. Having trouble getting along with other children or teenagers	______
g. Feeling like killing myself	______
h. Hating myself	______
i. Feeling like things don't matter anymore	______
j. Causing troublesome thought for everybody	______
k. Feeling tired all the time	______
l. Feeling listless often	______
m. Feeling easily upset	______
n. Getting down on myself easily	______
o. Feeling nervous and edgy	______
p. Having few friends	______
q. Feeling unusually fearful	______
r. Seeming too serious-minded	______
s. Unable to enjoy life	______
t. Feeling sad very often	______
u. Feeling sullen often	______
v. Not knowing how to have a good time	______
w. Lacking in self-confidence	______
x. Depending too much on others	______
y. Lacking in sense of humor	______
z. Feeling sick often	______
aa. Not liking to go to school	______
bb. Feeling lonely	______
cc. Spending a lot of time sleeping or lying around	______
dd. Thinking of myself as a failure	______

3. Why did you rank-order these behaviors they way you did? Please explain.

____

____

____

____

____

Homework: During the coming week, think about these behaviors and how you rank-ordered them. Perhaps the more you approach these behaviors instead of avoiding them, the easier it will be for you to forget about them and for them to have an effect on your behavior. Before going on with the next practice exercise, you need to answer these two questions in writing:

1. What will happen to you if you go on with the same sad and unhappy behaviors?

____

____

____

____

____

2. What would happen to you if you were to change these behaviors from sad to contented and from unhappy to pleasant?

____

____

____

____

____

Concluding Follow-Up Form for Depression Practice Exercise

Name______________________Sex________Date__________

The purpose of this form is to review whether this practice exercise was helpful to you or not.

1. Please select the answer that best fits how you feel about this practice exercise:

   a. I did not like working on this practice exercise at all. I wish I never saw it. _________
   b. I did not like this practice exercise at all, but I am glad I got to work on it. _________
   c. I am delighted I got a chance to work on this practice exercise._________
   d. I am not only delighted about working on this practice exercise, but I wish all children who suffer from the same painful experience had a chance to work on it. _________

2. How helpful was it to work on this practice exercise? Check the answer that applies to you:

a. Not helpful at all	________	c. Helpful	________
b. Somewhat helpful	________	d. Very helpful	________

3. Which practice exercise did you *like best or was it most helpful to you?* Please rank-order the practice exercises; rank as No. 1 the one you liked best or was most helpful to you, rank as No. 2 the one you liked next best, and so on; if there is one you did not like at all or that did not apply to you, mark it N/A.

Behaviors	*Rank-order*
a. Feeling like I am a bad	________
b. Feeling dumb and stupid	________
c. Thinking I am ugly	________
d. Thinking most other children or teenagers hate me	________
e. Wishing I could run away	________
f. Having trouble getting along with other children or teenagers	________
g. Feeling like killing myself	________
h. Hating myself	________
i. Feeling like things don't matter anymore	________
j. Causing troublesome thought for everybody	________
k. Feeling tired all the time	________
l. Feeling listless often	________
m. Feeling easily upset	________
n. Getting down on myself easily	________
o. Feeling nervous and edgy	________
p. Having few friends	________
q. Feeling unusually fearful	________
r. Seeming too serious-minded	________
s. Unable to enjoy life	________
t. Feeling sad very often	________
u. Feeling sullen often	________
v. Not knowing how to have a good time	________
w. Lacking in self-confidence	________
x. Depending too much on others	________
y. Lacking in sense of humor	________
z. Feeling sick often	________
aa. Not liking to go to school	________
bb. Feeling lonely	________
cc. Spending a lot of time sleeping or lying around	________
dd. Thinking of myself as a failure	________

4. Why did you rank-order the practice exercises the way you did? Please explain your reason(s) for your rank-order of practice exercises.

____
____
____
____
____

5. Feel free to write any comments that might improve this practice exercise.

____
____
____
____
____

Posttraumatic Stress

The purpose of this practice exercise is to help you deal with painful experiences and memories you experienced in the past. Very likely these painful experiences and memories are still effecting you in the present and may effect you in the future unless you can learn how to deal with them.

Practice Exercise 1. Definitions

Name______________________________Sex_____Date___________

This beginning practice exercise tries to help you learn more about the behaviors that were produced by past painful experiences.

____
____
____

1. Define each of the behaviors listed below by what each behavior means to you. To write these definitions, use a dictionary, ask the help of your parent(s), mental health professionals, close friends, or relatives. In most cases, however, you may not need a definition. Give two examples to make sure you understand the definition. It might take you more than a day to write down all these definitions. Take your time. After you have completed this list, go to item No. 2.

Behaviors and Definitions

Examples

a. Bad dreams ______ Example 1 ______

______ ______

______ Example 2 ______

______ ______

b. Upset by reminders Example 1 ______

______ ______

______ Example 2 ______

______ ______

c. Flashbacks (repetitive images) Example 1 ______

______ ______

______ Example 2 ______

______ ______

d. Upset by painful thoughts Example 1 ______

______ ______

______ Example 2 ______

______ ______

e. Avoidance of painful thoughts Example 1 ______

______ ______

______ Example 2 ______

______ ______

f. Avoidance of situations that remind you of painful experiences Example 1 ______

______

______ Example 2 ______

______ ______

g. Avoidance of painful feelings and emotions ______ Example 1 ______

______

______ Example 2 ______

______ ______

h. Numbness of emotions Example 1 ______

______ ______

______ Example 2 ______

______ ______

i. Emotional isolation/estrangement ____________________ Example 1 ____________________ Example 2 ____________________

j. Lack of pleasure ____________________ Example 1 ____________________ Example 2 ____________________

k. Easily startled ____________________ Example 1 ____________________ Example 2 ____________________

l. Body reactions and physical troublesome thought ____________________ Example 1 ____________________ Example 2 ____________________

m. Sleep troublesome thoughts ____________________ Example 1 ____________________ Example 2 ____________________

n. Repeating and being fearful most of the time ____________________ Example 1 ____________________ Example 2 ____________________

o. Attention troublesome thought ____________________ Example 1 ____________________ Example 2 ____________________

p. Memory/learning troublesome thoughts ____________________ Example 1 ____________________ Example 2 ____________________

2. Rank-order the behaviors defined above according to how painful they were for you, that is, according to how much they are still affecting your overall behavior now. Rank-order as No. 1 the most painful behavior, rank as No. 2 the next most painful behavior, and so on until you reach a behavior or behaviors that have not had any effect on you (N/A).

Behaviors	*Rank-order*	*Behaviors*	*Rank-order*
a. Bad dreams	________	i. Emotional isolation/ estrangement	________
b. Upset by reminders	________	j. Lack of pleasure	________
c. Flashbacks (repetitive images)	________	k. Easily startled	________
d. Upset by painful thoughts	________	l. Body reactions and physical troublesome thoughts	________
e. Avoidance of painful thoughts	________	m. Sleep troublesome thoughts	________
f. Avoidance of situations that remind you of past painful experiences	________	n. Fear of recurrence/ hypervigilance	________
g. Avoidance of painful feelings and emotions	________	o. Attention troublesome thoughts	________
h. Numbness of emotions	________	p. Memory/learning troublesome thoughts	________

3. Why did you rank-order these behaviors they way you did?

____

____

____

____

____

Homework: During the coming week, think about these behaviors and how you rank-ordered them. Perhaps the more you approach these behaviors instead of avoiding them, the easier it will be for you to forget about them and for them to have an effect on your behavior.

Standard Practice Exercise for Posttraumatic Stress

Practice Exercise No.____Title of behavior____________________

Name____________________________Sex______Date____________

The purpose of this practice exercise is to understand more about the behavior listed in the title above.

1. How does this behavior apply to you? Please explain in detail.

____
____
____
____
____

2. How often do you get this behavior?

a.	Practically every day	_______	e.	Once every 6 months	_______
b.	Once a week	_______	f.	Once a year	_______
c.	A couple of times a month	_______	g.	Once every few years	_______
d.	Once a month	_______			

Please explain further.

____
____
____
____
____

3. How did this behavior come about? Do you remember when it started? Check which answer fits best:

a. When I was a child (younger than 5 years of age) ______
b. When I was in elementary school ______
c. When I was in middle school ______
d. When I was in high school ______
e. After high school ______
f. Any other time ______

Please explain further if you remember any specific experience that started this behavior.

4. Is this behavior acceptable or unacceptable? Why is this symptom unacceptable to you? Please explain.

5. Give three specific examples of how this behavior effects you now.

   Example 1

   Ex.ample 2

   Example 3

Homework: The purpose of this homework is to help you achieve greater control over painful, past experiences. Next week, plan to bring about or repeat this behavior at preset times (for instance, at 8 a.m., 12 noon, 4 or 7 p.m.) on at least 3 days (Monday, Wednesday, and Friday, or Tuesday, Thursday, and Saturday). It may sound strange to you to be asked to repeat this behavior, especially when it is so painful to drudge it up. However, keep in mind that *if you can start it, you can control it.* If you can learn to control it, you may be able to let go of it. Otherwise, the behavior may come back when you least expect it; that is, the more you avoid this behavior now, the more it might haunt you in the future.

For each time you start this behavior, write down what happened in detail. Make sure to answer in writing the following four questions:

a. What happened that triggered this behavior?
b. How did you start it?
c. How did it end?
d. What did this symptom get you?

Time 1 (write the time you started__________)

a. ____
____
____

b. ____
____
____

c. ____
____
____

d. ____
____
____

Time 2 (write the time you started__________)

a. ____
____
____

b. ____
____
____

c. ____
____
____

d. ____
____
____

Time 3 (write the time you started__________)

a. ____
____
____

b. ____
____
____

c. ____
____
____

d. ____
____
____

Please check which of the following shows how you feel about this practice exercise:

a.	Completely useless	______	d.	Somewhat useful	______
b.	Somewhat useless	______	e.	Extremely useful	______
c.	So-so	______			

Explain in greater detail how you feel about this practice exercise and what you got out of it.

____
____
____
____
____

Concluding Follow-Up Form for Posttraumatic Stress

Name________________________________Sex____Date___________

The purpose of this form is to review whether this practice exercise was helpful to you or not.

1. Please select the answer that best fits how you feel about this practice exercise:

   a. I did not like working on this practice exercise at all. I wish I never saw it. ________
   b. I did not like this practice exercise at all, but I am glad I got to work on it. ________
   c. I am delighted I got a chance to work on this practice exercise. ________
   d. I am not only delighted about working on this practice exercise, but I wish all children who suffer from the same painful experience had a chance to work on it. ________

2. How helpful was it to work on this practice exercise? Check the answer that applies to you:

a. Not helpful at all	______	c. Helpful	______
b. Somewhat helpful	______	d. Very helpful	______

3. Which practice exercise did you *like* best? Please rank-order the practice exercises; rank as No. 1 the one you liked best or was most helpful to you, rank as No. 2 the one you liked next best, and so on; if there is one you did not like at all or that did not apply to you, mark it N/A.

Behaviors	*Rank-order*	*Behaviors*	*Rank-order*
a. Bad dreams	______	i. Emotional isolation/ estrangement	______
b. Upset by reminders	______	j. Lack of pleasure	______
c. Flashbacks (repetitive images)	______	k. Easily startled	______
d. Upset by painful thoughts	______	l. Body reactions and physical troublesome thoughts	______
e. Avoidance of painful thoughts	______	m. Sleep troublesome thoughts	______
f. Avoidance of situations that remind you of past painful experiences	______	n. Fear of recurrence/ hypervigilance	______
g. Avoidance of painful feelings and emotions	______	o. Attention troublesome thoughts	______
h. Numbness of emotions	______	p. Memory/learning troublesome thoughts	______

4. Why did you rank-order the practice exercises the way you did? Please explain your reason(s) for your rank order of practice exercises.

____

____

____

____

5. Feel free to write any comments that might improve this practice exercise.

____
____
____
____
____

Asperger's Disorder

Name________________________________Sex____Date___________

The purpose of this practice exercise is to learn more about the disorder that is affecting you and your family. Please answer all questions or instructions fully.

1. Next to each behavior, explain how it may apply to you. Give two examples of that behavior, whether it applies to you or not.

Behaviors	*Examples*
a. Impairment in social interaction	Example 1 ____________
____________	____________
____________	Example 2 ____________
____________	____________
b. Inability to look straight at others	Example 1 ____________
____________	____________
____________	Example 2 ____________
____________	____________
c. Fixed or frequently unusual body postures ____________	Example 1 ____________
	____________
____________	Example 2 ____________
____________	____________
d. Strange or unusual gestures ______	Example 1 ____________
____________	____________
____________	Example 2 ____________
____________	____________
e. Few if any friendships __________	Example 1 ____________
____________	____________
____________	Example 2 ____________
____________	____________

f. Inadequate enjoyment with others ______________
____
____

Example 1 ______________
____
Example 2 ______________
____

g. Little interest in others ______________
____
____
____

Example 1 ______________
____
Example 2 ______________
____

h. Lack of showing or pointing out objects to others ______________
____
____

Example 1 ______________
____
Example 2 ______________
____

i. Lack of social or emotional reciprocity ______________
____
____

Example 1 ______________
____
Example 2 ______________
____

j. Restricted and repetitive or stereotyped patterns of behavior
____
____

Example 1 ______________
____
Example 2 ______________
____

k. Limited interests or activities
____
____
____

Example 1 ______________
____
Example 2 ______________
____

l. Encompassing preoccupation with one or more patterns of interest
____
____

Example 1 ______________
____
Example 2 ______________
____

m. Focus on a few objects or ideas
____
____
____

Example 1 ______________
____
Example 2 ______________
____

n. Inflexible adherence to specific, nonfunctional routines or rituals
____
____

Example 1 ______________
____
Example 2 ______________
____

o. Stereotyped and repetitive motor mannerisms (hand or finger flapping or twisting) ______________ Example 1 ______________

Example 2 ______________

p. Complex whole-body movements ______________ Example 1 ______________

Example 2 ______________

q. Persistent preoccupation with parts of objects ______________ Example 1 ______________

Example 2 ______________

r. Impairment in social areas ______________ Example 1 ______________

Example 2 ______________

s. Impairment in occupational areas ______________ Example 1 ______________

Example 2 ______________

4 Please rank-order the behaviors listed below according to how much they apply to you, with No. 1 being the one the applies the most, No. 2 that applies second, No. 3 third, and so on; if there are some behaviors that do not apply at all, mark them N/A.

Behaviors	*Rank-order*
a. Impairment in social interaction	______
b. Inability to look straight at others	______
c. Fixed or frequently unusual body postures	______
d. Strange or unusual gestures	______
e. Few if any friendships	______
f. Inadequate enjoyment with others	______
g. Little interest in others	______
h. Lack of showing or pointing out objects to others	______
i. Lack of social or emotional reciprocity	______
j. Restricted and repetitive or stereotyped patterns of behavior	______
k. Limited interests or activities	______
l. Encompassing preoccupation with one or more patterns of interest	______

Behaviors	*Rank-order*
m. Focus on a few objects or ideas	________
n. Inflexible adherence to specific, nonfunctional routines or rituals	________
o. Stereotyped and repetitive motor mannerisms (hand or finger flapping or twisting)	________
p. Complex whole-body movements	________
q. Persistent preoccupation with parts of objects	________
r. Impairment in social areas	________
s. Impairment in occupational area	________

Adults

Depressive Personality

The purpose of this practice exercise is to help you become aware of certain personal characteristics that may put you at risk for unhappiness and make you depend too much on others. This practice exercise, however, may be useless unless you set appointments with yourself at predetermined times to complete each practice exercise.

Practice Exercise 1. What Makes Me So Unhappy?

Name____________________________Sex____Date__________

The purpose of this practice exercise is to find out which personal characteristics predispose you to depend so much on others.

1. How often do you feel sad, mad, or unhappy?

   a. Once a day or more ________
   b. Two or three times a week ________
   c. Once a week ________
   d. Once a month ________
   e. Once every 2 or 3 months ________
   f. Never or hardly ever ________

2. For how long do you feel sad, mad, or unhappy?

   a. Sometimes the whole day or more ________
   b. A couple of hours or half a day ________
   c. About an hour ________
   d. Less than 30 minute ________
   e. 1 minute at the most ________

3. How strong or intense do you feel when you are sad, mad, or unhappy?

   a. Very strong to the point of feeling like ending it all ________
   b. Very intense but without suicidal thoughts ________
   c. Strong enough to be worried about it ________
   d. Not very strong but lasting a long time ________
   e. Mostly moody or sad rather than depressed ________
   f. I am really never depressed, as far as I know ________
   g. Usually I am a very cheerful person ________
   h. Other (explain) ________

4. How do you begin feeling sad, mad, or unhappy?

   a. Usually something/somebody upsets me ________
   b. I really do not know ________
   c. Before I know it, I become sad, mad, or unhappy ________
   d. After an argument or a fight ________
   e. Other (explain) ________

5. How do you end feeling sad, mad, or unhappy?

   a. Suddenly I no longer feel sad, or mad, or unhappy ________
   b. I change my moods without being aware of this change ________
   c. I really do not know ________
   d. Other (explain) ________

6. Below is a list of characteristics usually associated with feeling sad, mad, or unhappy. These characteristics may make you depend on others to see whether you can become happier than you are. Define each characteristic by consulting a dictionary, a loved one, a friend, a teacher, or a professional helper, and give two examples of what you understand this characteristic means.

Characteristics and Definitions	*Examples*
a. Bitterness ________________	Example 1 ________________
________________	________________
________________	Example 2 ________________
________________	________________
b. Constricted ________________	Example 1 ________________
________________	________________
________________	Example 2 ________________
________________	________________

c. Counterdependent or denying dependency ______________________

Example 1 ______________________

Example 2 ______________________

d. Being critical of others ______________________

Example 1 ______________________

Example 2 ______________________

e. Finding it difficult to be critical of others ______________________

Example 1 ______________________

Example 2 ______________________

f. Feeling burdened ______________________

Example 1 ______________________

Example 2 ______________________

g. Given to worry ______________________

Example 1 ______________________

Example 2 ______________________

h. Gloomy ______________________

Example 1 ______________________

Example 2 ______________________

i. Introverted ______________________

Example 1 ______________________

Example 2 ______________________

j. Limited capacity for fun ______________________

Example 1 ______________________

Example 2 ______________________

k. Low self-esteem ______________________

Example 1 ______________________

Example 2 ______________________

l. Moralistic/judgmental ____________ Example 1 ____________
____________ ____________
____________ Example 2 ____________
____________ ____________

m. Negative reactivity ____________ Example 1 ____________
____________ ____________
____________ Example 2 ____________
____________ ____________

n. Talking too much ____________ Example 1 ____________
____________ ____________
____________ Example 2 ____________
____________ ____________

o. Overly dependent ____________ Example 1 ____________
____________ ____________
____________ Example 2 ____________
____________ ____________

p. Passive ____________ Example 1 ____________
____________ ____________
____________ Example 2 ____________
____________ ____________

q. Pessimistic ____________ Example 1 ____________
____________ ____________
____________ Example 2 ____________
____________ ____________

r. Quiet ____________ Example 1 ____________
____________ ____________
____________ Example 2 ____________
____________ ____________

s. Remorseful ____________ Example 1 ____________
____________ ____________
____________ Example 2 ____________
____________ ____________

t. Self-critical ____________ Example 1 ____________
____________ ____________
____________ Example 2 ____________
____________ ____________

u. Self-denying ________________ Example 1 ________________
________________ ________________
________________ Example 2 ________________
________________ ________________

v. Sensitive to rejection ________________ Example 1 ________________
________________ ________________
________________ Example 2 ________________
________________ ________________

w. Serious ________________ Example 1 ________________
________________ ________________
________________ Example 2 ________________
________________ ________________

x. Tense ________________ Example 1 ________________
________________ ________________
________________ Example 2 ________________
________________ ________________

y. Unassertive________________ Example 1 ________________
________________ ________________
________________ Example 2 ________________
________________ ________________

z. Underachiever ________________ Example 1 ________________
________________ ________________
________________ Example 2 ________________
________________ ________________

aa. Characteristic related to you that is not listed above (..................). Write what it is and give two examples of how it applies to you. Example 1 ________________
____
Example 2 ________________
____

7. Why do you become sad, mad, or unhappy? Below is the list of personality characteristics that are usually associated with depression. From this list, rank as No. 1 the strongest characteristic that may be related to being sad, rank-order as No. 2 the second strongest characteristic for feeling sad, mad, or unhappy, and so on; mark as N/A the characteristics that do not apply.

Characteristics	*Rank-order*
a. Bitterness	________
b. Constricted (tight)	________
c. Counterdependent or denying dependency	________

Characteristics	*Rank-order*
d. Critical of others	________
e. Difficulty being critical of others	________
f. Feeling burdened	________
g. Given to worry	________
h. Gloomy	________
i. Introverted	________
j. Limited capacity for fun	________
k. Low self-esteem	________
l. Moralistic	________
m. Negative reactivity	________
n. Talkative	________
o. Overly dependent	________
p. Passive	________
q. Pessimistic	________
r. Quiet	________
s. Remorseful	________
t. Self-critical	________
u. Self-denying	________
v. Sensitive to rejection	________
w. Serious	________
x. Tense	________
y. Unassertive	________
z. Underachiever	________
aa. Characteristic related to you that is not listed above (________________________)	________

8. State why you rank-ordered these characteristics the way you did.

____

____

____

____

Homework: During the coming week, think about your rank-order of characteristics that apply to you and change their rank-order if necessary. Discuss your completed practice exercise with whoever is helping you with this practice exercise.

Standard Format for Depressive Personality

Practice Exercise No._____Title of Characteristic______________________

Name_________________________Sex____Date________

The purpose of this practice exercise is to understand more about the characteristic listed in the title.

1. How did you start using this characteristic? Explain in detail.

____
____
____
____
____

2. How often do you use this characteristic? Check which answer applies to you:

a. Practically every day ______
b. Once a week ______
c. A couple of times a month ______
d. Once a month ______
e. Once every 6 months ______
f. Once a year ______
g. Once every few years ______

3. Explain further.

____
____
____
____
____

4. How did this characteristic come about? Do you remember when it started? Check which answer fits best:

a. When I was a child (younger than 5 years of age) ______
b. In elementary school ______
c. In middle school ______
d. In high school ______
e. Any other time ______

5. Explain further.

____
____
____
____
____

6. What does this characteristic get you? Please explain.

7. Give three specific examples of how using this characteristic is hurtful to you.

Example 1

Example 2

Example 3

8. Give three specific examples of how this characteristic is hurtful to others.

Example 1

Example 2

____
____
____
____
____

Example 3

____
____
____
____
____

9. Now that you have completed this practice exercise, write how you feel about it.

   Check which of these answers tells how you feel about it. There is also space for you to explain further, if you want to:

   a. I did not like it at all, a waste of time. I want to quit this stupid practice exercise. ________
   b. I did not like it very much, but I want to go on with this practice exercise. ________
   c. I liked it and I want to go on with this practice exercise. ________
   d. I liked it a lot and I wish I had something like this practice exercise earlier. ________
   e. I liked it so much that I wish all people with depressive personality characteristics could get something like this to work on. ________

10. Discuss your completed practice exercise with whoever has given it to you.

Homework: If you want to stop this undesirable characteristic, learn to start it. If you learn to start it, you will learn to stop it. Next week plan to repeat this characteristic at preset times (for instance, at 8 a.m., 12 noon, 4 or 7 p.m.) at least three times a week. Write down what happened in detail. For each time make sure to answer in writing the following four questions:

a. How did you start it?
b. What followed?
c. How did it end?
d. What did this behavior get you?

Time 1 (write the time you started__________)

a. ______________________________
____
____

b. ______________________________
____
____

c. ______________________________
____
____

d. ______________________________
____
____

Time 2 (write the time you started__________)

a. ______________________________
____
____

b. ______________________________
____
____

c. ______________________________
____
____

d. ______________________________
____
____

Time 3 (write the time you started__________)

a. ______________________________
____
____

b. ______________________________
____
____

c. ______________________________
____
____

d. ______________________________
____
____

Check which of the following shows what you got out of this homework practice exercise:

a. Completely useless ________
b. Somewhat useless ________
c. So-so ________
d. Somewhat useful ________
e. Extremely useful ________

Write down how you feel about this homework practice exercise and what you got out of it.

____
____
____
____
____

Concluding Feedback Form for Depressive Personality

Name__________________________Sex____Date____________

The purpose of this concluding feedback form is to understand what you learned from working on this practice exercise.

1. Please select the answer that best fits how you feel about this practice exercise:

   a. I did not like working on this practice exercise at all. I wish I never saw it. ________
   b. I did not like this practice exercise, but I am glad I got to work on it. ________
   c. I am happy I got a chance to work on this practice exercise. ________
   d. I am not only delighted with this practice exercise, but I wish depressed people could get it ________

2. How helpful was it to work on this practice exercise? Check the answer that applies to you:

   a. Not helpful at all ________
   b. Somewhat helpful ________
   c. Helpful ________
   d. Very helpful ________

3. Which practice exercise did you *like* best? Please rank-order the practice exercises; rank as No. 1 the one you liked best or was most helpful to you, rank as No. 2 the one you liked next best, and so on; if there is one you did not like at all or that did not apply to you, mark it N/A.

Characteristics	*Rank-order*
a. Bitterness	________
b. Constricted (tight)	________
c. Counterdependent or denying dependency	________
d. Critical of others	________
e. Difficulty being critical of others	________
f. Feeling burdened	________
g. Given to worry	________
h. Gloomy	________
i. Introverted	________
j. Limited capacity for fun	________
k. Low self-esteem	________
l. Moralistic	________
m. Negative reactivity	________
n. Oral	________
o. Overly dependent	________
p. Passive	________
q. Pessimistic	________
r. Quiet	________
s. Remorseful	________
t. Self-critical	________
u. Self-denying	________
v. Sensitive to rejection	________
w. Serious	________
x. Tense	________
y. Unassertive	________
z. Underachiever	________
aa. Characteristic related to you that is not listed above (____________________)	________

4. Now that you have completed this concluding form, write how you feel about it. Check which of these answers tells how you feel about it.

There is also space for you to explain further, if you want to:

a. I did not like it at all, a waste of time. ________
b. I did not like it very much, but I want to go on with working on practice exercises of this type. ________
c. I liked it and I want to go on with another practice exercise. ________
d. I liked it a lot and I wish I had received something like this practice exercise earlier in my life. ________
e. I liked it so much that I wish all people with depressive personality characteristics could get something like this practice exercise ________

5. How could this practice exercise be improved? Do you have any suggestions? Feel free to write whatever suggestion could improve this practice exercise.

Phobias

The purpose of this practice exercise is to help you achieve better control over fears or phobias that control you. However, before you start this practice exercise, you should have passed a complete physical examination, including an ear–nose-and-throat exam, to rule out the possibility that your phobias may arise from physical causes, such as an inner-ear malfunction. If no physical cause is found for your phobia(s), you can start this practice exercise.

Practice Exercise 1. The Nature of Phobias

Name____________________Sex________Date________

The purpose of this practice exercise is to understand what fears and phobias mean to you.

---

1. What do you mean by "fear" and "phobia," as you understand these words?

____
____
____
____
____

2. How are fears different from phobias? Answer this question in terms of at least three characteristics:

   a. Realistic versus unrealistic
   b. General versus specific
   c. Intense versus weak

3. Below is a list of common phobias. Rank them in order of the one(s) that apply directly to you to those that do not apply (N/A) to you at all. Write 1 for the phobia that bothers you the most, 2 for the phobia that bothers you second, and so on. Write NA if that phobia does not bother you at all.

Common Phobias	*Rank-order*	*Rating of Intensity (Strength)*
Blood	________	________
Boats or ships	________	________
Bridges	________	________

Common Phobias	*Rank-order*	*Rating of Intensity (Strength)*
Bright lights	________	________
Bugs	________	________
Buses	________	________
Cancer	________	________
Cars	________	________
Cats	________	________
Cemeteries	________	________
Choking	________	________
Closed spaces	________	________
Crossing the streets	________	________
Crowds	________	________
Dark	________	________
Dirt	________	________
Dogs	________	________
Driving	________	________
Elevators	________	________
Escalators	________	________
Fire	________	________
Flying	________	________
Germs and diseases	________	________
Getting fat	________	________
Heights	________	________
Homosexuals	________	________
Lightning	________	________
Loud noises	________	________
Mice	________	________
Motion	________	________
Needles or knives	________	________
Nuclear energy	________	________
Public speaking	________	________
Rape	________	________
School	________	________
Sex	________	________
Sleeping	________	________
Small enclosed places	________	________
Snakes	________	________
Sports	________	________
Stairs	________	________
Strangers	________	________
Suffocating	________	________
Technology (VCR, PC)	________	________
Telephones	________	________
Thunder	________	________

Common Phobias	*Rank-order*	*Rating of Intensity (Strength)*
Toxic waste	_________	_________
Trains	_________	_________
Traveling	_________	_________
Tunnels	_________	_________
Water (as in swimming)	_________	_________
Weather	_________	_________
Wide-open spaces	_________	_________
Any other phobia not listed above (______)	_________	_________

3. Now go back only to the phobias that you have ranked and not the phobias that you rated N/A. Next to each rated phobia, rate it according to the degree of intensity or strength that it has over you. Write a number that shows how much that phobia bothers you:

   (1) "Calm, as calm as can be"
   (2) "A little bit jittery"
   (3) "Uncomfortably uneasy"
   (4) "Decidedly uneasy"
   (5) "Jittery but still in control"
   (6) "Heart pounding and sweaty"
   (7) "Feeling of losing control"
   (8) "Feeling completely out of control"

4. How did your phobia(s) start? Check all that apply:

   a. Suddenly ______ versus slowly ______
   b. With trauma ______ without trauma ______ (trauma means any specific accident or event that brought about the phobia).
   c. With warning ______ without warning ______

5. What kind of physical feelings do you experience when you become overwhelmed by the phobia? Rank as No. 1 the feeling that applies to you the most. Rank as No. 2 the feeling that applies to you next, and so on. Mark feelings that do not apply to you at all as N/A.

Feelings	*Rank-order*
a. Fight versus flight	_________
b. Waves of anxiety	_________
c. Sense of dread	_________
d. Skipping or racing heart (palpitation)	_________
e. Tightness in the chest	_________
f. Difficulty in breathing (hyperventilation)	_________
g. Sweating	_________

Feelings	*Rank-order*
h. Shaking or trembling	________
i. Hot flushes	________
j. Cold chills	________
k. Light-headedness	________
l. Stomach distress	________
m. "Jelly legs"	________
n. Strange tingling	________
o. Feelings of unreality	________
p. Shortness of breath	________
q. Choking sensation	________
r. Feeling faint	________
s. Fear of going crazy or dying	________
t. Sudden stomach cramps	________
u. Sudden need to urinate	________
v. Coughing on your own spittle	________
w. "This is it. I can't think straight"	________
x. "Get me out of here!"	________
y. "My nerves are all shot"	________
z. "Nothing feels right"	________
Other ______ (Please write what sensations you feel that are not listed above)]	________

Homework: During the coming week, write down the time and duration of each phobia occurrence. Write what you think brought it about, what your reaction was, and how it ended. In addition start a separate sheet or diary in which you try to answer the following three questions in the next few weeks.

a. Why am I fearful?

____
____
____
____
____

b. What provokes my fearfulness?

____
____
____
____
____

c. Why do I anticipate or expect the worst rather than the best?

____
____
____
____
____

d. As thoughts about these three questions come into your mind, jot them down.

____
____
____
____
____

Practice Exercise 2. Learning More About Phobias

Name______________________________Sex____Date__________

The purpose of this practice exercise is to help you learn more about phobias so that you may become familiar with them.

____

1. There are at least seven kinds of phobias. See which of these relate to your particular phobia(s):

   A. Balance-related phobias:

      ii. Light-headedness
      iii. Feeling off-balance
      iv. Floating sensation
      v. Spinning or whirling sensation
      vi. "Magnetic tug" from the ground below
      vii. Falling
      viii. Fainting
      ix. Tipping or swaying

   B. Compass-related phobias:

      i. Disorientation
      ii. Confusion
      iii. Floating
      iv. Spaciness
      v. Feelings of unreality or dissociation from reality

C. Motor-related phobias

i. Trouble walking
ii. Trouble getting up from bed or chairs
iii. Trouble starting to walk

D. Visual phobias:

i. Not liking certain colors
ii. Not liking certain objects
iii. Not liking certain pictures

E. Auditory phobias

i. Not liking loud noises
ii. Not liking certain words
iii. Not liking certain music

F. Coordination phobias:

i. Not liking certain body positions
ii. Not liking standing erect
iii. Not liking sitting down
iv. Not liking lying down
v. Not liking certain sports

G. Feeling like a "guided missile" and not feeling in control:

i. Fear of escalators
ii. Fear of elevators
iii. Fear of tunnels
iv. Fear of bridges

2. Can you recognize any of these phobias in you? Which one(s)? Write about the one(s) that you recognize in yourself. Specify what the fear applies to. For instance, if you are fearful of loud noises, are there certain noises that you are more fearful of?

Homework: During the next week: (1) Continue to write down your answers to the three questions asked in the first practice exercise:

a. Why am I fearful?
b. What provokes my fearfulness?
c. Why do I anticipate the worst rather than the best?

(2) Become aware of which of the seven types of fears listed above seems to bother you. Write it down every time you become aware of this fear.

Standard Practice Exercise For Phobias

Practice Exercise No.____Title of Phobia________________________

Name____________________________Sex____Date_________

The purpose of this practice exercise and the following ones is to teach you to introduce "positive interference" every time you start to feel phobic. A positive interference is any positive activity that you will use every time you begin to feel phobic. This interference can be both physical and/or verbal. For instance, if you start to become phobic by feeling body sensations that indicate the beginning of your phobia, whichever phobia it may be, you need to start saying the word "relax." As soon as you say this word to yourself, you must immediately do two things. The first one you may not be able to perform except when you are at home. The second you can perform almost anywhere.

1. Relax physically: If possible, play a tape or radio station with pleasant music that you find soothing. Then lie down on a couch, sofa, bed, or floor. Start thinking about a very pleasant scene, such as a lake in the mountains, the seashore, etc. As you are thinking of this scene and pleasant music is also playing, tense up one extremity of your body at a time. Start with the lower part of your left leg, tense it as much as you can and let go when you say the word "relax." Go from one leg to the other, and then to the stomach, hips, chest (if you can), arms, and neck. If necessary, continue doing this exercise as long as necessary for you to feel relaxed and in control.

   After you are finished, record on a sheet of paper the time you exercised, for how long, and how many times you performed this exercise.

2. Relax verbally: Suppose you are talking with your boss or a customer, and all of a sudden, out of the blue, you start feeling phobic, for whatever reason. If you have a note pad in front of you, you could write the word "relax" on it. Instead of taking notes, you might start to write down words that begin with each of the five letters in the word "relax," such as "rest," "examine," "love," "almighty," "xylophone." You can do this exercise even when you are by yourself. However, you must be sure that all the words you use are positive and not negative. You might have a hard time finding positive words starting with "x," but this is another type of interference that will be useful to you instead of becoming phobic.

3. Here is a list of all the positive interferences you can apply to yourself whenever you start to feel phobic. Rank them in order of preference according to how comfortably you would apply it to yourself. Rank as No. 1 the positive interference that you want to apply most comfortably to yourself. Rank as No. 2. the next one, and so on; mark as N/A the interferences that you would not feel comfortable in applying to yourself.

Positive Interferences	*Rank-order*
a. Squeeze one hand with the other hand	________
b. Wiggle your big toe with your shoe on	________
c. Snap a rubber band encircling your wrist	________
d. Swat the back of your neck hard and fast ten times	________
e. Chew on a fresh stick of gum	________
f. Click your tongue against the roof of your mouth	________
g. Keep your eye on something real	________
h. Watch seconds go by on your watch or clock	________
i. Change the lighting	________
j. Sniff a handkerchief	________
k. Let your nose turn you on	________
l. Carry a menthol inhaler and use it when needed	________
m. Use of bottle of smelling salts when needed	________
n. Use a power light	________
o. Eat some comfort food	________
p. Lick a lollipop	________
q. Pick yourself up with a pickle	________
r. Turn up the volume of your radio when listening to music	________
s. Plug ears with headphones	________
t. Play a musical instrument	________
u. Give a little whistle	________
v. Listen to yourself	________
w. Memorize things to do or to buy	________
x. Do a crossword puzzle or any puzzle	________
y. Pull the lobe of your left ear three times	________
z. Concentrate on your breathing for at least 5 minute	________

4. Can you think of any other type of positive interference not listed above that you would feel comfortable in using? What is it?____________________

5. How would you rate it in comparison to the positive interferences listed above?

Homework: Select which positive interference you would feel comfortable in using, and during the coming week(s) keep track of how many times you have used it. Make sure to write down how many times you have used this positive interference during the coming week(s) and what kind of results you got. Bring this list to your professional helper for discussion and feedback.

Next-to-the-Last Practice Exercise: Learning to Start your Phobia(s)

Name______________________________Sex____Date___________

Now comes the hard part. The purpose of this practice exercise is to find out whether you have learned to control your phobia(s) or whether it or them still control you. The principle behind this practice exercise is that if you have learned to control your phobia(s), you can start it whenever you want to and not when the phobia wants to. If you can start your phobia, you can stop it. If you can control it without being bothered by it, that means that you have won the battle of control over your phobia.

Consequently, during the next week, set up specific times and places when and where you will start your phobia. If possible, see if you can start some of the physical sensations that go together with your phobia(s). For example, you may want to start the phobia on Monday, Wednesday, and Friday at 9 p.m. in your family room. It is important that you set this appointment with yourself beforehand (at least 24 h in advance) when you will start your phobia, because this appointment will put you in control of your phobia. Make sure that you record every time you have started your phobia(s).

Make sure you bring your record of your appointments to your professional helper for discussion, feedback, and recommendations.

Last Practice Exercise for Phobia

Name______________________________Sex____Date____________

Check on homework and if necessary retest if any instrument was administered before this practice exercise. If results are negative, and your phobias are still present 3–4 weeks after starting this practice exercise, and the phobias are still bothering you, you may need to consult (1) another behavioral therapist–psychologist–specialist, or (2) a psychiatrist for possible medication. The important thing is not to give up on yourself. If this approach does not work, try something else. Remember that Rome was not built in a day! Thank you for trying!

Procrastination

The purpose of this practice exercise and its practice exercises is to help you deal with procrastination in your work or study habits.

Practice Exercise 1. Defining Procrastination

Name______________________________________Sex____Date__________

The purpose of this practice exercise is to help you define what procrastination means to you and how it affects your life. Please answer the following questions to the best of your ability.

1. What does procrastination mean to you? Please write how you tend to procrastinate.

____

____

____

____

____

2. How much does it affect you personally?

   a. A great deal, most of the time __________
   b. Sometimes, but not all the time __________
   c. Never __________

3. How does it affect your routines?

   a. A great deal, most of the time __________
   b. Sometimes, but not all the time __________
   c. Never __________

4. How does (or did) it affect your studies?

   a. A great deal, most of the time __________
   b. Sometimes, but not all the times __________
   c. Never __________

5. How does it affect your personal relationships?

   a. A great deal, most of the time __________
   b. Sometimes, but not all the time __________
   c. Never __________

6. Does procrastination affect some parts of your personality or does it pervade all of your personaliy?

   a. All my personality __________
   b. Parts of my personality __________
   c. No part of my personality __________

7. Who has reacted to your procrastination? Check more than one.

   a. Your parents ________
   b. Your relatives ________
   c. Your brothers and sisters ________
   d. Your best friend ________
   e. Your teachers ________
   f. Your boss ________
   g. Your coworkers ________
   h. Your friends ________

8. Please specify what reactions you received from whom.

____
____
____
____
____

9. How intense (strong) is your tendency to procrastinate?

   a. Very strong ________
   b. Strong ________
   c. Somewhat strong ________
   d. Weak ________
   e. Very weak ________

10. Explain in greater detail how strong this tendency to procrastinate is for you.

____
____
____
____
____

Homework: During the next week try to become more aware of how procrastination controls your life, especially in three areas:

a. Studies (if it applies)
b. Relationships with people you care about
c. Work (if it applies)
d. Any other area not covered by the three previous items

If you have not yet figured out why you keep putting things off, spend some time trying to figure it out. Make an appointment with yourself, sit in a comfortable chair with a notebook, and start to write down all the possible reasons, causes, and past events that may be responsible for your procrastination. Was it your toilet training? Was it your mother's habit to delay completing anything? Was it your father's? Did you receive more attention by not completing tasks than by completing them? Write down as many possibilities as come to mind, no matter how outlandish they may be. Do not try to write well; just write down what circumstances may have existed for your putting things off. Put your notes where you can find them. Wait at least 48 h to make another appointment with yourself and go back to your original notes. See whether more thoughts come to you as you read them. Is the possible cause still valid now, or does it appear less plausible or valid than it appeared when you wrote it down? Once your list is restricted to two or three conclusions, bring it to your counseling or therapy session and discuss your conclusions with your professional helper.

Practice Exercise 2. The Causes of Procrastination

Name____________________________________Sex____Date________

The purpose of this practice exercise is to find the possible causes of your procrastination.

1. Among the many causes of procrastination listed below, rank as No. 1 the ones that are most troublesome to you. Rank as No. 2 the causes that are the next most troublesome to you, and so on, so that the least troublesome ones would be ranked last:

Possible Causes	*Rank*
a. Delay	________
b. Irrationality	________
c. Weak personality	________
d. Depression	________
e. Anxiety	________
f. Low self-esteem	________
g. Guilt and shame	________
h. Incorrect thinking	________
i. Other cause (_______________)	________

2. Now that you have ranked these causes, start concentrating on the most troublesome cause, by writing about it in detail. What is it?_______________

   a. How did this type of procrastination start?

   ____

   ____

   ____

b. How did you keep it up?

____

____

____

c. What are the results of this type of procrastination?

____

____

____

3. What did you do to avoid procrastinating, if at all?

____

____

____

____

4. What were the results?

____

____

____

____

5. Do you want to learn to control procrastination or do you want it to control you? If you choose to have procrastination continue to control you, you do not need to complete this practice exercise or this practice exercise. However, if you want to learn to control your procrastination, do complete this homework.

Homework: During the next week become aware of how much this procrastination is controlling you and how it affects you by lowering your level of functioning or performance. Make sure you write down any instance of procrastination. As you are completing this part of the homework, answer the following questions:

1. What are my overall goals in life?
2. What are my most immediate goals?
3. How am I going to differentiate most immediate from least immediate goals?
4. How am I going to reach my most immediate goal?

After you have answered questions 1–3, answer question 4 by developing a plan of small steps that will allow to reach your most immediate goal without failure. Discuss this plan with whoever helps you with this practice exercise.

Practice Exercise 3. Learning to Control Procrastination

Name________________________________Sex____Date__________

The purpose of this practice exercise is to help you learn to control your procrastination.

1. If you want to learn to control your procrastination, there are many ways of achieving control over it. This practice exercise suggests a variety of steps that you should try. Perhaps one of them will work for you.

   Step 1. Plan when you will start procrastinating by setting a time when you will start and a time when you will end procrastinating.

   The principle behind this step is that if you want to end something, you have to learn to start it. If you have the power to start procrastinating, eventually you will have the power to end it.

   Step 2. Write down how you feel when you are procrastinating. Do you feel blue, sad, happy, angry, or something else? How much of these feelings are behind your tendency to procrastinate?

   Step 3. Make a list of everything you need to do. After you have completed this list, rank all your items according to two criteria: (1) importance, and (2) urgency. You have to ask yourself how each item is important to you and how urgent it is. After you have rank-ordered your items according to both criteria, write down what the consequences will be if you delay implementing that item. Divide the consequences into positive and negative ones. Then decide which item would give you the greatest grief or discomfort if you were to delay its completion. Ask yourself if you want to subject yourself to grief and discomfort, or whether you would be better off if you were to complete the item after all.

   Hence, you now have three criteria to rank-order your items:

   (1) Importance to your survival
   (2) Urgency in terms of what is expected of you by those who would be affected by your delay
   (3) Long-term consequences that would take place if you were to delay completion

   Step 4. Pick the item that seems to be the most important to your survival and pleasure, the most urgent in terms of what is expected of you, and in the long-term consequences to you if you were to delay completion. If the task to be completed is too large or complicated, to the point that even talking about it is scary or anxiety-provoking to you, start to break it down into smaller steps by writing down what each step is and how you are going to complete it.

Step 5. Go back to Step 1 and start all over again.

Homework: During the next week, write down how you feel when you have completed a task, no matter how small and mundane it may be. For instance, how do you feel after you have brushed your teeth, gone to the bathroom, washed, or completed a meal? Similarly, write down how you feel when you do not complete a task. It is very important that you begin to discriminate how you feel after completion and after noncompletion, because these feelings are going to be the major determinants of whether you complete or do not complete a task.

Practice Exercise 4. Practicing Your Plan

Name________________________________Sex____Date_________

The purpose of this practice exercise is to start practicing a plan to control your procrastination.

1. If you have completed last week's homework practice exercise, by now you should have been able to discriminate between "good" feelings after completion and not-so-good feelings after noncompletion. Which feelings do you like best. If you like your feelings after noncompletion, you do not need to go any further in this practice exercise. You do need to speak with your professional helper about these feelings. If, however, you do not like the feelings that result from noncompletion and want to go on with this program, go right ahead!

2. Pick another task, job, responsibility, or whatever you have procrastinated about and follow all the steps outlined in the previous practice exercise. Write down what the consequences, positive or negative, would be of your delaying completion of that task. If positive consequences are greater than the negative ones, go ahead, if you can, and tackle the task. Again, if the task is too complex or difficult, break it down into small steps and attack each step, one at time.

3. If you have trouble in getting started, ask yourself whether you expect perfection from yourself and therefore you need to be perfect in even completing this homework practice exercise. If perfection is one of the causes of your delay, make yourself do or complete some task in a very sloppy way. Allow yourself to be imperfect. If you cannot accept your imperfection, you need to discuss this inability with your professional helper. If you can accept your imperfection, do go on.

4. Some people are unable to even get started because they are equating their performance and production to their personality: "What I do or have is what I am." If their performance or production is inadequate or incomplete, their own self is going to be inadequate or incomplete. What is the error in such an equation? If we are what we do or have, who are we? Hence, it could be that by equating what you do or have with yourself, you have been unable to separate your performance or production from your own self. Who you are is separate and independent from what you do and what you have. You may need to discuss this issue with your professional helper. How much does this possibility apply to you?

   a. A great deal, most of the time __________
   b. Sometimes, but not all the time __________
   c. Never __________

5. If you answered "a" or "b," you will need to discuss this with your professional helper. If you answered "c," this practice exercise may not be relevant to your needs.

Homework: During the next week, force yourself not to complete anything well or adequately. You need to practice being a human being (by definition imperfect) rather than trying to be a perfect piece of machinery. Write down what you left undone and how you felt afterwards.

Practice Exercise 5. Checking on Your Progress (If There Is Any)

Name______________________________Sex____Date_________

The purpose of this practice exercise is to check on your progress in following the plan you have devised in the previous practice exercise.

1. Assuming that you have kept lists of what you have accomplished or not accomplished during the last few weeks, look over your lists and try to determine whether there is any pattern in the tasks you have completed successfully and in those that you have not. If there is one, can you find it? If you cannot find a pattern, go on with this practice exercise. If you have found a pattern, discuss it with your professional helper and then decide whether you need to go on with this practice exercise or not.

2. What happens when you give yourself deadlines? Are deadlines something to avoid because they cause too much anxiety, or are they to be kept because they make you more effective? However, if you are about to set deadlines, make sure they are realistic and feasible.

3. If you are unable to stick with deadlines, do you know why? If you do not know, do you need to know? Can you keep deadlines even if you do not know

why you cannot keep them? There is such a thing as going overboard with deadlines. Where is the happy medium for you? Answer these questions to the best of your knowledge and, if necessary, discuss your answers with your professional helper.

4. Behind any procrastination looms the whole issue of what time means for you. Is time something to squander and waste, or is time something precious that we need to preserve and use to its fullest? Does time control you or are you in control of your time? Answer these questions and go on to the next question.

5. You may need to start keeping more notice of how much time you need to brush your teeth, bathe, dress, cook or have breakfast, get to work, and so on, until the end of the day.

Homework: Next week, keep a running diary of exactly how much time it takes for completion of any activity or task, starting from brushing your teeth, washing, eating breakfast, going to work, etc. Coming home from work, you need to write down how long it took to cook and finish dinner, how long it took to read the paper or go through your mail, etc., including how long it took to take your clothes off and preparing to go to bed. Without this knowledge it may very hard for you to appreciate time and to learn to control it for your purposes.

Practice Exercise 6. Looking Back and Looking Forward

Name______________________________Sex____Date_________

The purpose of this practice exercise is to reflect on what you have done or not done to control and use your procrastination to your advantage.

1. It is time to take stock of whether you have learned anything from this practice exercise. How much did you learn?

   a. A great deal ________ c. Not at all ________
   b. Some ________

2. Not all practice exercises like this can be helpful to all people. If you have checked "c," then this practice exercise failed to help you. You will need to discuss this failure with your professional helper. If you have checked "a" or "b," write down in detail how this practice exercise was helpful to you.

____
____
____
____
____

3. What did you like about this practice exercise? Was there any practice exercise that was particularly more helpful than others? Why?

____
____
____
____
____

4. What did you dislike about the practice exercise? Was there any practice exercise that was particularly useless to you? Why?

____
____
____
____
____

5. How could this practice exercise be improved? Your suggestions for any improvement will be very welcome. Feel free to write any suggestion that you think would improve this program.

____
____
____
____
____

6. The success of any practice exercise is indicated by whether you would recommend it to anyone you know who suffers from procrastination. Would you recommend it to someone?

   a. Highly ________ c. Not at all ________
   b. Possibly ________

7. Your reasons for your above choice would be greatly appreciated.

____
____
____
____
____

Anxiety

The purpose of this practice exercise is to help you learn to live with and possibly control and lower your anxiety level. To achieve this goal, you will need to make an appointment with yourself to work on each practice exercise at a preset time. For instance, you may set your time at 7 p.m. on Wednesdays. That means that every Wednesday, no matter what, you will set aside time to work on your anxiety at 7 p.m. If something happens that you cannot control that does not allow you to meet at this preset time, give yourself at least 24 h' notice, so that you learn to control anxiety when you want, rather than having anxiety control you.

Practice Exercise 1. Defining Anxiety

Name______________________________________Sex____Date____________

The purpose of this practice exercise is to help you understand what anxiety means to you and how it controls you. In this way, you can learn more from it, rather than going around in circles and not being able to control what you do not understand.

1. What is anxiety for you? Please define it as it applies especially to you.

____
____
____
____
____

2. How often do you experience these feelings?

a. All the time __________ d. Seldom __________
b. Often __________ e. Other (please explain)
c. Occasionally __________

3. How long do they last?

a. Years __________ d. Days __________
b. Months __________ e. Hours __________
c. Weeks __________ f. Other (please explain) __________

4. How intense are these feelings?

a. Extreme __________ c. Mild __________
b. Moderate __________ d. Other (please explain) __________

5. Anxiety is made up by a variety of feelings. Define each feeling as you understand it, and give two examples of or explain how each feeling applies to you.

Feelings and Definitions	*Examples*
a. Tension (shaky, restless, tight muscles or tired) ______ ______	Example 1 ______ ______ Example 2 ______ ______
b. Heart pounding or palpitations ______ ______ ______	Example 1 ______ ______ Example 2 ______ ______
c. Shortness of breath ______ ______ ______	Example 1 ______ ______ Example 2 ______ ______
d. Nausea, diarrhea, or abdominal distress ______ ______	Example 1 ______ ______ Example 2 ______ ______
e. Sweating or clammy hands ______ ______ ______	Example 1 ______ ______ Example 2 ______ ______
f. Other physical troublesome thoughts ______ ______ ______	Example 1 ______ ______ Example 2 ______ ______
g. Sleep troublesome thoughts ______ ______ ______	Example 1 ______ ______ Example 2 ______ ______
h. Worrying ______ ______ ______	Example 1 ______ ______ Example 2 ______ ______

i. Trouble concentrating ______________________ Example 1 ______________________
______________________ Example 2 ______________________
______________________ ______________________

j. Fear of losing my mind Example 1 ______________________
______________________ ______________________
______________________ Example 2 ______________________
______________________ ______________________

k. Fear of not making it in life Example 1 ______________________
______________________ ______________________
______________________ Example 2 ______________________
______________________ ______________________

l. Fear of losing my job Example 1 ______________________
______________________ ______________________
______________________ Example 2 ______________________
______________________ ______________________

m. Fear of failing in school Example 1 ______________________
______________________ ______________________
______________________ Example 2 ______________________
______________________ ______________________

n. Fear of losing my friends Example 1 ______________________
______________________ ______________________
______________________ Example 2 ______________________
______________________ ______________________

o. Irritability Example 1 ______________________
______________________ ______________________
______________________ Example 2 ______________________
______________________ ______________________

p. Other fears (name them) and define ______________________ Example 1 ______________________
______________________ Example 2 ______________________
______________________ ______________________

6. Rank those feelings, emotions, or troublesome thoughts in the order of most troublesome to least troublesome according to how you feel. Rank-order the feeling, emotion, or troublesome thought that is generally the worst as number 1, the next worst as number 2, the next worst as number 3; mark as N/A the feelings that do not apply to you.

Feelings	*Rank-order*
a. Tension (shaky, restless, tight muscles, or tired)	________
b. Heart pounding or palpitations	________
c. Shortness of breath	________
d. Nausea, diarrhea, or abdominal distress	________
e. Sweating or clammy hands	________
f. Other physical troublesome thoughts	________
g. Sleep troublesome thoughts	________
h. Worrying	________
i. Trouble concentrating	________
j. Fear of losing my mind	________
k. Fear of not making it in life	________
l. Fear of losing my job	________
m. Fear of failing in school	________
n. Fear of losing my friends	________
o. Irritability	________
p. Other fears	________

Homework: During the coming week, think more about all these feelings and how you rank-ordered them. Change the rank order if you feel it needs to be changed.

Now you must make up your mind. Do you want to learn to control your anxiety, or do you want your anxiety to control you? If you want your anxiety to control you, do nothing and go on as you have always done in the past. If you want to learn to control your anxiety, the following homework may be of help to you.

During the next week, make an appointment with yourself (at least 24 h from now) every other day at regular times for regular periods of time, for instance, Tuesday, Thursday, and Saturday at 9 p.m. for 30–60 minute. During these times make sure that you can work on your anxiety without anyone or anything disturbing you. Remember that if you want to learn to stop your anxiety, you need to start it at preset, regular times. In this way, you will learn to achieve control over your anxiety.

During each of these appointments, pay attention to the feeling you selected to write about during this week's practice exercise. Go back to a time when you strongly felt this emotion (you may feel it in the present). As soon as you feel this feeling, begin to write down whatever you feel or whatever comes into your mind that relates to it or that is brought forth by your experiencing and staying with the feeling. Try to make yourself stay with the feeling during the length of the practice exercise.

Discuss your notes with your professional helper each week after you complete your practice exercise. After you finish with this anxiety feeling, use the same procedure for the next anxiety feeling. (Try to stay with the same feeling for the entire week. Switch to another feeling the next week if you can.)

Standard Practice Exercise for Anxiety

Practice Exercise No. Title of Symptom.

Name______________________________Sex_____Date______________

The goal of this practice exercise and the following ones is to help you learn to control your anxiety rather than having your anxiety control you. To achieve this goal, write in the title of this practice exercise the feeling you have ranked as being the most troublesome to you, that is, No. 1. In future practice exercises, write in the title of each practice exercise the feeling that was next in rank order, until you have completed all the feelings you rank-ordered that apply to you.

1. Why did you select the feeling or troublesome thought that you rated as the most uncomfortable? What makes this feeling or troublesome thought seem so bad?

2. How did this feeling or troublesome thought develop? What events and thoughts have contributed to this feeling or troublesome thought developing in your life?

3. How old were you when you became aware of this feeling?

4. How has your family contributed to this feeling or troublesome thought? Are there other family members who share the same feeling?

5. What does this feeling or troublesome thought do to you?

6. What does this feeling or troublesome thought do to your family?

7. What does this feeling do to people you are attracted to?

8. How does this feeling or troublesome thought upset other areas of your life? (i.e., friends, work, leisure, school)

9. What memories do you have of experiencing this troublesome thought or feeling? What was happening? Do you remember?

Homework: At least twice or three times during the coming week, make appointments for yourself at preset times to start feeling the way you have just written about in this practice exercise. The rule to follow is that if you can learn to start it on your own, you will be able to have control over it, and eventually, if and when you learn to start it, you will learn how to stop it. Start it if you want to stop it! However, make sure you write down what you are feeling during this practice exercise.

Concluding Follow-Up Form

Name____________________________________Sex____Date________

The purpose of this form is to find out whether the practice exercises of this practice exercise helped you or not. Feel free to be as open and honest as you can because only in this way will you be helped if further help is needed.

1. Please select the answer that best fits how you feel about this practice exercise:

   a. I did not like working on this practice exercise at all. I wish I never saw it. _________
   b. I did not like this practice exercise, but I am glad I got to work on. _________
   c. I am happy I got a chance to work on this. _________
   d. I am not only delighted about this practice exercise, but I wish all people who are very anxious could get it. _________

2. How helpful was it to work on this practice exercise? Check the answer that applies to you:

   a. Not helpful at all _________ c. Helpful _________
   b. Somewhat helpful _________ d. Very helpful _________

3. Which practice exercise did you like best? Please rank-order the practice exercises; rank as No. 1 the one you liked best or was most helpful to you, rank as No. 2 the one you liked next best, and so on; if there is one you did not like at all or that did not apply to you, mark it N/A.

Practice Exercises	*Rank-order*
a. Tension (shaky, restless, tight muscles, or tired)	_________
b. Heart pounding or palpitations	_________
c. Shortness of breath	_________
d. Nausea, diarrhea, or abdominal distress	_________
e. Sweating or clammy hands	_________
f. Other physical troublesome thoughts	_________
g. Sleep troublesome thoughts	_________
h. Worrying	_________

Practice Exercises	*Rank-order*
i. Trouble concentrating	________
j. Fear of losing my mind	________
k. Fear of not making it in life	________
l. Fear of losing my job	________
m. Fear of failing in school	________
n. Fear of losing my friends	________
o. Irritability	________
p. Other fears	________

4. Please explain why you rank-ordered the practice exercises the way you did.

____
____
____
____
____

5. Any suggestions on how to improve this practice exercise will be greatly appreciated.

____
____
____
____
____

Depression

The purpose of this practice exercise is to help you learn to control depression rather than having depression control you.

Practice Exercise 1. Defining Signs of Depression

Name________________________________Sex____Date__________

The purpose of this practice exercise is to define depression as you understand it. There are many definitions of depression and it is important that you define it as you see it.

1. What does depression mean to you?

2. Define and give two examples of how each sign that applies to you. Use a dictionary or online information to define a sign if you need to.

Signs and Definitions	Examples
a. Finding little or no pleasure in life	Example 1 Example 2
b. Feeling worthless or extremely guilty	Example 1 Example 2
c. Crying a lot for no reason	Example 1 Example 2
d. Withdrawing from other people	Example 1 Example 2
e. Experiencing severe anxiety, panic, and fear	Example 1 Example 2
f. Having bad mood swings	Example 1 Example 2

g. Experiencing a change in eating or sleeping patterns

Example 1 ______________________________

Example 2 ______________________________

h. Having very low energy

Example 1 ______________________________

Example 2 ______________________________

i. Losing interest in hobbies and pleasurable activities

Example 1 ______________________________

Example 2 ______________________________

j. Having too much energy, having trouble concentrating or following through on plans

Example 1 ______________________________

Example 2 ______________________________

k. Feelings easily irritated or angry

Example 1 ______________________________

Example 2 ______________________________

l. Experiencing racing thoughts or agitation

Example 1 ______________________________

Example 2 ______________________________

m. Hearing voices or seeing images that other people do not experience

Example 1 ______________________________

Example 2 ______________________________

n. Believing that others are plotting against you

Example 1 ______________________________

Example 2 ______________________________

o. Wanting to harm yourself or someone else

Example 1 ______________________________

Example 2 ______________________________

5. After you have defined these signs of depression, rank them according to how closely each of them resembles your depression. Rank-order the most familiar or applicable to you as No. 1, the second most familiar as No. 2, and so on; mark as N/A the least familiar to you.

Signs of Depression	*Rank-order*
a. Finding little or no pleasure in life	_________
b. Feeling worthless or extremely guilty	_________
c. Crying a lot for no reason	_________
d. Withdrawing from other people	_________
e. Experiencing severe anxiety, panic, and fear	_________
f. Having bad mood swings	_________
g. Experiencing a change in eating or sleeping patterns	_________
h. Having very low energy	_________
i. Losing interest in hobbies and pleasurable activities	_________
j. Having too much energy, having trouble concentrating or following through on plans	_________
k. Feelings easily irritated or angry	_________
l. Experiencing racing thoughts or agitation	_________
m. Hearing voices or seeing images that other people do not experience	_________
n. Believing that others are plotting against you	_________
o. Wanting to harm yourself or someone else	_________

4. Explain why you rank-ordered these sign the way you just did.

____
____
____
____
____

Homework: During the next few days, keep on thinking about these signs and whether you want to keep their rank order as is or whether you want to change it.

Standard Practice Exercise for Signs of Depression

Name of Sign____________________Practice Exercise No.______

Name______________________________Sex____Date______

The purpose of this practice exercise is to learn more about the sign of depression listed in the title of this practice exercise.

1. How does this sign trouble you? Please explain in detail.

____

____

____

____

____

2. How often does this sign trouble you? Check which answer applies to you:

a. Practically every day	_____	e. Once every 6 months	_____
b. Once a week	_____	f. Once a year	_____
c. A couple of times a month	_____	g. Once every few years	_____
d. Once a month	_____		

3. Please explain further.

____

____

____

____

____

4. How did this sign come about? Do you remember when you started feeling it? Check which answer fits best:

a. When I was a child (younger than 5 years of age) _________
b. When I was in elementary school _________
c. When I was in middle school _________
d. When I was in high school _________
e. After high school _________
f. Any other time _________

5. Please explain further.

____

____

____

____

____

6. Give three specific examples of how this sign troubles you.

   Example 1

   ____
   ____
   ____
   ____
   ____

   Example 2

   ____
   ____
   ____
   ____
   ____

   Example 3

   ____
   ____
   ____
   ____
   ____

Homework: Next week, in order for you to learn to control this sign ("Start it if you want to stop it!"), plan to repeat it at preset times (for instance, at 8 a.m., 12 noon, 4 or 7 p.m.), on at least 3 days (Monday, Wednesday, and Friday, or Tuesday, Thursday, and Saturday). Write down what happened in detail. For each time make sure to answer in writing the following four questions:

a. How did you start this sign?
b. What followed after you felt this sign?
c. How did this sign end?
d. What did this sign get you?

Time 1 (write the time you started__________)

a. ____
____
____

b. ____
____
____

c. ____
____
____

d. ____
____
____

Time 2 (write the time you started__________)

a. ____
____
____

b. ____
____
____

c. ____
____
____

d. ____
____
____

Time 3 (write the time you started__________)

a. ____
____
____

b. ____
____
____

c. ____
____
____

d. ____
____
____

Please check which of the following shows what you got out of this practice exercise:

a. Completely useless _______
b. Somewhat useless _______
c. So-so _______
d. Somewhat useful _______
e. Extremely useful _______

Explain how you feel about this homework practice exercise and what you got out of it.

____
____
____
____
____

Concluding Feedback Form for Signs of Depression

Name________________________________Sex____Date______

The purpose of this form is to find out how you feel about the practice exercises you completed in this practice exercise.

1. Please select the answer that best fits how you feel about this practice exercise:

   a. I did not like working on this practice exercise at all. I wish I never saw it. ________
   b. I did not like this practice exercise at all, but I am glad I got to work on it. ________
   c. I am delighted I got a chance to work on this practice exercise. ________
   d. I am not only delighted about this practice exercise, but I wish all depressed people had a chance to work on it. ________

2. How helpful was it to work on this practice exercise? Check the answer that applies to you:

   a. Not helpful at all ________ c. Helpful ________
   b. Somewhat helpful ________ d. Very helpful ________

3. Rank-order the practice exercises you have completed. Rank-order each practice exercise according to how much you liked it. Rank-order as No. 1 the practice exercise you liked the most. Rank as No. 2 the practice exercise that you liked second best, and so on; mark as N/A the practice exercises you did not like at all or that you do not feel you can rank with the others.

Signs of Depression	*Rank-order*
a. Finding little or no pleasure in life	________
b. Feeling worthless or extremely guilty	________
c. Crying a lot for no reason	________
d. Withdrawing from other people	________
e. Experiencing severe anxiety, panic, and fear	________
f. Having bad mood swings	________

Signs of Depression | *Rank-order*

g. Experiencing a change in eating or sleeping patterns ________
h. Having very low energy ________
i. Losing interest in hobbies and pleasurable activities ________
j. Having too much energy, having trouble concentrating or following through on plans ________
k. Feelings easily irritated or angry ________
l. Experiencing racing thoughts or agitation ________
m. Hearing voices or seeing images that other people do not experience ________
n. Believing that others are plotting against you ________
o. Wanting to harm yourself or someone else ________

4. Why did you rank-order the practice exercises the way you did?

____
____
____
____
____

6. Which practice exercise was the most helpful to you? Sometimes what we like most is not necessarily the most helpful. Consequently, could you rank the practice exercises according to their helpfulness to you? Rank as No. 1 the most helpful, No. 2 the next most helpful, and so on until the least helpful practice exercise.

Signs of Depression | *Rank-order*

a. Finding little or no pleasure in life ________
b. Feeling worthless or extremely guilty ________
c. Crying a lot for no reason ________
d. Withdrawing from other people ________
e. Experiencing severe anxiety, panic, and fear ________
f. Having bad mood swings ________
g. Experiencing a change in eating or sleeping patterns ________
h. Having very low energy ________
i. Losing interest in hobbies and pleasurable activities ________
j. Having too much energy, having trouble concentrating or following through on plans ________
k. Feelings easily irritated or angry ________
l. Experiencing racing thoughts or agitation ________
m. Hearing voices or seeing images that other people do not experience ________
n. Believing that others are plotting against you ________
o. Wanting to harm yourself or someone else ________

6. Why did you rank-order the practice exercises the way you did?

____
____
____
____
____

7. Feel free to write any comments that might improve this practice exercise.

____
____
____
____
____

Posttraumatic Stress Disorder

The purpose of this practice exercise is to help you understand the nature of your disorder. You will be asked to answer in writing many practice exercises containing a great many questions about the many behaviors that make up your condition. Of course, you do not have to answer any question or complete any practice exercise. Participation in working on this practice exercise is completely voluntary, and you do not have to answer any questions or complete any practice exercise if you do not want to do it. It is completely up to you whether you want to learn more about yourself and whether you want the professionals interested in your welfare to learn more about you. If you complete this practice exercise, it means that you do want to learn more about yourself and that you are interested in improving your condition.

Practice Exercise 1. Understanding Your Behavior

Name____Sex____Date_____

The purpose of this practice exercise is to understand more about your behavior and how it affects you.

To learn more about yourself, you will need to define what the behaviors listed below mean to you. Behaviors make up your disorder. To understand how they apply to you, you will need the help of a dictionary, of your attending professional, your relatives, your friends (or staff members, if you are at the present time in a medical or psychiatric facility). Make sure you explain briefly how each behavior applies to you. Give two examples of how this behavior applies to you as you understand it.

Behaviors	Examples
a. Intrusive memories	Example 1 ______
	Example 2 ______
b. Distressing dreams	Example 1 ______
	Example 2 ______
c. Reliving/flashbacks	Example 1 ______
	Example 2 ______
d. Distress over cues/signals	Example 1 ______
	Example 2 ______
e. Reacting to signals	Example 1 ______
	Example 2 ______
f. Avoiding thoughts/feelings	Example 1 ______
	Example 2 ______
g. Avoiding people/places	Example 1 ______
	Example 2 ______
h. Amnesia	Example 1 ______
	Example 2 ______
i. Diminished interest	Example 1 ______
	Example 2 ______

j. Detached from others ____________ Example 1 ____________

Example 2 ____________

k. Restricted range of emotions ____________ Example 1 ____________

Example 2 ____________

l. Not paying attention to the future ____________ Example 1 ____________

Example 2 ____________

m. Disturbed sleep ____________ Example 1 ____________

Example 2 ____________

n. Anger outbursts ____________ Example 1 ____________

Example 2 ____________

o. Poor concentration ____________ Example 1 ____________

Example 2 ____________

p. Extreme alertness ____________ Example 1 ____________

Example 2 ____________

q. Extreme sudden ____________ Example 1 ____________

Example 2 ____________

2. Now that you have completed these definitions, it is important to find out how they apply to you. Next to each behavior that you have defined, rank-order each behavior according to how much that behavior applies to you. Rank as No. 1 the behavior that applies to you the most. Rank as No. 2 the behavior that applies to you next, and so on; mark as N/A the behaviors that do not apply to you at all.

Behaviors	*Rank-order*
a. Intrusive memories	________
b. Distressing dreams	________
c. Reliving/flashbacks	________
d. Distress over cues	________
e. Reacting to cues	________
f. Avoiding thoughts/feelings	________
g. Avoiding people/places	________
h. Amnesia	________
i. Diminished interest	________
j. Detached from others	________
k. Restricted range of affect	________
l. Foreshortening future	________
m. Disturbed sleep	________
n. Anger outbursts	________
o. Poor concentration	________
p. Hypervigilance	________
q. Exaggerated startle	________

3. Write why you ranked your behaviors the way you just did.

____
____
____
____
____

4. Now that you have completed this practice exercise, check which of these answers describes how you felt about it. There is also space for you to explain further, if you want:

   a. I did not like this practice exercise at all. I want to quit this stupid practice exercise. ________
   b. I did not like this practice exercise very much, but I want to go on with this practice exercise. ________
   c. I liked this practice exercise and I want to go on with this practice exercise. ________
   d. I liked this practice exercise a lot and I wish I had something like this practice exercise years ago. ________
   e. I liked it so much that I wish all people in need of professional help could get something likes this practice exercise to work on. ________

4. Discuss your completed practice exercise with whoever has given it to you.

Homework: During the coming week, think more about the behaviors covered by these words and whether you want to change the rank-order of these behavior as listed above, or start working on the next practice exercise.

Concluding Follow-Up Form for Posttraumatic Stress Disorder

Name________________________________Sex____Date________

The purpose of this form is to review whether this practice exercise was helpful to you or not.

1. Please select the answer that best fits how you feel about this practice exercise:

   a. I did not like working on this practice exercise at all. I wish I never saw it. ________
   b. I did not like this practice exercise at all, but I am glad I got to work on it. ________
   c. I am delighted I got a chance to work on this practice exercise. ________
   d. I am not only delighted about working on this practice exercise, but I wish all people with painful experiences had a chance to work on it ________

2. How helpful was it to work on this practice exercise? Check the answer that applies to you:

   a. Not helpful at all ________ c. Helpful ________
   b. Somewhat helpful ________ d. Very helpful ________

3. Which practice exercise did you like best? Please rank-order the practice exercises; rank as No. 1 the one you liked best or was most helpful to you, rank as No. 2 the one you liked next best, and so on; if there is one you did not like at all or that did not apply to you, mark it N/A.

Behaviors	*Rank-order*
a. Intrusive memories	________
b. Distressing dreams	________
c. Reliving/flashbacks	________
d. Distress over cues	________
e. Reacting to cues	________
f. Avoiding thoughts/feelings	________
g. Avoiding people/places	________
h. Amnesia	________

Behaviors	*Rank-order*
i. Diminished interest	________
j. Detached from others	________
k. Restricted range of affect	________
l. Foreshortening future	________
m. Disturbed sleep	________
n. Anger outbursts	________
o. Poor concentration	________
p. Hypervigilance	________
q. Exaggerated startle	________

4. Why did you rank-order the behaviors the way you did? Please explain.

____
____
____
____
____

5. Sometimes what we like most is not necessarily the most helpful. Which practice exercise was the most helpful to you? Could you rank the practice exercises according to their helpfulness to you? Rank as No. 1 the most helpful, No. 2 the next most helpful, and so on to the least helpful; mark as N/A the practice exercises that did not apply to you.

Behaviors	*Rank-order*
a. Intrusive memories	________
b. Distressing dreams	________
c. Reliving/flashbacks	________
d. Distress over cues	________
e. Reacting to cues	________
f. Avoiding thoughts/feelings	________
g. Avoiding people/places	________
h. Amnesia	________
i. Diminished interest	________
j. Detached from others	________
k. Restricted range of affect	________
l. Foreshortening future	________
m. Disturbed sleep	________
n. Anger outbursts	________
o. Poor concentration	________
p. Hypervigilance	________
q. Exaggerated startle	________

6. Why did you rank-order the behaviors the way you did? Please explain.

____

____

____

____

____

7. Write any comments you have that might improve this practice exercise.

____

____

____

____

____

Loneliness

Ideally, before starting on this practice exercise, you should have answered a questionnaire especially written to check on your loneliness. This questionnaire should be given to you again on completion of this practice exercise to evaluate whether this practice exercise was helpful to you.

The purpose of this practice exercise is to help you learn from your loneliness to your advantage rather than to your disadvantage. This program is made up of six practice exercises. The first practice exercise deals with the meaning and nature of your loneliness. The second practice exercise deals with possible explanations for loneliness. The third practice exercise deals with how to use loneliness to your advantage. The fourth practice exercise helps you to think about loneliness in different ways. The fifth practice exercise helps you cope with loneliness in different ways. The sixth practice exercise helps you review how you have dealt with loneliness.

Practice Exercise 1. The Meaning of Loneliness

Name________________________________Sex____Date___________

Please note: During the course of completing practice exercises in this practice exercise, make appointments with yourself at specific, preset times (9 a.m., 8 p.m.) when you will complete the practice exercises of this practice exercise. *Do not work on this practice exercise when you feel lonely.* Write only at preset, prearranged times, whether you feel lonely or not. Write the time next to the date of the practice exercise you are completing. Do not work on each practice exercise for longer than 1 h. If necessary to write more, make another appointment with yourself at least 24 h ahead to complete each practice exercise.

1. What does loneliness mean to you? In your own words write down what this word means to you.

____

____

____

____

____

2. How often do you feel lonely? Check the answer that fits your loneliness best:

a.	Once a day	_______	d.	More than once a week	_______
b.	More than once a day	_______	e.	Once a month	_______
c.	Once a week	_______	f.	More than once a month	_______

3. How long does your loneliness last? Check the answer that fits your loneliness best:

a.	A few minutes a day	_______	g.	Many (2–5) hours a month	_______
b.	At least 1 h a day	_______	h.	Many (more than 5) hours a month	_______
c.	More than 1 h a day	_______	i.	Most of the time	_______
d.	Many hours a day	_______			
e.	At least 1 h a week	_______			
f.	More than 1 h a month	_______			

4. How strong is your loneliness? Check which answer fits your loneliness best:

a.	Pretty strong	_______	d.	Extremely strong	_______
b.	Somewhat strong	_______	e.	So strong I cannot bear it	_______
c.	Very strong	_______			

5. How does loneliness *affect* you? Check as many answers as fit your loneliness best:

a.	Not at all	_______	h.	In my relationship with my coworkers	_______
b.	At home	_______	i.	In my relationship with my neighbors	_______
c.	At work	_______	j.	In my relationship with my friends	_______
d.	In my free time	_______	k.	In my relationship with my relatives	_______
e.	In my relationships with my partner	_______	l.	Any other area not covered above	_______
f.	In my relationship with my family	_______			
g.	In my relationship with my boss	_______			

(Write what this area is: ___________)

6. Since when do you remember being effected by your loneliness? Check which answer(s) fits your loneliness best:

a.	Before kindergarten	_______	d.	During high school	_______
b.	During elementary school	_______	e.	After high school	_______
			f.	During college	_______
c.	During middle school	_______	g.	After college	_______

7. How has your loneliness effected the following situations? Check as many as apply to your loneliness:

a.	Finances	_______	e.	Friendships	_______
b.	Education	_______	f.	Social life	_______
c.	Occupation	_______	g.	Religion	_______
d.	Marriage	_______	h.	Health	_______

8. What feelings are associated with your loneliness? Check as many as apply to your loneliness:

a.	Desperation	_______	m.	Melancholy	_______
b.	Emptiness	_______	n.	Alienation	_______
c.	Panic	_______	o.	Longing	_______
d.	Helplessness	_______	p.	Impatience	_______
e.	Fear	_______	q.	Boredom	_______
f.	Sadness	_______	r.	Uneasiness	_______
g.	Hopelessness	_______	s.	Anger	_______
h.	Abandonment	_______	t.	Inability to concentrate	_______
i.	Vulnerability	_______	u.	Shame	_______
j.	Depression	_______	v.	Insecurity	_______
k.	Isolation	_______	w.	Negative about self	_______
l.	Sorrow	_______	x.	Any other feeling not listed above:	_______

9. Write about how the feelings that you have checked affect you.

____

____

____

____

____

10. Check as many of the behaviors listed below in response to your loneliness as apply to you:

a.	Cry	________	l.	Exercise	________
b.	Sleep	________	m.	Walk	________
c.	Sit and think	________	n.	Work on a hobby	________
d.	Do nothing	________	o.	Go to a movie	________
e.	Overeat	________	p.	Read	________
f.	Take tranquilizers	________	q.	Play music	________
g.	Watch television	________	r.	Spend money	________
h.	Drink or get "stoned"	________	s.	Go shopping	________
i.	Study or work	________	t.	Call a friend	________
j.	Write	________	u.	Visit someone	________
k.	Listen to music	________			

11. Below is a list of different meanings of loneliness. Rank these meanings according to how they apply to you. Rank as No. 1 the meaning that is closest and applies to your experience the most. Rank as No. 2 the meaning that applies secondarily to your experience, and so on, with the last meaning ranked as No. 13. If all these meanings apply equally to you just rank them as 1 and 2.

Loneliness Means	*Rank-order*
a. Being all alone and lost in the world	________
b. Being alone in a crowd of people	________
c. Being distant and isolated from other people	________
d. Being very distressed and hurt	________
e. Not being intimate with those I love and who love me	________
f. Not having satisfying relationships with anybody	________
g. Not having close relationships with anybody	________
h. Being aware of how I am separated from others	________
i. Feeling very bad about not being able to connect with others	________
j. Wanting to be close to other people who count in my life	________
k. Being deprived of the warmth of human relationships	________
l. Feeling completely cut off from those who matter to me	________
m. Feeling immobilized by fatigue and overwhelming tiredness	________

12. If none of the meanings listed above applies to you, write down why they do not.

____

____

____

____

____

Homework: During the next week become extremely aware of (1) how often, (2) how long, and (3) how strongly you feel lonely. Keep a daily diary (journal, log) of how lonely you have felt each day. Discuss this diary with whoever is working with you on this practice exercise.

Practice Exercise 2. Explanations for Loneliness

Name________________________________Sex____Date___________

The purpose of this practice exercise is to help you find a positive rather than negative explanation for your loneliness, because loneliness means different things to different people.

1. Below is a list of possible reasons, all negative, for feeling lonely and possibly (but not necessarily) keeping away from others. Please rank them according to how they apply to you. Rank as No. 1 the main reason for keeping away, rank as No. 2 the second reason all the way to the last reason.

Reasons for Feeling Lonely	*Rank-order*
a. Rejection	_________
b. Criticism and disapproval	_________
c. Being hurt even more	_________
d. Being subjected to further abuse	_________
e. Being ridiculed and being made fun of	_________
f. Receiving more physical abuse	_________
g. Receiving more verbal abuse	_________
h. Being called names	_________
i. Not being attractive enough	_________
j. Not being socially acceptable	_________
k. Making a fool of myself in a group	_________
l. Not being able to say anything witty or intelligent	_________
m. Any other reason not listed above	_________
Write what this reason is: (_____________)	

2. If none of these reasons applies to you, write your specific reasons for keeping away from others. For instance, you may not keep away from others, but you may still feel very lonely. Other general reasons may be:

   a. Being unattached (without a partner, or loss of mate, partner, or lover)
   b. Alienation (feeling unattractive, misunderstood, unneeded, no friends)
   c. Being alone (coming home to an empty house)
   d. Forced isolation (being housebound or hospitalized, or having no transportation)
   e. Dislocation (away from home, new job or school, moving too often, traveling too much)

Write about any of these if they apply to you.

____
____
____
____
____

Homework: As you can readily see, all of the reasons listed above are negative. Now you need to start thinking about all the possible positive reasons for feeling lonely. The reason for thinking positively about loneliness is to allow you to learn to control and use your loneliness for your advantage rather than being controlled by it. To learn to control it, you need to start thinking positively about it. During the coming week, write down positive reasons for profiting from loneliness.

Discuss These Reasons With Whoever is Helping you with This Pracatice Exercise

Practice Exercise 3. Positive Reasons for Loneliness

Name______________________________Sex____Date___________

The purpose of this practice exercise is to help you think through all the positive reasons for loneliness.

1. If you have done your homework from the previous practice exercise and you have shared and discussed it with someone, check on how your answers compare and contrast with the positive reasons given below.

Positive Reasons About Loneliness	*Rank-order*
a. Being able to feel and think for myself	_________
b. Having a private life of my own	_________
c. Having time to spend with myself	_________
d. Allowing myself to reflect on my life	_________
e. Having an inner life that belongs to me and to no one else	_________
f. Being different from other people	_________
g. Allowing myself to examine and study myself	_________
h. Loneliness gives me an awareness of feelings I would not have otherwise	_________
i. Loneliness allows me to see other people in ways that would not be possible otherwise	_________
j. Loneliness may be a gift that very few people have	_________
k. An unexamined life is not worth living	_________
l. Another positive reason not listed above	_________
Write what this reason may be:	_________

2. Rank-order as No. 1 the positive reason among those listed above that appeals to you the most. Rank as No. 2 the reason that appeals to you next, and so on until you have ranked all the reasons.

3. Write down why you rank-ordered the positive reasons the way you did.

____
____
____
____
____

Homework: During the coming week, keep a daily diary and, in addition to keeping a log of how long, how often, and how strongly you feel lonely, pick the negative reason that you have ranked No. 1 and pair it with a positive reason. Why did you rate both as No. 1? Write about them together, and then pick the reasons you ranked as No. 2 and write about them together, until you have written about as many as you can during the times you have scheduled for yourself during this week. Discuss these writings with whoever is helping you with this practice exercise.

Practice Exercise 4. Making Loneliness a Friend

Name______________________________Sex____Date___________

The purpose of this practice exercise is to teach you how to control and use your loneliness to your advantage rather than to your disadvantage. You do have a choice, however. Do you want to learn to control and use your loneliness or do you want loneliness to control you and learn nothing as a result? If you want loneliness to control you, you do not need to go any further. You can stop right now. However, if you want to learn to control and use your loneliness to your advantage, please go on. You may learn something new about yourself.

1. Make an appointment with yourself as you have done with the two previous practice exercises, at preset, prearranged times. This time, however, you need to make sure that you allow yourself to feel as lonely as possible during this time. You may ask: "How is it possible for me to feel lonely when I want to get rid of my loneliness?" This is a perfectly good question. Reasons for you to make yourself feel lonely at preset times are as follows:

    a. If you want to learn to control your loneliness you need to learn to start it. Sounds crazy? No. If you learn to start your loneliness, you will learn to stop it. Control means being able to start as well as to stop. *If you want to learn to stop it, start it.* Your employer/boss controls you because he tells you when to start working and when to stop. He also tells you what to do in between starting and stopping. Consequently, your employer/boss has control over you. Does he not?

b. If you want to control your loneliness, you will have to learn to behave like an employer/boss of your loneliness; that is, start your loneliness but control beforehand when to stop it. You should not stay lonely longer than 1 h. Therefore, set the length of how long (15, 20, 30, 60 minute) you are going to be lonely by using a timer or alarm clock. Choose also how often you are going to start feeling lonely (once a week, twice a week, three times a week, every other day, every day). By setting the time, how often, and how long you are going to feel lonely, you will learn to control your loneliness.

c. You need to learn from your loneliness in between starting and stopping it. During the time set to be lonely, write down everything that comes into your mind when you set yourself to be lonely. Keep these notes and discuss them with whoever is working with you on this program.

Homework: Keep repeating setting tim'es for you to be lonely and writing about what comes into your mind during preset times for at least 3 weeks. Discuss what you have written with whoever is working with you on this practice exercise.

Practice Exercise 5. Using Loneliness to Your Advantage

Name________________________________Sex____Date___________

The purpose of this practice exercise is to help you think more about your loneliness in ways that you may have not done thus far.

1. Below is a list of ways you can think of to overcome your loneliness. Some of these ways may have been already implemented in the previous practice exercise.

   a. Think about things you can do to overcome your loneliness. Write down what these things are.

   ____
   ____
   ____
   ____

   b. Remind yourself that you actually do have good relationships with other people. Write down what your good relationships are and then write down what you think are the bad relationships.

   ____
   ____
   ____
   ____

c. Write down a plan to change your bad relationships into good ones. If necessary, ask the help of a friend to make this change.

____
____
____
____

d. Try to figure out why you are lonely. You already have gone over the reasons for your loneliness. Perhaps by now you may have thought more about those reasons and come up with a more specific and valid reason. What is it?

____
____
____
____

e. Think about all the positive qualities that you have (being warm, intelligent, sensitive, caring, self-sufficient, etc.). Write down these good qualities and then write down what you think are your negative qualities. Are you going to let the negative qualities cancel your good qualities?

____
____
____
____

f. Tell yourself that your loneliness would not last forever, that things will be better. Write down how things could be better and develop a plan (in writing) of how things could be better if you were to change your attitude.

____
____
____
____

g. Think about things you can do extremely well. List them and write down things you do not do well. Will you allow what you do not do well to destroy what you do well?

____
____
____
____

h. Tell yourself that most other people are lonely at one time or another. This may not be too helpful to you at the moment. However, you may want to ask others about their loneliness and learn more from them about it. Why don't you call people you can talk with and ask them? Write down what they say.

____

____

____

____

i. Take you mind off feeling lonely by deliberately thinking about other things (anything other than your loneliness). This may distract you from feeling lonely, but it will not make your loneliness go away. Allow yourself to feel lonely. However, do it under your control, as recommended in the previous practice exercise, rather than under the control of your loneliness. Write down what happens when you shift your focus.

____

____

____

____

j. Tell yourself that you are overreacting, that you shouldn't be so upset. By the same token, feeling lonely is a perfectly human feeling and you are entitled to feel lonely all you want. Think about how under certain situations you may have overreacted and under other circumstances you may have underreacted. Write down both types of situations.

____

____

____

____

k. Think about the possible benefits of your experience of loneliness (such as telling yourself that you were learning to be self-reliant, that you would grow from the experience, etc.). This in a way is a continuation of the previous practice exercise. Perhaps now you may be ready to appreciate all the good that there is in feeling lonely. What is it?

____

____

____

____

l. Change your goals for social relationships (such as telling yourself that it is not that important to be popular, that at this point in your life it's right not to have a boyfriend or girlfriend, etc.). Write down what your priorities are and how they fit in relationship to your loneliness. Discuss your answer and all the other answers to points made above with whoever is working with you on this program.

____
____
____
____

Homework: Rank-order from 1 to 12 the ways you like to think about your loneliness. During the first week work on the one that you have ranked No. 1. During the second week work on the one you have rated No. 2, and so on, until you feel in better control of your loneliness. Discuss what you have written with whoever is working with you on this practice exercise.

Reasons	*Rank-order*	*Reasons*	*Rank-order*
a.	________	g.	________
b.	________	h.	________
c.	________	i.	________
d.	________	j.	________
e.	________	k.	________
f.	________	l.	________

Practice Exercise 6. Things to Do About Loneliness

Name____________________________Sex____Date___________

If making loneliness a friend does not work, perhaps there are other things that you can do that may help. The purpose of this practice exercise is to help you do and try new things that you may have not done or tried before.

1. Below is a list of things you can do to minimize your loneliness:

   a. Try harder to be friendly with other people (such as making an effort to talk to people at home, work, and other places).
   b. Take your mind off feeling lonely through some mental activity (such as reading, watching TV, listening to the radio or records, going to a movie).
   c. Work particularly hard to succeed at some activity (studying harder for an exam, putting extra time into practicing a musical, athletic, or mechanical skill).
   d. Do something helpful for someone else (such as helping or volunteering in a charitable organization).

e. Do something you are very good at (hobby, avocation, etc.).
f. Take your mind off feeling lonely through some physical activity (jogging, shopping, artwork, etc.).
g. Try new ways of meeting people (joining a health club, the historical society, symphony orchestra auxiliary, hospital volunteer, church singles group, etc.).
h. Do something to make yourself more physically attractive (going on a diet and sticking to it, buying new clothes, changing your hairstyle, asking a beauty professional for help with makeup or a barber for help with your hairstyle).
i. Do something to improve your social skills (learning to dance, learning to be more assertive, improving conversational skills; *Hint:* Look up Dale Carnegie courses or similar organizations in the Yellow Pages).
j. Talk to a friend or relative about ways to overcome your loneliness.
k. If none of the above has helped you, consider talking with a professional counselor to overcome your loneliness. What is holding you up?

Homework: Rank the list of things to do above in order of how feasible they are and how willing you are to pursue them. Rank as No. 1 the activity that is both feasible and that you are willing to do, and during the next week follow the suggestion given there. Then rank No. 2 the activity that is second and follow it for 1 week, and so on. Stop only when you think you have a handle on your loneliness. Discuss what you have written with whoever is working with you on this practice exercise.

Things To Do	*Rank-order*	*Things To Do*	*Rank-order*
a.	________	g.	________
b.	________	h.	________
c.	________	i.	________
d.	________	j.	________
e.	________	k.	________
f.	________		

Practice Exercise 7. What Did You Learn About Your Loneliness?

Name________________________________Sex____Date____________

Perhaps there are parts of your loneliness that were not touched in the previous practice exercises. The purpose of this practice exercise is to help you think even more about your loneliness, especially if you have not been able to control and use it heretofore.

Being Alone Means	*Rank-order*
a. Being discontented with being alone	________
b. Having low self-esteem	________
c. Being anxious about social relationships	________
d. Feeling awkward socially	________

Being Alone Means *Rank-order*

e. Not trusting others not to hurt you ________
f. Being unable to share your loneliness with anyone else ________
g. Having troublesome thoughts in selecting a partner ________
h. Being unable to be close and intimate with another person ________
i. Expecting rejection ________
j. Being very anxious about your sexual performance ________
k. Being anxious about a long-term emotional commitment with another person ________
l. Feeling insecure and unable to assert yourself in social situations ________
m. Being unrealistic in what to expect from yourself and others ________
n. Any other reason not covered in the course of this program ________
(Write what this reason is__________) ________

Homework: During the next week write at will and at length (but always by appointment!) about the reason you have ranked No 1. During the second week write at will about the reason you have ranked No. 2, and so on. Discuss what you have written with whoever is helping you with this practice exercise.

At this point, after completing a standard final feedback form, you should receive the same questionnaire given to you before starting this practice exercise. Complete it and give it back to whoever gave it to you. If necessary, ask for a written report of the results to see whether there was an improvement in your loneliness.

Disruptive Developmental Disorders

Hyperactive/Attention Deficit

The following practice exercise is to be administered to the child and/or to the major attachment figure(s).

Name ________________________________Sex____Date_________

The purpose of this practice exercise is to learn more about the disorder that is afflicting your child and your family. Please answer all questions or instructions fully.

Instructions: Please rank-order the behaviors listed below according to how much they apply to your child, with No. 1 being the one the applies the most, No. 2 that applies second, No. 3 third, and so on; mark as N/A the behaviors that do not apply at all.

Behaviors	*Rank-order*
a. Inattention or no paying attention to others or to instructions	________
b. Failure to pay close attention to details or making careless mistakes in school	________
c. School work or other activities	________
d. Difficulty in sustaining attention in tasks or play activities	________
e. Not seeming to listen when spoken to directly	________
f. Not following through on instructions	________
g. Failing to finish schoolwork, chores, or assigned duties in home.	________
h. Difficulty in organizing tasks or activities	________
i. Avoiding, disliking, or being reluctant to engage in tasks requiring sustained mental efforts	________
j. Losing things necessary for tasks or activities (e.g., toys, school practice exercises, pencils, books, or tools)	________
k. Often distracted by external stimuli	________
l. Forgetfulness in daily activities	________
m. Hyperactivity or being continuously in motion with few occasional stops	________
n. Fidgeting with hands or feet or squirming while sitting	________
o. Unable to seat down for long periods of time (classroom, church)	________
p. Running about or climbing when either behavior is inappropriate	________
q. Restlessness	________
r. Unable to be quiet	________
s. Being noisy	________
t. Always on the go or "driven by a motor"	________
u. Excessive talking	________
v. Impulsivity or quick, immediate response to a situation	________
w. Blurting out answers before a question has been completed	________
x. Difficulty waiting one's turn	________
y. Interrupting or intruding on others (e.g., butting into conversations or games)	________
z. Verbal fluency	________
aa. Confrontational communication	________
bb. Unbalanced effort allocation (putting time or energy in tasks or activities that do not warrant it)	________
cc. Trouble in developing, applying, and self-monitoring organizational skills	________
dd. Internal dialogue within yourself	________
ee. Inability to adhere to restrictive instructions	________

Anger

The purpose of this practice exercise is to help you with your anger and the hurtful behaviors that go with it. The purpose of this practice exercise is to learn more about how you express your anger to help you deal with it in better ways than you did in the past.

Practice Exercise 1. How I Deal with My Anger

Name________________________________Sex____Date_____

The purpose of this practice exercise is to help you learn how to deal with your anger more constructively than in the past.

1. Check which of these behaviors apply to you, and how often.

Reactions	*Most of the Time*	*Sometimes*	*Never*
a. Hurting animals	______	______	______
b. Attacking others	______	______	______
c. Bothering others	______	______	______
d. Swearing	______	______	______
e. Fire setting	______	______	______
f. Being spiteful	______	______	______
g. Being touchy	______	______	______
h. Running away	______	______	______
i. Stealing	______	______	______
j. Blaming others	______	______	______
k. Temper tantrums	______	______	______
l. Being cruel to others	______	______	______
m. Destroying property	______	______	______
n. Fighting	______	______	______
o. Arguing	______	______	______
p. Truant from the law	______	______	______
q Lying	______	______	______
r. Hitting others	______	______	______
s. Defying others	______	______	______
t. Being stubborn	______	______	______
u. Breaking rules	______	______	______
v. Bullying, threatening	______	______	______
w. Doing the opposite of what you are told	______	______	______
x. Drinking, smoking, using drugs	______	______	______
y. Being angry	______	______	______
z. Breaking things	______	______	______
aa. Being uncooperative	______	______	______

Reactions	*Most of the Time*	*Sometimes*	*Never*
bb. Talking back	______	______	______
cc. Being irritable, hot tempered, easily angered	______	______	______
dd. Arguing and quarreling	______	______	______
ee. Sulking and pouting	______	______	______
ff. Denying mistakes	______	______	______
gg. Pushing limits, persisting	______	______	______
hh. Nagging, and not taking no for an answer	______	______	______
ii. Picking on others to get attention	______	______	______
jj. Bragging and boasting	______	______	______
kk. Teasing others	______	______	______
ll. Not sharing with others	______	______	______
mm. Other (write what it is)	______	______	______

2. Now that you have checked how these behaviors apply to you, it is important for you to rank-order the angry behaviors that apply to you most of the time or sometimes. This rank-order, of course, depends on whether you want to change those angry behaviors or not. If you do not want to change any angry behavior, then you are wasting your time going on with practice exercise. You may as well quit now. However, if you do want to change angry behaviors that apply to you most of the time or sometimes, rank as No. 1 the angry behavior you want to change the most, rank as No. 2 the angry behavior you want to change next, and so on, until all the angry behaviors that apply to you have been rank-ordered according to how much you want to change them.

3. Now that you have finished this rank-order, explain why you rank-ordered the angry behaviors the way you did.

____

____

____

____

____

Homework: During the coming week, think more about your angry behaviors and what they get you. Think also whether you want to change the rank-order of angry behaviors you want to change.

Concluding Feedback Form for Anger

Name__________________________________Sex____Date______

The purpose of this practice exercise is to review whether this practice exercise was helpful to you or not.

1. Please select the answer that best fits how you feel about this practice exercise:

   a. I did not like working on this practice exercise at all. I wish I never saw it. _______
   b. I did not like this practice exercise at all, but I am glad I got to work on it. _______
   c. I am delighted I got a chance to work on this practice exercise. _______
   d. I am not only delighted about working on this practice exercise but I wish all angry or aggressive people had a chance to work on it. _______

2. How helpful was it to work on this practice exercise? Check the answer that applies to you:

a. Not helpful at all _________ c. Helpful _________
b. Somewhat helpful _________ d. Very helpful _________

3. Which practice exercise did you like best? Please rank-order the practice exercises; rank as No. 1 the one you liked best or was most helpful to you, rank as No. 2 the one you liked next best, and so on; if there is one you did not like at all or that did not apply to you, mark it N/A.

Angry Behaviors	*Rank-order*
a. Hurting animals	_________
b. Attacking others	_________
c. Bothering others	_________
d. Swearing	_________
e. Fire setting	_________
f. Being spiteful	_________
g. Being touchy	_________
h. Running away	_________
i. Stealing	_________
j. Blaming others	_________
k. Temper tantrums	_________
l. Being cruel to others	_________
m. Destroying property	_________
n. Fighting	_________
o. Arguing	_________
p. Truant from the law	_________

Angry Behaviors	*Rank-order*
q. Lying	________
r. Hitting others	________
s. Defying others	________
t. Being stubborn	________
u. Breaking rules	________
v. Bullying, threatening	________
w. Doing the opposite of what you are told	________
x. Drinking, smoking, using drugs	________
y. Being angry	________
z. Breaking things	________
aa. Being uncooperative	________
bb. Talking back	________
cc. Being irritable, hot tempered, easily angered	________
dd. Arguing and quarreling	________
ee. Sulking and pouting	________
ff. Denying mistakes	________
gg. Pushing limits, persisting	________
hh. Nagging, and not taking no for an answer	________
ii. Picking on others to get attention	________
jj. Bragging and boasting	________
kk. Teasing others	________
ll. Not sharing with others	________
mm. Other (write what it is)	________

4. Liking and helpfulness may not go together. Which practice exercises were most helpful to you? Rank as No. 1 the one that was most helpful to you, rank as No. 2 the one that was next helpful, and so on; mark as N/A the practice exercises that were not at helpful.

Angry Behaviors	*Rank-order*
a. Hurting animals	________
b. Attacking others	________
c. Bothering others	________
d. Swearing	________
e. Fire setting	________
f. Being spiteful	________
g. Being touchy	________
h. Running away	________
i. Stealing	________
j. Blaming others	________
k. Temper tantrums	________
l. Being cruel to others	________
m. Destroying property	________
n. Fighting	________

Angry Behaviors		*Rank-order*
o.	Arguing	________
p.	Being truant from the law	________
q.	Lying	________
r.	Hitting others	________
s.	Defying others	________
t.	Being stubborn	________
u.	Breaking rules	________
v.	Bullying, threatening	________
w.	Doing the opposite of what you are told	________
x.	Drinking, smoking, using drugs	________
y.	Being angry	________
z.	Breaking things	________
aa.	Being uncooperative	________
bb.	Talking back	________
cc.	Being irritable, hot tempered, easily angered	________
dd.	Arguing and quarreling	________
ee.	Sulking and pouting	________
ff.	Denying mistakes	________
gg.	Pushing limits, persisting	________
hh.	Nagging, and not taking no for an answer	________
ii.	Picking on others to get attention	________
jj.	Bragging and boasting	________
kk.	Teasing others	________
ll.	Not sharing with others	________
mm.	Other (write what it is)	________

5. Please explain why you rank-ordered the practice exercises the way you did.

____
____
____
____
____

6. Feel free to write any comments that might improve this practice exercise.

____
____
____
____
____

Conduct Disorder

Practice Exercise 1. Conduct Disorder

Name________________________________Sex____Date______

The purpose of this practice exercise is to learn more about the disorder that is affecting you and your family.

Please answer all questions or instructions fully.

Instructions: Please rank-order the behaviors listed below according to how much they apply to your child, with No. 1 being the one the applies the most, No. 2 that applies second, No. 3 third, and so on; mark as N/A the behaviors that do not apply at all.

Angry Behaviors	*Rank-order*
a. Aggression against people or animals	________
b. Bullying, threatening, or intimidating others	________
c. Starting fights	________
d. Using weapons that may cause serious physical injury (bat, brick, broken bottle, knife, gun)	________
e. Being physically cruel to people	________
f. Being physically cruel to animals	________
g. Stealing while confronting a victim (e.g., mugging, purse snatching, extortion, armed robbery)	________
h. Forcing someone into sexual activity	________
i. Destruction of property	________
j. Deliberately engaging in fire setting with intention to cause serious damage	________
k. Deliberately destroying others' property	________
l. Deceitfulness or theft	________
m. Breaking into someone's house, building, or car	________
n. Lying to obtain goods or favors or to avoid obligations; conning others	________
o. Stealing objects of some value without confronting the victim (shoplifting without breaking or entering, forgery)	________
p. Serious violation of rules	________
q. Staying out at night despite parental prohibition	________
r. Running away from home overnight at least twice	________
s. School truancy	________
t. Poor social functioning	________
u. Poor academic functioning	________
v. Poor occupational functioning	________

Oppositional Defiant

Name________________________________Sex____Date___________

The purpose of this practice exercise is to learn more about the disorder that is affecting you and your family.

Please answer all questions or instructions fully.

Instructions: Please rank-order the behaviors listed below according to how much they apply to your child, with No. 1 being the one the applies the most, No. 2 that applies second, No. 3 third and so on; mark as N/A the behaviors that do not apply at all.

Behaviors	*Rank-order*
a. Negativism	__________
b. Hostility	__________
c. Defiance	__________
d. Losing temper	__________
e. Arguing with adults	__________
f. Defying or refusing to comply with adults' requests or rules	__________
g. Deliberately annoying people	__________
h. Blaming others for mistakes or misbehavior	__________
i. Being touchy or easily annoyed by others	__________
j. Being angry and resentful	__________
k. Being spiteful or vindictive	__________
l. Social impairment	__________
m. School impairment	__________
n. Occupational impairment	__________

After signing the Informed Consent Form (Appendix A), participants can be administered the Standard Practice Exercise Form (Appendix B) according to the rank-order given above until all rank-ordered practice exercises have been completed. On completion of practice exercises, administer the Standard Concluding Feedback Form (Appendix C).

Troublemaking

The purpose of this practice exercise is to help you learn more about behaviors that have gotten you in trouble in the past. These behaviors might get you into more trouble or even in jail in the future. If you do not want to learn about these behaviors, you do not have to go on with this practice exercise, especially if you like or enjoy getting into trouble.

Practice Exercise 1. Behaviors that Got You or Might Get You into Trouble with the Law

Name________________________________Sex____Date_______

If you want to (1) learn more about behaviors that have gotten you into trouble (and possibly in jail), and (2) avoid getting into trouble in the future, please complete this practice exercise. The purpose of this practice exercise is to learn more about which behaviors might get you into trouble with the law.

1. Below is a list of behaviors that get many young people in trouble with the law. Define each behavior as you understand it and give two examples of that behavior. You may want to check in a dictionary, ask your friends, adults, parents, brothers and sisters, or relatives. It may take you a week or longer to complete these definitions. Feel free to use any examples from your experience to define these behaviors. Take your time. It is important that you understand what these behaviors are and how they might get you in trouble with the law.

What do you understand by the following? Define and give two examples.

a. Glibness/superficial charm — Example 1 ________ Example 2 ________

b. Pathological lying — Example 1 ________ Example 2 ________

c. Conning/manipulative — Example 1 ________ Example 2 ________

d. Lack of remorse or guilt — Example 1 ________ Example 2 ________

e. Shallow feelings — Example 1 ________ Example 2 ________

f. Callousness/lack of empathy

Example 1 ______________________

Example 2 ______________________

g. Failure to accept responsibility for your own actions

Example 1 ______________________

Example 2 ______________________

h. Parasitic lifestyle

Example 1 ______________________

Example 2 ______________________

i. Poor behavioral control

Example 1 ______________________

Example 2 ______________________

j. Lack of plans

Example 1 ______________________

Example 2 ______________________

k. Impulsivity

Example 1 ______________________

Example 2 ______________________

l. Irresponsibility

Example 1 ______________________

Example 2 ______________________

m. Criminal versatility

Example 1

Example 2 ______________________

2. Now that you have completed the first part of this practice exercise, here comes the hard part: Below are listed the 13 behaviors that you have defined during the past week or so. Rank-order each of them according to how each (mis)

behavior applies to you. Rank-order as No. 1 the (mis)behavior that applies to you the best (or most!). Rank as No. 2 the (mis)behavior that applies to you next best. Rank as No. 3 the behavior that applies to you next. Mark as N/A (not applicable) the (mis)behaviors that do not apply to you at all.

Behaviors	*Rank-order*
a. Glibness/superficial charm	_________
b. Pathological lying	_________
c. Conning/manipulative	_________
d. Lack of remorse or guilt	_________
e. Shallow affect	_________
f. Callousness/lack of empathy	_________
g. Failure to accept responsibility for tour own actions	_________
h. Parasitic lifestyle	_________
i. Poor behavioral control	_________
j. Lack of plans	_________
k. Impulsivity	_________
l. Irresponsibility	_________
m. Criminal versatility	_________

3. Write down why you rank-ordered these behaviors the way you did.

____
____
____
____
____

4. Now that you have completed this practice exercise, check which of these answers tells how you felt about it. There is also space for you to explain further, if you want to:

   a. I did not like it at all, a waste of time. I want to quit working on this stupid practice exercise. _________
   b. I did not like it very much, but I want to go on with this practice exercise. _________
   c. I liked it and I want to go on with this practice exercise. _________
   d. I liked it a lot and I wish I had something like this practice exercise earlier. _________
   e. I liked it so much that I wish all children could get something like this practice exercise to work on. _________

Homework: During the coming week, think more about the behaviors that got you into trouble and whether you want to change the rank-order of these behaviors as listed above, or start working on the next practice exercise.

Standard Practice Exercise for Troublemaking

Practice Exercise No.____Title:________________________

Name____________________________Sex____Date______

The purpose of this practice exercise is to understand more about the behavior listed in the title.

1. How did this behavior get you into trouble? Please explain in detail.

____
____
____
____

2. How often did this behavior get you into trouble? Check which answer applies to you:

a.	Practically every day	_______	d.	Once a month	_______
b.	Once a week	_______	e.	Once every 6 months	_______
c.	A couple of times a month	_______	f.	Once a year	_______
			g.	Once every few years	_______

3. Please explain further.

____
____
____
____

4. How did this behavior come about? Do you remember when you started it? Check which answer fits best:

a. When I was a child (younger than 5 years of age) _______
b. In elementary school _______
c. In middle school _______
d. In high school _______
e. Any other time _______

5. Please explain further.

____
____
____
____

6. How did this behavior get you in trouble? Please explain.

7. Give three specific examples of how this behavior got you in trouble in the past.

Example 1

Example 2

Example 3

8. Give three specific examples of how this behavior got you in trouble now.

Example 1

Example 2

Example 3

9. Give three specific examples of how this behavior will get you in trouble in the future.

Example 1

Example 2

Example 3

Homework: Next week, plan to repeat this behavior at preset times (for instance, at 8 a.m., 12 noon, 4 or 7 p.m.) on at least 3 days. Write down what happened in detail. For each time, make sure to answer in writing the following four questions:

a. How did you start it?
b. What followed?
c. How did it end?
d. What did this behavior get you?

Time 1 (write the time you started__________)

a. ____
____
____

b. ____
____
____

c. ____
____
____

d. ____
____

Time 2 (write the time you started__________)

a. ____
____
____

b. ____
____
____

c. ____
____
____

d. ____
____

Time 3 (write the time you started__________)

a. ____
____
____

b. ____
____
____

c. ____
____
____

d. ____
____
____

Check which of the following shows what you got out of this homework practice exercise:

a. Completely useless _______
b. Somewhat useless _______
c. So-so _______
d. Somewhat useful _______
e. Extremely useful _______

Write down how you feel about this homework practice exercise and what you got out of it.

____
____
____
____
____

Concluding Feedback Form for Troublemaking

Name______________________________ Sex ____Date ______

The purpose of this concluding feedback form is to review whether practice exercises in this practice exercise were helpful to you.

1. Please select the answer that best fits how you feel about this practice exercise:

   a. I did not like working on this practice exercise at all. I wish I never saw it. _______
   b. I did not like this practice exercise, but I am glad I got to work on it. _______
   c. I am happy I got a chance to work on this practice exercise. _______
   d. I am not only delighted about this practice exercise, but I wish all people in trouble (with the law) had a chance to work on it. _______

2. How helpful was it to work on this practice exercise? Check the answer that applies to you:

   a. Not helpful at all _______
   b. Somewhat helpful _______
   c. Helpful _______
   d. Very helpful _______

3. Which practice exercise did you like best? Please rank-order the practice exercises; rank as No. 1 the one you liked best or was most helpful to you, rank as No. 2 the one you liked next best, and so on to the one you did not like at all (No. 13).

Behaviors	*Rank-order*
a. Glibness/superficial charm	_______
b. Pathological lying	_______
c. Conning/manipulative	_______
d. Lack of remorse or guilt	_______
e. Shallow affect	_______
f. Callousness/lack of empathy	_______
g. Failure to accept responsibility	_______
h. Parasitic lifestyle	_______
i. Poor behavioral control	_______
j. Lack of plans	_______
k. Impulsivity	_______
l. Irresponsibility	_______
m. Criminal versatility	_______

4. Which practice exercise was the most helpful to you? Sometimes what we like most is not necessarily the most helpful. Therefore, rank-order the practice exercises according to their helpfulness to you. Rank as No. 1 the most helpful, rank as No. 2 the next most helpful, and so on until you reach the least helpful (either No. 13 or not applicable [N/A]).

Behaviors	*Rank-order*
a. Glibness/superficial charm	_______
b. Grandiose sense of self-worth	_______
c. Need for stimulation/proneness to boredom	_______
d. Pathological lying	_______
e. Conning/manipulative	_______
f. Lack of remorse or guilt	_______
g. Shallow affect	_______
h. Callous/lack of empathy	_______
i. Parasitic lifestyle	_______
j. Poor behavioral control	_______
k. Promiscuous sexual behavior	_______
l. Impulsivity	_______
m. Irresponsibility	_______
n. Failure to accept responsibility for your own actions	_______

5. Now that you have completed this practice exercise, write how you feel about it. Check which of these answers tells how you felt about it. There is also space for you to explain further, if you want to:

   a. I did not like it at all, a waste of time. I want to quit this stupid practice exercise. _______
   b. I did not like it very much, but I want to go on with this practice exercise. _______

c. I liked it and I want to go on with this practice exercise. ________
d. I liked it a lot and I wish I had something like this practice exercise earlier. ________
e. I liked it so much that I wish all juvenile could get something like this practice exercise to work on. ________

6. Feel free to write any comments that might improve this practice exercise.

____
____
____
____
____

7. Discuss this completed lesson with whoever has given it to you.

____
____
____
____
____

Adults

The practice exercises in this section include disorders in which patients tend to blame others for their behavior, not taking responsibility for themselves, and acting out against whoever is perceived as a threat or as an enemy.

Anger

The purpose of this practice exercise is to help you understand the nature of your anger, hostility, and aggression, and how these behaviors may control you and others hurtfully and possibly destructively.

Practice Exercise 1.

Name____Sex____Date_________

The purpose of this first practice exercise is to find whether and how you want to change your anger, hostility, and aggression for the better.

1. Below is a list of four areas in which anger, hostility, and aggression are felt and expressed through a variety of reactions. Check how often each reaction applies to you.

Reactions That Apply to Me	*Most of the Time*	*Sometimes*	*Never*
Anger			
a. Increased heart rate	________	________	________
b. Increased general muscle tension or increased tension in specific muscles, such as clenched hands or jaws	________	________	________
c. Trembling or shaky feelings	________	________	________
d. Sweaty or clammy hands	________	________	________
e. Rapid breathing	________	________	________
f. Reddening of the skin or hot sensations	________	________	________
g. Restlessness or agitation	________	________	________
h. Jumpiness or exaggerated startle reactions	________	________	________
i. Feeling hyper aroused, keyed up, or on edge	________	________	________
j. Stomach pain or nausea	________	________	________
k. Other (write what they are)	________	________	________

2. Which of these reactions would you like to change, if any? If you do not want to change any reactions, then stop and do not go any further in this practice exercise. On the other hand, if you do want to change some angry or aggressive reactions, rank-order them according to which reactions you want to change among all those listed below. Rank as No. 1 the reaction you want to change the most. Rank as No. 2 the reaction you want to change next, and so on; mark as N/A the reactions that you do not want to change.

Reactions	*Rank-order*
a. Increased heart rate	________
b. Increased general muscle tension or increased ension in specific muscles, such as clenched hands or jaws	________
c. Trembling or shaky feelings	________
d. Sweaty or clammy hands	________
e. Rapid breathing	________
f. Reddening of the skin or hot sensations	________
g. Restlessness or agitation	________
h. Jumpiness or exaggerated startle reactions	________
i. Feeling hyper aroused, keyed up, or on edge	________
j. Stomach pain or nausea	________
k. Other (write what they are)	________

3. Please explain why you rank-ordered these reactions the way you did.

____
____
____
____
____

Practice Exercise 2. Your Thinking about Anger, Hostility, and Aggression

Name____________________________Sex____Date_________

The purpose of this first practice exercise is to find whether and how you want to change your anger, hostility, and aggression for the better.

1. Below is a list of four areas in which anger, hostility, and aggression are felt and expressed through a variety of reactions. Check how often each reaction applies to you.

Reactions That Apply to Me	*Most of the Time*	*Sometimes*	*Never*
a. Strong belief that you have been treated unfairly, trespassed on, or violated in some way	______	______	______
b. Rigid demands that others or situations should be as be as you want them to be	______	______	______
c. Demanding that you should not be or have been exposed to or have to endure any provocation	______	______	______
d. Blaming others or external situations for your troublesome thoughts, angry feelings, and/or reactions	______	______	______
e. Negative labeling (like cursing) of people or situations involved	______	______	______
f. Belief that your anger or aggression is justified because of the nature of outside situations	______	______	______
g. Thoughts and/or images of harm to, revenge on or retaliation against the source of provocation	______	______	______
h. Brooding or angry ruminations about provocations	______	______	______
i. Racing thoughts or concentrations difficulties	______	______	______
j. Other (write what they are)	______	______	______

2. Which of these reactions would you like to change, if any? If you do not want to change any reactions, then stop and do not go any further in this practice exercise. On the other hand, if you do want to change some angry or aggressive reactions, rank-order them according to which reactions you want to change among all those listed below. Rank as No. 1 the reaction you want to change the most. Rank as No. 2 the reaction you want to change next, and so on; mark as N/A the reactions that you do not want to change.

Reactions	*Rank-order*
a. Strong belief that you have been treated unfairly, trespassed on, or violated in some way	________
b. Rigid demands that others or situations should be as you want them to be	________
c. Demanding that you should not be or have been supposed to or have to endure any provocation	________
d. Blaming others or external situations for your troublesome thoughts, angry feelings, and/or reactions	________
e. Negative labeling (like cursing) of people or situations involved	________
f. Belief that your anger or aggression is justified because of the nature of outside situations	________
g. Thoughts and/or images of harm to, revenge on, or retaliation against the source of provocation	________
h. Brooding or angry ruminations about provocations	________
i. Racing thoughts or concentrations difficulties	________
j. Other (write what they are)	________

3. Please explain why you rank-ordered these reactions the way you did.

____
____
____
____

Hostility

The purpose of this practice exercise is to help you understand the nature of your anger, hostility, and aggression, and how these behaviors may control you and others hurtfully and possibly destructively.

Practice Exercise 1.

Name____Sex____Date_________

The purpose of this first practice exercise is to find whether and how you want to change your anger, hostility, and aggression for the better.

1. Below is a list of four areas in which anger, hostility, and aggression are felt and expressed through a variety of reactions. Check how often each reaction applies to you.

Reactions That Apply to Me	*Most of the Time*	*Sometimes*	*Never*
a. Negative attitudes toward others	_______	_______	_______
b. Negative judgments about others	_______	_______	_______
c. Negative evaluation of others	_______	_______	_______
d. Dislikes for many people	_______	_______	_______
e. Discounting and denigration of others	_______	_______	_______
f. Blame and punishment of others	_______	_______	_______
g. Easily provoked by others	_______	_______	_______
h. Put downs and criticisms of others	_______	_______	_______
i. Seeing people as threatening to self	_______	_______	_______
j. Ridicule (making fun) of others	_______	_______	_______
k. Repeated sarcasm, cutting verbal remarks, or hostile humor	_______	_______	_______
l. Holding grudges	_______	_______	_______
m. Other (write what they are)	_______	_______	_______

2. Which of these reactions would you like to change, if any? If you do not want to change any reactions, then stop and do not go any further in this practice exercise. On the other hand, if you do want to change some angry or aggressive reactions, rank-order them according to which reactions you want to change among all those listed below. Rank as No. 1 the reaction you want to change the most. Rank as No. 2 the reaction you want to change next, and so on; mark as N/A the reactions that you do not want to change.

Reactions	*Rank-order*
a. Negative attitudes toward others	_______
b. Negative judgments about others	_______
c. Negative evaluation of others	_______
d. Dislikes for many people	_______
e. Discounting and denigration of others	_______
f. Blame and punishment of others	_______
g. Easily provoked by others	_______
h. Put downs and criticisms of others	_______
i. Seeing people as threatening to self	_______
j. Ridicule (making fun) of others	_______
k. Repeated sarcasm, cutting verbal remarks, or hostile humor	_______
l. Holding grudges	_______
m. Other (write what they are)	_______

3. Please explain why you rank-ordered these reactions the way you did.

____
____
____
____
____

Aggression

The purpose of this practice exercise is to help you understand the nature of your anger, hostility, and aggression, and how these behaviors may control you and others hurtfully and possibly destructively.

Practice Exercise 1.

Name______________________________Sex____Date________

The purpose of this first practice exercise is to find whether and how you want to change your anger, hostility, and aggression for the better.

1. Below is a list of four areas in which anger, hostility, and aggression are felt and expressed through a variety of reactions. Check how often each reaction applies to you.

Reactions That Apply to Me	*Most of the Time*	*Sometimes*	*Never*
a. Loud verbal outbursts, yelling, and screaming	______	______	______
b. Being or becoming verbally threatening, insulting, intimidating, or highly argumentative	______	______	______
c. Acting in a physically threatening or intimidating manner	______	______	______
d. Physically assaultive behaviors toward others (as in hitting, kicking, slapping, punching, grabbing, shoving, throwing things, etc	______	______	______
e. Destructive behaviors against property, like throwing, slamming, banging on, pounding on, breaking etc	______	______	______
f. Actively seeking out or provoking verbally aggressive confrontations	______	______	______
g. Belligerent or stubborn refusal to cooperate with reasonable requests in dealing with provocations or difficulties	______	______	______

Reactions That Apply to Me	*Most of the Time*	*Sometimes*	*Never*
h. Sullen or sulky withdrawal, like pouting or icy stares	_______	_______	_______
i. Other (write what they are)	_______	_______	_______

2. Which of these reactions would you like to change, if any? If you do not want to change any reactions, then stop and do not go any further in this practice exercise. On the other hand, if you do want to change some angry or aggressive reactions, rank-order them according to which reactions you want to change among all those listed below. Rank as No. 1 the reaction you want to change the most. Rank as No. 2 the reaction you want to change next, and so on; mark as N/A the reactions that you do not want to change.

Reactions	*Rank-order*
a. Loud verbal outbursts, yelling, and screaming	_________
b. Being or becoming verbally threatening insulting, intimidating, or highly argumentative	_________
c. Acting in a physically threatening or intimidating manner	_________
d. Physically assaultive behaviors toward others(as in hitting, kicking, slapping, punching, grabbing, shoving, throwing things, etc	_________
e. Destructive behaviors against property, like throwing, slamming, banging on, pounding on, breaking etc	_________
f. Actively seeking out or provoking verbally aggressive confrontations	_________
g. Belligerent or stubborn refusal to cooperate with reasonable requests in dealing with provocations or difficulties	_________
h. Sullen or sulky withdrawal, like pouting or icy stares	_________
i. Other (write what they are)	_________

3. Please explain why you rank-ordered these reactions the way you did.

____
____
____
____
____

Antisocial Behavior

The purpose of this practice exercise is to help you understand the behavior that may have gotten you in trouble (with the law) in the past and that may get you in trouble in the future.

Practice Exercise 1. Life Is a Power Struggle

Name____Sex____Date_____

The purpose of the first practice exercise is to help you understand whether life is a power struggle or whether life is what you make it. It can be a power struggle if you want to make it that way, or it can be more peaceful if that is what you want to make it. It is up to you. Do you want to make life a power struggle or more peaceful? If you want to go on making life a power struggle, you do not need to work on this practice exercise or this practice exercise. If you want to make life more peaceful for yourself, go on and answer the questions in this practice exercise.

1. A "power struggle" means that in any human relationship there are winners and losers. As a result, life becomes a struggle to win and avoiding losing, where defeating others seems necessary to survive. How much is life a power struggle for you?

   a. A great deal ________ c. Not at all ________
   b. Often times ________

2. If you have checked "a" or "b," go ahead with this practice exercise. If you checked "c," you may not be ready or willing to undertake this and other practice exercises, and a different practice exercise or approach may be necessary for you.

3. How did life begin as a power struggle for you?

   a. Write as much as you can remember about how victories and losses became part of your life.

____

____

____

____

   b. Who won at whose expense?

____

____

____

____

   c. Who lost and lost again?

____

____

____

____

d. How did you learn to defeat others before they defeated you?

e. Do not limit yourself to answering the above questions; write as much as you can.

4. Would you say that you learned to lose by defeating others?

a. How did you learn to do that?

b. Write about the situations where you lost by defeating others.

5. Did you ever win by defeating others?

a. Write about the situations where you felt you won by defeating others.

b. Who were they and how did you do it?

____

____

____

____

____

6. Do you want to go on with this power struggle, or do you want to give it up? If you want to go on with it, you do not need to complete this lesson and you can quit right now. If you want to give up this power struggle, what kind of life do you want to lead for yourself? Rank-order all the statements below according to what you want the most (No. 1) to the statement that you want the least (No. 7).

Life Goals	*Rank-order*
a. I want a peaceful life	________
b. I want a self-enhancing life	________
c. I want to learn to give up the power struggle	________
d. I do not know what I want	________
e. I want to learn to win rather than to defeat myself and others	________
f. I want to learn to win at no one else's expense	________
g. (Write here what you want that is not stated above)	________

Homework: During the next week, write down how you would like to achieve the life goals you have just ranked. Write first about the goal ranked No. 1, then goal No. 2, and so on, until you have written about all the life goals you want to achieve. Make sure you receive feedback from a professional about what you have written.

Practice Exercise 2. "I Know Better Than Anybody Else"

Name________________________________Sex____Date______

The purpose of this practice exercise is to help you understand an attitude that seems to be at the bottom of most behavior that may get you into trouble.

1. As part of this life struggle, many of us, in order to survive, develop an attitude of "knowing better" than others, knowing better than our parents, knowing better than our teachers, knowing better than authority figures, and knowing better than our mate or partner. How does this attitude apply to you?

   a. A great deal _____
   b. Often times _____
   c. Not at all _____

2. If you answered "a" or "b," go ahead with this practice exercise. If you answered "c," this practice exercise may not apply to you and a different practice exercise or practice exercise may be necessary.

3. Write down how this attitude of knowing better has helped you survive in life.

   a. How did you develop it?

____
____
____
____
____

   b. Be as specific and detailed as you can be. You may need more than one sitting to answer this statement.

____
____
____
____
____

4. How was this attitude destructive to you (if at all)? Write down the situations where this attitude of knowing better got you in trouble. Be as specific and detailed as you can be. You may need more than one sitting to answer this statement.

____
____
____
____
____

5. What has this attitude gotten you in life? Do you want to keep it or do you want to give it up? Complete the statement that applies to you.

   a. I want to keep it because …

____
____
____
____
____

b. I want to give it up because …

____

____

____

____

____

6. If you completed "a," you may need a different practice exercise or approach. If you completed "b," go on with this practice exercise.

7. If you are willing to give this attitude up, rank the attitudes you want to develop in your life. Rank as No. 1 the attitude that you want the most, rank as No. 2 the attitude you want next, and so on, to the one you want the least:

Attitudes	*Rank-order*
a. I want to learn to respect others' opinions	_________
b. I want to realize my limitations	_________
c. I want to recognize my strengths as well as my weaknesses	_________
d. I want to forgive my mistakes so that I can forgive the mistakes of others	_________
e. I want to assert my importance without putting anyone else down	_________
f. I do not know better	_________
g. I want to learn how to enhance myself without destruction	_________
h. (Write down an attitude you want that was not included above)	_________

Homework: During the next week, write down how you would like to achieve the attitudes you have just ranked. Write first about the attitude ranked No. 1, then about No. 2, and so on, until you have written about all the life goals you want to achieve. Make sure you receive feedback from a professional about what you have written.

Practice Exercise 3. "I Am More Important Than Anybody Else"

Name____Sex____Date______

The purpose of this practice exercise is to help you deal with another destructive attitude that may determine a great deal of your behavior, and that is that you have to show all the time to everybody how important you are, and that you will not allow anybody to put you down, cheat, swindle, or lie to you. You may do it to others, but you will not allow others to do it to you. You are going to show to everybody how tough and smart you are. No one will take the upper hand with you.

You win no matter what happens to anybody else. Since life is a struggle, you may as well try to win rather than lose.

1. How true are the statements made above? Check the answer that applies to you:

   a. Completely false; these statements have nothing to do with me ______
   b. There may be some truth to them ______
   c. They may apply to me sometimes but not all the time ______
   d. True; they apply to me most of the time ______
   e. Completely true; they apply to me all the time ______

2. What has this attitude gotten you in your life? Check those answer(s) that apply to you:

   a. Got me what I wanted when I wanted it ______
   b. Lets me get by the best I can ______
   c. I like to win at someone else's expense ______
   d. Better me that the other guy ______
   e. Got me a lot of grief ______

3. How did you develop this attitude? Check any answer that applies to you:

   a. This is the best way I know how to survive ______
   b. This is the only way to live my life ______
   c. Better winning that losing ______
   d. What else is there? ______
   e. I do not like to lose ______
   f. I may not like to lose, but why did I end up in jail? Is this a way to win? ______
   g. Am I winning here? ______
   h. In life we either win or lose, there is no in between ______

4. In your own words, write down how this attitude developed as one way to survive:

   a. In your family

____
____
____
____
____

b. With your parents (or parent-substitutes)

c. With your brothers and sisters

d. With other relatives

e. With your friends

f. With your teachers

g. With the authorities

h. With your partner (if you have any)

____
____
____
____
____

i. With anybody else (name who)..............................:

____
____
____
____
____

5. How did you win at someone else's else expense? Check all that apply to you:

a. By taking their life	_____	f. By abusing them physically	_____
b. By taking their money	_____	g. By abusing them sexually	_____
c. By taking their goods	_____	h. By cheating them	_____
d. By attacking them	_____	i. By __________	
e. By hurting them	_____	(specify, if not listed above)	

6. Is it possible that your victories were really short-term and that in the long run you lost? In your own words, explain how that is possible.

____
____
____
____
____

7. Is it possible that any victory made at anyone else's expense is a hollow, short-lived victory? In the long run, when you win at someone else's expense you are going to lose as well. Is that possible?

____
____
____
____

Homework: During the next week, write down in greater detail how winning at someone else's expense got you in trouble (or in jail). Try to recall or remember specific events in your life where you lost by having someone else lose as well.

Practice Exercise 4. "I Will Not Be Caught"

Name____Sex____Date______

The purpose of this practice exercise is to help you understand that you may be in trouble because you think that this time (whenever you did what got you in trouble) you would get away with it and you won't be caught. How often have you been able to get away with it and not be caught? What made you think that you could outsmart everybody else, especially the law?

1. Many people who are in jail thought that they could get away with hurtful behaviors that involve putting others down, through violence, theft, lying, murder, and other types of hurtful behaviors. How much of this attitude about "not being caught" is part of your thinking?

    a. A great deal _____
    b. Often times _____
    c. Not at all _____

2. If you checked "a" or "b," go ahead with this practice exercise. If you checked "c," you may need another practice exercise or practice exercise.

3. Write down how this attitude of thinking that you will not be caught has helped you survive in life. How did you develop it? Be as specific and detailed as you can be. You may need more than one sitting to answer this statement.

____
____
____
____
____

4. How was this attitude destructive to you (if at all)? Write down the situations where this attitude of thinking that you will not be caught got you into trouble. Be as specific and detailed as you can be. You may need more than one sitting to answer this statement.

____
____
____
____
____

5. What has this attitude gotten you in life? Do you want to keep it or do you want to give it up? Complete the statement that applies to you.

   a. I want to keep it because ...

____
____
____
____
____

   b. I want to give it up because ...

____
____
____
____
____

If you completed "a," you may need a different practice exercise or approach. If you completed "b," go on with this practice exercise.

6. If you are willing to give this attitude up, check the attitudes that you want to develop in your life. Rank as No. 1 the attitude that you want the most, rank as No. 2 the attitude you want next, and so on, until all the attitudes are ranked.

	Attitude	*Rank-order*
a.	There are always consequences to my behavior	________
b.	In the long run, I have to live with the consequences of my behavior, destructive or constructive	________
c.	I have to choose whether I want to be caught or whether I want to behave in ways that do not entail being caught	________
d.	I have paid every time I did something destructive	________
e.	I want to learn to behave in ways that do not entail being caught	________
f.	I have been caught in spite of my thinking otherwise	________
g.	I do not like being caught	________
h.	(Write down an attitude you want that was not included above)	

Homework: During the coming week, think about the attitudes you have just ranked. Write first about the attitude ranked No. 1, then No. 2, and so on, until you have written about all the attitudes you want to achieve. Make sure you receive feedback from a professional about what you have written.

Practice Exercise 5. Reject Others Before They Reject Me

Name________________________________Sex____Date______

The purpose of this practice exercise is to help you understand that as long as you think that you are more important than others, they will reject you and you will not be accepted, including by those who love you.

1. In a life where power is the major struggle, rejection is a major outcome. How much has this outcome, that is, rejection by or of others, been present in your past?

   a. A great deal _____
   b. Often times _____
   c. Not at all _____

2. If you checked "a" or "b," go on with this practice exercise. If you checked "c," you may need a different practice exercise or practice exercise.

3. Write down how this outcome (rejecting and being rejected) has helped you survive in life.

   a. How did you develop it?

   ____
   ____
   ____
   ____

   b. Be as specific and detailed as you can be. You may need more than one sitting to answer this statement.

   ____
   ____
   ____
   ____

4. How was this outcome helpful or hurtful to you (if at all)? Write down the situations where this was the outcome of your relationships with others. Be as specific and detailed as you can be. You may need more than one sitting to answer this question.

____
____
____
____

5. What has this outcome gotten you in life?

   a. Do you want to keep it or do you want to give it up? Why?

____
____
____
____

   b. Complete the statement that applies to you.

   a. I want to keep it because …

____
____
____
____

   b. I want to give it up because …

____
____
____
____

6. If you completed "a," you may need a different practice exercise or approach. If you completed "b," go on with this practice exercise.

7. If you are willing to give up this behavior, that is, rejection, rank the behaviors you want to develop in your life. Rank as No. 1 the behavior that you want the most, rank as No. 2 the behavior you want next, and so on until the behavior you want the least.

Behaviors	*Rank-order*
a. I want to give up rejecting others and being rejected	________
b. I do not know how to learn giving up rejection	________
c. I want to learn to accept others as they are	________
d. I need to forgive those I rejected in the past	________
e. I need to be forgiven by those I have rejected in the past	________
f. I do not know how to forgive myself or others	________
g. I do not need to forgive myself or others	________
h. Rejection is a natural part of life and all of us reject or are rejected at times	________
i. (Write down an attitude you want that was not included above)	

Homework: During the coming week, write down how you would like to achieve the behaviors you have just ranked. Write first about the behavior ranked No. 1, then No. 2, and so on, until you have written about all the behaviors you want to achieve. Make sure you receive feedback from a professional about what you have written.

Practice Exercise 6. Dealing with Hurts

Name____Sex____Date______

The purpose of this practice exercise is to help you learn more about hurts, both your own and those of others you may have hurt in the past. If you deny hurts inside yourself, you will also continue to hurt others.

1. We cannot live and not be hurt or hurt others. How much were you hurt in your life?

   a. A great deal _____
   b. Often times _____
   c. Not at all _____

2. If you checked "a" or "b," go on with this practice exercise If you checked "c," you may need a different practice exercise or practice exercise.

3. List the hurts that you have received in your life.

____
____
____
____
____

4. List the hurts that you have produced in others.

____
____
____
____
____

5. How are your hurts related to rejections? Write how hurts and rejections were related in your life (if at all).

____
____
____
____
____

6. How did you learn to deal with your hurts in the past? Rank as No. 1 the most painful hurt that you received in your life, rank as No. 2 the next most painful, and so on until the least painful hurt to you.

Hurts	*Rank-order*
a. Seeing my father or mother drunk (circle which parent)	________
b. Seeing my parents fight	________
c. Not having a father or mother	________
d. Being physically abused by my mother or father	________
e. Being sexually abused by my mother or father	________
f. Being abused by my brothers or sisters	________
g. Being abused by a relative, sexually or otherwise	________
h. Being put down by members of my family	________
i. Being put down by my friends	________
j. No matter what I did, I was always put down	________
k. No one ever recognized my importance as a person	________
l. No matter what I did, it was never good enough	________
m. Being verbally abused by my father and mother	________
n. Being verbally abused by my brothers and sisters	________
o. Being verbally abused by a relative	________
p. (Write down any other hurt not listed above)	

Homework: During the coming week, take 15 minute a day for 4 days in a row to write down all the hurts you received in your life. Make sure you make an appointment with yourself ahead of time and keep your set appointments as much as possible. If you do not set appointments with yourself at a preset and prearranged time, it will be very hard to learn to have control of your life.

Practice Exercise 7. Saying One Thing and Doing Another

Name________________________________Sex____Date______

The purpose of this practice exercise is to help you become aware of how saying and doing do not always go together. If and when that happens, one may learn to lie and cheat, by saying one thing and doing another.

1. To survive, many of us have developed a habit of saying one thing and doing another. How much does this habit apply to you?

   a. A great deal _____
   b. Often times _____
   c. Not at all _____

2. If you checked "a" or "b," go on with this practice exercise. If you checked "c," you may need a different practice exercise or practice exercise.

3. Write down how saying one thing and doing another has helped you survives in life. How did you develop it? Be as specific and detailed as you can be. You may need more than one sitting to answer this statement.

4. How was this habit destructive to you (if at all)?

5. Write down the situations where this habit got you into trouble. Be as specific and detailed as you can be. You may need more than one sitting to answer this statement.

6. What has this habit gotten you in life? Has it been helpful to you? Write down the situations where this habit was helpful to you:

7. Do you want to keep it or do you want to give it up? Complete the statement that applies to you.

   a. I want to keep it because …

b. I want to give it up because …

____
____
____
____
____

8. If you completed "a," you may need a different practice exercise or approach. If you completed "b," go on with this practice exercise.

9. If you are willing to give this habit up, rank the habits you want to develop in your life. Rank as No. 1 the habit that you want the most, rank as No. 2 the habit you want next, and so on until the habit you want the least.

Habit	*Rank-order*
a. Saying one thing and doing another	________
b. Talking our of one side of my mouth	________
c. Being straight with myself and others	________
d. Telling the truth even if it hurts	________
e. Saying what I feel without putting others down	________
f. Saying what I think without putting others down	________
g. Being respectful of myself and others	________
h. Being positive about myself and others	________
i. Being helpful rather than being hurtful	________
j. (Any other habit not listed above; specify)	________
k. (Any other habit not listed above; specify)	________

Homework: Now that you have ranked your habits, during the coming week, take the habit you ranked No. 1 and answer the following questions about it:

a. What did this habit get you in the past?

____
____
____
____
____

b. What did this habit get you in the present?

____
____
____
____

c. What will this habit get you in the future?

____

____

____

____

After you have completed answering these questions about the No. 1 ranked habit, do the same for habit ranked No. 2. Repeat this for all the habits you have ranked.

Practice Exercise 8. Push the Limits to the Limit

Name____Sex____Date______

The purpose of this practice exercise is to for you to understand that most of the behavior that got you into trouble consisted of your pushing the limits until you got caught and/or punished.

1. Many of us push the limits in order to get what we want or to have our way, no matter what the results would be for others. "Pushing the limits" means doing whatever it takes, including murder, to get what we want. How does this statement apply to you?

   a. A great deal _____
   b. Often times _____
   c. Not at all _____

2. If you checked "a" or "b," go on with this practice exercise. If you checked "c," you may need a different practice exercise or practice exercise.

3. Write down how pushing the limits has helped you survive in life. How did you develop this behavior? Be as specific and detailed as you can be. You may need more than one sitting to answer this statement.

____

____

____

____

4. Was pushing the limits destructive to you (if at all)? How? Write down the situations where pushing the limits got you into trouble. Be as specific and detailed as you can be. You may need more than one sitting to answer this statement.

____

____

____

____

5. What has pushing the limits gotten you in life? Do you want to keep it or do you want to give it up? Complete the statement that applies to you.

   a. I want to keep it because …

____
____
____
____

   b. I want to give it up because …

____
____
____
____

6. If you completed "a," you may need a different practice exercise or approach. If you completed "b," go on with this practice exercise.

7. If you are willing to give up pushing the limits, rank the positive behaviors you want to develop in your life. Rank as No. 1 the behavior that you want to do the most, rank as No. 2 the behavior you want to do next, and so on, until the behavior you want to do the least is rated last:

Limits	*Rank-order*
a. Taking advantage of others	________
b. Lying, stealing, and cheating others	________
c. Getting whatever I want no matter who gets hurt	________
d. I do not want to take advantage of others	________
e. If I take advantage of others, they will take advantage of me	________
f. I want to quit pushing limits to get what I want	________
g. I need to learn to consider the rights of others	________
h. Others are just as important as I am	________
i. I want to treat others the way I want to be treated	________
j. If I do not respect others, they will not respect me	________
k. Others have the same rights as I do	________
l. If I hurt others, they will do their best to hurt me	________

m. (Any other positive behavior not listed above, write it down)

____
____
____

n. (Any other positive behavior not listed above, write it down)

____
____
____

Homework: Now that you have ranked your limits, during the coming week, take the limit you ranked No. 1 and answer the following questions about it:

a. What did this limit get you in the past?

____
____
____
____
____

b. What did this limit get you in the present?

____
____
____
____
____

c. What will this limit get you in the future?

____
____
____
____
____

After you have completed answering those questions about the No. 1 ranked limit, do the same for the limit ranked No. 2, and so on.

Practice Exercise 9. Avoid Thinking at All Costs

Name______________________________Sex____Date______

The purpose of this practice exercise is to help you realize that if you do not think in terms of the Golden Rule, "Do unto others as you would have them do unto you," you will always be in trouble.

1. Many people act before thinking about what the consequences of their actions will be. How does this statement apply to you?

   a. A great deal ______
   b. Often times ______
   c. Not at all ______

2. If you checked "a" or "b," go on with this practice exercise. If you checked "c," you may need a different practice exercise or practice exercise.

3. Write down how this avoidance of thinking before acting has helped you survive in life. How did you develop it? Be as specific and detailed as you can be. You may need more than one sitting to answer this statement.

____

____

____

____

____

4. Was acting before thinking destructive to you (if at all)? Write down the situations where acting before thinking got you into trouble. Be as specific and detailed as you can be. You may need more than one sitting to answer this statement.

____

____

____

____

____

5. What has acting before thinking gotten you in life? Do you want to keep doing it or do you want to give it up? Complete the statement that applies to you.

   a. I want to keep it because …

____

____

____

____

____

   b. I want to give it up because …

____

____

____

____

____

6. If you completed "a," you may need a different practice exercise or approach. If you completed "b," go on with this practice exercise.

7. If you willing to give up acting before thinking, rank the behaviors you want to develop in your life. Rank as No. 1 the behavior that you want to develop the most, rank as No. 2 the behavior you want to develop next, and so on until the behavior you want to develop the least.

Behavior		*Rank-order*
a.	I want to learn to think before I act	________
b.	Acting before thinking has always gotten me into trouble	________
c.	I do not know how to think before I act	________
d.	Thinking before acting is for sissies	________
e.	I do not know how to think in helpful ways	________
f.	I do not know how to think	________
g.	I wish I could learn how to think in more positive ways	________
h.	Thinking is very hard for me to do	________
i.	I am so used to acting that I doubt whether I can learn to think	________
j.	Thinking too much may make me crazy	________
k.	I want help in learning how to think in helpful ways	________
l.	(Any other positive behavior not listed above, write it down)	________
m.	(Any other positive behavior not listed above, write it down)	________

Homework: Now that you have ranked your behaviors, during the coming week, take the behavior you ranked No. 1 and answer the following questions about it:

a. What did this behavior get you in the past?

____
____
____
____
____

b. What did this behavior get you in the present?

____
____
____
____
____

c. What will this behavior get you in the future?

____
____
____
____
____

After you have completed answering these questions about the No. 1 ranked behavior, do the same for the behavior ranked No. 2, and so on.

Practice Exercise 10. Follow-Up

Name_______________________________________Sex____Date______

The purpose of this practice exercise is to review whether this practice exercise was helpful to you or not.

1. Please select the answer that best fits how you feel about this practice exercise:

   a. I did not like working on this practice exercise at all. I wish I never saw it. _________
   b. I did not like this practice exercise at all, but I am glad I got to work on it. _________
   c. I am delighted I got a chance to work on this practice exercise. _________
   d. I am not only delighted about this practice exercise, but I wish all people at risk for incarceration had a chance to work on it _________

2. How helpful was it to work on this practice exercise? Check the answer that applies to you:

   a. Not helpful at all _________ c. Helpful _________
   b. Somewhat helpful _________ d. Very helpful _________

3. Which practice exercise did you like best? Please rank-order the practice exercises; rank as No. 1 the one you liked best or was most helpful to you, rank as No. 2 the one you liked next best, and so on, to the one you did not like at all (No. 9).

Practice Exercise	*Rank-order*
a. Life is a power struggle	_________
b. I know better	_________
c. I am more important than anybody else	_________
d. I will not be caught	_________
e. Reject others before they reject me	_________
f. Dealing with hurts	_________
g. Saying one thing and doing another	_________
h. Push the limits to the limit	_________
i. Avoid thinking at all costs	_________

4. Which practice exercise was the most helpful to you? Sometimes what we like most is not necessarily the most helpful. Consequently, rank the practice exercises according to their helpfulness to you? Rank as No. 1 the most helpful, rank as No. 2 the next most helpful, and so on until the least helpful (No. 9).

Practice Exercise		*Rank-order*
a.	Life is a power struggle	_________
b.	I know better	_________
c.	I am more important than anybody else	_________
d.	I will not be caught	_________
e.	Reject others before they reject me	_________
f.	Dealing with hurts	_________
g.	Saying one thing and doing another	_________
h.	Push the limits to the limit	_________
i.	Avoid thinking at all costs	_________

5. Explain why you rank-ordered the practice exercises the way you did.

____
____
____
____
____

6. Feel free to write any comments that might improve this practice exercise.

____
____
____
____
____

Troublemaking

This practice exercise is intended for incarcerated felons or individuals at high risk for incarceration. The purpose of this practice exercise is to help you learn more about behaviors that have gotten you in trouble (and possibly in jail) in the past or in the present. These behaviors, if they persist, might get you into trouble (and in jail) again in the future. If you do not want to learn about these behaviors, you do not have to go on with this practice exercise. However, if you do want to (1) learn more about behaviors that have gotten you into trouble with the law, and (2) avoid getting into trouble with the law in the future, please complete this practice exercise.

Practice Exercise 1. Behaviors that Got You in Trouble (and Perhaps in Jail?)

Name_________________________________Sex____Date_______

The purpose of this practice exercise is to learn more about which behaviors get you into trouble.

1. Below is a list of behaviors that get many people in trouble with the law. You need to define each behavior as you understand it. You may want to check in a dictionary, ask your cellmate, a guard, relatives, or friends. It may take you a week or longer to complete these definitions. Use two examples from your experience to define each behavior. Take your time. It is important that you understand what these behaviors are why they landed you in jail.

What do you understand by the following items?

Give a definition and two examples.

a. Glibness/superficial charm — Example 1 ______ Example 2 ______

b. Grandiose sense of self-worth — Example 1 ______ Example 2 ______

c. Need for stimulation/proneness to boredom — Example 1 ______ Example 2 ______

d. Pathological lying — Example 1 ______ Example 2 ______

e. Conning/manipulative — Example 1 ______ Example 2 ______

f. Lack of remorse or guilt — Example 1 ______ Example 2 ______

g. Shallow affect (feelings) — Example 1 ______ Example 2 ______

h. Callousness/lack of empathy

Example 1 ______________________

____

Example 2 ______________________

____

i. Parasitic lifestyle

Example 1 ______________________

____

Example 2 ______________________

____

j. Poor behavioral control

Example 1 ______________________

____

Example 2 ______________________

____

k. Promiscuous sexual behavior

Example 1 ______________________

____

Example 2 ______________________

____

l. Impulsivity

Example 1 ______________________

____

Example 2 ______________________

____

m. Irresponsibility

Example 1 ______________________

____

Example 2 ______________________

____

n. Failure to accept responsibility for your actions

Example 1 ______________________

____

Example 2 ______________________

____

2. Now that you have completed the first part of this practice exercise, here comes the hard part: Below are listed the 14 behaviors that you have defined during the past week or so. Rank each of them according to how each (mis)behavior applies to you. Rank as No. 1 the (mis)behavior that applies to you the most, rank as No. 2 the (mis)behavior that applies to you next best, and so on; mark as N/A (not applicable) the (mis)behaviors that do not apply to you at all.

Behaviors	*Rank-order*
a. Glibness/superficial charm	_________
b. Grandiose sense of self-worth	_________
c. Need for stimulation/proneness to boredom	_________
d. Pathological lying	_________
e. Conning/manipulative	_________
f. Lack of remorse or guilt	_________
g. Shallow affect	_________
h. Callous/lack of empathy	_________
i. Parasitic lifestyle	_________
j. Poor behavioral control	_________
k. Promiscuous sexual behavior	_________
l. Impulsivity	_________
m. Irresponsibility	_________
n. Failure to accept responsibility for my own actions	_________

3. Why did you rank-order these behaviors the way you did? Write the reason(s) here:

____
____
____
____
____

4. Now that you have completed this practice exercise, write how you felt about it. Check which of these answers tells how you felt about it. There is also space for you to explain further, if you want to:

   a. I did not like it at all. I want to quit this stupid practice exercise. ______
   b. I did not like it very much, but I want to go on with this practice exercise. ______
   c. I liked it and I want to go on with this practice exercise. ______
   d. I liked it a lot and I wish I had something like this practice exercise years ago. ______
   e. I liked it so much that I wish all people in jail could get something like this practice exercise to work on. ______

5. Discuss your answers with whoever has given you this practice exercise.

Homework: During the coming week, think more about the behaviors that got you into trouble and whether you want to change the rank-order of these behaviors as listed above, or start working on the next practice exercise.

Standard Practice Exercise No.____

Title of Behavior:................................

Name____Sex____Date______

The purpose of this practice exercise is to understand more about the behavior listed in the title.

1. How did this behavior get you into trouble (and perhaps in jail)? Please explain in detail:

____
____
____
____
____

2. How often did this behavior get you into trouble? Check which answer applies to you:

   a. Practically every day _____
   b. Once a week _____
   c. A couple of times a month _____
   d. Once a month _____
   e. Once every six 6 months _____
   f. Once a year _____
   g. Once every few years _____

3. Please explain further:

____
____
____
____
____

4. How did this behavior come about? Do you remember when you started it? Check which answer fits best:

   a. When I was a child (younger than 5 years of age) ______
   b. When I was in elementary school ______
   c. When I was in middle school ______
   d. When I was in high school ______
   e. After high school ______
   f. Any other time ______

5. Please explain further:

6. How did this behavior get you in trouble (and perhaps in jail)? Please explain:

7. Give three specific examples of how this behavior got you in trouble.

Example 1

Example 2

Example 3

Homework: Next week, in order for you to learn to control this behavior ("Start it if you want to stop it!"), plan to repeat this behavior at preset times (for instance, at 8 a.m., 12 noon, 4 or 7 p.m.) on at least 3 days. Write down what happened in detail. For each time make sure to answer in writing the following four questions:

a. How did you start it?
b. What followed?
c. How did it end?
d. What did this behavior get you?

Time 1 (write the time you started__________):

a.

b.

c.

d.

Time 2 (write the time you started__________):

a.

b.

c.

d.

Time 3 (write the time you started__________):

a.

b.

c.

d.

Please check which of the following shows what you got out of this lesson:

a. Completely useless _____ d. Somewhat useful _____
b. Somewhat useless _____ e. Extremely useful _____
c. So-so _____

Feel free to explain how you feel about the homework practice exercise and what you got out of it.

____
____
____
____
____

Concluding Feedback Practice Exercise

Name_______________________________________Sex____Date______

The purpose of this practice exercise is to review whether this practice exercise was helpful to you or not.

1. Please select the answer that best fits how you feel about this practice exercise:

   a. I did not like working on this practice exercise at all. I wish I never saw it. ____
   b. I did not like this practice exercise at all, but I am glad I got to work on it. _____
   c. I am delighted I got a chance to work on this practice exercise. _______
   d. I am not only delighted about this practice exercise, but I wish all people at risk for incarceration had a chance to work on it. _____

2. How helpful was it to work on this practice exercise? Check the answer that applies to you.

   a. Not helpful at all _____ c. Helpful _____
   b. Somewhat helpful _____ d. Very helpful _____

3. Which practice exercise did you like best? Please rank-order the practice exercises; rank as No. 1 the one you liked best or was most helpful to you, rank as No. 2 the one you liked next best, and so on, to the one you did not like at all (No. 14).

Practice Exercises/Behaviors	*Rank-order*
a. Glibness/superficial charm	________
b. Grandiose sense of self-worth	________
c. Need for stimulation/proneness to boredom	________
d. Pathological lying	________
e. Conning/manipulative	________
f. Lack of remorse or guilt	________
g. Shallow affect	________
h. Callous/lack of empathy	________
i. Parasitic lifestyle	________
j. Poor behavioral control	________
k. Promiscuous sexual behavior	________
l. Impulsivity	________
m. Irresponsibility	________
n. Failure to accept responsibility for my own actions	________

4. Explain why you have ranked these practice exercises the way you did.

____

____

____

____

____

5. Which practice exercise was the most helpful to you? Sometimes what we like most is not necessarily the most helpful. Consequently, rank the practice exercises according to their helpfulness to you? Rank as No. 1 the most helpful, No. 2 the next most helpful, and so on, until the least helpful practice exercise (No. 14).

Practice Exercises/Behaviors	*Rank-order*
a. Glibness/superficial charm	________
b. Grandiose sense of self-worth	________
c. Need for stimulation/proneness to boredom	________
d. Pathological lying	________
e. Conning/manipulative	________
f. Lack of remorse or guilt	________
g. Shallow affect	________
h. Callous/lack of empathy	________
i. Parasitic lifestyle	________
j. Poor behavioral control	________
k. Promiscuous sexual behavior	________
l. Impulsivity	________
m. Irresponsibility	________
n. Failure to accept responsibility for own actions	________

6. Explain why you have ranked these practice exercises the way you did.

____
____
____
____

7. Feel free to write any comments that might improve this practice exercise.

____
____
____
____

Psychological Problems

Even though overdependency and sexual abuse may not seem as severe as mood swings, both conditions are very resistant to change, especially when change is attempted only through talk therapy. Hence, both conditions are included here because both are difficult to treat through talk therapy. Both conditions lead to severe consequences not only for patients but also for their significant others.

Overdependency

The purpose of this practice exercise is to help you learn more about overdependency or codependency, which entails being unusually attached to someone who is physically and verbally abusive, or someone who is addicted to gambling, or is abusing alcohol, drugs, or medications.

Practice Exercise 1. The Meaning of Overdependency

Name________________________________Sex____Date______

The purpose of this practice exercise is to help you understand and change a pattern of overdependency on individual(s) who themselves are addicted to substances (drugs or alcohol), work, gambling, or other behaviors.

1. There are many definitions of "overdependency" or "codependency." What do they mean to you? Write your definition in words that are specific and particular to your experience.

____
____
____
____

2. Among the many meanings of "overdependency" or "codependency" given below, give two examples of how that meaning applies specifically to your experience.

Meanings	*Examples*
a. Any behavior that controls one's life at the expense of other parts of one's life ______	Example 1 ______ ______ Example 2 ______ ______
b. Allowing another person to influence oneself ______ ______	Example 1 ______ ______ Example 2 ______ ______
c. Being obsessed (and therefore controlled) with controlling another person's behavior ______	Example 1 ______ ______ Example 2 ______ ______
d. An emotional, psychological, and behavioral condition that develops as a result of an individual's past abuses ______	Example 1 ______ ______ Example 2 ______ ______
e. Prolonged contact with a set of strong and rigid rules that control your behavior ______	______ Example 1 ______ ______ Example 2 ______
f. Practice of strong and rigid rules ______ ______ ______	Example 1 ______ ______ Example 2 ______ ______
g. Avoidance of open expression of feelings ______ ______	Example 1 ______ ______ Example 2 ______ ______
h. Avoidance of the direct discussion of personal and family troublesome thoughts ______ ______	Example 1 ______ ______ Example 2 ______ ______

i. Following rules that "should" be followed by everybody, especially your partner, your parents, or your children

Example 1 ______________________

Example 2 ______________________

j. A dysfunctional pattern of living and of problem solving that is reinforced by a set of rules within the family unit

Example 1 ______________________

Example 2 ______________________

k. A pattern of extreme dependency on another person

Example 1 ______________________

Example 2 ______________________

l. Spending a long period of time in association with anyone who is abusive or neglectful

Example 1 ______________________

Example 2 ______________________

m. Self-defeating, learned behaviors patterns or character defects

Example 1 ______________________

Example 2 ______________________

n. A decreased ability to start or to participate in loving relationships

Example 1 ______________________

Example 2 ______________________

o. A personality pattern found within most members of abusive or neglectful families

Example 1 ______________________

Example 2 ______________________

p. An addictive behavioral pattern that is openly supported by an addictive society

Example 1 ______________________

Example 2 ______________________

q. Other (write what it is): ____________________ Example 1 ____________________

____________________ Example 2 ____________________

____

3. Rank-order the meanings that apply to you. Rank as No. 1 the meaning that applies to you the most, rank as No. 2 the meaning that applies to you next, and so on; mark as N/A the meanings that do not apply to you at all.

Meanings	*Rank-order*
a. Any behavior that controls one's life at the expense of other parts of one's life	________
b. Allowing another person to influence oneself	________
c. Being obsessed (and therefore controlled) with controlling another person's behavior	________
d. An emotional, psychological, and behavioral condition that develops as a result of an individual's past abuses	________
e. Prolonged contact with a set of strong and rigid rules that control your behavior	________
f. Practice of strong and rigid rules	________
g. Avoidance of open expression of feelings	________
h. Avoidance of the direct discussion of personal and social troublesome thoughts	________
i. Following rules that "should" be followed by everybody, especially your partner, your parents, or your children	________
j. A dysfunctional pattern of living and of problem solving that is reinforced by a set of rules within the family system	________
k. A pattern of extreme dependency on another person	________
l. Spending a long period of time in association with anyone who is abusive or neglectful	________
m. Self-defeating, learned behaviors patterns or character defects	________
n. A decreased ability to start or to participate in loving relationships	________
o. A personality pattern found within most members of abusive or neglectful families	________
p. An addictive behavioral pattern that is openly supported by our addictive society	________
q. Other (write what it is): (____________________)	________

4. Write in detail about three of the meanings above that you have checked in order of greatest importance to you, numbered 1–3:

1. ____
____
____

2. ____
____
____

3. ____
____
____

5. Which of the following rules apply to the way you were brought up? Rank them according to how much they apply to you. Rank as No. 1 the rule that applied the most, rank as No. 2 the rule that applied next, and so on; mark as N/A the rules that did not apply to you at all.

Rule	*Rank-order*
a. It is not acceptable to talk about one's troublesome thoughts	________
b. Feelings should not be expressed openly	________
c. Communication is best if indirect, with one person acting as messenger between two others	________
d. Be strong, good, right, and perfect, whatever is meant by these words	________
e. Make us proud of your performance, at the expense of your sense of importance and self-esteem	________
f. Don't be selfish; other people are more important than you are	________
g. Do as we say, not as we do	________
h. It's not acceptable to play or be playful, laugh, and enjoy life; life is grim and not to be enjoyed	________
i. Keep things as they are and do not "rock the boat"	________
j. Do not admit to any shortcomings and certainly not to troublesome thoughts or personal failures in our family	________
k. "Cry on your own time" and do not bother us with your troublesome thoughts and tears	________
l. Make a good appearance no matter what, never show your true feelings, smile and say "thank you"	________
m. Other rule(s) peculiar to your family background that were not listed above (write rule):	________

6. Write in detail about three rules that you have ranked as the most important to your experience, numbered 1–3:

1. ____
____
____

2. ____
____
____

3. ____
____
____

7. How much have these experiences hurt you? List as many hurts as you can remember and explain them in detail.

____
____
____
____

8. How have all of these hurts influenced your behavior? What kind of person have you become because of these hurtful experiences? Answer as fully as you can.

____
____
____
____

Homework: During the coming week, think about what you wrote in this practice exercise and discuss it with your professional helper.

Practice Exercise 2. Changing Major Troublesome thoughts in the Relationship

Name______________________________Sex____Date______

The purpose of this practice exercise is to start planning to control your life and not being controlled by your partner's abusive behavior.

1. List all of the troublesome thoughts you have had or are having with your partner.

____
____
____
____

2. Of the many troublesome thoughts listed above, pick the three major ones, and write about them in detail.

____
____
____
____
____

3. Major differences found in abusive-codependent couples, no matter what the nature of the abuse or addiction may be, are listed below. Check which of these differences apply to you and which to your partner:

Differences Between Two Styles in Overly Dependent Relationships

Partner		*Overdependent*	
Denial of personal errors	______	Acceptance or admission of personal errors	______
More able to receive than to give love	______	More able to give than to receive love	______
Spoiled (picky)	______	Neglected	______
Self-indulgent	______	Self-sacrificing or self-neglectful	______
More critical of others than of self	______	More critical of self than others	______
Blaming others rather than self	______	Blaming self rather than others	______
Committed to self more than to others	______	Committed to others more than to self	______
Decisive (very certain)	______	Indecisive (very uncertain)	______
Dominant–authoritarian	______	Submissive–permissive	______
Rigid (unbending)	______	All too flexible (pliable)	______
Neither trusting nor trustworthy	______	Naively trusting, gullible	______
Unconventional	______	Conventional	______
Uses anger to manipulate others	______	Uses fear, anxiety, worry, and sadness to manipulate self	______
Driven	______	Pushed	______
Unreflective and/or impulsive (not worried) about consequences	______	Overanxious, worried about consequences	______
Dominant	______	Submissive	______

3. Explain in detail those characteristics that apply to you and how they have led you to defeat yourself and your sense of self-importance.

____
____
____
____
____

4. In overly dependent relationships, closeness and intimacy between partners and among family members may be impossible unless there is equality of importance and of reciprocity in giving and getting. What are your reactions to this statement?

____
____
____
____
____

5. Do you want to change self-defeating characteristics or are you satisfied with the way you are? If you are satisfied, you do not need to do anything else. Drop this program. If you are not satisfied, you may want to put your energy into changing into a winning person. What is your decision? Please write down what is that you want for yourself.

____
____
____
____
____

Homework: if you want to change, here are some guidelines that you may need to follow from now on:

a. Plan to do something new that you have never done before: Doing something new means doing something new for yourself. Something new means finding a different behavior, such as shopping for yourself before shopping for others; insisting on watching a favorite TV program, rather than allowing everybody else in the family to watch theirs; or going out with friends. In other words, "doing something new" means to affirm, assert, and insist that you are important and that no one will be allowed to put you down. If they do, as they inevitably will, they are going to do it at their peril! You need to get used to the idea that buying things, or watching a TV program, or going out with friends are all things and activities that can be discussed. What cannot be discussed is your sense of self-importance and your love for those who love you. You will talk things over provided there is equality of importance between you and your partner and reciprocity in what you give, or give up, and what you receive. Please write down your reactions to the above statements.

b. Do something new that is also positive: Something is positive when it does not put anybody else down or is not done at anybody's expense, including our own. You need to ask yourself: "Will anybody suffer or feel put down for or from this behavior? Will somebody become frightened if I assert my importance?" If you are convinced that whatever you are doing enhances yourself, would make you feel proud and pleased, would bring a new perspective to yourself and to the relationship, and does not hurt anyone else, then that behavior is positive and can be executed or implemented. Please write down your reactions to the above statements.

c. Use the rule of three: Very likely your partner will react negatively to a new and positive behavior on your part. S/he will object to almost anything new and positive that you do. Consequently, you do not need his/her permission nor that of anybody else to do something new and positive. If your partner gets mad, you may well be on the right track, because usually abusive or addicted individuals are afraid of anything that may threaten the status quo, especially any behavior that may show that you want to behave like a grown-up person in his/her own right. When this negative reaction takes place, your partner should be asked to come up with at least three reasons why this new, positive behavior should not take place. Here, the rule of three should be practiced; that is, we need to have three relevant and positive reasons for doing what we want to do, provided no one else is hurt by this behavior, including ourselves. You (and your partner) need to come up with at least three reasons for doing something new and positive:

"I like it because ________________________"
"It makes me feel good because ________________"
"I want it because ______________________"
"I need it because _____________________"

Homework: Do something new, positive, and strong: "Strong" means doing whatever one needs to do to express one's personal importance and strong commitment to change. Something new and positive has to be strong and powerful enough to make a difference in your life and perhaps in the relationship with your partner. Remember that the more you change and work for change, the greater the resistance from your partner will be. What could you do that is new, positive, and strong enough to make a difference in your life? Discuss your results with your professional helper.

Practice Exercise 3. Drawing Lines

Name____________________________________Sex____Date________

The purpose of this practice exercise is for you to learn to set clear, definite limits to protect yourself from abuse or neglect.

1. What does drawing lines mean to you? Please write down your definition and give one or two examples of how drawing lines applies to your experience.

____
____
____
____
____

2. As a result of past and present training, the overly dependent person is usually unable to draw lines to assert her or his importance. How does this conclusion apply to your experience? Were you ever able to draw lines on your partner's behavior?

   a. If no, why not? Explain in detail.

____
____
____
____
____

   b. If yes, how were you able to do it? Explain in detail.

____
____
____
____
____

3. If the experience of not being able to draw lines concerning your partner's behavior does not apply to you, skip this lesson, unless you feel you still would like to learn how to draw lines with your partner or anybody else. Perhaps you may need another practice exercise or a different way of helping you. Please respond to the above statement.

4. Drawing boundary lines as to what you will or will not put up with from your partner refers to what is acceptable and not acceptable to you. If you do not know what will be acceptable or unacceptable to you, how will you be able draw lines? How do we learn to set boundaries? Setting lines or boundaries in a sexual relationship can be related to using condoms. If a woman, for instance, does not know how to set a boundary to protect herself and her body from the very outset of a relationship, she has lost it. By the same token, a man should use a condom to protect both himself and his partner. Lines need to be drown before sexual intercourse in either a casual or a committed relationship to avoid either an unwanted pregnancy or serious diseases. If one cannot set boundaries at this point, it is doubtful whether one can or will be able to set firm and

clear boundaries on any other issues from then on in the relationship. Selfish partners usually could not care less. They want to get what they can get when they can get it, and how they get it is not important! Their immediate needs are more important than their partner's needs! If you does not care about your importance, why should your partner care? What do you think about the above statements?

5. Below is a list of different ways a codependent may be unable to draw lines with the partner from the very beginning of the relationship, perhaps because of giving more importance to the partner rather than to oneself. This first line of defense (the "condom line") deals with how one protects and safeguards one's body during courtship or after marriage. Read this list and check which of these statements applies to your experience.

Relationships Between Abusive and Overly Dependent Individuals

Partner		*Overdependent*	
1. Not taking "precautions" during intercourse before marriage	________	Allowing it to happen	________
2. Not taking responsibility if and when one's sexual partner gets pregnant	________	Allowing it to happen	________
3. Not holding a steady job and to be taken care of by others, including spouse, partner, or live-in companion	________	Allowing it to happen	________
4. Using work or work pressures to avoid taking responsibilities in the home	________	Allowing it to happen	________
5. Not sharing in household chores	________	Allowing it to happen	________
6. Watching TV or drinking while partner is still working	________	Allowing it to happen	________
7. Not taking initiative in child's care	________	Allowing it to happen	________
8. Having to be reminded of duties and responsibilities relevant to the role of partner and caregiver	________	Allowing it to happen	________
9. Spending leisure time away from home, with friends or in projects that are not related to the family and home	________	Allowing it to happen	________
10. Being or becoming addicted to work, TV, alcohol, or gambling	________	Allowing it to happen	________

Partner		*Overdependent*	
11. Verbally, sexually, or physically abusing of partner and/or children	________	Allowing it to happen	________
12. Running around with other "friends")	________	Allowing it to happen	________
13. Buying more clothes than the rest of the family to look good and make a good impression at work	________	Allowing it to happen	________
14. Any other behavior that takes place at the other's expense, write what it is:	________	Allowing it to happen	________

6. After you have checked them, pick the three most important statements and write in detail how they apply to you and what was the outcome for you as a person and as a partner.

a. ____
____
____

b. ____
____
____

c. ____
____
____

d. ____
____
____

7. In addition to the above list, are there other abusive or neglectful behaviors that you were not able to deal with in your partner? List as many as you can remember.

____
____
____
____
____

8. Which of these abusive or neglectful behaviors in your partner are similar to behaviors in either of your parents? Explain how they are or are not.

9. Which of the abusive behaviors listed in the table above are the opposite of behaviors in either of your parents? Explain how they are or are not.

10. Would you conclude (from everything that has been presented thus far in these practice exercises) that one of the major troublesome thoughts with your relationship is an inability to draw lines? If you agree, write down why. If you disagree write down your reason for disagreeing.

11. Does your partner match your inability to draw lines by his or her ability to push the limits? How is it done (pushing the limits, that is)? Describe all the ways your partner pushes the limits, if indeed s/he does.

12. Whether you agree or disagree with the conclusion, are you willing to learn how to draw lines to safeguard yourself? Please write your answer.

13. How and when do we draw lines? First, to draw lines verbally with an addicted partner means that "words are cheap," and are often useless. Words, most of the time, lead to escalations and to explosive arguments and fights. Before speaking and trying to talk sense with your partner, you must avoid engaging him or her in another round of useless and destructive arguments, unless you have thought an issue through and the rule of three has been used successfully. If you cannot come up with at least three good (appropriate, relevant, positive, helpful, etc.) reasons, it means that not enough thought has been given to the issue at hand. What are your reactions to the statements above?

14. If you are ready to learn how to draw lines, read the instructions in the list below. Using a blank, unlined, piece of paper, draw these lines using a yellow or red pen or pencil for lines 1–3 and a black pencil or pen for lines 4 and 5.

    Learning to Draw Lines
    1. Draw two straight, parallel, uninterrupted, yellow or red lines
    2. Draw two straight, parallel yellow or red lines with one (just one!) break in between
    3. Draw one straight uninterrupted yellow or red line
    4. Draw one straight uninterrupted black line
    5. Draw one straight, interrupted, dotted black line, like this: ---------------

15. What do these lines remind you of? If your answer is "Highway" or "Road" signs, you are absolutely correct. Applied to your life these lines indicate what you will put up with and what you will not put up with.

Line No. 1: What would you put up with? Infidelity? Violence? Rape? Incest? What would your partner need to do for you to draw a line? Commit murder? Is anything and everything your partner does acceptable or unacceptable? Are you trying to make excuses for his/her behavior and allow him/her to get away with murder? Here, list all of the behaviors that you find completely unacceptable under any conditions and that you will not put up with:

Line No. 2: What behavior would you put up with just once, not to be repeated ever again? Running around with other people? Rape? Incest? Violence? Physical and verbal abuse? Getting drunk or hitting you? Just because you failed to draw a firm line the first time, it does not mean that you cannot draw a firm line now. Write down exactly what you would do if your partner were to do something to you that legally, morally, emotionally, and personally would be hurtful to you or to those you love. Make it very clear that the first time you were hurt, it was the responsibility of your partner. However, if you are hurt again, then the responsibility belongs to you to protect oneself. We have only two cheeks!

Line No. 3: What would you put up with over an extended period of time? Everyday decisions? Who is going to take care of the house? What chores should be taken up by whom? Who is going to clean what? Who is responsible for doing what? Who will draw up a budget? Who will follow it? How are disagreements going to be settled? By fighting? By sitting down at a table at a preset time with an agenda? How are purchases to be made? Separately? Jointly? Should vacations be taken with relatives or away from relatives? How is money to be spent? Ideally, both of you should be working, talking, and solving troublesome thoughts without blaming, and without using abusive behaviors.

Line No. 4: What is still unclear in the relationship that would require further, continued, and prolonged discussion? Some of these troublesome thoughts may have been dealt with under line No. 3. Other troublesome thoughts are still unresolved and are still affecting the relationship. Here you may find troublesome thoughts that need upgrading to either line No. 3, to keep in line No. 4, or to downgrade to line No. 5.

Line No. 5: What troublesome thoughts are taken for granted by both of you that are already set up, accepted, and that do not require talking over? Here you may list things that have already been solved, or that do not need any discussion. They do not present a troublesome thought to either one of you.

Homework: Once this practice exercise is completed, put it aside and sleep on it for one or more nights. Then go back to it and see whether it needs any improvement, changing whatever needs to be changed. Once you have a final draft, you should make at least two copies, one for yourself and one for your counselor (or friend). Discuss your answers with your counselor (or another significant individual in your life) and change whatever needs to be changed on the basis of your discussion. Make three copies of your final draft.

Practice Exercise 4. Watch Your Language!

Name________________________________Sex____Date__________

The purpose of this practice exercise is for you to use language that will not be used against you as an excuse for your partner to use foul language. This is how he or she want to "hook" you, that is, to get you mad enough or upset enough to justify his or her abuse.

1. If you want to avoid getting upset whenever you talk with your partner, you need to remember that your partner is used to (and probably likes) having you upset, because then s/he is in control of the situation. Please write your reaction to this statement.

2. Do you need to set some guidelines on how you are going to behave whenever you talk with your partner? It would be good if your partner were to follow the same guidelines, but one cannot expect that much.

   a. If your answer is yes, explain why.
   b. If your answer is no, explain why.

3. To be in charge of yourself (and not of your partner, because no one can control others), you may need to avoid the seven deadly, abusive, and suicidal ways (errors, that is) of talking. These ways are so deadly that they will be called the "seven deadly errors." They kill our sense of self-importance. You may need to memorize them, or to keep them in front of you while you talk with your partner, making sure you do not make these errors:

Deadly error No. 1: Using the "You" instead of the "I" or "We" pronouns. If and when you find yourself using the "You" pronoun, you are getting hooked to your partner and you are becoming abusive. Use the "I" or "We" pronoun when it is appropriate to use it, but avoid using "You." If you do use it, you are starting to lose the most important part of yourself: your identity as a person and as a partner. This identity is expressed by our use of the pronoun "I." Please write your comments on this guideline.

Deadly error No. 2: Avoid using and making general statements, such as "never" and "always." If you find yourself saying. "You never ..." or "You always ..." you have already lost it! What are your reactions to this guideline?

Deadly error No. 3: Do not bring up the past, and when your partner does, say, "I cannot change the past mistakes I have made. However, I can change the present, what I am doing now, and what I plan to do for the future." What are your reactions to this guideline?

Deadly error No. 4: Avoid reading your partner's mind, telling him or her what she or he should or shouldn't do, think, or feel. How would you like it if your partner reads your mind? When your partner does read your mind, answer, "I am responsible for what I do, say, think, and feel. You are responsible for what you do, say, think, and feel." If your partner pushes the issue, remind him/her that you will not stand for any mind-reading. What do you feel about this guideline?

Deadly error No. 5: Do not use emotional blackmail or bribery, for instance: "If you do not do as I want, I will ..." Part of this blackmail is setting ultimatums, using sex as part of the blackmail. Please respond to this guideline.

Deadly error No. 6: Do not make up or use excuses to justify your behavior. If you goofed, you goofed; what else is new? Can you forgive yourself and accept that mistakes prove that we are human beings? If you wanted to be as perfect as your partner, an individual who makes no mistakes, you would have married someone else! When your partner starts making excuses for his/her behavior, say: "We cannot change the mistakes we have made in the past. However, we can learn from them, and try to avoid making them again." What is your reaction to this guideline?

Deadly error No. 7: This pattern needs to be discovered from how you and your partner talk with each other. One of the most frequent and destructive patterns among related partners is distraction or use of irrelevant behavior (for instance, talking about the price of eggs in China) or computer-like reactions devoid of feelings. What is your reaction to this guideline?

4. Are there other deadly patterns that have not been covered by the guidelines above? Please write down a pattern not listed above.

____
____
____
____
____

Homework: If there are going to be meetings with your partner to talk things over, you must follow three other guidelines. If these guidelines are not followed, it is questionable whether any progress will be possible.

a. Meetings with your partner need to be made by appointment, at least 24 h in advance. How does the rest of the world get things done? By appointment and by the written record. Why should we not follow the same practices used by everybody else in the world? What makes us think that intimate relationships should follow different practices than the rest of the world? Thus, through weekly meetings at a time that is mutually agreeable and through written records, partners may learn to work together. After you both have made up a list of issues, whatever they may be, both should rank them in order of importance, for instance, how we talk with each other about (1) money, (2) sex, (3) children, (4) in-laws, (5) friends, (6) work, etc. Divide these issues in terms of special interests. For instance, if one partner takes (1), (4), and (5), the other partner takes (2), (3), and (6). What are your reactions to the above guideline?
b. During the next week and before the next meeting, you and your partner need to write down a proposal on how to solve or resolve each particular issue on your agenda. If possible, each partner should give three reasons for suggested solutions. At the next meeting, if there is one, partners should avoid talking as much as possible. Instead, they need to exchange their written proposals, add whatever new issues each may have thought of during the preceding week, and end the meeting, even if it lasts only a few minutes. Talking should be kept to the barest minimum. Both of you have done enough talking in the past; did it help? What are your reactions to the above statements?
c. Keep a written record of what has been talked over in your meetings. The goals of this first meeting, of course, are to see whether the partner can understand and accept (1) your codependent's position; (2) working out an agenda, including issues that are important to both of you; and (3) working on solving those issues for the long haul by negotiating and problem solving together. It would be helpful if at this meeting both of you were to start listing the various troublesome thoughts facing you, such as (1) what rules of conduct should be followed with each other, like doing the opposite of the seven deadly sins; and (2) how both partners are going to work out these troublesome thoughts: by exploding at each other, by command, by instant decisions without prior discussion? Or, are they going to start working together by making regular weekly or biweekly appointments with each other? What are your reactions to the above?

Practice Exercise 5. Talking Things Over with Your Partner

Name______________________________________Sex____Date________

The purpose of this practice exercise is to help you learn to control yourself and start to control your life instead of giving controls to your partner.

1. An appointment with your partner should be made at least 24 h in advance, because one needs to discuss things that are important by appointment. In asking for an appointment, avoid making it look like an ambush and do not, under any conditions, give in to the partner's inevitable request for immediate explanations. You need to present a copy of your paper about drawing lines to the partner because you need his or her feedback. However, no immediate reaction is desired or needed. Allow time for your partner to read it in comfort (at least 24 h) and decide at what time both of you can get together to talk about it. Then, you must listen to the partner's reactions, assuming that they are positive, and write down whatever helpful suggestions s/he may make to improve clarifying drawing lines. What are your reactions to the above?

2. If the reaction you get is one of angry put-down, criticism, and negativity, talk about the destructive aspects of this behavior and express how you feel about it: "It makes me very unhappy (sad, desolate, hurt) to see that you do not approve of my efforts to improve our relationship." If your partner is not willing to sit down and talk at an agreed upon time, then s/he is failing to behave like a partner. However, your partner should not be allowed to control the relationship any more than you should. You need to keep cool and avoid reacting and escalating to your partner's provocation (remember the seven deadly errors listed above). What are your reactions to the above?

3. You need to learn setting boundaries and drawing lines with your partner. This learning means behaving as much as possible at your very best regardless of your partner's worst behavior. Just because your partner robs banks, does this behavior excuse you for robbing banks also? Setting boundaries means not getting "hooked" into the partner's provocations and setups. Your partner is just as involved in getting you to behave (like a "bitch" or like a "bastard") to prove to himself/herself that s/he is justified in behaving the way s/he does (like a bitch or like a bastard). In other words, your partner is set to make a "monster" out of you. S/he will do whatever s/he can to prove himself/herself right! S/he will push you to the limit. Once you explode, your partner will receive the greatest gift of all—s/he will be in control of the relationship! Will you allow him/her to control you and push you to the point of explosion? If and when you lose control, your partner has won! Very likely, that is the way s/he has learned to behave with his/her mother or father to have his or her own way. Why should s/he not do it with you? What are your reactions to the above?

4. If you start to set boundaries and draw lines, one can predict that your partner will escalate (push limits) immediately. S/he will not tolerate any change in the direction of self-assertion and initiative on your part. Your changing for the better will be extremely threatening to your partner. Consequently, you need to be very careful about how to go about drawing lines. Your partner will become very upset whenever you do something that is new, positive, and strong. One would hope that your partner may not escalate. However, if and when s/he does, and this suggestion does not work, one may need to go on to the next, more difficult lesson. What are your reactions to the above?

5. This practice exercise has consisted of discussion rather than step-by-step items. What are your reactions to the whole practice exercise?

Homework: Next week, go over the previous lessons and review what you have learned and applied and what you have not applied.

a. What have learned and applied that worked for your and the relationship?
b. What did you apply that did not work?
c. Discuss your practice exercise and homework with your professional helper.

Practice Exercise 6. Dealing with Denials and Resistance to Change

Name______________________________Sex____Date__________

The purpose of this practice exercise is to help you deal with the resistance to change that you will find in your partner. If you find resistance, it means that he or she is afraid of it, that is, "the devil I know is better than the devil I don't know."

1. If you are unable to get your partner to cooperate with any of the previous suggestions, asking for professional help as a couple may be an issue. This issue may come up at any time during your working on this practice exercise. Your partner typically will continue his/her denial and avoidance of change and confrontation, refusing to see a professional helper, and using all sorts of excuses, tricks, and rationalizations to support this avoidance, for instance:

Statement 1: "I am not crazy and I don't need any help (or a crazy doctor)."

Answer: "Being in trouble does not mean being crazy, it means being human."

____

____

____

Statement 2: "Those guys need to be crazy to work in that field."

Answer: "It may take one to cure one!" Finding targets outside of the self is another form of distraction, among the many.

___

___

___

Statement 3. "I knew someone who did go and it did not help a bit."

Answer: "How about the flip side of this statement, those who have been helped?" Is your partner strong enough to ask for help? It takes strong people to ask for help. He or she must feel very weak and vulnerable to use denial and resisting change in his or her life.

___

___

___

Statement 4: "All they are interested in is money."

Answer: "A professional should work for charity? Why?" Again, this is another form of distraction that focuses on something that has nothing to do with wanting help, like the price of eggs in China!

___

___

___

Statement 5: "I don't need any help from anybody. I know better than anybody else."

Answer: "How does anything, including your car, fix itself without help from outside? Does your car fix itself? How are we human being different from other physical things?" Can we fix ourselves or our relationships by ourselves? Where is the evidence?

___

___

___

Statement 6: "What could those guys tell me that I don't know already."

Answer: "Of course, s/he knows better! Who is going to tell him/her anything? Knowing something is one thing, changing it is another. You may know your car needs fixing, but that does not tell you how to fix it."

___

___

___

Statement 7. "I knew somebody who went to see one of those head doctors (or shrinks!) and they put him/her in the hospital for life."

Answer: Your partner may have forgotten that that somebody had such a serious breakdown (and probably delayed getting professional help) that it was impossible for that individual to return to society.

___

___

___

Statement 8. "I can quit (name of addiction or habit) anytime I want if I really put my mind to it."

Answer: When is the last time s/he quit?

___

___

___

Statement 9. "You need to go, because if it wasn't for you I would be OK."

Answer: This is another way to avoid responsibility, by shoving it outside of the self and on the closest target, you!

___

___

___

Statement 10. "I wouldn't get anything out of it."

Answer: How would s/he know if this route was never tried?

___

___

___

Statement 11. "It's too expensive."

Answer: If one really wants help, it can be gotten almost anywhere. Where there is a will there is a way. If there is no will, there is no way. Furthermore, the addiction is more expensive than anything else.

___

___

___

Statement 12. Write your partner's excuse (defense) that is different from any of the above.

Answer: Think of an appropriate answer and write it below.

2. If your try to talk over the self-destructive nature of these excuses, you need to remember that all of them show only one thing, and that is a tremendous fear of the unknown and of breaking down, possibly going "crazy," and losing control. All of these excuses come from a strong sense of helplessness that your partner (and you!) may not want to admit. Seeing professional help as a negative is part of the process of denial that controls the life of most addicted or abusive individuals. What is your reaction to the above?

3. Throughout this program, and at any point within it, it is important for you to learn how to cope nonreactively but not passively to the inevitable ambushes and attacks from your partner. To avoid getting "hooked" into your partner, you need to develop a written plan on how s/he will behave when your partner attacks you. An example of such a plan is found in the list below. In spite of this plan, you may fail to maintain a nonreactive stance in front of the onslaught of abusive and manipulative behavior from your partner. Remember s/he wants to see you upset and lose control of yourself! Reaching a nonreactive level is especially important in trying to implement the next step in this program. Remembering and applying suggestions made in this list may be helpful. These suggestions are given to help you get "unhooked" from your partner, whenever s/he is trying to draw you out, by pushing your button, so to speak, and trying to get you to lose control of yourself.

How to Avoid Getting "Hooked" into Provocations by Partner

1. Avoid using the seven suicidal and homicidal patterns: (1) blaming ("You always…You never…"); (2) bringing up the past; (3) mind-reading; (4) ultimatums; (5) threats; (6) blackmail or bribery; and (7) distracting or computing.

2. Instead, use all the opposite patterns consistently: (1) use pronoun "I" or "We" only; (2) stay in the present; (3) deal with what it is said or done in front of your eyes; (4) suggest possible consequences of destructive behavior; (5) use natural, real consequences of what *will* happen and not what *could* happen; (6) be mindful that even unconditional love has limits on the behavior (i.e., we can love a person but we do not like what s/he is doing); (7) stay on the topic of discussion and make sure it is important and relevant to the relationship.

3. Respond to the feelings rather than to the behavior. For instance, reflect the feelings of hurt, helplessness, and frustration that your partner may experience even if he or she denies them.

4. Rather than react in kind, muse on what would happen if you were to indulge in the same behavior. For instance: "If I were to bring up the past, we would be both unable to deal with the present, even if the present is even worse than the past."

5. Consider alternatives in how to respond by asking for more information and suggesting possible solutions, even if the solutions are rejected. In that case, comment to the effect that "I guess that the only solution possible is for me to lose and for you to win. I wonder whether we can ever win together. I guess that's too much to ask."

6. When he or she asks "hooking" questions, designed to upset the codependent, make her or him lose control; if you do not how to answer, say, "I will have to think about it before I give you an answer," or "I am not ready to give you an answer right now, so let me sleep on it," or "I doubt I can come up with a helpful answer when I am upset. Let me calm down and I'll get back to you."

7. When your partner accuses or criticizes you, avoid defending yourself; instead say, "You may be right about that," or "I am not perfect and I am entitled to make mistakes."

8. When the attack goes on, suggest the following: "Since we are both upset, wouldn't it be better if we stop this discussion and postpone it until we have both calmed down?" or "I do not think well when I am under attack, please give me a break," or "I really need some time to think about what you said. If you'll excuse me, I'll go for a walk."

9. When an ambush is sudden and unexpected, excuse yourself to go to the bathroom. While there, review possible strategies to use, without reacting or overreacting as your partner wants you to do. Your overreaction will give him or her more ammunition to avoid confrontation, and, therefore, power.

10. If all of the previous strategies fail, and you are at the point of "losing it," get on the phone and call your doctor (therapist, minister, friends, relatives) for support and suggestions.

11. Make it clear that you will not stand for any verbal or physical abuse: "That is completely unacceptable."

12. If there is a threat or danger to you in the form of physical abuse, leave the house immediately. Do not come back until you are sure that you are perfectly safe and that no harm will come to you. If promises are made to make you come back, make sure that these promises are made in writing and in front of a witness.

4. Which of these suggestions has been helpful for you and how?

____
____
____
____
____

5. Which suggestions were useless to you in dealing with your partner?

____
____
____
____
____

Homework: Expect to make mistakes, to fall down, to fall for your partner's provocations, to lose your cool, and "lose it." This is a process that needs to be experienced little by little. There are not going to be giant steps, only small ones. What is your reaction to this statement? Discuss this practice exercise and your reactions with your professional helper.

Practice Exercise 7. Writing a Bill of Rights for Overdependency

Name____Sex____Date__________

The purpose of this practice exercise is for you to learn and practice writing a Bill of Rights for yourself to learn to protect yourself and to learn to control your life.

1. Writing a Bill of Rights is a process rather than a task to be accomplished in a few easy lessons. It will take some time to complete this process. It needs to be broken down into three separate steps: (a) learning to write a Bill of Rights; (b) introducing it to the partner; and (c) learning to deal with the consequences of attempting to change a rather entrenched and rigid relationship.

2. Learning how: Writing a Bill of Rights is based on one single principle, the same principle of boundaries discussed under the previous lesson of drawing lines. Write down various areas of troublesome thought to you, that is, behaviors about which you have not been able to draw lines in the past. After you have identified these behaviors, and it may take some time for you to do so, write down how you plan and intend to behave in relation to those behaviors. Whatever the behavior you choose, it should follow the rule of three presented in an earlier exercise. You need to think of three positive, relevant, and realistic reasons for the new behavior. An example of a Bill of Rights written by a codependent individual, the wife of the alcoholic, is shown in the table below:

Example of a Bill of Rights for Codependent or Overly Dependent Relationships

A. I will not allow myself to
   1. ARGUE when my partner has been drinking (or is angry, upset, strung out, etc.), because
      a. When I argue, it causes me to become defensive and to justify myself
      b. Arguments when we are upset accomplish absolutely nothing
      c. Arguments cause me to become sad and/or mad
      d. During arguments we say things we regret later
   2. BE PUT DOWN and be abused verbally or otherwise, because
      a. I am human and I am entitled to make mistakes
      b. Put-downs cause me to become defensive. I do not need to defend myself. I am a responsible, caring, and loving individual
      c. I cannot use put downs. They do not give me any helpful information about me or anybody else. However, I can use support and guidance if this is a reciprocal process and my support and guidance are listened to
      d. Put-downs cause me to become sad and/or mad, and lose control of myself, and I do not like myself when I lose control of myself, even when my partner provokes it
   3. ACCEPT more than my share of responsibilities, because
      a. Eventually, I would become resentful and angry
      b. Then I feel used and abused
      c. It would increase the stress I am under
      d. I already have more responsibilities than I can handle. The more responsibilities I have taken on in the past, the greater the chances of my having been criticized, put-down, and abused. Therefore, I shall only assume responsibilities that enhance me and that will not debase my partner and my relationships with him or her
      e. If I accept more than my share of responsibilities, I would not have energy and time left for myself first and others second
   4. "HOLD IN" my emotions, because
      a. I could become physically sick
      b. I am entitled to express my feelings, provided I do not put anybody else down

c. If I hold my feelings in, I could "build them up" to the point of a "blow-up"
d. Expressing my feelings lets other people know that my feelings are important, because they are *my* feelings, and I am important
e. Feelings are to be discussed with those I love and who love me. If someone does not care about my feelings, maybe they do not care about me
f. Sharing my feelings with those I love will give them a chance to discuss their feelings with me also
g. Sharing my feelings will help people I love learn to know me better and appreciate me for what I am – an important person

B. I will not allow anybody to
  1. Keep me from doing the positive things I enjoy doing, because
    a. I deserve some enjoyment out of life
    b. My family is part of my life. I enjoy being with them and I should be able to spend time with them, without feeling guilty
    c. It makes me happy and content to do things I enjoy, including doing absolutely nothing! (I am important even when I am doing nothing)

3. You do not have to follow this example to the letter. You can and should write a Bill of Rights that applies specifically to you and to no one else. However, this example can be used as a model to improve on. Go over several drafts, paying special attention to the use of language. For instance, you need to avoid accusations, put-downs, and name calling. Use the "I" position, referring to your thoughts and feelings and not attempting to read your partner's mind nor making negative comments about him/her, avoiding the use of the seven deadly errors from a previous lesson. Complaints should be kept strictly to the behavior and not to the person. This Bill of Rights is to be written for how you are going to behave, not about how your partner is going to behave. You cannot control your partner's behavior, you can only learn to control yours. Give up fantasies or hopes that your are going to change your partner. Concentrating instead on how you are going to change. Comment on the above statements.

Homework: There is another important step that needs to be undertaken here. If you look up most of the points made in the table above, you will readily see that all of these points are written in a negative fashion, *what* the codependent will allow herself/himself *not to do.* You need to stress the flip side of this negativity, giving support and permission to think about *what to do positively.* Thus, for each negative point on the table above, think of some positive behavior you want to start. Again write down at least three reasons why you want and need to do it. Think of the rule of three: (a) Are you doing what you want to do? (b) Are you doing what you need to do? (c) Are you doing what you wish or like to do? Does it hurt anyone else? Why? After a reasonable document has been completed, with various drafts and revisions, make three copies, one for you, one for your partner, and one for your records or a friend or your counselor (therapist). Write down whatever has happened throughout this process.

Practice Exercise 8. Presenting the Bill of Rights to your Partner

Name____________________________________Sex____Date__________

The purpose of this practice exercise is to confront your partner with your Bill of Rights. Expect a tremendously negative reaction with putdowns of you, of whatever you have written, and whoever suggested it

1. This step is not as easy as it may seem at first glance. You might become anxious, wondering fearfully about your partner's reactions, and perhaps thinking that this Bill of Rights should not be shown at all. This is an option that is still open to you. You do not need to show this document. You can keep it to yourself and act accordingly. However, you must have at least three good reasons for choosing this course of *no action*.

   Reason a

   ____
   ____
   ____

   Reason b

   ____
   ____
   ____

   Reason c

   ____
   ____
   ____

2. Think of at least three good reasons for presenting your Bill of Rights to your partner.

   Reason a

   ____
   ____
   ____

Reason b

Reason c

---

3. If you choose to show your partner your Bill of Rights, be prepared to receive a predictably angry, if not explosive, reaction. Thus, it may help to put an introduction at the top of the page, such as: "I know that this paper is going to upset you a great deal. However, it is important for me to learn to control myself, regardless of how you behave. Go ahead and respond the way you usually do (get mad, stamp your feet, holler, have a temper tantrum, etc.). After you have finished, I would like to set a time (at least 24 h from now) to discuss this paper with you, if you are interested in our welfare and in our relationship." Please comment on the above:

---

4. In case you have written down different reasons, we need to stress the purpose of presenting your Bill of Rights to your partner. There are at least three reasons for doing it: (a) you need to make a strong statement about being an independent human being in charge of herself or himself; (b) your partner needs to know that you (1) no longer want to behave like a doormat, (2) have a will of your own, (3) are interested in making things better for yourself, and (4) no one can win at your expense, unless you let them, nor do you want to win at your partner's expense. You both need to win. If one wins, you both win. If one loses, you both lose. Presenting the Bill of Rights is the first step in the process of learning how to win, preferably for *both* partners. Please comment on the above.

---

5. Keep in mind, however, that your partner wants to "win" and see you lose by losing your control. Please comment:

6. There is another and most important reason for presenting the Bill of Rights: to start a dialogue between you two that will lead to a helpful outcome. What would this helpful outcome consist of? That outcome cannot be predicted at this point of the program because it depends on so many factors. One successful outcome, for instance, would be for both of you to come up with a conjugal contract that would direct both of you to work as real partners, and not as enemies. This contract must be in writing, to avoid distortions and deletions (forgetting, misunderstanding, etc.). Thus, the major reason for presenting a Bill of Rights is to have both partners start talking with each other as friends and not as adversaries. Please comment:

7. If you let your partner get into an argument with you right then and there, when the paper is presented, then the whole purpose of writing this Bill of Rights is lost. You must be very clear and firm that you want your partner to read this paper first and then think about it before discussing it: "I want you to have time to think it through." You may need to practice not allowing your partner to bully or bulldoze you into an instant replay of past fights: "I am not ready to discuss it now. We will need to talk about it whenever we are both calm." If the partner persists or goes off half cocked, you may need to walk out of the room, or if necessary leave the house. At worst, if the partner becomes violent or abusive, one should call the police. Please comment:

8. The issue here is one of control: who controls whom? If you lose your cool because of your partner's inevitable and predictable provocations (verbal and physical abuse, put-downs, blames, accusations, criticisms, etc.), you are giving

up control of the situation. That is what your partner wants the most, namely, to have you at his/her beck and call, to dominate, manipulate, and bully you at will. If you give up the time of the stated appointment and give in, by responding immediately to provocation, on the spot, when a copy of the Bill of Rights is given, control is lost on both sides. Both of you must negotiate when and where you will have the proposed meeting. The time and place may be negotiable. However, having a meeting is not negotiable. You need to watch out, because after the meeting has been set, your partner may try other tricks to get you to lose your cool. Please comment:

____

____

____

____

____

Homework: This is a very crucial time that may make or break anything that you have been trying to do. Your partner cannot stand your becoming more detached, more in control of situations, and more "reasonable" instead of being what oftentimes you may have been accused of being, and that is volatile, capricious, and "irrational," or even worse. If you are no longer reacting to your partner as s/he wants you to, this change may be very frightening for both. Your partner may try anything, including threats of suicide and/or murder, for you to go back to the way you were. Under these circumstances, you must set clear, firm, and nonnegotiable limits: "I am sorry, but I am not ready to talk about it now. I am too upset to think rationally. Let's set a time for us to talk about it calmly." You may need to refer to behaviors suggested in earlier practice exercises.

Practice Exercise 9. Holding a Meeting Together

Name____________________________________Sex____Date__________

If you have reached this stage in your relationship, you and your partner are doing great. The purpose of this practice exercise is to try to discuss issues like adults, with a plan, rather than like children, with no plan.

1. If and when you both meet, you must be prepared accordingly. The first step to maintain control is to write down what is going on between you two on a pad of paper. Even better, you could use a tape recorder ("My memory plays tricks on me, and I want to be sure I record everything we say."). Why record what is going on at this meeting? For three reasons: (a) to help you keep your cool and in control of yourself; (b) memory, especially during critical situations, plays tricks on us, we tend to forget, distort, and delete whatever might have been said; and (c) writing or tape recording starts a record that needs to be kept for future meetings (if there are going to be others!). This record will allow both

of you to go back and see whether any change or improvement has taken place over time. Please comment:

____
____
____
____

2. In addition, a time limit for this meeting must be set, preferably no longer than 1 h. The kitchen timer should be set for 1 h and this limit should be kept, in spite of the partner also pushing these time limits, like everything else. If these time limits are not kept, control is lost. Instead of running over, a time for another meeting should be set, at least 24 h later. Why should this limit be set beforehand? For three reasons: (a) time limits are a form of control, and we achieve control by setting clear space (where you are meeting) and time (when and how long) boundaries; (b) if you go beyond the preset time, you will start losing controls and boundaries; consequently, this meeting would deteriorate into a shouting match or a fight, an outcome we do not suggest or support; (c) not much might be settled in 1 h; however, you both will need to set a weekly "relationship hour" on a preset, agreed-upon basis. The written or recorded record will allow the therapist to follow what areas in the relationship need improvement. Please comment:

____
____
____
____

Practice Exercise 10. Problem Solving Together (If Possible!)

Name ____________________________ Sex____ Date ________

The purpose of this practice exercise is to practice problem solving about your troublesome thoughts together. This is a very hard step to accomplish. However, if you and your partner have reached this stage, you both are doing extremely well.

1. Issues between you two are not going to be solved by arguing. If either one of you loses control, the meeting should end immediately, but a time for a future appointment should be agreed upon ("We are not ready to solve troublesome thoughts when we are upset. We can negotiate only when we are calm and have thought through how to solve troublesome thoughts."). Please comment:

____
____
____
____

2. During the next week, each of you should look over the other partner's suggested proposals for solutions. Each should write down whatever pro's and cons they see in this proposal. On the basis of these criticisms (not insults!), a counterproposal should be written. These counterproposals should be presented at the next meeting and exchanged. The partners should look these proposals over and decide whether they are now ready to write down a final solution that would be acceptable to both of them. For instance, let's take one single issue first:

Troublesome thoughts: How should we treat each other and solve problems together?

Goals: (a) to treat each other with the utmost respect and care, (b) to assert each other's importance, (c) to enhance each other and our relationship; (d) to work as partners and not as enemies.

Proposed solutions: (a) to meet regularly at preset, clearly stated times; (b) to keep most of our discussions in written form, to avoid distortions and deletions and our getting more upset, as we have done in the past; (c) to avoid using the suicidal seven errors listed above, relying instead on their opposites; (d) to end our meetings when we become upset; and (e) set another meeting at our earliest convenient time, 24 h after this meeting. Please comment:

____

____

____

____

____

Homework: During the coming week, follow the same process for each point, that is: (a) definition of problem areas; (b) how each of you feels about the problem; (c) set goal(s) to achieve in that area; and (d) proposed solutions. The resulting paper may be your final contract. Allow 3 months to see how this contract is working or not working and what changes are needed to improve it. Remember that if you want to achieve your goals you need to solve problem through the written word. If you rely mainly or only on the spoken word, you are going to lose control of yourselves and of your relationship.

Practice Exercise 11. Going on Strike

Name ______________________________ Sex____ Date ________

The purpose of this practice exercise is to teach you how to give up doing anything for anybody, something that goes against what you have done all your life, thinking more of others than of yourself. It is time that you start thinking about yourself and not about others. Taking care of oneself is a full-time job. At this time in your life you do not need to care of anybody else but yourself.

1. If whatever has been suggested above does not work, you may need to work toward the very last step in the process of possible change, and that is, going on strike. Going on strike may well be the most difficult thing you have ever done in your life. It requires you to give up being the overresponsible, overnurturing, overcompetent, and overcaring person you wanted to be all along. Does not your sense of importance stem from what you do – cooking, cleaning, washing, driving, buying, and working for the benefit of everybody (especially your partner) except yourself! Now you are being asked to quit doing everything. Very likely, you will not be able to do it right off the bat. You may be as addicted to chores and responsibilities as your partner is addicted to something else. Before you go on strike, you need to consider if you are willing to do it as a last resort. Write down at least three reasons why you would be better off going on strike than to keep things as they are.

   Reason a

   ___
   ___
   ___

   Reason b

   ___
   ___
   ___

   Reason c

   ___
   ___
   ___

2. Write down what would happen if you did not do something to change the relationship.

   ___
   ___
   ___
   ___
   ___

3. Going on strike is new, positive, and powerfully change-producing. By going on strike you are telling anyone who cares that (a) you are important, (b) you want change for the better, and (c) you are willing to work for it. Going on strike may not be the best term to call what you need to do. For instance, you may choose to call it "having a nervous breakdown" instead of going on strike, as a way of telling your partner and the rest of your family about your inability

to take care of all of them as you have done in the past ("I am at the end of my rope and I cannot cope any more. Either I just care for myself or I may need to go to a hospital."). Please comment:

____
____
____
____
____

4. What are the goals of going on strike? As usual, you must have at least three reasons for doing it: (a) to bring attention to a problem, that is, (1) lack of change in the relationship, (2) being taken for granted, (3) being treated as not unimportant, (4) assuming too much responsibility, etc.; (b) to make your partner (or the rest of the family) understand that without talking things over, that is, without cooperation in efforts to change, the relationship is doomed; (c) to bring your partner to the table and start putting some order in the relationship through problem solving. Without talking things over, there is no hope that things will change for the better. Please comment:

____
____
____
____
____

5. Think through why and how you are going to do it, planning it step by step. Expect a strong and usually negative reaction from everybody in the family, especially your partner. For once, a family member, that is, you, is now acting instead of just talking! Once your partner or your family is assembled together, after a 24-h notice has been given, announce your decision to quit doing anything for anybody else, since doing for everybody thus far has not brought about any change. Keep a pad of paper and write down the answers of your partner or other family members. Your partner and other family members will not like what you propose to do (or not do!). They will have to think about what they are going to do to eat, to get things washed, to take care of the house, to buy whatever is needed in the home, etc. You might give your partner or family options: "Would you like me to go to bed or would you like for me to go to a motel?" or "Would you like me to have a nervous breakdown at home or should I wait until things are so bad that I will need to go to the hospital?" Please comment:

____
____
____
____
____

6. If you choose to stay home, it should be made clear that you will not play the part of consultant, telling your partner and other family members what they have to do and how they have to do it. Act as if you were sick, letting them find out how to deal with all these issues by themselves. Once the announcement about what is going to happen is made, you must follow this path, unless it becomes a useless threat. Write down your partner's and family members' reactions, reading your notes afterwards to see whether anything new has been learned. Avoid getting into any arguments with any of your family members and especially your partner. If you get into an argument, you are again going to lose control. Please comment:

____
____
____
____

7. If going on strike works, go back to the Bill of Rights steps. If it does not work, you may need to see a lawyer! If seeing an attorney works (and it may not), one may keep in mind that marriage is slavery when the possibility of divorce does not exist. Before seeking a divorce, however, ask yourself if you have changed enough, feeling proud and pleased of yourself, to warrant taking this final step. Please comment:

____
____
____
____

Homework: If going on strike works, in addition to learning to talk things over, go on to the next practice exercise and do both, talking things over and joining other people who are in the same trouble as you are.

Practice Exercise 12. Forming or Joining a Study or Support Group

Name________________________________Sex____Date________

The purpose of this practice exercise is to start taking leadership steps to make a life for yourself separate from your partner.

1. You may invite your partner to take active participation in such a course. Now you need to make up your mind as to whether you want to join a support group or a study group. Examples of support groups are Alcoholic Anonymous, Adult Children of Alcoholics (ACOA), Al-Anon if the troublesome thought is alcohol, Nar-Anon or Narateen if the troublesome thought is drug abuse, Gamblers Anonymous if the troublesome thought is gambling, Codependents of Sexual Addictions, or groups that focus on domestic violence, or sexual or

physical abuse. Check the phone book or Internet or ask your friends, clergyman, physician, or lawyer for where you would find such a support group. These groups may not give you skills but may help you find enough confidence in yourself to take more steps to advance yourself. Please comment:

2. Study groups focus on learning self-help skills. There are a great many courses and study groups on many topics, such as parenting, marital fitness, relationship enhancement, etc. Some of these courses are formal and some are informal. Especially in large metropolitan areas, there are courses and workshops on marital and parental relationships. Usually these courses include some practical "hands-on" experiential, not book-based, training between partners or with their children. Most universities have faculty members who are qualified and eager to give these courses. Search and ask. Doing nothing is not going to change anything. Please comment:

3. If you cannot find any support or study group, then start a support group by asking around and checking how many people there are in the neighborhood, church, community, etc. who have the same troublesome thought as you do. This task means getting on the phone and calling potential study group members by passing the word around with friends and acquaintances. If you do start a study/support group, make sure that whoever joins is committed to coming at a regular time and for a definite number of sessions. Before starting this group, write down a tentative outline of topics or subjects that might be of interest and of use to the group. During the first session of the group, set specific times and durations for weekly, biweekly, or monthly meetings. Let the group decide about the number of meetings you are going to have. Work out a specific agenda of topics the group needs to follow. Even though you may be the founder of the group, do not take responsibility for the whole process. Each member of the study group is responsible for leading at least one session of the series, deciding on topics to be discussed beforehand, and distributing phone numbers so that each member of the group can get in touch with the others. Please comment:

Homework: Another approach is to ask your church's director of education or other church members about organizing such a study group. Or you may be able to do start such a study group with coworkers with a supervisor's approval and/or assistance.

Practice Exercise 13. Conclusion (Optional)

Name______________________________Sex____Date__________

This practice exercise gives some suggestions on how you can reach a higher level of functioning. Comment with your reactions to any or all the points made below.

1. Very likely, obtaining this higher level of functioning may destroy your relationship.
2. Your partner may not be able to tolerate change for the better.
3. How can s/he cope without an always available partner, a caring friend, a sex object, a purchasing agent, etc.?
4. While any changes you may have made for the betterment of the relationship may motivate your partner to do better, such changes may possibly produce a deterioration in your partner, and, possibly, in the relationship.
5. Improving yourself may incur the risk of possibly losing your partner.
6. Is change worth that kind of price?
7. Some people are so afraid of losing their partners that they prefer to stay the same and avoid changing just to please the other, to avoid conflict, or "for the children's sake."
8. Other people feel that the financial security they enjoy is too valuable to jeopardize it in any way.
9. If that is the price you want to pay, to be stepped on and demeaned every day, you can continue doing what you have been doing all along.
10. Avoid changing for the better, and do not apply any of the suggestions made in this practice exercise.
11. What did you get out of this practice exercise? Please comment:

____
____
____
____
____

Sexual Abuse

The purpose of this practice exercise is to help victims of sexual abuse come to terms and deal with their past hurts in this painful area of their lives.

Practice Exercise 1. Acknowledgment of the Problem

Name____Sex____Date_______

The purpose of this practice exercise is to help you remember hurts related to your past sexual abuse.

1. When did you first begin to face that you had a problem? Describe in detail how this realization took place.

____
____
____
____
____

2. What did the abuse consist of?

   a. What was the nature of the abuse (what was done to you)?

____
____
____
____
____

   b. Where did it take place?

____
____
____
____
____

   c. Who was the abuser or abusers?

____
____
____
____
____

d. How long did it last?

e. How old were you?

3. Most of us tend to deny painful or hurtful experience. How did you deal with your experience of abuse over the years? Explain in terms of years.

   a. While the abuse was going on:

   b. After the abuse stopped:

   c. Immediately after the abuse:

   d. How long did it take for you to face the abuse after it stopped?

e. Later on, months or years after the abuse:

4. Once you began to face these abuses, what did you do? Write in detail.

5. How and how much did this abuse influence you?

6. What did you do to cope with the abuse?

7. What did the abuser say to you to keep you from talking about it to anybody else?

8. What did the abuser(s) tell you during and after the abuse took place?

9. Any other comment that you think is important for you to write down at this point:

____
____
____
____

Homework: During the coming week, make sure you seat down in a safe place, as free as possible from distractions and interruptions, and write for 15 minute a day for at least 4 days and more (possibly or preferably at a preset time), about all the hurts that you have experienced from this abuse, including those you never discussed with anybody. Discuss your notes about past hurts with whoever is working with you on this practice exercise.

Practice Exercise 2. Awareness of Feelings About Past Abuse

Name____Sex____Date______

The purpose of this practice exercise is to make sure that you let go of all the past hurts related to your abuse. Very likely these memories are so painful that you would like to avoid dealing with them. Avoiding remembering them, however, will not help you get rid of them. We need to approach and face them squarely because you have avoided these memories and they are still controlling if not dominating you. Let's see if we can get rid of them.

Remembering painful memories is always very hard. However, to keep all of those painful memories all stored up inside of you is even more painful in the long run. What do you think about this issue? Do you want to get it out of yourself or do you want to keep it and let it fester inside of you? Please answer one way or another. If writing about painful memories is too hard for you, you can skip this practice exercise and come back to it when you feel more comfortable about it.

1. How did you feel while this experience was taking place?

____
____
____
____

2. How did you feel afterwards?

____
____
____
____

3. How did you feel after the abuse stopped (if ever)?

4. How do you feel about it now?

5. How did you feel about yourself as a child?

6. How did you feel about yourself as a person?

7. How did you feel about yourself as a (wo)man?

8. How do you feel now about the abuser?

Homework: During the coming week, allow yourself to experience all the painful feelings that may come to you. You do not need to be afraid of these feelings. We need to face them in order to get rid (if we can) of them. It would be helpful if you wrote down these feelings anytime they came to mind. Discuss your notes with whoever is working with you on this practice exercise.

Practice Exercise 3. Flashbacks from Past Experience

Name________________________________Sex____Date_______________

The purpose of this practice exercise is to help you deal with flashbacks from your experience of past abuse.

1. Did you ever have any flashbacks of this experience? If so, write about them:

   a. When did you experience your first flashback?

   b. What happen to make you remember what happened in the past?

   c. How often did you experience these flashbacks?

   d. How long did each flashback last?

e. How intense was each flashback?

2. What kind of relationship did you keep with the abuser(s)?

3. How do you feel about the abuser(s) now?

4. What would you like to see happen to your abuser(s)?

5. Any other comments relating to your remembering the abuse:

Homework: During the coming week, as soon as you experience a flashback, make sure to write the time and place it came to you and whether there was anything about your surroundings that brought it about. Wait until you have made an appointment time beforehand to write about that flashback in greater detail. Do not write about the flashback when it happens, because if you do, the flashbacks will start to control you. If you want to learn to control your flashbacks, you need to write about them by appointment only.

Practice Exercise 4. Sharing Feelings and Experiences with Trusted People

Name________________________________Sex____Date______

The purpose of this practice exercise is to help you learn how to discuss painful feelings and experiences with people you love and who love you.

1. Discussing experiences of this kind may be even more painful than recalling them. On the other hand, if we do not discuss painful experiences with people we love and trust, then we do not make it possible for them to do the same with us. The result is isolation and lack of trust and eventually of intimacy. How can others trust us if we do not trust them? If intimacy means discussing hurts, then we can achieve it if and when we show our trust by discussing our hurts with selected others. What do you think about the above statement? Have you ever discussed your abuse with anyone? Write what happened:

2. With whom? List the people with whom you have discussed this experience.

3. What happened when you told of your experience?

4. Would you be willing to discuss this experience with someone you trust now?

5. Who would you choose and why?

____

6. Who would be your first choice?

____

7. Who would be your second choice?

____

Homework: If you are still fearful of discussing your feelings and experiences with anyone, think about writing a letter where you discuss these feelings and experiences with someone you love and who loves you. Talk it over with whoever is helping you with his practice exercise; discuss whether and why you could mail this letter to more than one person.

Practice Exercise 5. Acceptance of Self and of Others

Name______________________________Sex____Date_______

The purpose of this practice exercise is to allow you to accept yourself and selected others unconditionally, without any requirements for performance, production, perfection, or problem solving.

1. There is always the danger that a person who has been abused may think of herself or himself as "soiled," "dirty," "shameful," and therefore not worthy of love from self or from others. Write what your experience has done to your self-esteem and self-confidence.

____

2. The act of sexual abuse in and of it self means that you were not important and that the abuser's immediate pleasure was more important than your pain. You pain was never considered in the act. If your pain was unimportant, then you as a person may also be unimportant. How do you react to this statement?

3. What can be done to restore your acceptance of yourself as an important person?

4. Since the abuser did not think that you were very important, then perhaps you must have concluded that you were not important. You might have left to the abuser to define your own sense of importance. Did you do this, and should you continue to give the abuser so much power to define you?

5. Who is ultimately responsible for defining you and what kind of person you are?

6. Why?

7. Any other thoughts that you may have about the above issues:

____

____

____

____

____

Homework: During the coming week, think and write about how you are the one that defines how important you are to yourself and to those you love and who love you. Discuss your thoughts with whoever is helping you with this practice exercise.

Practice Exercise 6. Realizing How Much the Abuse Influenced the Self

Name________________________________Sex____Date________

The purpose of this practice exercise is to help you realize how much you let the abuse influence and affect who you are and what you do.

1. How did the experience of abuse influence you?

   a. Emotionally:

____

____

____

____

   b. Intellectually:

____

____

____

____

   c. Interpersonally:

____

____

____

____

   d. Sexually:

____

____

____

____

e. In intimate relationships:

____
____
____
____
____

f. In any other respects:

____
____
____
____
____

2. How did this experience influence the reactions of others towards you?

____
____
____
____
____

Homework: During the coming week, think about how much you let the abuse influence you and determine how you feel about yourself and others. Write down whatever thoughts come into your mind and discuss them with your professional helper.

Practice Exercise 7. Understanding Why Abusers Abuse

Name ______________________ Sex____ Date_______

The purpose of this practice exercise is to help you make sense of why abusers abuse.

1. We do not want to excuse or condone whatever abuse took place in your life. The abuse is unforgivable. We may need, however, to understand why the abuser took advantage of you. Among the various possibilities there are the following:

   a. The abuser did not know any better.
   b. The abuser was after pleasure for himself or herself regardless of what harm resulted to others.
   c. The abuser sought closeness and love in the only way he or she knew how.
   d. This was the only way the abuser knew how to get pleasure and closeness.
   e. Write about other possibilities that may come to mind:

2. Which of these possibilities make sense to you and why?

3. Very likely it will be impossible for you to forget this painful experience. However, will it be possible for you to forgive the abuser?

    a. Why should you?

    b. How would you?

    c. Can you?

    d. Why not?

4. List the pros and cons of not forgiving. What will happen to you and to your sense of importance if you do not forgive?

5. What does forgiveness mean to you?

____
____
____
____
____

6. Could you consider the possibility that one way to define forgiveness is to give up expecting perfection from others as well as ourselves? How do you feel about this definition?

____
____
____
____
____

Homework: You may not want to forgive your abuser just right now. However, during the coming week think and write some more about the pros and cons of forgiveness in terms of your well-being rather than the well-being of the abuser?

Practice Exercise 8. Learning and Integrating Experiences

Name_______________________________Sex____Date_______

The purpose of this practice exercise is to help you put together all the pieces from the past and present that will allow you to go on and enjoy life rather than just surviving.

1. What did you learn from working on this practice exercise?

____
____
____
____
____

2. What did you learn from working on this practice exercise with the help of a group of other survivors of sexual abuse?

____
____
____
____
____

3. What did you learn from relating to your professional helper?

____
____
____
____

4. What did you learn from others? Was anyone more helpful than the others?

____
____
____
____

5. How did you put together this experience?

____
____
____
____

6. What has this work meant to you?

____
____
____
____

Homework: How can you go on living in better and better ways? Write down the concrete and specific plans you may have to ensure that your past experience and all the work you have put into changing yourself and on this practice exercise will multiply for yourself and those who love you. Discuss your notes with your group or your professional helper, if you have one.

Psychological Problems

The purpose of this practice exercise is to help you learn to control your psychological problems rather than having them control you.

Practice Exercise 1. Defining Psychological Problems

Name________________________________Sex____Date__________

The purpose of this practice exercise is to define psychological problems as you understand them. There are many definitions of psychological problems, and it is important that you define them as you see them

1. What do psychological problems mean to you?

2. In case you do not know, below there is a list of psychological problems. Explain what each sign means to you, and give two examples of how each sign applies to you.<COMP: Please set the sentences and dotted lines under heading "Signs of Psychological Problems and Definitions" and Examples 1 AND 2 under heading "Examples" SHOULD BE ALIGNED equally in 2 columns as in sample book.>

Signs of Psychological Problems and Definitions	*Examples*
a. Delusions	Example 1 Example 2
b. Hallucinations	Example 1 Example 2
c. Disorganized speech	Example 1 Example 2
d. Grossly disorganized behavior	Example 1 Example 2

e. Inability to express feelings and emotions

Example 1 ______

Example 2 ______

f. Work disturbances

Example 1 ______

Example 2 ______

g. Social disturbances

Example 1 ______

Example 2 ______

h. Educational disturbances

Example 1 ______

Example 2 ______

i. Disturbances in self-care

Example 1 ______

Example 2 ______

j. Preoccupation with one or more delusions (to the exclusion of reality)

Example 1 ______

Example 2 ______

k. Inability to move or talk (maintenance of a rigid posture)

Example 1 ______

Example 2 ______

l. Excessive motor activity

Example 1 ______

Example 2 ______

m. Extreme negativism

Example 1 ______

Example 2 ______

n. Lack of motivation ______ Example 1 ______ Example 2 ______

o. Resistance to authority ______ Example 1 ______ Example 2 ______

p. Peculiarities in thinking ______ Example 1 ______ Example 2 ______

q. Bizarre (strange) postures or prominent mannerisms ______ Example 1 ______ Example 2 ______

r. Repeating what other people say ______ Example 1 ______ Example 2 ______

s. Repeating what other people do ______ Example 1 ______ Example 2 ______

t. Confusion in thinking ______ Example 1 ______ Example 2 ______

u. Confusion in reality testing ______ Example 1 ______ Example 2 ______

v. Confusion in behavior ______ Example 1 ______ Example 2 ______

w. Thinking that another person is in love with you

Example 1

Example 2

x. Loving someone at a distance (writing love letters to someone)

Example 1

Example 2

y. Fear of being followed

Example 1

Example 2

z. Stalking someone

Example 1

Example 2

aa. Thinking someone or some organization has it in for you

Example 1

Example 2

bb. Thinking you are a very powerful person, like God, Jesus, or the Virgin Mary

Example 1

Example 2

cc. Thinking your partner is unfaithful to you without evidence

Example 1

Example 2

dd. Imaginary health problems

Example 1

Example 2

ee. Inability to deal with feelings and emotions

Example 1

Example 2

ff. A sign not included in the list above (write what it is): ______________________________ ______________________________ Example 1 ______________________________ Example 2 ______________________________

gg. A sign not included in the list above (write what it is): ______________________________ ______________________________ Example 1 ______________________________ Example 2 ______________________________

3. After you have defined these signs of psychological problems, rank them according to how closely each of them applies to you. Rank-order the most applicable to you with No. 1. Rank-order the second most applicable with No. 2, and so on; mark as N/A the signs tat are not applicable to you.

Signs of Severe Troublesome thoughts	*Rank-order*	*Signs of Severe Troublesome thoughts*	*Rank-order*
a. Delusions	________	q. Bizarre postures and prominent mannerisms	________
b. Hallucinations	________	r. Repeating what other people say	________
c. Disorganized speech	________	s. Repeating what other people do	________
d. Grossly disorganized behavior	________	t. Confusion in thinking	________
e. Inability to express feelings and emotions	________	u. Confusion in reality testing	________
f. Work disturbances	________	v. Confusion in behavior	________
g. Social disturbances	________	w. Thinking that another person is in love with you	________
h. Educational disturbances	________	x. Loving someone at a distance (writing love letters to someone)	________
i. Disturbances in self-care	________	y. Fear of being followed	________
j. Preoccupation with one or more delusions	________	z. Stalking someone	________
k. Inability to move or talk (maintenance of a rigid posture)	________	aa. Thinking someone or some organization has it in for you	________
l. Excessive motor activity	________	bb. Thinking you are a very powerful person	________
m. Extreme negativism	________		
n. Lack of motivation	________		
o. Resistance to authority	________		
p. Peculiarities in thinking	________		

Signs of Severe Troublesome thoughts	*Rank-order*	*Signs of Severe Troublesome thoughts*	*Rank-order*
cc. Thinking your partner is unfaithful to you without evidence	________	ff. A sign not included in the list above (__________)	________
dd. Imaginary health problems	________	gg. A sign not included in the list above (__________)	________
ee. Unable to deal with feelings and emotions	________		

4. Explain why you rank-ordered these signs the way you did.

____

____

____

____

____

Homework: During the next few days keep on thinking about these signs and whether you want to keep their rank-order as is or whether you want to change it.

Standard Practice Exercise for Signs of Psychological Problems

Title of Sign____________________Practice Exercise No.______

Name________________________________Sex____Date______

The purpose of this practice exercise is to learn more about the sign of psychological problems listed in the title of this practice exercise.

1. How does this sign trouble you? Please explain in detail.

____

____

____

____

____

2. How often does this sign trouble you? Check which answer applies to you:

a. Practically every day	_____	d. Once a month	_____
b. Once a week	_____	e. Once every six 6 months	_____
c. Couple of times a month	_____	f. Once a year	_____
		g. Once every few years	_____

3. Please explain further:

____
____
____
____
____

4. How did this sign come about? Do you remember when you started feeling? it? Check which answer fits best:

   a. When I was a child (younger than 5 years of age) ________
   b. When I was in elementary school ________
   c. When I was in middle school ________
   d. When I was in high school ________
   e. After high school ________
   f. Any other time ________

5. Please explain further:

____
____
____
____
____

6. Give three specific examples of how this sign troubles you:

   Example a

____
____
____
____

   Example b

____
____
____
____

   Example c

____
____
____
____

Homework: Next week, in order for you to learn to control this sign ("Start it if you want to stop it!"), plan to repeat it at preset times (for instance, at 8 a.m., 12 noon, 4 or 7 p.m.) on at least 3 days (Monday, Wednesday, and Friday, or Tuesday, Thursday, and Saturday). Write down what happened in detail. For each time make sure to answer in writing the following four questions:

a. How did you start this sign?
b. What followed after you felt this sign?
c. How did this sign end?
d. What did this sign get you?

Time 1 (write the time you started__________)

a. ____
____
____

b. ____
____
____

c. ____
____
____

d. ____
____
____

Time 2 (write the time you started__________)

a. ____
____
____

b. ____
____
____

c. ____
____
____

d. ____
____
____

Time 3 (write the time you started__________)

a. ____
____
____

b. ____
____
____

c. ____
____
____

d. ____
____
____

Check which of the following shows what you got out of this practice exercise:

a. Completely useless ________
b. Somewhat useless ________
c. So-so ________
d. Somewhat useful ________
e. Extremely useful ________

Explain how you feel about this homework practice exercise and what you got out of it.

____
____
____
____
____

Concluding Feedback Form for Psychological Problems

Name________________________________Sex____Date______

The purpose of this concluding feedback form is to find out how you feel about the practice exercises you completed in this practice exercise.

1. Please select the answer that best fits how you feel about this practice exercise:

   a. I did not like working on this practice exercise at all. I wish I never saw it. ________
   b. I did not like this practice exercise at all, but I am glad I got to work on it. ________
   c. I am delighted I got a chance to work on this practice exercise. ________
   d. I am not only delighted about this practice exercise, but I wish all people with severe problems had a chance to work on it. ________

2. How helpful was it to work on this practice exercise? Check the answer that applies to you:

a. Not helpful at all	________	c. Helpful	________
b. Somewhat helpful	________	d. Very helpful	________

3. Rank-order the practice exercises you have completed. Rank-order each practice exercise according to how much you liked it. Rank-order as No. 1 the practice exercise you liked the most. Rank as No. 2 the practice exercise that you liked second best, and so on; mark as N/A the practice exercises you did not like at all or that you did not feel you could rank with the others.

Signs of Psychological Problems	*Rank-order*
a. Delusions	________
b. Hallucinations	________
c. Disorganized speech	________
d. Grossly disorganized behavior	________
e. Inability to express feelings and emotions	________
f. Work disturbances	________
g. Social disturbances	________
h. Educational disturbances	________
i. Disturbances in self-care	________
j. Preoccupation with one or more delusions	________
k. Inability to move or talk (maintenance of a rigid posture)	________
l. Excessive motor activity	________
m. Extreme negativism	________
n. Lack of motivation	________
o. Resistance to authority	________
p. Peculiarities in thinking	________
q. Bizarre postures and prominent mannerisms	________
r. Repeating what other people say	________
s. Repeating what other people do	________
t. Confusion in thinking	________
u. Confusion in reality testing	________
v. Confusion in behavior	________
w. Thinking that another person is in love with you	________
x. Loving someone at a distance (writing love letters to someone)	________
y. Fear of being followed	________
z. Stalking someone	________
aa. Thinking someone or some organization has it in for you	________
bb. Thinking you are a very powerful person	________

Signs of Psychological Problems	*Rank-order*	*Signs of Psychological Problems*	*Rank-order*
cc. Thinking your partner is unfaithful to you without evidence	________	ff. A sign not included in the list above (__________)	________
dd. Imaginary health problems	________		
ee. Unable to deal with feelings and emotions	________	gg. A sign not included in the list above (___________)	________

4. Why did you rank-order the practice exercises the way you did?

____
____
____
____
____

5. Which practice exercise was the most helpful to you? Sometimes what we like most is not necessarily the most helpful. Consequently, rank the practice exercises according to their helpfulness to you. Rank as No. 1 the most helpful, rank as No. 2 the next most helpful, and so on, until the least helpful practice exercise.

Signs of Psychological Problems	*Rank-order*	*Signs of Psychological Problems*	*Rank-order*
a. Delusions	________	j. Preoccupation with one or more delusions	________
b. Hallucinations	________	k. Inability to move or talk (maintenance of a rigid posture)	________
c. Disorganized speech	________	l. Excessive motor activity	________
d. Grossly disorganized behavior	________	m. Extreme negativism	________
e. Inability to express feelings and emotions	________	n. Lack of motivation	________
f. Work disturbances	________	o. Resistance to authority	________
g. Social disturbances	________	p. Peculiarities in thinking	________
h. Educational disturbances	________	q. Bizarre postures and prominent mannerisms	________
i. Disturbances in self-care	________		

Signs of Psychological Problems	*Rank-order*	*Signs of Psychological Problems*	*Rank-order*
r. Repeating what other people say	________	aa. Thinking someone or some organization has it in for you	________
s. Repeating what other people do	________	bb. Thinking you are a very powerful person	________
t. Confusion in thinking	________	cc. Thinking your partner is unfaithful to you without evidence	________
u. Confusion in reality testing	________	dd. Imaginary health problems	________
v. Confusion in behavior	________	ee. Unable to deal with feelings and emotions	________
w. Thinking that another person is in love with you	________	ff. A sign not included in the list above (________)	________
x. Loving someone at a distance (writing love letters to someone)	________	gg. A sign not included in the list above (________)	________
y. Fear of being followed	________		
z. Stalking s omeone	________		

6. Why did you rank the practice exercises the way you did?

____
____
____
____
____

7. Feel free to write any comments that might improve this practice exercise.

____
____
____
____
____

Mood Swings

The purpose of this practice exercise is to help you learn to control your mood swings rather than having them control you.

Practice Exercise 1. Defining Mood Swings

Name______________________________Sex____Date__________

The purpose of this practice exercise is to define mood swings as you understand them. There are many definitions of mood swings, and it is important that you define them as you see them.

1. What do mood swings mean to you?

____

____

____

____

____

2. Here are some signs of mood swings. Explain what each sign means to you and give two examples of how each sign applies to you.

Signs and Definitions	*Examples*
a. Euphoria	Example 1 __________
__________	__________
__________	Example 2 __________
__________	__________
b. Grandiosity	Example 1 __________
__________	__________
__________	Example 2 __________
__________	__________
c. Depression	Example 1 __________
__________	__________
__________	Example 2 __________
__________	__________
d. Loss of interest	Example 1 __________
__________	__________
__________	Example 2 __________
__________	__________

e. Sleeping too much

Example 1 ______

Example 2 ______

f. Sleeping too little

Example 1 ______

Example 2 ______

g. Racing thoughts

Example 1 ______

Example 2 ______

h. Full of energy

Example 1 ______

Example 2 ______

i. Doing too many things

Example 1 ______

Example 2 ______

j. Highly distractible

Example 1 ______

Example 2 ______

k. Suicidal thoughts

Example 1 ______

Example 2 ______

l. Easily fatigued

Example 1 ______

Example 2 ______

m. Unable to concentrate

Example 1 ______

Example 2 ______

n. Irritability ______ Example 1 ______ Example 2 ______

o. Feeling worthless ______ Example 1 ______ Example 2 ______

p. Taking big or unusual risks ______ Example 1 ______ Example 2 ______

q. Feeling wired ______ Example 1 ______ Example 2 ______

r. High level of anxiety ______ Example 1 ______ Example 2 ______

s. Feeling slowed down ______ Example 1 ______ Example 2 ______

t. Feeling speeded up ______ Example 1 ______ Example 2 ______

u. Overly goal-driven ______ Example 1 ______ Example 2 ______

v. Aggressive impulses ______ Example 1 ______ Example 2 ______

w. Hopelessness

____

____

____

Example 1 ______________________________

____

Example 2 ______________________________

____

x. Passivity

____

____

____

Example 1 ______________________________

____

Example 2 ______________________________

____

y. A sign not listed above (______________________)

____

____

Example 1 ______________________________

____

Example 2 ______________________________

____

z. A sign not listed above (______________________)

____

____

Example 1 ______________________________

____

Example 2 ______________________________

____

3. After you have defined these signs of mood swings, rank them according to how closely each of them resembles your experience and is applicable to you. Rank the most familiar or applicable to you as No. 1. Rank-order the second most familiar as No. 2, and so on, until the least familiar; mark as N/A the signs that are not applicable to you.

Signs of Mood Swings	*Rank-order*	*Signs of Mood Swings*	*Rank-order*
a. Euphoria	________	o. Feeling worthless	________
b. Grandiosity	________	p. Taking big or unusual risks	________
c. Depression	________		
d. Loss of interest	________	q. Feeling wired	________
e. Sleeping too much	________	r. High level of anxiety	________
f. Sleeping too little	________	s. Feeling slowed down	________
g. Racing thoughts	________	t. Feeling speeded up	________
h. Full of energy	________	u. Overly goal-driven	________
i. Doing too many things	________	v. Aggressive impulses	________
		w. Hopelessness	________
j. Highly distractible	________	x. Passivity	________
k. Suicidal thoughts	________	y. A sign not listed above (__________)	________
l. Easily fatigued	________		
m. Unable to concentrate	________		
		z. A sign not listed above (__________)	________
n. Irritability	________		

4. Explain why your rank-ordered these signs the way you did.

____
____
____
____
____

Homework: During the next few days, keep on thinking about these signs and whether you want to keep their rank order as is or whether you want to change it.

Standard Practice Exercise for Signs of Mood Swings

Title of Sign____________________Practice Exercise No.______

Name______________________________Sex____Date______

The purpose of this practice exercise is to learn more about the sign of mood swings listed in the title of this practice exercise.

1. How do this sign trouble you? Please explain in detail.

____
____
____
____
____

2. How often does this sign trouble you? Check which answer applies to you:

   a. Practically every day _______
   b. Once a week _______
   c. A couple of times a month _______
   d. Once a month _______
   e. Once every six 6 months _______
   f. Once a year _______
   g. Once every few years _______

3. Please explain further:

____
____
____
____
____

4. How did this sign come about? Do you remember when you started feeling it? Check which answer fits best:

   a. When I was a child (younger than 5 years of age) ________
   b. When I was in elementary school ________
   c. When I was in middle school ________
   d. When I was in high school ________
   e. After high school ________
   f. Any other time ________

5. Please explain further:

____
____
____
____
____

6. Give three specific examples of how this sign troubles you.

   Example a

____
____
____
____
____

   Example b

____
____
____
____
____

   Example c

____
____
____
____
____

Homework: Next week, in order for you to learn to control this sign ("Start it if you want to stop it!"), plan to repeat it at preset times (for instance, at 8 a.m., 12 noon, 4 or 7 p.m.), on at least 3 days (Monday, Wednesday, and Friday, or Tuesday, Thursday, and Saturday). Write down what happened in detail. For each time make sure to answer in writing the following four questions:

a. How did you start this sign?
b. What followed after you felt this sign?
c. How did this sign end?
d. What did this sign get you?

Time 1 (write the time you started__________)

a. ______________________________
____
____

b. ______________________________
____
____

c. ______________________________
____
____

d. ______________________________
____
____

Time 2 (write the time you started__________)

a. ______________________________
____
____

b. ______________________________
____
____

c. ______________________________
____
____

d. ______________________________
____
____

Time 3 (write the time you started__________)

a. ______________________________
____
____

b. ______________________________
____
____

c. ______________________________
____
____

d. ____
____
____

Check which of the following shows what you got out of this practice exercise:

a. Completely useless ________
b. Somewhat useless ________
c. So-so ________
d. Somewhat useful ________
e. Extremely useful ________

Feel free to explain how you feel about this homework practice exercise and what you got out of it.

____
____
____
____
____

Concluding Feedback Form for Mood Swings

Name______________________________Sex____Date______

The purpose of this last concluding feedback form is to find out how you feel about the practice exercises you completed in this practice exercise.

1. Please select the answer that best fits how you feel about this practice exercise:

   a. I did not like working on this practice exercise at all. I wish I never saw it. _____
   b. I did not like this practice exercise at all, but I am glad I got to work on it. _____
   c. I am delighted I got a chance to work on this practice exercise. ________
   d. I am not only delighted about this practice exercise, but I wish all people with bipolar disorder had a chance to work on it. _____

2. How helpful was it to work on this practice exercise? Check the answer that applies to you:

   a. Not helpful at all _____
   b. Somewhat helpful _____
   c. Helpful _____
   d. Very helpful _____

3. Rank-order the practice exercises you have completed. Rank-order each practice exercise according to how much you liked it. Rank-order as No. 1 the practice exercise you liked the most. Rank as No. 2 the practice exercise that you liked second best, and so on, until you reach an practice exercise you did not like at all or that you did not feel you could rank with the others (N/A).

Signs of Mood Swings	*Rank-order*	*Signs of Mood Swings*	*Rank-order*
a. Euphoria	________	o. Feeling worthless	________
b. Grandiosity	________	p. Taking big or unusual risks	________
c. Depression	________	q. Feeling wired	________
d. Loss of interest	________	r. High level of anxiety	________
e. Sleeping too much	________	s. Feeling slowed down	________
f. Sleeping too little	________	t. Feeling speeded up	________
g. Racing thoughts	________	u. Overly goal-driven	________
h. Full of energy	________	v. Aggressive impulses	________
i. Doing too many things	________	w. Hopelessness	________
j. Highly distractible	________	x. Passivity	________
k. Suicidal thoughts	________	y. A sign not listed above (________)	________
l. Easily fatigued	________	z. A sign not listed above (________)	________
m. Unable to concentrate	________		
n. Irritability	________		

4. Why did you rank-order practice exercises the way you did?

____
____
____
____
____

5. Which practice exercise was the most helpful to you? Sometimes what we like most is not necessarily the most helpful. Consequently, could you rank the practice exercises according to their helpfulness to you? Rank as No. 1 the most helpful, rank as No. 2 the next most helpful, and so on, until the least helpful practice exercise.

Signs of Mood Swings	*Rank-order*	*Signs of Mood Swings*	*Rank-order*
a. Euphoria	________	g. Racing thoughts	________
b. Grandiosity	________	h. Full of energy	________
c. Depression	________	i. Doing too many things	________
d. Loss of interest	________	j. Highly distractible	________
e. Sleeping too much	________	k. Suicidal thoughts	________
f. Sleeping too little	________		

Signs of Mood Swings	*Rank-order*	*Signs of Mood Swings*	*Rank-order*
l. Easily fatigued	________	t. Feeling speeded up	________
m. Unable to concentrate	________	u. Overly goal-driven	________
n. Irritability	________	v. Aggressive impulses	________
o. Feeling worthless	________	w. Hopelessness	________
p. Taking big or unusual risks	________	x. Passivity	________
q. Feeling wired	________	y. A sign not listed above (__________)	________
r. High level of anxiety	________	z. A sign not listed above (__________)	________
s. Feeling slowed down	________		

6. Why did you rank the practice exercises the way you did?

____
____
____
____
____

7. Feel free to write any comments that might improve this practice exercise.

____
____
____
____
____

Section 2
Relational Self-Help Practice Exercises for Couples and Families in Conflict

Couples

Complaints

The purpose of this practice exercise is to improve your relationship with your partner.

Answer each practice exercise individually and get together with your partner at predetermined times (set up at least 24 h ahead) to discuss your completed practice exercises for no longer than 1 h. If you get upset during this time, end the discussion and make another appointment for another time at least 24 h ahead.

Practice Exercise 1. Defining Complaints

Name ________________________________ Sex __________ Date ________

The purpose of this practice exercise is to help you define more clearly the nature of complaints most couples make about their relationships. Make sure that you understand and discuss with each other the meaning of each complaint that makes up this practice exercise.

L. L'Abate, *Sourcebook of Interactive Practice Exercises in Mental Health*, DOI 10.1007/978-1-4419-1354-8_12,

1. Below are listed various complaints that cover a range of possibilities. If you have a complaint not found in this list, add it at the end; there is room for additional complaints. Define each complaint, and give two examples of how that complaint manifests itself in your relationship.

Complaints and Definitions	*Examples*
a. Trouble with children ________	Example 1 ________
________	________
________	Example 2 ________
________	________
b. Trouble with in-laws ________	Example 1 ________
________	________
________	Example 2 ________
________	________
c. Different social needs ________	Example 1 ________
________	________
________	Example 2 ________
________	________
d. Conflicts about children ________	Example 1 ________
________	________
________	Example 2 ________
________	________
e. Division of responsibilities ________	Example 1 ________
________	________
________	Example 2 ________
________	________
f. Partner does not understand me ____	Example 1 ________
________	________
________	Example 2 ________
________	________
g. Financial disagreements ________	Example 1 ________
________	________
________	Example 2 ________
________	________
h. Frequent arguments ________	Example 1 ________
________	________
________	Example 2 ________
________	________

i. Difficulty discussing problems ____ Example 1 ____

Example 2 ____

j. Less interested in talking to each other ____ Example 1 ____

Example 2 ____

k. Too little time spent together ____ Example 1 ____

Example 2 ____

l. Boredom ____ Example 1 ____

Example 2 ____

m. Physical attacks by partner ____ Example 1 ____

Example 2 ____

n. Being blamed for everything that goes wrong ____ Example 1 ____

Example 2 ____

o. Sexual dissatisfaction ____ Example 1 ____

Example 2 ____

p. Partner's alcoholism ____ Example 1 ____

Example 2 ____

q. Partner's drug use ____ Example 1 ____

Example 2 ____

r. Partner's chronic or recurrent illness ____________	Example 1 ____________ Example 2 ____________
s. Partner's actual or suspected infidelity ____________	Example 1 ____________ Example 2 ____________
t. Partner's stubbornness ____________	Example 1 ____________ Example 2 ____________
u. Partner depends on me too much ____________	Example 1 ____________ Example 2 ____________
v. Lack of partner's ambition ____________	Example 1 ____________ Example 2 ____________
w. Partner's sloppiness ____________	Example 1 ____________ Example 2 ____________
x. Partner's excessive neatness ____________	Example 1 ____________ Example 2 ____________
y. Partner does not fill my emotional needs ____________	Example 1 ____________ Example 2 ____________
z. Partner does not respect me ____________	Example 1 ____________ Example 2 ____________

aa. A complaint not listed above ____	Example 1 ____________
____________	____________
____________	Example 2 ____________
____________	____________
bb. A complaint not listed above	Example 1 ____________
____________	____________
____________	Example 2 ____________
____________	____________
cc. A complaint not listed above	Example 1 ____________
____________	____________
____________	Example 2 ____________
____________	____________

2. Now that you have defined the meaning of these complaints, you need to rank-order them according to how troublesome they are to you in this relationship. Rank as No. 1 the complaint that is the most troublesome to you, rank as No. 2 the complaint that is next most troublesome to you, and so on; mark as N/A (not applicable) the complaints that are not troublesome to you or that do not apply to this relationship.

	Rank-orders		
Complaints	*Mine*	*Partner*	*Joint*
a. Trouble with children	______	______	______
b. Trouble with in-laws	______	______	______
c. Different social needs	______	______	______
d. Conflicts about children	______	______	______
e. Division of responsibilities	______	______	______
f. Partner does not understand me	______	______	______
g. Financial disagreements	______	______	______
h. Frequent arguments	______	______	______
i. Difficulty discussing problems	______	______	______
j. Less interested in talking to each other	______	______	______
k. Too little time spent together	______	______	______
l. Boredom	______	______	______
m. Physical attacks by partner	______	______	______
n. Being blamed for everything that goes wrong	______	______	______
o. Sexual dissatisfaction	______	______	______
p. Partner's alcoholism	______	______	______
q. Partner's drug use	______	______	______
r. Partner's chronic or recurrent illness	______	______	______

Complaints	*Rank-orders* Mine	*Partner*	*Joint*
s. Partner's actual or suspected infidelity	________	________	________
t. Partner's stubbornness	________	________	________
u. Partner depends on me too much	________	________	________
v. Lack of ambition of partner	________	________	________
w. Partner's sloppiness	________	________	________
x. Partner's excessive neatness	________	________	________
y. Partner does not fill my emotional needs	________	________	________
z. Partner does not respect me	________	________	________
aa. A complaint not listed above	________	________	________
bb. A complaint not listed above	________	________	________
cc. A complaint not listed above	________	________	________

3. Why did you rank-order these complaints the way you did?

____

____

____

____

____

Homework: During the coming week, make an appointment with your partner and go over your definitions and your rank-orders. Record your partner's rank-orders in the appropriate column and add both to achieve a joint rank-order. Take notes of your discussion while you are comparing and contrasting your answers. Give your completed practice exercises and your notes to the professional who is assisting you with this practice exercise.

Whatever joint rank-order you agree on will determine the order of future practice exercises. The next practice exercise must be given the title of the joint complaint that has been rated jointly as No. 1. After that practice exercise, all other practice exercises should follow the joint rank-order given above.

____

____

____

____

____

Standard Practice Exercise for Couple Complaints

Practice Exercise No. ______Title of Complaint: ________________

Name ________________________Sex __________Date ________

The purpose of this practice exercise is to understand more about the complaint listed in the title.

1. How did this complaint start? Please explain in detail.

____
____
____
____
____

2. How often does this complaint take place? Check which answer applies to you:

   a. Practically every day ______
   b. Once a week ______
   c. A couple of times a month ______
   d. Once a month ______
   e. Once every 6 months ______
   f. Once a year ______
   g. Once every few years ______

3. Please explain further.

____
____
____
____
____

4. What generated this complaint? Do you remember how it started? Check which answer fits best:

   a. As we met for the first time ______
   b. During courtship or while dating ______
   c. Before marriage or before we started living together ______
   d. During the honeymoon or as we were moving in together ______
   e. Right after the honeymoon or right after we moved in together ______
   f. A few months after the marriage or after we moved in together ______
   g. 1 year after the marriage or when we moved in together ______
   h. Years after marriage or when we moved in together ______

5. Please explain further.

6. What does this complaint get you? Please explain.

7. Give three specific examples of how this complaint is hurtful to you.

Example 1:

Example 2:

Example 3:

8. Give three specific examples of how this complaint is hurtful to those you love and who love you.

Example 1:

____
____
____
____
____

Example 2:

____
____
____
____
____

Example 3:

____
____
____
____
____

Homework: Next week, plan to repeat the behavior that caused the complaint, if it belongs to you, or remind you partner to repeat it if it belongs to him or her. Make sure it is repeated at preset times (for instance, at 8 a.m., 12 noon, 4 or 7 p.m.) on at least 3 days. Write down what happened in detail. In case you wonder why this behavior should be started, keep in mind that if you or your partner start it, whoever starts it will acquire the power to end it.

For each time make sure to answer in writing the following four questions:

(a) How did it start?
(b) What followed?
(c) How did it end?
(d) What did this behavior get you or your partner?

Time 1 (write the time when it started __________)

a. ____
____
____

b. ____
____
____

c. ____
____
____

d. ____
____
____

Time 2 (write the time when it started __________)

a. ____
____
____

b. ____
____
____

c. ____
____
____

d. ____
____
____

Time 3 (write time it started __________)

a. ____
____
____

b. ____
____
____

c. ____
____
____

d. ____
____
____

Check which of the following shows what you got out of this practice exercise:

a. Completely useless _____
b. Somewhat useless _____
c. So-so _____
d. Somewhat useful _____
e. Extremely useful _____

Write down how you feel about this homework practice exercise and what you got out of it.

____
____
____
____
____

Concluding Follow-Up Form for Couple Complaints

Name ______________________ Sex ______ Date ________

The purpose of this final practice exercise is to review whether the practice exercises in this practice exercise were helpful to you.

1. Which answer best fits how you feel about this practice exercise?

   a. I did not like working on this practice exercise at all. I wish I never saw it. ________
   b. I did not like this practice exercise, but I am glad I got to work on it. ________
   c. I am happy I got a chance to work on this. ________
   d. I am not only delighted about this practice exercise, but I wish all couples with difficulties could get it. ________

2. How helpful was it to work on this practice exercise? Please check the answer that applies to you:

   a. Not helpful at all ______ c. Helpful ______
   b. Somewhat helpful ______ d. Very helpful ______

3. Which practice exercise did you like best that was the most helpful to you? Please rank-order the practice exercises from the one that you liked best (Rank No. 1) to the one you liked next best (Rank No. 2) and so on; mark as N/A the ones you did not like at all or did not apply to you.

Complaints	*Rank-orders* *Mine*	*Partner*	*Joint*
a. Trouble with children	________	________	________
b. Trouble with in-laws	________	________	________
c. Different social needs	________	________	________
d. Conflicts about children	________	________	________
e. Division of responsibilities	________	________	________
f. Partner does not understand me	________	________	________
g. Financial disagreements	________	________	________

h. Frequent arguments	________	________	________
i. Difficulty discussing problems	________	________	________
j. Less interested in talking to each other	________	________	________
k. Too little time spent together	________	________	________
l. Boredom	________	________	________
m. Physical attacks by partner	________	________	________
n. Being blamed for everything that goes wrong	________	________	________
o. Sexual dissatisfaction	________	________	________
p. Partner's alcoholism	________	________	________
q. Partner's drug use	________	________	________
r. Partner's chronic or recurrent illness	________	________	________
s. Partner's actual or suspected infidelity	________	________	________
t. Partner's stubbornness	________	________	________
u. Partner depends on me too much	________	________	________
v. Lack of ambition of partner	________	________	________
w. Partner's sloppiness	________	________	________
x. Partner's excessive neatness	________	________	________
y. Partner does not fill my emotional needs	________	________	________
z. Partner does not respect me	________	________	________
aa. A complaint not listed above	________	________	________
bb. A complaint not listed above	________	________	________
cc. A complaint not listed above	________	________	________

4. Explain why you have rank-ordered the practice exercises the way you did.

____
____
____
____
____

5. Make an appointment with your partner at least 24 h ahead and write down in the appropriate column your partner's rank-orders. Discuss (compare and contrast) whatever differences you may find in your individual rank-orders.
6. After completion of this practice exercise, write how you feel about it. Check which of these answers tells how you felt about it. There is also space for you to explain further, if you want to:

   a. I did not like it at all, a waste of time. I wish I never saw this stupid practice exercise. ________
   b. I did not like it very much, but I want to go on with another practice exercise. ________

c. I liked it and I want to go on with another practice exercise. ________
d. I liked it a lot and I wish I had something like this practice exercise earlier. ________
e. I liked it so much that I wish all couples could get something like this practice exercise to work on. ________

7. How could this practice exercise be improved? Do you have any suggestions? Feel free to write whatever could improve this practice exercise.

____
____
____
____
____

Sexuality

The purpose of this practice exercise is to improve your skills in your sexual presence and performance.

Practice Exercise 1. Description

Name ________________________Sex __________Date ____________

The purpose of this practice exercise is to get more information about your sleeping patterns and how they relate to your sexuality.

Please answer the following questions:

1. What time do you usually get up in the morning?

a. 5–6:30 a.m. _____
b. 6:30–7:45 a.m. _____
c. 7:45–9:45 a.m. _____
d. 9:45–11 a.m. _____
e. 11 a.m.–noon _____

2. How easy is it for you to get up in the morning?

a. Not at all easy _____
b. Not very easy _____
c. Fairly easy _____
d. Very easy _____

3. How tired do you feel the first half-hour after getting up?

a. Very tired _____
b. Fairly tired _____
c. Fairly refreshed _____
d. Very refreshed _____

4. If you have to take a test or examination, at what time do you think you will perform best?

   a. From 8 to 10 a.m. ____
   b. From 10 a.m. to 1 p.m. ____
   c. From 1 to 5 p.m. ____
   d. From 5 to 7 p.m. ____
   e. From 7 to 9 p.m. ____

5. One night you must remain awake between 4 and 6 a.m. to take your turn on a night-watch patrol. You have no commitments the next day. How would you prepare for it?

   a. I would not go to bed until the watch is over ____
   b. I would take a nap before and sleep after ____
   c. I would sleep before and a nap after ____
   d. I would get all the sleep I could before the watch ____

6. A friend invites you to jog between 7 and 8 a.m. How do you think you would perform?

   a. Well ____
   b. Reasonably well ____
   c. Would find it hard to do ____
   d. Would find it very hard to do ____

7. If you have to wake up at a specific time every morning, how dependent are you on an alarm clock?

   a. Not at all dependent ____
   b. Slightly dependent ____
   c. Fairly dependent ____
   d. Very dependent ____

8. At what time in the evening do you feel tired and need sleep?

   a. 8–9 p.m. ____
   b. 9–10:15 p.m. ____
   c. 10:15 p.m.–12:45 a.m. ____
   d. 12:45–2 a.m. ____
   e. 2–3 a.m. ____

Scoring:

1. Give yourself 5 points for a, 4 for b, 3 for c, 2 for d, and 1 for e.
2. Give 1 point for a, 2 for b, 3 for c, and 4 for d.
3. Give 1 point for a, 2 for b, 3 for c, and 4 for d.
4. Give 6 points for a, 4 for b, 2 for c, and 0 for d.
5. Give 1 point for a, 2 for b, 3 for c, and 4 for d.
6. Give 4 points for a, 3 for b, 2 for c, and 1 for d.
7. Give 4 points for a, 3 for b, 2 for c, and 1 for d.
8. Give 5 points for a, 4 for b, 3 for c, 2 for d, and 1 for e.

A 15 high score means positive sleep habits, while a 14 low score means negative sleep habits. What is important here is that you and your partner have compatible sleep habits with each other, so that you can get together sexually in a reasonable frame of mind and with a relaxed body.

9. Compare and contrast your answers and scores with your partner to see whether you are either a night owl or a morning lark or neither. What do you conclude about your sleep patterns and those of your partner?

10. How do you experience time in terms of (a) your interest and involvement in the past, the present, or the future; and (b) your experiencing it as slow or fast:

a. ____
____
____

b. ____
____
____

11. How often do these differences in sleep patterns and time involvement cause conflicts between you and your partner?

a. More than once a day	____	e. Every couple of weeks	____
b. Once a day	____	f. Once a month	____
c. Two or three times a week	____	g. Other (explain):	____
d. Once a week	____		

____
____
____
____
____

12. How strong are these differences?

a. Very strong, causing a lot of conflict between us	____	d. Moderate	____
b. Very strong, but we manage to handle them	____	e. Hardly strong at all	____
c. Strong enough	____	f. Other (explain):	____

____
____
____
____
____

13. What areas of your relationship are most affected by differences considered in Questions 1 and 3? Rank the most troublesome 1, the second 2, down to the least troublesome:

a.	Chores around the house	____	e.	Relationships with others	____
b.	Schedules	____	f.	Children and child rearing	____
c.	Sex	____	g.	Health	____
d.	Money use and budgeting	____	h.	Other (explain):	____

____
____
____
____
____

14. Do the different speeds at which you and your partner work affect your relationship? Please explain:

____
____
____
____
____

15. What have you done to solve and resolve some of these differences?

____
____
____
____
____

16. Of the troublesome areas listed in Questions 6, pick the one that you would like to change the most. Explain why.

____
____
____
____
____

17. How does the past affect this problem area?

____
____
____
____
____

18. How does the present affect this area?

____
____
____
____
____

19. How does the future affect this area?

____
____
____
____
____

Homework: Get together with your partner by making an appointment at least 24 h in advance and discuss with each other various ways of dealing with this problem area. Write down possible solutions.

____
____
____
____
____

Practice Exercise 2. Explanations

Name ______________________ Sex _____ Date _________

The purpose of this practice exercise is to explain in greater detail how you see your sexuality.

1. The following is a list of what different experiences of time do for families (in this case spouses or partners) with regard to sex and sexuality. Get together for at least 1 h and discuss which of the following explanations applies specifically to your relationship.

____
____
____

Experiences	*Rank-order*
a. Experiencing sex at a slow pace is a way of relishing the event and making me feel cared about	________
b. Experiencing sex at a fast pace is a way of feeling passion that is much stronger	________
c. Bringing up past sexual experiences is a way of affirming our current relationship; people don't compare relationships unless these relationships are very important to them	________
d. Sexual problems are a good opportunity to discuss important issues that otherwise might not get brought up; these kinds of discussions are important to a relationship because they offer a chance to grow	________
e. Different speeds are very useful in different situations; going at different speeds is a good way of expressing individuality	________
f. Experiencing the present only is a good way of enjoying the moment and the sensual pleasure of the moment; not worrying about the past or the future is a good way of expressing complete interest in your mate	________
g. Fantasizing about the future is a good way of finding out what you wish for; this is important for setting goals and acting upon them	________
h. Having differences in your experience of time that upset you is proof that you care deeply about one another; people who don't love each other don't care and don't get upset	________
i. Going very slowly as you experience sex and refusing to speed it up is a way of saying how important your mate is because you want this experience to last for a long time	________
j. Not having time for sex could be due to the intense schedules you keep to take care of your family	________

2. Now that you have read and discussed whether or not these explanations apply to you, rank them from 1 (most important) to 10 (least important).

3. If none of these apply to you, write down what you think is the most likely explanation for the problem(s) you have.

____

____

____

____

____

4. Compare and contrast your rank-orders with those of your partner, by making an appointment 24 h in advance. Discuss what differences are present and what you could do to reconcile them.

Homework: During the coming week, think about how different experiences of time in dealing with your sexuality can be improved. Explain in detail.

____

____

____

____

____

Then go back to what you have written at the end of the first practice exercise and write down in detail your own (not your partner's) step-by-step plan to deal with these issues.

____

____

____

____

____

Homework: Make an appointment 24 h in advance. See if the two plans can be put together. Each of you should then write down what possible solutions could be worked out by putting both plans together. Do not talk about these plans. Do all of the communication in writing if you want to find a solution. If you do not want a solution, keep on talking and see if you come up with one.

Practice Exercise 3. Prescriptions

Name ________________________________ Sex ________ Date _______

The purpose of this practice exercise is to help you achieve greater control over your sexuality.

If you do not want to resolve your time differences in the area of sexuality, then you should ignore these guidelines. Although they may seem strange, just consider them steps toward your goal of a better sex life. You have been putting so much energy into having a positive sexual experience. Now put your energies in planning and having a bad sexual experience. In this way you may become free to have a better experience.

1. Be sure to set an appointment at least 24 h in advance to fail in your sexual experience. *It is important that you do everything you can to make this experience not work.* It needs to be planned in the future as well so that you can prepare for it. Set a time when sex would most likely occur naturally. Make sure that you will not be interrupted by the phone or by children. Set a timer for 30 minute. Then go ahead and begin to use completely different speeds and other time factors, such as bringing up the past and fantasizing about the future or

whatever will most likely cause failure. It might seem strange or weird to you, but if you can fail on purpose, you may succeed on purpose.

2. Follow these instructions without talking about this project. Do this as naturally as you can. However, do pay attention to what is happening so that you can discuss it afterward. Be sure to support each other so that one of you will not give in and fail this project by having a good sexual experience. It is important that neither of you give up.
3. You may even make this experience more extreme by exaggerating the time elements that cause you to fail.
4. Plan to do this experience at least three times during the next 2 weeks. You may discontinue this project only if the problem disappears. If this problem comes back when you are not trying to fail, implement the same procedure immediately. Go ahead and make that experience as unsuccessful as possible.
5. Take notes on the conversations that you have about your experience as well as of what happened in the experience. Discuss these notes with whoever has given you these practice exercises.

Note: If these homework practice exercises did not work for you, you need to consult with a specialist in the area of sexuality. Do not give up; keep in mind that people who care for themselves are the ones who ask for help.

Depression

The purpose of this practice exercise is to teach you how to deal with depression and depressive feelings.

Practice Exercise 1. Terrific Triangles: The Family Drama

Name ________________________________ Sex ______ Date _______

The purpose of this practice exercise is to learn more about destructive patterns that interfere with living with loved ones.

1. To keep the couple or family together and to protect it from change, we often create a triangle in which we, in one way or another, play all three parts at different times. The three parts are the victim, the persecutor, and the rescuer. These basic parts have variations within themselves. For instance, we may play the judge of other family members, and, on the basis of this part, we may then become jury and executioner. Below you will find three lists that relate to the three basic parts. Read them.

Persecutor	*Victim*	*Rescuer*
Judge	Criminal	Therapist
Parent	Defendant	Know-it-all
Juror	Invalid (sick)	Expert (teacher, preacher, consultant)
Policeman	Child	Big Daddy
Patriot	Drug addict	Tycoon
Detective	Servant	Peacemaker
Hellfire-and-brimstone preacher	Martyr	Caretaker Red Cross nurse or paramedic
Executioner	Sinner	Meddler
Inquisitor	Culprit	Saint/Missionary
Oppressor	"Poor little me"	Superman/Superwoman
Inspector general	Oppressed	Wholesaler
Interrogator	Innocent	Advice giver

2. Circle the part and the variations on the part that you recognize in yourself. Then indicate which of these parts you play best (a), second best (b), and third best(c). Write in detail how you play each part.

   a. ______________________________

   b. ______________________________

   c. ______________________________

3. What happens to your partner or the rest of the family when you play these parts? Explain in detail.

____

4. Do you need to play these parts and what do you get out from playing them? Explain in detail.

____

5. Who is responsible for your playing these parts?

____

____

____

____

____

6. How do you get yourself set up to play these parts? Explain in detail.

____

____

____

____

____

7. Unless you like playing these parts and you do get something positive out of playing them, how can you avoid setting yourself up to play them? Explain in detail.

____

____

____

____

____

Homework: During the coming week, you must continue to play these three parts as you have done in the past. However, from now on jot down and log every time you find yourself playing one of these parts. In addition, since keeping logs is usually not enough, make an appointment with yourself or your partner (if you have one) at specific, prearranged times (e.g., 8 o'clock p.m. on Tuesdays) to play these parts and learn to control them, rather than these parts controlling you. The purpose of these meetings is for you to become aware of how these parts are played within and without the family. If necessary you may need more than one meeting to play these parts until these parts no longer effect you and the family (unless, of course, the family wants to continue playing these parts). Keep notes of these meetings to discuss with your professional helper.

Practice Exercise 2. Terrific Triangles: Distance in the Family

Name ______________________ Sex ______ Date _______

The purpose of this practice exercise is to learn about another destructive pattern that increases depression in families.

Another terrific triangle we often play to keep the family together and protect it from change has three parts: the pursuer, the distancer, and the distance regulator.

For instance, a distancer may avoid emotional closeness but become a pursuer sexually. An emotional pursuer, by the same token, may become a sexual distancer. The distance regulator may want people to come close, but when they do, they are put off or even rejected. Write your responses below.

1. Which of these parts do you play best?
2. How do you play it?
3. Which of these parts do you play second best?
4. How do you play it?
5. Which of these parts do you play third best?
6. How do you play it?
7. What happens to you and to the rest of the family when you play these parts? Please explain in detail.
8. How do you set yourself up to play these parts?
9. Unless you like playing them and you get something out of playing them, how can you avoid setting yourself up to play them?

Homework: Make sure to continue playing theses parts until each family member is completely aware of how destructive these parts are. Discuss (compare and contrast) your answers with your partner/family members and keep notes about the discussion. Discuss these notes with your professional helper.

Practice Exercise 3. Defining Depression

Name ________________________________ Sex ______ Date ________

The purpose of this practice exercise is to define depression as you understand it. There are many definitions of depression and it is important that members of the family define it as they see it.

1. What does depression mean to you?
2. Are you willing to consider the following explanations of depression? (For this step it is sufficient to read the opinions listed below):

Definitions	*Rank-order*
a. Depression is a valuable signal that we could use other people's help and support in our lives	_________
b. Being depressed is a sign of our strength and willingness to recognize what we are feeling; many people are unwilling or unable to recognize their depression!	_________
c. Depression is a feeling that all of us experience to some degree; we cannot live and not be depressed because all of us, as human beings, are vulnerable to hurts	_________

Definitions	*Rank-order*
d. Saying that we are depressed indicates that we know how we feel inside and that therefore we can begin to do something about it; if we did not know how we felt or if we did not admit to feeling depressed, we might do something destructive, such as drinking, abusing drugs, gambling, etc.	________
e. Depression can be a useful feeling and one that, used correctly, may eventually lead us to understand and appreciate its importance	________
f. Instead of being considered an enemy and a foe, depression can be thought of as a friend: something we are able to join, use well, and, eventually, something we learn to live with and even enjoy	________
g. Depression is the royal road to self and selfhood; it allows us to have time to ourselves, to be by ourselves, to listen to ourselves, and thus to learn more about ourselves	________
h. When we experience our depression fully, we are being honest and real with ourselves; when we deny or reject our depression, we are being phony, essentially withdrawing from our emotional selves	________
i. Depression is a choice; up to now, depression has controlled you, your life, and perhaps your marriage and your family; perhaps you can choose whether you allow it to control you or you will learn how to control it	________

3. After you have read these explanations of depression, rank them from 1 to 9, according to how closely each of them resembles you in your depression; rank the most familiar or applicable with No. 1; rank the second most familiar with No. 2, and so on, ranking the least familiar to you with No. 9.
4. If none of the preceding descriptions fit you in any way, please explain why.
5. Even if none of the descriptions seems to fit you, try choosing three that seem as if they might be useful to you as a way of describing depression.
6. If any of the descriptions do fit you, please explain how.

Homework: During the next few days, choose three of the most applicable, or useful, descriptions of depression and notice carefully how well (or how poorly) these descriptions apply to depression during the coming week.

Practice Exercise 4. The Positive Element

Name ______________________________Sex _____Date __________

The purpose of this practice exercise is to help you see that there may even be some good in what at first seems to be such a bad, negative experience of depressed feelings.

1. We need to check last week's homework. How well did the descriptions you chose apply to your depression during the week?
2. As you may have noticed, depression often contains a positive element that is helpful to the person who is depressed. Write down two of the positive or useful aspects of your depression – however small or insignificant they appear to be.
3. Because depression may contain some useful and valuable ingredients, it would not make sense (nor would it be possible) to try to eliminate depression. We cannot be alive and not be depressed. It may, however, be useful to learn from it and to control it by deciding when to experience depression.

Homework: During the coming week, allow yourself to be depressed. Now, on three separate occasions, pay attention to the positive and valuable aspects of your depression. Notice the subtle, perhaps small, but real benefits of this experience. Write down the results of this homework practice exercise. In addition, during the week, decide whether the depression is controlling you and your family or whether you and the family want to control the depression.

Practice Exercise 5. Achieving Control

Name ________________________________Sex ____Date ________

The purpose of this practice exercise is to help you achieve greater control over depression. You must make up your mind whether depression is going to control you and your family or whether you and your family are going to control it. One way to learn greater control is to make sure that regular, preset meetings will take place for the family members to share what they are learning from these homework practice exercises.

1. a. We need to check last week's homework. What positive or useful aspects of your depression were you able to find?
   b. Did you find that you controlled the depression, or was the depression controlling you?

2. Despite the usefulness of depression, most people seem to allow their depression to control and overwhelm them. You will learn that you can choose to allow your depression to control you, or you can learn how to begin to control it. If you are interested in learning how to control your depression,

proceed to the next step. If not, stop here and list the many ways that depression is controlling your life and how you are going to let it control you and your family.

3. Although depression is a valuable and useful method of learning about ourselves, it is not enough simply to recognize this fact. It is important to achieve some control over when we choose to experience depression. To achieve some control over depression, we may begin by learning and practicing how to start being depressed. Thus, if you want to stop it, start it! Most people don't realize that they have the freedom to start a depression on command. We can start a depression by controlling its content. For example, we can start being depressed in the following ways:

   a. By thinking negative thoughts about ourselves
   b. By thinking negatively about the world around us
   c. By thinking negatively about our future

4. Which method can you use to start to make yourself feel depressed? Which one works best for you? Do you have your own creative and effective ways of becoming depressed?
5. Although depression can often be a valuable and useful experience, it is helpful to learn to control it in order to use it at our leisure. We can control depression by starting it in a specific place at a specific time. Where do you most often tend to feel depressed? At home? At work? Outside?

   a. At what times do you tend to feel most depressed? In the morning, the afternoon, the evening, or before going to bed?

Homework: During the coming, week begin practicing to control depression by starting it two times during the week. However, make sure that you remain alone and isolated during these first depression practice sessions. It is important to be free of distractions so that you can allow yourself to experience your depression fully. In addition, start the depression at a prearranged time (e.g., 8 p.m.) and not when you most often feel depressed. Do, however, place a time limit on these depressive times. Do it for 20–30 minute at the most. Remember not to go over the agreed time limit. It may even be useful to set an alarm clock to remind you when the time is up. Finally, in addition to concentrating on being depressed, it is important that you write down all the thoughts and feelings that come to your mind during the controlled depression practice sessions. You can use the experience to learn more about yourself by reviewing your written notes. Good luck in taking this important step.

Practice Exercise 6. Flexible Control

Name ______________________________ Sex _____ Date _______

The purpose of this practice exercise is to learn better ways to control your depression.

1. We need to check on last week's practice exercise. Describe your two controlled depressive episodes. Review your notes on the main thoughts and feelings you had during these episodes.
2. What did you learn about yourself through these experiences?
3. If you didn't perform this homework practice exercise, do you feel somewhat depressed about that? If so, write down your thoughts and feelings on this matter. If not, make note of your growing ability not to have to perform perfectly at all times in order to feel OK.
4. Part of learning the art of control is acquiring flexibility and adapting to life's changing conditions. To improve your control of your depression, you may have to arrange to be depressed at different times, for different periods of time, and under varying situations. In this way, you can begin to master your depressive episodes and to learn to observe and study them in all kinds of situations.

   a. At what time do you tend to feel somewhat less depressed?
   b. In what places (home, work, etc.) do you tend to feel less depressed?
   c. Under what conditions (working, socializing, exercising, etc.) do you tend to feel somewhat less depressed?

Homework: To acquire further control over your depression, during the coming week practice getting depressed three times, for 20 minute each time. However, arrange these periods to take place (a) at times that are prearranged at least 24 h ahead, and (b) in places where you often tend to feel less depressed. Write down everything you think and feel at the time of the appointment. Make sure you keep a written record. Discuss your notes with your professional helper. Remember to recall and write down for later review what you experience during these controlled depressive times.

Practice Exercise 7. Letting Others Help

Name ______________________________________ Sex ___ Date _____

The purpose of this practice exercise is to use depression to allow others to help you without your rejecting them in order to be miserable all by yourself.

1. Did you do your homework on arranging three depressive times this week? What new insights (if any) did you have about your inner depressive processes?

2. As we mentioned in an earlier lesson, depression can be viewed as an ally, a friend who reminds us that we could use other people's help and support. Who do you most often discuss your depression with?
3. To further increase your control over your depression, it would be useful to enlist the help of these people. Which of the people you listed could you ask to help you to control your depression? If there is no one, try to think of someone who might be willing to help you out (a friend, family member, coworker, professional helper).
4. Sometimes it is difficult to find the energy to remember to schedule a depression a specific number of times during the week. A friend can help by reminding you to do so.

Homework: During this coming week, find someone who will be willing to remind you to schedule some controlled depressive times during the week. That person can even help you to decide which days and how long to be depressed. (Make sure, however, that you practice at least three times this week. It is important to maintain your skill level.) In addition, your helper can check on your progress during the week to make sure that you are doing your homework correctly. Again, remember to record, in writing, your experience of these controlled depressions.

Practice Exercise 8. Using Depression

Name ______________________________ Sex ________ Date ________

The purpose of this practice exercise is to make sure that you have learned to use and even enjoy depression, by learning more about yourself.

1. Did you find someone to help you to schedule your depressions last week? Were you able to follow through and complete your practice exercise fully?
2. Review your notes on your depressions. Were you able to learn anything more about yourself during your self-initiated depressions?
3. What have you concluded about your growing ability to control your depression at will? Have you noticed any change in your feelings about yourself and that gold mine of potential self-knowledge – your depression?
4. Learning how to schedule, initiate, time, record, and review one's own depressions is clearly a difficult skill to master. Those who are willing and able to practice this skill usually feel more confident and feel better about themselves. They realize that they have truly accomplished something special. They have learned a new skill and have been able to use the depression, at their own leisure, to learn more about themselves. What was your experience of this process?
5. You are entitled to feel proud of yourself for having mastered this new skill. On the other hand, there is no need to feel depressed or to belittle yourself for not having completely mastered this skill. If, after completion of all these

lessons, you continue to feel uncomfortable depressed, stop and consider the following step. Pay attention to your depression; remember that it can be a signal reminding us that we need to ask others for help. Are you strong enough to ask for help? Only the strong can give themselves permission to seek help from others.

Depression Feedback Form

Name ______________________________Sex ______Date _________

The purpose of this form is to receive your feedback about the helpfulness and usefulness of this practice exercise to help control depression. Now that you have completed this practice exercise, respond to the following questions concerning the use of these written homework practice exercises.

1. Using a scale of 1–8, rank the practice exercises according to their usefulness in coping with depression. Rank the most useful task as No. 1. Rank the second most useful as No. 2, and so on until you rank the least useful as No. 8.

Practice Exercise	*Rank*	*Practice Exercise*	*Rank*
Drama triangle	______	Achieving control	______
Distance triangle	______	Flexible control	______
Defining depression	______	Letting others help	______
The positive element	______	Using depression	______

2. How useful did you find this practice exercise in understanding and coping with depression?

a. Very useful	______	d. Slightly useful	______
b. Quite useful	______	e. Not at all useful	______
c. Somewhat useful	______		

3. How useful would you rate this practice exercise in terms of developing or improving your attitude toward yourself in general?

a. Very useful	______	d. Slightly useful	______
b. Quite useful	______	e. Not at all useful	______
c. Somewhat useful	______		

4. How likely would you be to recommend this practice exercise to other people you know who might be depressed?

a. Very likely	______	d. Slightly likely	______
b. Quite likely	______	e. Not likely at all	______
c. Somewhat likely	______		

5. your own words, what did you find useful about this practice exercise?
6. comments could you give that could improve this practice exercise? We would appreciate any suggestions that would make this practice exercise better.

Difficulties

The purpose of this practice exercise is to improve your relationship with your partner, either in the marriage or in a committed couple relationship. Answer each practice exercise individually and get together with your partner at preset times (arranged at least 24 h ahead) to share and discuss your completed practice exercises for no longer than 1 h. If you get upset during this time, end the discussion to cool off, and make another appointment for another time at least 24 h ahead.

Practice Exercise 1. Defining Difficulties

Name ______________________ Sex __________ Date __________

The purpose of this practice exercise is to help you define more clearly the nature of difficulties most couples encounter in their relationships. Make sure that you understand and discuss with each other the meaning of each difficulty that makes up this practice exercise.

1. Below are listed various difficulties that cover a range of possibilities. If you have a difficulty not found in this list, add it at the end (there is room for additional difficulties). Define each difficulty, and give two examples of how that difficulty is shown concretely in your relationship.

Difficulties and Definitions	*Examples*
a. Doubts about the relationship's future (divorce; separation) ______ ______ ______	Example 1 ______ ______ Example 2 ______ ______
b. Disrespectful behavior (intentional rudeness, contemptuous remarks, blatant disregard for partner's desires, lying) ______	Example 1 ______ ______ Example 2 ______ ______
c. Extramarital intimacy boundary issues (jealousy, use of pornography, dancing with other people) ______	Example 1 ______ ______ Example 2 ______ ______

d. Excessive or inappropriate displays of anger (innocuous or innocent situation leads to partner getting angry; unfair accusation; yelling or attacking) ____________________

Example 1 ____________________

Example 2 ____________________

e. Sexual interaction (initiation, arousal, frequency, interest) ____________________

Example 1 ____________________

Example 2 ____________________

f. Lack of communication (refusal to talk, not sharing feelings, not expressing desires) ____________________

Example 1 ____________________

Example 2 ____________________

g. In-laws and extended family (conflict with in-laws, time spent with relatives, spouse's behavior around extended family) ____________________

Example 1 ____________________

Example 2 ____________________

h. Confusing, erratic, or emotional behavior (suddenly becoming upset, sudden change of mind, behavior that contradicts a previous plan) ____________________

Example 1 ____________________

Example 2 ____________________

i. Criticism (correcting, blaming, explaining how partner should have done something, challenging partner's viewpoint) ____________________

Example 1 ____________________

Example 2 ____________________

j. Poor communication skills (being unclear or hard to understand, failure to negotiate) ____________________

Example 1 ____________________

Example ____________________

k. Child-rearing issues (discipline, expectations, partner's behavior in front of children) ______________

Example 1 ______________

Example 2 ______________

l. Finances (how to spend money, dealing with bills, shopping) ______________

Example 1 ______________

Example 2 ______________

m. Lack of follow-through (disregarding previous plans or commitments with partner, not doing something as agreed, forgetting to keep a promise ______________

Example 1 ______________

Example 2 ______________

n. Showing support in public or social situations (contradicting spouse in front of others, not standing up to others on spouse's behalf) ______________

Example 1 ______________

Example 2 ______________

o. Showing affection (lack of comfort, not showing affection, lack of romance) ______________

Example 1 ______________

Example 2 ______________

p. Lack of listening (poor listening, not listening, problem solving instead of understanding, defensive listening) ______________

Example 1 ______________

Example 2 ______________

q. Annoying behavior (unconventional behavior, wishing partner would change a habit, use of undesirable language, bothersome idiosyncrasies, lack of punctuality, etc. ______________

Example 1 ______________

Example 2 ______________

r. Important decisions (major purchases, vacations, where to live, job change, retirement, education plans) ______________

Example 1 ______________

Example 2 ______________

s. Extent or quality of time together (wanting more intimate time together, time for quality communication, being too tired or too busy to do activities together) ________

Example 1 ________

Example 2 ________

t. Careless or unthinking behavior (mistakes that cause inconvenience, forgetting something) ________

Example 1 ________

Example 2 ________

u. Household tasks (chores, cleanliness, responsibilities, standards and methods of household maintenance) ________

Example 1 ________

Example 2 ________

v. Showing recognition or appreciation (failure to notice or appreciate something, failure to acknowledge skills and competencies) ________

Example 1 ________

Example 2 ________

w. Outside frustration or potential stress (worries about the job or having a bad day) ________

Example 1 ________

Example 2 ________

x. Social and entertainment activities (whether to attend something) ________

Example 1 ________

Example 2 ________

y. A difficulty not listed above ________

Example 1 ________

Example 2 ________

z. A complaint not listed above ________

Example 1 ________

Example 2 ________

2. Now that you have defined the meaning of these difficulties, you need to rank-order them according to how troublesome they are to you in this relationship. Rank as No. 1 the difficulty that is the most troublesome to you, rank as No. 2 the difficulty that is next troublesome to you, and so on; mark as N/A the difficulties that may not be troublesome to you at all or that does not apply to this relationship.

	Rank-Orders		
Difficulties	*Mine*	*Partner*	*Joint*
a. Doubts about the relationship's future	________	________	________
b. Disrespectful behavior	________	________	________
c. Extramarital intimacy boundary	________	________	________
d. Excessive or inappropriate displays of anger	________	________	________
e. Sexual interaction	________	________	________
f. Lack of communication	________	________	________
g. In-laws and extended family	________	________	________
h. Confusing, erratic, or emotional behavior	________	________	________
i. Criticism	________	________	________
j. Poor communication skills	________	________	________
k. Child-rearing issues	________	________	________
l. Finances	________	________	________
m. Lack of follow-through	________	________	________
n. Showing support in public or social situations	________	________	________
o. Showing affection	________	________	________
p. Lack of listening	________	________	________
q. Annoying behavior	________	________	________
r. Important decisions	________	________	________
s. Extent or quality of time together	________	________	________
t. Careless or unthinking behavior	________	________	________
u. Household tasks	________	________	________
v. Showing recognition or appreciation	________	________	________
w. Outside frustration or potential stress	________	________	________
x. Social and entertainment activities	________	________	________
y. A difficulty not listed above	________	________	________
z. A complaint not listed above	________	________	________

Homework: During the coming week, make an appointment with your partner and go over your definitions and your rank-orders of your difficulties as you see them Record your partner's rank-orders in the appropriate column and add both to achieve a joint rank-order. Take notes of your discussion while you are discussing (comparing and contrasting) your answers. Give your completed practice exercises and your notes to the professional who is assisting you with this practice exercise. If you do not have a professional helping you with this practice exercise, ask the advice of a friend to break any deadlock you both may have reached.

Whatever joint rank-order you agree with will determine the order of future practice exercises. The next practice exercise must be given the title of the joint complaint that has been rated together as No. 1. After that practice exercise, all other practice exercises should follow the joint rank-order given above.

Standard Practice Exercise for Couple Difficulties

Practice Exercise No. ____Title of Difficulty ____________________

Name ________________________________Sex ____Date _______

The purpose of this practice exercise is to understand more about the difficulty listed in the title.

1. How did this difficulty start? Explain in detail.

____
____
____
____
____

2. How often does this difficulty take place? Check which answer applies to you:

   a. Practically every day _____
   b. Once a week _____
   c. A couple of times a month _____
   d. Once a month _____
   e. Once every 6 months_____
   f. Once a year _____
   g. Once every few years_____

3. Please explain further.

____
____
____
____
____

4. How did this difficulty come about? Do you remember how it started? Check which answer fits best:

   a. As we met for the first time ______
   b. During courtship or while dating ______
   c. Before marriage or before we started living together ______
   d. During the honeymoon or as we were moving in together ______

e. Right after the honeymoon or right after we moved in together ______
f. Few months after the marriage or after we moved in together ______
g. 1 year after the marriage or when we moved in together ______
h. Years after marriage or when we moved in together ______

5. Please explain further.

____
____
____
____
____

6. What does this difficulty get you? Please explain.

____
____
____
____
____

7. Give three specific examples of how this difficulty is hurtful to you.

Example 1:

____
____
____
____
____

Example 2:

____
____
____
____
____

Example 3:

____
____
____
____
____

8. Give three specific examples of how this difficulty is hurtful to those you love and who love you.

Example 1:

___

___

___

___

___

Example 2:

___

___

___

___

___

Example 3:

___

___

___

___

___

Homework: Next week, plan to repeat this difficulty, if it belongs to you, or remind you partner to repeat it if it belongs to him or her. Make sure it is repeated at pre-set times (for instance, at 8 a.m., 12 noon, 4 or 7 p.m.), at least three times. Write down what happened in detail. In case you wonder why this difficulty should be started, keep in mind that if you or your partner start it, whoever starts it on time, will acquire the power to end it. For each time make sure to answer in writing the following four questions:

(a) How did it start?
(b) What followed?
(c) How did it end?
(d) What did this behavior get you or your partner?

Time 1 (write the time when it started ________)

a. ___
b. ___
c. ___
d ___

Time 2 (write the time when it started__________)

a. ____________________
b. ____________________
c. ____________________
d. ____________________

Time 3 (write time it started__________)

a. ____________________
b. ____________________
c. ____________________
d. ____________________

Check which of the following indicates what you got out of this practice exercise:

a. Completely useless ______
b. Somewhat useless ______
c. So-so ______
d. Somewhat useful ______
e. Extremely useful ______

Write down how you feel about this homework practice exercise and what you got out of it.

____
____
____
____
____

Concluding Follow-Up Form for Couple Difficulties

Name ____________________ Sex ______ Date ________

The purpose of this final practice exercise is to review whether the practice exercises in this practice exercise were helpful to you.

1. How do you feel about this practice exercise?

    a. I did not like working on this practice exercise at all. I wish I never saw it. ________
    b. I did not like this practice exercise, but I am glad I got to work on. ______
    c. I am happy I got a chance to work on this. ________
    d. I am not only delighted about this practice exercise, but I wish all husbands who use abusive or violent thinking could get it. ________

2. How helpful was it to work on this practice exercise? Please check the answer that applies to you:

a. Not helpful at all	_____	c. Helpful	_____
b. Somewhat helpful	_____	d. Very helpful	_____

3. Which practice exercise did you like best that was the most helpful to you? Rank-order the practice exercises. Rank as No. 1 the one that you liked best, rank as No. 2 the one you liked next best, and so on; mark as N/A the ones you did not like at all or did not apply to you.

	Rank-Orders		
Difficulties	*Mine*	*Partner*	*Joint*
a. Doubts about the relationship's future	_______	_______	_______
b. Disrespectful behavior	_______	_______	_______
c. Extramarital intimacy boundary	_______	_______	_______
d. Excessive or inappropriate displays of anger	_______	_______	_______
e. Sexual interaction	_______	_______	_______
f. Lack of communication	_______	_______	_______
g. In-laws and extended family	_______	_______	_______
h. Confusing, erratic, or emotional behavior	_______	_______	_______
i. Criticism	_______	_______	_______
j. Poor communication skills	_______	_______	_______
k. Child-rearing issues	_______	_______	_______
l. Finances	_______	_______	_______
m. Lack of follow-through	_______	_______	_______
n. Showing support in public or social situations	_______	_______	_______
o. Showing affection	_______	_______	_______
p. Lack of listening	_______	_______	_______
q. Annoying behavior	_______	_______	_______
r. Important decisions	_______	_______	_______
s. Extent or quality of time together	_______	_______	_______
t. Careless or unthinking behavior	_______	_______	_______
u. Household tasks	_______	_______	_______
v. Showing recognition or appreciation	_______	_______	_______
w. Outside frustration or potential stress	_______	_______	_______
x. Social and entertainment activities	_______	_______	_______
y. A difficulty not listed above	_______	_______	_______
z. A complaint not listed above	_______	_______	_______

4. Explain why you have rank-ordered the practice exercises the way you did.

____
____
____
____
____

5. Make an appointment with your partner and write down in the appropriate column your partner's rank-orders. Discuss (compare and contrast) whatever differences you may find in your individual rank-orders.

6. After completion of this practice exercise, write how you feel about it. Check which of these answers tells how you felt about it. There is also space for you to explain further, if you want to:

   a. I did not like it at all, a waste of time. I wish I never saw this stupid practice exercise. ________
   b. I did not like it very much, but I want to go on with another practice exercise. ________
   c. I liked it and I want to go on with another practice exercise. ________
   d. I liked it a lot and I wish I had something like this practice exercise earlier. ________
   e. I liked it so much that I wish all couples could get something like this practice exercise to work on. ________

7. How could this practice exercise be improved? Do you have any suggestions? Feel free to write whatever could improve this practice exercise.

____
____
____
____
____

Arguing or Fighting

The purpose of this practice exercise is to help you stop arguing and fighting in favor of negotiating over your differences. However, before learning how to negotiate, you need to give up arguing and fighting as a way of connecting with each other. It will not be easy but you should to give it a good try.

Practice Exercise 1. Description

Name ________________________________ Sex ____ Date _______

The purpose of this practice exercise is for each of you, independently of the other partner, to write about your arguing or fighting. After you have answered this practice exercise individually, set up an appointment at least 24 h ahead to discuss your answers with each other. If you get too angry during this discussion, take time out and get together within 24–48 h.

1. Define what an argument or fight is for you.

____

____

____

____

____

2. How does it take place in your home?

____

____

____

____

____

3. How often do you have these arguments or fights?

   a. Once a day or more ______
   b. Two or three times a week ______
   c. Once a week ______
   d. Once a month ______
   e. Once every 2 or 3 months ______
   f. Never or hardly ever ______

4. How long do these arguments or fights last?

   a. Sometimes the whole day or more ______
   b. A couple of hours or half a day ______
   c. About an hour or more ______
   d. Less than 30 minute ______
   e. 1 minute at the most ______

5. How heated, strong, or intense are these arguments or fights?

a. Very strong to the point of physical violence ______
b. Very intense but without physical violence ______
c. Strong and verbally abusive ______
d. Not very strong ______
e. We get excited but we calm down soon ______
f. Usually we keep cool and rational ______
g. We never lose our cool, we just avoid each other ______
h. We do not argue or fight, we just bicker ______
i. Other (explain): ______

____
____
____
____

6. How do these arguments or fights get started?

a. I usually start them ______
b. My partner usually starts them ______
c. Sometimes I start them, sometimes my partner starts them ______
d. I don't know ______
e. Other (explain): ______

____
____
____
____

7. How do these arguments or fights end?

a. We kiss and make up ______
b. We stay mad for hours ______
c. We stay mad for days ______
d. We stay mad for weeks on end ______
e. We stay away from each other until we have another argument or fight ______
f. Other (explain): ______

____
____
____
____

8. What are the major problems that start the argument or fight? Rank 1 for the most troublesome problem, 2 for second, etc. down to the least troublesome problem.

a.	Money	______	e.	Parents or in-laws	______
b.	Sex	______	f.	Friends	______
c.	Working hours and schedule	______	g.	Neighbors	______
d.	Children	______	h.	Other (explain):	______

____
____
____
____
____

9. Add whatever information you feel is important to better understand your arguments or fights. After you have answered these questions make an appointment (at least 24 h in advance) with your partner to look over your answers and to talk about them together. If possible, keep notes of your discussion and bring this completed practice exercise and your notes to your professional helper.

Practice Exercise 2. Explanations

Name ________________________________ Sex _____ Date _______

The purpose of this practice exercise is to find out what explanations you have for your arguing or fighting. If you do not like the explanations given below, come up with your own. After you have completed this practice exercise, get together (by preset appointment only) with your partner to compare and discuss your answers. If you get too angry, take time out and set up another appointment 24 or 48 h ahead.

A. Here is a list of what arguments or fights usually do for couples. Read them carefully on your own and think about which of the following explanations applies specifically to your relationship or family.

Arguments	*Rank-order*
1. Arguments are a good way of being involved, because as long as we spend energy on each other, we do not have to waste this energy either on our selves or outside of the family	_________
2. Arguments are one way of showing we care passionately about our family; usually we do not argue or fight with strangers or people we do not really care about	_________

Arguments	*Rank-order*
3. Arguments can be a good form of distraction; as long as we argue we do not need to worry about bills to be paid, how to set limits on each other, etc.	______
4. Arguments can also be a form of protection; we keep each other busy arguing so that the other one will not get depressed or leave the home or do more destructive things	______
5. Arguments are good ways of finding out how far we can go with each other and other members of the family; every time we have an argument, we test the limits of each other's endurance and patience	______
6. Arguments are a good way of blowing off steam and expressing oneself and letting other(s) in the family know how we feel about what we argue about	______
7. Arguments can be good way of providing excitement where there is nothing but boredom and apathy; they are a good way of proving we are alive	______
8. Arguments are one way of showing we are attracted to someone we love; we usually avoid people we do not like; therefore, arguments are better than withdrawing and avoiding contact by leaving the house	______
9. Arguments are one form of confrontation that indicate the need for change and progress in the family; without these confrontations, there would not be any improvement	______
10. Arguments are one form of conflict that is necessary in all families to settle accounts and to even scores among the various parties; without conflict, family members would not know how and where everybody stands on any problem	______

B. Now that you have read whether or how these explanations apply to you and to your relationship, rank-order them from the one that seems to apply the best to the one that applies the least to your arguments/fights. Rank as No. 1 the one that applies the most to you, rank as No. 2 the one that applies to you next best, and so on, down the line to the one that does not apply to you at all (No. 10).

C. If none of these explanations applies to you, disregard them and write down what you think is the most likely explanation for these arguments or fights.

____

____

____

____

____

D. What have you (personally, not your partner) done to improve these arguments or fights?

____

____

____

____

____

E. What could you (personally, not your partner) do to improve these arguments or fights? Explain in detail.

____

____

____

____

____

F. What could your partner do to improve these arguments or fights?

____

____

____

____

____

G. How are your present arguments or fights similar to or different from those your parents had (or failed to have)?

____

____

____

____

____

Homework: Make an appointment (at least 24 h ahead of time) to discuss (compare and contrast) your individual answers. It would help if you kept written notes of your discussion to bring to your professional helper.

Practice Exercise 3. Prescriptions

Name ______________________ Sex ________ Date ______

The purpose of this practice exercise is to show you how to argue or fight dirty. Have you ever had a clean argument or fight? If you have, more power to you. The more aware you become of how you argue or fight, the better will you be able to give it up. However, you will not be able to give it up until you are completely aware of how wasteful these arguments or fights are.

Here are guidelines on how to argue or fight really dirty. Note that if you want ensure that both of you and the whole family will lose, disregard completely these guidelines. You may also follow part of these guidelines and ignore other parts or withdraw completely and avoid confrontation and conflict. If you do not want to learn anything, keep on avoiding having any argument or fighting. In this way you will ensure that these arguments will go on. If you are interested in both you and your partner failing at arguments, as well as in other areas of your life, you may not only ignore these guidelines but also find something wrong with the author of these guidelines (He also is no darn good!)

A. Be sure to set an appointment date for the fight or argument at least 24 h in advance. It would be most helpful if you could agree (although it may be impossible) for you to argue on a regular schedule, like at a specific time on Mondays, Wednesdays, and Fridays, or Tuesdays, Thursdays, and Saturdays, or just on weekends, 8 o'clock, 9 o'clock, etc.
B. Choose a comfortable setting, preferably at the dining room or kitchen table or in the living room. You will need a table to take notes. Make sure that you sit as close to each other as possible.
C. Just before the argument or fight is to start, set a timer or alarm clock for just 1 h. Stop the argument as soon as the alarm rings. If your argument is not finished, reschedule the time for another argument at least 24 h in advance, then separate and go as far away from each other as your house (and your partner) will allow. If or when you meet again for a second argument, make sure you set the timer for 1 h.
D. Make a tape recording of your argument or fight. This recording is absolutely necessary. If you do not have a recording device, borrow or rent one. Also keep detailed written notes of what happened during and after the argument. Write down what you think or feel went on during the argument.
E. Follow as much as you can the following six destructive patterns that take place in most couple difficulties. If you follow a destructive pattern not contained in these instructions, make detailed notes of this pattern, describe it in detail, and bring it up the next time you meet with your counselor. In arguing, be sure to follow these seven destructive patterns as closely as possible:

    1. Use "You" statements exclusively, accusing, blaming, and name-calling each other as much as you can. For instance, use "You never_" and "You always_" statements as much as possible. Do not use either "I" or "We" statements under any conditions.
    2. Keep bringing up the painful past in as much negative detail as possible. Keep remembering dates, places situations, and occasions where you were hurt deeply. Keep on hurting each other by reliving as much as possible all of your past painful experiences in this relationship, which were obviously

the fault of your partner. See if each of you can top the other in remembering as many painful details as possible. Do not forget (or let alone forgive!) any single possible past hurt!

3. Read each other's mind. Try to tell each other what you think or feel. Disclose to each other all of the many evil intentions each of you knows the other one harbors. Bring up all of the possible nasty and guilty thoughts or feelings that your partner is guilty of thinking and feeling, let alone doing.
4. Use emotional blackmail and bribery, such as, "If you do not do what I want, I will leave you," or "If you do not give me what I want, I will call the lawyer," or "Either you quit (drinking, gambling, etc.) or I will take the children away," etc.
5. As part of point 4, give each other ultimatums. Threaten each other with the worst possible consequences that will follow from your partner's behavior. Make sure to specify dates and circumstances when you will make good on your ultimatum.
6. Make as many excuses as you can to justify your own behavior, especially by using your partner's behavior as an excuse: "I did such and such because you did such and such." Do not allow your partner to make any excuses for his or her behavior. Follow the principle that it is perfectly acceptable to behave miserably as long as your partner behaves miserably as well! Have a really dirty argument. Bring the recording to the next meeting.
7. Try to distract your partner from the major issue you are arguing about. Change the topic, sidetrack to another argument, find other issues to talk about that are not connected to the one you are arguing or fighting about.

Have a Good Dirty Argument or Fight!

Practice Exercise 4. Instructions

Name ______________________________Sex _______Date _________

The purpose of this practice exercise is for you to become painfully aware of, and perhaps give up, the destructive patterns that take place more often without you even knowing about them. The sooner you become aware of each destructive pattern, the better off you and your partner will be.

After recording the argument or fight prescribed in Practice Exercise No. 3 on a tape recorder, go back by yourself alone to listen to the recording of the argument or fight, without your partner. Below, there is list of the seven destructive patterns your were told to follow, plus whatever other pattern you have discovered that is peculiar to your arguing or fighting. Listen to the recording carefully and note each time you (not your partner) are indulging in any one of these patterns:

1. "You" statements: Total ______
2. Bringing up the painful past: Total ______
3. Mind-reading: Total ______
4. Blackmail or bribery: Total ______
5. Ultimatums or threats: Total ______
6. Excuses: Total ______
7. Distracting: Total ______
8. Your peculiar pattern: Total ______

Show and discuss these results with your partner after s/he has completed the same practice exercise. Then bring them with a written summary of your discussion to your next meeting with your professional helper. You will receive practice exercises that are specifically geared to deal with destructive patterns in the order of the highest total scores first, moving down to the lowest.

Instructions to professional helper: Administer the next practice exercises to each partner according to the number of times each partner has scored on each particular pattern. For instance, if one partner has the highest number of "you" statements, he or she should be administered the "you" statements practice exercise. By the same token, if the other partner has the highest number of statements on "mind-reading," he or she should receive the "mind-reading" practice exercise. Continue to administer practice exercises according to the scores given in Practice Exercise No. 4 in a descending order from most frequent to least frequent, or until they are no longer necessary.

Practice Exercise About Making "You" Statements

Name __________________________ Sex ________ Date __________

The purpose of this practice exercise is for you to become aware of how hurtful and destructive "you" statements are to you, to your partner, and to your relationship, so that perhaps you can stop using them.

1. How often do you think and speak about your partner?

   a. All the time ______
   b. Quite often (more than twice a week) ______
   c. Often enough (at least once a week) ______
   d. Sometimes (once or twice as month) ______

2. When do you think about your partner? Check which answer applies best:

   a. Only when I am angry ______
   b. Only when I am sad ______
   c. Only when I hurt ______
   d. Only when I am upset ______
   e. Only when (please complete this sen tence): ______

____
____
____
____
____

3. What is that you think about your partner?

   a. All negative ______
   b. More negative than positive ______
   c. More positive than negative ______
   d. All positive ______

4. Why do you think so much or so negatively about your partner? (Check more than one if appropriate):

   a. It keeps me busy and alive ______
   b. It distracts me from becoming sad ______
   c. It shows how much I care for my partner ______
   d. It takes away from my worries ______
   e. As long as I think and worry about my partner I do not have to worry about myself ______
   f. Give your own reason: . ______

____
____
____
____
____

5. What are your reactions to the possibility that thinking about your partner takes away from you and weakens your identity, hurting yourself?

____
____
____
____
____

6. What do you think about this other possibility: "I do not have to take responsibility for my behavior, because as long as I focus my energy on my partner, it leaves very little energy left for me to take care of myself and possibly change my behavior."

7. What do you think about the possibility that thinking excessively or negatively about your partner puts the whole burden of change on your partner rather than on you?

8. Now think about the usual result of your thinking too much and/or negatively about your partner:

    a. What does it do to you?

    b. What does it do to the relationship?

    c. What does it do to your partner?

d. What is the result, then, of your thinking excessively and/or negatively about your partner?

9. What would be the result if your partner were to do exactly what you are doing (that is, thinking excessively and/or negatively about you)?

10. Our language has mutually exclusive pronouns. If and when we use "you," it will be impossible for us to use the "I" or "we" pronouns. What do you think about this statement?

11. What are your reactions to the statement that using the "you" pronoun, that is, thinking and talking about your partner excessively and/or negatively, is the cancer of relationships?

12. Think of one or more positive reasons for continuing to use the "you" pronoun in thinking and talking about your partner:

13. Sometimes we can think of destructive patterns (described in Practice Exercise No. 4) as "suicidal" patterns. Why would this be so? What does the term "suicidal" mean to you?

____

____

____

____

____

14. "Suicidal" means to kill oneself. What do you think about using any behavior of this kind as destructive rather than suicidal?

____

____

____

____

____

Homework: Next week, see what happens to you and to your partner when you use the pronoun "You" instead of the "I" or "We" pronouns. Make sure you use "You" at least three times. Describe in detail what happened and what the outcome was.

Time No. 1 How did you use the "You?"

____

____

____

Outcome

____

____

____

Time No. 2 How did you use the "You?"

____

____

____

Outcome

____

____

____

Time No. 3 How did you use the "You?"

Outcome

Homework: If your want to have a miserable relationship, or if you want your relationship to end, all you have to do is continue thinking excessively and/or negatively about your partner by using the pronoun "You." Next week, write down three times when you used the pronouns "I" or "We" instead of the pronoun "You." Describe in detail what happened before, during, and after you used them.

Time No. 1 Before

During

After

Time No. 2 Before

During

After

Time No. 3 Before

During

After

After you have completed this practice exercise, make an appointment at least 24 h in advance with your partner to show and discuss your answers and their implications for the future of your relationship. Keep notes of your discussion and bring them to your professional helper with your completed practice exercises.

Practice Exercise About Bringing Up the Painful Past

Name ______________________________ Sex ________ Date __________

The purpose of this practice exercise is for you to become aware of how hurtful to yourself, to your partner, and to your relationship bringing up the past is, so that perhaps you will learn to stop doing it.

1. How often do you bring up the painful past when dealing with your partner?

   a. Almost every day ______
   b. At least once or twice a week ______
   c. Once every 2 or 3 weeks ______
   d. Once a month or less ______
   e. Once in a blue moon ______
   f. Never ______

If "f" is your answer, then this practice exercise must have been given to you in error. Check with your partner and your professional helper to find out why you were given this practice exercise.

2. When do you bring up the painful past?

   a. Only when we are fighting ______
   b. Only when we make love ______
   c. Anytime I feel bad, mad, or sad ______
   d. When (please complete as you see fit):

____
____
____
____

3. What does it get you to bring up hurts from the past? (Check more than one if appropriate):

   a. It makes me feel better about myself ______
   b. It makes my partner look bad ______
   c. I enjoy it ______
   d. It makes my partner feel bad ______
   e. Give your own reason:

____
____
____
____

4. What things (memories, events, episodes, hurts, etc.) from the past do you enjoy bringing up?

   a. Always pleasant ______
   b. Sometime pleasant ______
   c. Mostly hurtful ______
   d. Mostly unpleasant ______
   e. Always unpleasant ______
   f. None of the above ______

____
____
____
____
____

5. What does bringing up the painful past do to:

   a. You?

   b. Your relationship?

   c. Your partner?

6. What do you think about this statement: "As long as we keep on bringing up the painful past we have no time or energy left for a pleasant present or a better future?"

7. Suppose your partner kept on bringing up the painful past in the same way you do. What would happen:

   a. To you?

b. To your relationship?

c. To your partner?

Homework: During the coming week, note how often you keep bringing up the painful past and write down what happened for at least three of the times:

a. To you:

Time No. 1

Time No. 2

Time No. 3

b. To your relationship:

Time No. 1

Time No. 2

Time No. 3

c. To your partner:

Time No. 1

Time No. 2

Time No. 3

____

After you have completed this practice exercise, make an appointment with your partner at least 24 h in advance to show, discuss, and compare your answers to the questions above. Summarize and record your discussion.

Practice Exercise About Mind Reading

Name ________________________ Sex ________ Date __________

The purpose of this practice exercise is to make you aware of how hurtful mind reading is to you, to your relationship, and to your partner.

As part of your caring for and committing to your relationship, you might be spending a great deal of time and energy wondering what your partner feels, thinks, and does. Often you may even be sure that you know exactly beforehand, without asking or checking it out, what your partner feels, thinks, or does. This kind of behavior is frequent in couples who care a great deal about each other but who cannot separate one's self from the other's self. Does this behavior apply to you? If your answer is no, stop this exercise. If your answer is yes, go on.

1. How often do you wonder about your partner's feelings, thinking, motives, and behavior?

   a. All the time ______
   b. Very often ______
   c. Often enough ______
   d. Rarely ______
   e. Almost never ______

2. What do you wonder about or really know about your partner? Describe in detail:

   a. His/her feelings

____

b. His/her attitudes

____
____
____
____
____

c. His/her thinking

____
____
____
____
____

d. His/her motives

____
____
____
____
____

e. His/her behavior

____
____
____
____
____

f. Any other area or topic not covered by questions asked above:

____
____
____
____
____

3. Are there special or particular times when you wonder and know what your partner is feeling or thinking?

   a. When we fight ______
   b. When we make love ______
   c. When we are apart ______

d. When I feel sad ______
e. When I am angry ______
f. Any other occasion or situation not covered by the above items: ______

____
____
____
____
____

4. What does reading your partner's mind do for you?

a. It makes me happier ______
b. It makes my partner happier ______
c. It keeps me busy ______
d. It makes him/her mad ______
e. It makes me sad ______
f. It makes me feel better about myself ______
g. Any other result not included in the above items: ______

____
____
____
____
____

5. What does reading your partner's mind do for your relationship?

a. It improves it considerably ______
b. It keeps it exciting ______
c. It renews it ______
d. It makes it worse ______
e. It's the pits! ______

6. Describe in greater detail what reading your partner's mind does for you and for your relationship:

____
____
____
____
____

7. What would happen to your relationship if your partner read your mind the way you read your partner's?

8. Why do you think mind reading is a suicidal pattern in any close and prolonged relationship?

9. What would happen to you if you did not read your partner's mind?

10. What would happen to your relationship if you did not read your partner's mind?

Homework: During the coming week, write down every time you find yourself reading your partner's mind; keep track of at least three times. Record what happens to you and to your relationship when you read your partner's mind.

Time No. 1 What did your mind reading consist of?

What was the result of your mind reading?

Time No. 2 What did your mind reading consist of?

What was the result of your mind reading?

Time No. 3 What did your mind reading consist of?

What was the result of your mind reading?

Write down three times when you did *not* read your partner's mind and instead you asked and checked out what s/he was feeling, thinking, or planning to do. What happened?

Time No. 1

Time No. 2

Time No. 3

___

___

___

Homework: After you have finished answering this practice exercise, make an appointment with your partner at least 24 h in advance to discuss your answers to the questions above. Keep notes of your discussion and bring them with your completed practice exercises to your professional helper.

Practice Exercise About Blackmail/Bribery

Name ______________________ Sex ______ Date _________

The purpose of this practice exercise is to make you aware of how hurtful blackmail or bribery is to you, to your partner, and to your relationship, so that perhaps you can stop doing it.

Most examples of this suicidal/homicidal pattern are emotional, and they are usually proceeded by an "If," as in, "If you do not do what I want, I will leave you." In other words, emotional blackmail or bribery is an abusive form of control, coercion, and manipulation in order to get one's way.

1. Do you use this pattern in your relationship? If your answer is no, you may stop this practice exercise. If your answer is yes, continue.

2. How often do you use it?

   a. Very often (once a day) ______
   b. Often (two or three times a week) ______
   c. Sometimes (once every 2 weeks) ______
   d. Seldom (once every 2 or 3 months) ______

3. How and when do you use blackmail? Describe in detail:

___

___

___

___

___

4. How and when do you use bribery?

5. What do you get out of using either blackmail or bribery?

6. How does this pattern affect your relationship?

7. How does this pattern affect your partner?

8. What happens or what would happen if or when your partner were to use this pattern with you?

9. Can you remember how you learned this pattern? When did you start using it?

10. Are you ready to give it up? If your answer is no, don't go any further. Keep on using this pattern and see what it gets you in the long run. If your answer is yes, then read on and do the following homework practice exercise.

Homework: During all of next week, use this pattern at least three times. Remember that: if you want to stop it, you have to learn to start it. Write in detail what specific kind of blackmail you used and the situation in which you used it. What was the result?

Time No. 1 Use

Result

Time No. 2 Use

Result

Time No. 3 Use

Result

Also during the next week record three times when you used bribery. How did you use it and what was the result?

Time No. 1 Use

Result

Time No. 2 Use

Result

Time No. 3 Use

Result

____

____

____

After completing this homework, make an appointment with your partner at least 24 h ahead of time to show and discuss your answers to this practice exercise. Bring your completed practice exercises and notes to your professional helper.

Practice Exercise About Excuses

Name __________________________ Sex ________ Date ____________

The purpose of this practice exercise is to show you how hurtful excuses are to you, to your partner, and to your relationship.

Often excuses are used to explain or justify one's behavior. For instance, you may use your partner's (rotten!) behavior to justify your own actions: "I did this and that because you did this and that." In other words, we make excuses for our (rotten!) behavior on the basis of our partner's behavior. Usually, however, we do not accept the same pattern of excuses from our partner. The premise behind this pattern is that it is perfectly acceptable to behave miserably as long as our partner behaves miserably as well!

1. How often do you use this pattern?
   a. Very often (almost every day) _____
   b. Often (once or twice a week) _____
   c. Sometimes (once or twice a month) _____
   d. Seldom (once every 2 or 3 months) _____
   e. Never _____

If you never use excuses, then this practice exercise was given to you by mistake. Discuss this possibility with your partner and your professional helper. If either one (partner or helper) feels that you do use excuses while you do not feel you do, let them record your excuses in writing and present them to you after 1 or 2 weeks. Only then will you be able to go on with this practice exercise.

2. How do you make excuses? Describe in detail:

____

____

____

____

____

3. What does this pattern mean? Check more than one if necessary:
   a. I am unable to take responsibility for myself and my behavior ____
   b. I behave better than my partner ____
   c. My partner is wrong and I am right ____
   d. My behavior is excusable, but my partner's behavior is not ____
   e. As long as my partner behaves miserably I have the same right ____
   f. Write your own explanation: ____

____

____

____

____

____

4. How do you react to the following statement: "Children find excuses for their behavior; adults need to take responsibility for their actions?"

____

____

____

____

____

5. What do you get out of making excuses for your behavior?

____

____

____

____

____

6. What would happen to your relationship if both you and your partner made excuses about your behavior?

____

____

____

____

____

7. How did you learn to make excuses? Explain in detail:

Homework: If you want to learn to stop this pattern, follow these instructions. Next week, try to find at least three situations where you can make excuses for your behavior. Write below each situation in detail and report on the results.

Situation No. 1 Excuse used

What happened?

Situation No. 2 Excuse used

What happened?

____
____
____
____

Situation No. 3 Excuse used

____
____
____

What happened?

____
____
____

____
____
____

Homework: After you have completed this practice exercise, make an appointment with your partner at least 24 h in advance. Show and discuss your answers with your partner. See whether together you can come up with more helpful ways to take responsibility for your behavior than just finding excuses. Make notes of your discussion and bring them to your professional helper.

Practice Exercise About Ultimatums

Name ________________________________ Sex ______ Date _____

The purpose of this practice exercise is to become aware of how hurtful ultimatums are to you, to your partner, and to your relationship.

1. What does the word "ultimatum" mean to you? Check one:

   a. A meaningless foreign word _____
   b. One of those big words doctors use to make themselves feel important _____
   c. Another form of bribery/blackmail _____
   d. One of those words your partner uses to be one up on you _____

e. Find your own definition (you may use your dictionary if you want): _____

2. Would you agree that an ultimatum consists of a deadline or of a consequence that would have negative results for your partner? Please comment:

3. How often do you use ultimatums?

a. Practically every day _____
b. Once a week _____
c. Once a month
d. Once in a blue moon _____
e. Other (explain): _____

4. When do you use ultimatums?

a. When my partner makes me mad _____
b. When I make my partner mad _____
c. When I am under pressure _____
d. When I don't know what else to do _____
e. When I (complete it you rself):

5. What kind of ultimatums do you give your partner? Give at least three examples:

   Example 1:

   ____

   ____

   ____

   ____

   ____

   Example 2:

   ____

   ____

   ____

   ____

   ____

   Example 3:

   ____

   ____

   ____

   ____

   ____

6. Why do you give ultimatums? Check as many as apply:

   a. Because I enjoy it _____
   b. Because it makes me feel good _____
   c. Because it gives me a sense of satisfaction _____
   d. Because in this way I can control my partner _____
   e. Because it worked for my parents _____
   f. Because (give a reason not listed above): _____

   ____

   ____

   ____

   ____

   ____

7. What do ultimatums do

   a. To you?

   b. To your relationship?

   c. To your partner?

8. How did you learn to use ultimatums?

9. What would happen to your relationship if your partner were to give you ultimatums?

Homework: Next week, try to use as many ultimatums as you can. List at least three of them below. Write

a. What kind of ultimatum you used
b. With whom
c. What kind of result you got out of it

Ultimatum No. 1

a. ______________________________
____
____

b. ______________________________
____
____

c. ______________________________
____
____

Ultimatum No. 2

a. ______________________________
____
____

b. ______________________________
____
____

c. ______________________________
____
____

Ultimatum No. 3

a. ______________________________
____
____

b. ______________________________
____
____

c. ______________________________
____
____

Homework: After completing this practice exercise show and discuss it with your partner after setting an appointment at least 24 h ahead of time. Discuss what you learned from it and write down what you two discussed about it. Bring this practice exercise and your notes to your professional helper.

Practice Exercise About Your Own Peculiar Pattern

Name ______________________________ Sex ______ Date __________

The purpose of this practice exercise is for you to become aware of any pattern that may be hurtful to you, to your partner, and to your relationship, so that perhaps you can stop doing it.

By listening to the recording of your last fight, in addition to reviewing the seven destructive patterns listed in Practice Exercise No. 3, you might have been able to find a peculiar destructive pattern that is specific to how you two argue or fight. For instance, another common destructive pattern is "Distracting," that is, changing the subject or introducing extraneous or irrelevant arguments. If you find another pattern, congratulations! Not many partners can. Do you want to replace it or do you want to keep it?

1. Define and describe in detail this peculiar pattern. What does it consist of?

____

____

____

____

____

2. Write down the advantages and disadvantages of this pattern.

   a. Advantages

____

____

____

____

____

   b. Disadvantages

____

____

____

____

____

3. How often do you use it?

   a. Very often (almost every day) ______
   b. Often enough (once or twice a week) ______
   c. Occasionally (once every 2 or 3 weeks) ______
   d. Once in a while (once every 2 or 3 months) ______

4. When does it take place?

____
____
____
____
____

5. What does it get either one of you? Check more than one answer if necessary:

   a. It shows we love each other ______
   b. It keeps us busy ______
   c. It allow us to make contact ______
   d. It keeps us excited ______
   e. It keeps us from being bored ______
   f. Give your explanation for using this pattern: ______

____
____
____
____
____

6. Do you enjoy it? In what way?

____
____
____
____
____

7. If you enjoy it, keep it up, and stop answering these questions. If you do not enjoy it and you want to replace it with a more positive pattern, complete the following homework practice exercise.

Homework: During the coming week, make sure that either one of you will use this peculiar pattern at least three times. If necessary, flip a coin to decide which of you should use it first. Write down how this pattern was used and what the result was.

Time No. 1 Use

____
____
____
____

Result

____
____
____
____

Time No. 2 Use

____
____
____

Result

____
____
____

Time No. 3 Use

____
____
____

Result

____
____
____

Homework: After completing this practice exercise, make an appointment with your partner, at least 24 h in advance, and discuss how you could replace this peculiar pattern with a more positive one. Make notes of your discussion and bring them to your professional helper.

Violence

The purpose of this practice exercise is to help couples at risk for violence in their relationship confront and control thoughts that may lead them to violence.

Practice Exercise 1. Defining Thoughts About Violence in the Relationship

Name ______________________________ Sex ______ Date __________

The purpose of this practice exercise is to understand what thoughts of partner violence consist of in your particular case.

1. Below there is a list of violent or abusive thoughts that may come to mind when you are angry. You will find some of these words about your thoughts rather strange and unusual. If you do not understand what the thought listed below means, consult a dictionary or ask your partner, a friend, or whoever is helping you learn to control your violence. After you have defined each thought, give two examples for each specific thought listed.

Definitions of Violent Thoughts	*Examples*
a. Placing hostile blame on partner	Example 1 ________
________	________
________	Example 2 ________
________	________
b. Magnification	Example 1 ________
________	________
________	Example 2 ________
________	________
c. Either/or thinking	Example 1 ________
________	________
________	Example 2 ________
________	________
d. Arbitrary inference	Example 1 ________
________	________
________	Example 2 ________
________	________
e. Demandingness	Example 1 ________
________	________
________	Example 2 ________
________	________
f. Anger-control statements	Example 1 ________
________	________
________	Example 2 ________
________	________
g. Personalization	Example 1 ________
________	________
________	Example 2 ________
________	________

h. "Awfulizing" Example 1 ____________________
______________________________ ____________________
______________________________ Example 2 ____________________
______________________________ ____________________

i. Overgeneralization Example 1 ____________________
______________________________ ____________________
______________________________ Example 2 ____________________
______________________________ ____________________

j. Negative self-thoughts Example 1 ____________________
______________________________ ____________________
______________________________ Example 2 ____________________
______________________________ ____________________

k. Low frustration tolerance Example 1 ____________________
______________________________ ____________________
______________________________ Example 2 ____________________
______________________________ ____________________

2. Check whether each thought applies to you not at all, sometimes, or most of the time:

Violent Thoughts	*Applies* *Not at all*	*Sometimes*	*Most of the time*	*Rank-order*
a. Placing hostile blame on partner	______	______	______	______
b. Magnification	______	______	______	______
c. Either/or thinking	______	______	______	______
d. Arbitrary inference	______	______	______	______
e. Demandingness	______	______	______	______
f. Anger-control statements	______	______	______	______
g. Personalization	______	______	______	______
h. "Awfulizing"	______	______	______	______
i. Overgeneralization	______	______	______	______
j. Negative self-thoughts	______	______	______	______
k. Low frustration tolerance	______	______	______	______

3. Now rank-order these thoughts according to how frequent, serious, or strong they are in your relationship with your partner. Rank as No. 1 the thought that is the strongest or most frequent, rank as No. 2 the thought that is second

strongest or most frequent, and so on; mark as N/A the thoughts that may not apply to your relationship.

4. Which of these thoughts were present in your family of origin? Please check whether they applied to your mother (or mother substitute), father (or father substitute), brothers, or sisters, if present. Check all that apply:

Violent Thoughts	*Mother*	*Father*	*Brothers*	*Sisters*
a. Placing hostile blame on wife/husband	_____	_____	_____	_____
b. Magnification	_____	_____	_____	_____
c. Either/or thinking	_____	_____	_____	_____
d. Arbitrary inference	_____	_____	_____	_____
e. Demandingness	_____	_____	_____	_____
f. Anger-control statements	_____	_____	_____	_____
g. Personalization	_____	_____	_____	_____
h. "Awufulizing"	_____	_____	_____	_____
i. Overgeneralization	_____	_____	_____	_____
j. Negative self-thoughts	_____	_____	_____	_____
k. Low frustration tolerance	_____	_____	_____	_____

Homework: During the next few days write down all of the advantages and disadvantages you get from thinking violent thoughts.

Standard Practice Exercise for Violence in a Relationship

Practice Exercise No. ____Title: ________________________________

Name ________________________________Sex _____Date _______

The purpose of this practice exercise is to understand more about the thought listed in the title.

1. How did you start using this thought? Please explain in detail:

____

____

____

____

____

2. How often do you use this thought? Check which answer applies to you:

a.	Practically every day	_____	e.	Once every 6 months	_____
b.	Once a week	_____	f.	Once a year	_____
c.	A couple of times a month	_____	g.	Once every few years	_____
d.	Once a month	_____			

3. Please explain further:

____

____

____

____

____

4. How did this thought come about? Do you remember when you started thinking it?
Check the answer that fits best:

a. When I was a child (younger than 5 years of age) _____
b. In elementary school _____
c. In middle school _____
d. In high school _____
e. Any other time _____

5. Please explain further:

____

____

____

____

____

6. What does this thought do for you or get you? Please explain:

____

____

____

____

____

7. Give three specific examples of how this thought was hurtful to you in the past:

   Example 1:

   Example 2:

   Example 3:

8. Give three specific examples of how this thought is hurtful to you in the present:

   Example 1:

   Example 2:

Example 3:

9. Give three specific examples of how this thought will be hurtful to you in the future:

Example 1:

Example 2:

Example 3:

10. Give three specific examples of how this thought was hurtful to those you love and who love you:

Example 1:

Example 2:

____
____
____
____
____

Example 3:

____
____
____
____
____

Homework: Next week plan to repeat this thought at preset times (for instance, at 8 a.m., 12 noon, 4 or 7 p.m.), at least three times. Write down what you thought in detail. *If you can start it, you can stop it.* For each time this thought comes to mind, make sure to answer in writing the following four questions:

(a) How did you start it?
(b) What followed?
(c) How did it end?
(d) What did this behavior get you?

Time 1 (write time you started __________)

a. ____
____
____

b. ____
____
____

c. ____
____
____

d. ____
____
____

Time 2 (write time you started __________)

a. ____
____
____

b. ____
____
____

c. ____
____
____

d. ____
____
____

Time 3 (write time you started__________)

a. ____
____
____

b. ____
____
____

c. ____
____
____

d. ____
____
____
____

Check which of the following shows what you got out of this practice exercise:

a.	Completely useless	_____	d.	Somewhat useful	_____
b.	Somewhat useless	_____	e.	Extremely useful	_____
c.	So-so	_____			

Write down how you feel about this practice exercise and what you got out of it:

____
____
____
____
____

Final Follow-Up Form for Violence in a Relationship

Name ________________________________ Sex ____ Date ______

The purpose of this form is to review whether the practice exercises in this practice exercise were helpful to you.

1. Which answer best fits how you feel about this practice exercise?

   a. I did not like working on this practice exercise at all. I wish I never saw it. ________

   b. I did not like this practice exercise, but I am glad I got to work on it. ________

   c. I am happy I got a chance to work on this. ________

   d. I am not only delighted about this practice exercise, but I wish all husbands who use abusive or violent thinking could get it. ________

2. How helpful was it to work on this practice exercise? Please check the answer that applies to you:

   a. Not helpful at all ______
   b. Somewhat helpful ______
   c. Helpful ______
   d. Very helpful ______

3. Which practice exercise did you like best? Rank as No. 1 the one that you liked best, rank as No. 2 the one you liked next best, and so on; mark as N/A the ones you did not like at all or did not apply to you.

Violent Thoughts	*Rank-order*
a. Placing hostile blame on partner	________
b. Magnification	________
c. Either/or thinking	________
d. Arbitrary inference	________
e. Demandingness	________
f. Anger-control statements	________
g. Personalization	________
h. “Awfulizing”	________
i. Overgeneralization	________
j. Negative self-thoughts	________
k. Low frustration tolerance	________

4. Now that you have completed this practice exercise, check which of these answers describes how you feel about it. There is also space for you to explain further, if you want to:

   a. I did not like it at all, a waste of time. I wish I never saw this stupid practice exercise. ________
   b. I did not like it very much, but I want to go on with another practice exercise. ________
   c. I liked it and I want to go on with another practice exercise. ________
   d. I liked it a lot and I wish I had something like this practice exercise earlier. ________
   e. I liked it so much that I wish all partners with violent or abusive thoughts could get something like this practice exercise to work on. ________

5. How could this practice exercise be improved? Do you have any suggestions? Feel free to write whatever could improve this practice exercise.

____
____
____
____
____
____

Controlling Violence

The purpose of this practice exercise is to help partners at risk for violence confront and control their tendencies toward violence. The purpose of this practice exercise is to understand what violence consists of in your particular case.

Practice Exercise 1. Defining Violence in a Relationship

Name ______________________ Sex ______ Date ________

1. Below is a list of violent or abusive behaviors. Please check whether each behavior applies to you not at all, sometimes, or most of the time:

	Applies			
Abusive or Violent Behaviors	*Not at all*	*Sometimes*	*Most of the time*	*Rank*
a. Insulting or swearing	______	______	______	______
b. Sulking or refusing to talk	______	______	______	______
c. Stomping out	______	______	______	______
d. Crying	______	______	______	______
e. Doing or saying something to spite	______	______	______	______

f. Threatening to hit or throw	____	____	____	____
g. Throwing an object	____	____	____	____
h. Throwing object at partner	____	____	____	____
i. Pushing-grabbing-shoving partner	____	____	____	____
j. Slapping partner	____	____	____	____
k. Kicking-biting-hitting with fist	____	____	____	____
l. Hitting with object	____	____	____	____
m. Beating up	____	____	____	____
n. Choking or strangling	____	____	____	____
o. Threatening with knife or gun	____	____	____	____
p. Using knife or gun	____	____	____	____
q. Any other physical violence	(____)	____	____	____

2. Now rank-order these behaviors according to how frequent, serious, or strong they are in your relationship. Rank as No. 1 the behavior that is the strongest or most frequent, rank as No. 2 the behavior that is second strongest or most frequent, and so on; mark as N/A the behaviors that may not apply to your relationship.

3. Which of these behaviors were present in your family of origin? Please check whether they applied to your mother (or mother substitute), father (or father substitute), brothers or sisters if present. Check all that apply:

	Applies			
Abusive or Violent Behaviors	*Mother*	*Father*	*Brother*	*Sister*
a. Insulting or swearing	____	____	____	____
b. Sulking or refusing to talk	____	____	____	____
c. Stomping out	____	____	____	____
d. Crying	____	____	____	____
e. Doing or saying something to spite	____	____	____	____
f. Threatening to hit or throw	____	____	____	____
g. Throwing an object	____	____	____	____
h. Throwing object at partner	____	____	____	____
i. Pushing-grabbing-shoving partner	____	____	____	____
j. Slapping partner	____	____	____	____
k. Kicking-biting-hitting with fist	____	____	____	____
l. Hitting with object	____	____	____	____
m. Beating up	____	____	____	____
n. Choking or strangling	____	____	____	____
o. Threatening with knife or gun	____	____	____	____
p. Using knife or gun	____	____	____	____
q. Any other physical violence	(____)	____	____	____

Homework: During the next few days write down all of the advantages and disadvantages you get from behaving in an abusive or violent fashion.

Standard Practice Exercise for Violence in a Relationship

Practice Exercise No. ____Title: ______________________________

Name ______________________________Sex ________Date ______

The purpose of this practice exercise is to understand more about the behavior listed in the title.

1. How did you start to use this behavior? Please explain in detail:

____
____
____
____
____

2. How often do you use this behavior? Check which answer applies to you:

   a. Practically every day ______
   b. Once a week ______
   c. A couple of times a month ______
   d. Once a month ______
   e. Once every 6 months ______
   f. Once a year ______
   g. Once every few years ______

3. Please explain further:

____
____
____
____
____

4. How did this behavior come about? Do you remember when you started it? Check which answer fits best:

   a. When I was a child (younger than 5 years of age) ______
   b. In elementary school ______
   c. In middle school ______
   d. In high school ______
   e. Any other time ______

5. Please explain further:

6. What does this behavior get you?
Please explain:

7. Give three specific examples of how this behavior was hurtful to you. Please explain:

Example 1:

Example 2:

Example 3:

8. Give three specific examples of how this behavior was hurtful to those you love and who love you.

Example 1:

____
____
____
____
____

Example 2:

____
____
____
____
____

Example 3:

____
____
____
____
____

Homework: Next week plan to repeat this behavior at preset times (for instance, at 8 a.m., 12 noon, 4 or 7 p.m.), at least three times. Write down what happened in detail. For each time make sure to answer in writing the following four questions:

(a) How did you start it?
(b) What followed?
(c) How did it end?
(d) What did this behavior get you?

Time 1 (write time you started __________)

a. ____
____
____

b. ____
____
____

c. ____
____
____

d. ____
____
____

Time 2 (write time you started __________)

a. ____
____
____

b. ____
____
____

c. ____
____
____

d. ____
____
____

Time 3 (write time you started __________)

a. ____
____
____

b. ____
____
____

c. ____
____
____

d. ____
____
____

Check which of the following shows what you got out of this practice exercise:

a. Completely useless ______
b. Somewhat useless ______
c. So-so ______
d. Somewhat useful ______
e. Extremely useful ______

Write down how you feel about this homework practice exercise and what you got out of it:

____

____

____

____

____

Concluding Feedback Form for Violence in a Relationship

Name ______________________________ Sex ______ Date __________

The purpose of this form is to review whether practice exercises in this practice exercise were helpful to you.

1. Which answer fits how you feel about this practice exercise?

   a. I did not like working on this practice exercise at all. I wish I never saw it. ______
   b. I did not like this practice exercise, but I am glad I got to work on. ______
   c. I am happy I got a chance to work on it. ______
   d. I am not only delighted with this practice exercise, but I wish all people who use abusive or violent behavior could get it. ______

2. How helpful was it to work on this practice exercise? Please check the answer that applies to you.

   a. Not helpful at all ______
   b. Somewhat helpful ______
   c. Helpful ______
   d. Very helpful ______

3. Which practice exercise did you like best? Rank as No. 1 the one that you liked best, rank as No. 2 the one you liked next best, and so on; mark as N/A the ones you did not like at all or did not apply to you.

Abusive or Violent Behaviors *Rank-order*

a. Insulting or swearing ______
b. Sulking or refusing to talk ______
c. Stomping out ______
d. Crying ______
e. Doing or saying something to spite ______

f. Threatening to hit or throw ________
g. Throwing an object ________
h. Throwing object at partner ________
i. Pushing-grabbing-shoving partner ________
j. Slapping partner ________
k. Kicking-biting-hitting with fist ________
l. Hitting with object ________
m. Beating up ________
n. Choking or strangling ________
o. Threatening with knife or gun ________
p. Using knife or gun ________
q. Any other physical violence (________)

4. Now that you have completed this practice exercise, check which of these answers indicates how you feel about it. There is also space for you to explain further, if you want to:

   a. I did not like it at all, a waste of time. I wish I never worked on this stupid practice exercise. ________
   b. I did not like it very much, but I want to go on with working on practice excercises of this type. ________
   c. I liked it and I want to go on with another practice exercise. ________
   d. I liked it a lot and I wish I had received something like this practice exercise earlier in my life. ________
   e. I liked it so much that I wish all violent or abusive individuals could get something like this practice exercise to work on. ________

5. How could this practice exercise be improved? Do you have any suggestions? Feel free to write whatever could improve this practice exercise.

____
____
____
____
____

Families

When Parents Argue: From the Eyes of a Child

Instructions to the professional: Make sure both parents sign an informed consent form. Parents should make an appointment with each other at prestated, prearranged times. They are to complete each practice exercise individually and then compare, contrast, and discuss with each other their answers to each practice exercise by appointment. They should not meet for longer than 1 h (by preset timer). If they get too angry, should call time out, go to opposite corners, and reschedule another appointment at least 24 h ahead.

The second and subsequent practice exercises should be administered according to the combined rank-orders of arguments given by both parents. The practice exercise that receives the lowest combined score should be administered first. The one that receives the second lowest combined score should be administered second, and so on. The title and number of each practice exercise should be written on top of each practice exercise. The number of practice exercises to be administered depends on the number of items parents agree or disagree about. The more virulent the arguments, the greater should be the number of practice exercises to be administered.

To parents: The purpose of this practice exercise is to help you both have better arguments, that is, instead of arguing, learning how to negotiate by "proacting" with each other rather than reacting to each other. If you both have agreed to work together on this practice exercise, it means that you love each other enough to make things better for both and your children. This practice exercise, however, may be useless unless you set appointments with each other at predetermined, agreed-upon times to discuss your individually completed practice exercises. If, during one of these appointments you find yourself getting too angry, call for time out and reschedule another appointment at least 24 h ahead. This postponement will allow you to cool off and process what is going on between you two. Keep in mind that indifference is the opposite of love. If you get upset with each other, it means you still care.

Practice Exercise 1. What Do You Argue About?

Name ______________________________ Sex _____ Date ________

The purpose of this practice exercise is to find out how you see the seriousness of your arguments:

1. How often do you have these arguments or fights?

   a. Once a day or more ______
   b. Two or three times a week ______
   c. Once a week ______
   d. Once a month ______
   e. Once every 2 or 3 months ______
   f. Never or hardly ever ______

2. How long do these arguments or fights last?

   a. Sometimes the whole day or more ______
   b. A couple of hours or half a day ______
   c. About an hour ______
   d. Less than 30 minute ______
   e. 1 minute at the most ______

3. How heated, strong, or intense are these arguments or fights?

   a. Very strong to the point of physical violence ______
   b. Very intense but without physical violence ______
   c. Strong and verbally abusive ______
   d. Not very strong ______
   e. We get excited but we calm down soon ______
   f. Usually we keep cool and rational ______
   g. We never lose our cool, we just avoid each other ______
   h. We do not argue or fight, we just bicker ______
   i. Other (explain) ______

4. How do these arguments or fights get started?

   a. I usually start them ______
   b. My partner usually starts them ______
   c. Sometimes I start them, sometimes my partner starts them ______
   d. I don't know ______
   e. Other (explain) ______

5. How do these arguments or fights end?

   a. We kiss and make up ______
   b. We stay mad for hours ______
   c. We stay mad for days ______
   d. We stay mad for weeks on end ______
   e. We stay away from each other until we have another argument or fight ______
   f. Other (explain): ______

6. Why do you argue or fight? Rank as No. 1 the most troublesome reason for arguing, rank as No. 2 the second most troublesome reason for arguing, and so on; mark as N/A the reasons that do not apply.

Reasons for Arguing	*Your Rank-order*	*Partner's Rank-order*	*Combined Rank-order*
a. It's our fault when we do it	________	________	________
b. One partner wants things one way and the other wants them another way	________	________	________
c. Work	________	________	________
d. We do not know how to get along	________	________	________
e. We do not understand each other	________	________	________
f. Money	________	________	________
g. Our children misbehave and do something wrong	________	________	________
h. One partner is worried about something	________	________	________
i. Chores or jobs around the house	________	________	________
j. One partner had a bad day	________	________	________
k. The other partner had a bad day	________	________	________
l. People outside the family, relatives/friends	________	________	________
m. One partner is worried about something	________	________	________
n. One partner does not feel good	________	________	________
o. It's our children's fault	________	________	________
p. One partner does not feel well	________	________	________
q. The kind of person one partner is	________	________	________
r. Our children are bad	________	________	________
s. It's one partner's fault	________	________	________
t. One partner is the kind of person who likes to argue	________	________	________
u. The kind of person the partner is	________	________	________
v. We really do not like each other	________	________	________
w. It's the other partner's fault	________	________	________
x. The other partner is the kind of person who likes to argue	________	________	________
y. State your own reason (____________________)	________	________	________

7. Now state why you rank-ordered these reasons for arguing the way you did it.

____
____
____
____
____

Homework: By preset appointment, compare, contrast, and discuss with each other your answers to this practice exercise. Write down the respective rank-orders of your partner on your sheet and combine the two rankings in the last column above. Give copies of your completed practice exercises to whoever is helping you with this practice excercise.

Standard Practice Exercise for Arguing and Fighting

Practice Exercise No.____Title of Practice Exercise________________

Name__________________________________Sex_____Date________

The purpose of this practice exercise is to understand more about the reason for arguing listed in the title.

1. How did you start to use this reason this way? Please explain in detail:

____
____
____
____
____

2. How often do you use this reason? Check which answer applies to you:

a.	Practically every day	_____	e.	Once every 6 months	_____
b.	Once a week	_____	f.	Once a year	_____
c.	A couple of times a month	_____	g.	Once every few years	_____
d.	Once a month	_____			

3. Please explain further:

____
____
____
____
____

4. How did this reason come about? Do you remember when you started it? Check which answer fits best:

a. When I was a child (younger than 5 years of age) ______
b. In elementary school ______
c. In middle school ______
d. In high school ______
e. Any other tim ______

5. Please explain further:

____
____
____
____
____

6. What does this reason get you? Please explain:

____
____
____
____
____

7. Give three specific examples of how using this reason is hurtful to you.

Example 1:

____
____
____
____
____

Example 2:

Example 3:

8. Give three specific examples of how this reason is hurtful to your partner.

Example 1:

Example 2:

Example 3:

Homework: If you want to stop undesirable behavior, learn to start it. If you learn to start it, you will learn to stop it. Next week plan to repeat it using this reason at preset times (for instance, at 8 a.m., 12 noon, 4 or 7 p.m.) at least three times. Write down what happened in detail. For each time make sure to answer in writing the following four questions:

(a) How did you start it?
(b) What followed?
(c) How did it end?
(d) What did this reason get you?

Time 1 (write the time you started __________)

a. ____
____
____

b. ____
____
____

c. ____
____
____

d. ____
____
____

Time 2 (write the time you started __________)

a. ____
____
____

b. ____
____
____

c. ____
____
____

d. ____
____
____

Time 3 (write the time you started __________)

a. ____
____
____

b. ____
____
____

c. ____
____
____

d. ____
____
____

Check which of the following shows what you got out of this practice exercise:

a. Completely useless _____
b. Somewhat useless _____
c. So-so _____
d. Somewhat useful _____
e. Extremely useful _____

Write down how you feel about this homework practice exercise and what you got out of it.

____
____
____
____
____

Concluding Feedback Form

Name____________________________Sex______Date_____________

The purpose of this form is to understand what you learned from working on this practice excercise.

1. Which answer fits how you feel about this practice excercise?

    a. I did not like working on this practice excercise at all. I wish I never saw it. _____
    b. I did not like this practice excercise, but I am glad I got to work on it. _____
    c. I am happy I got a chance to work on this practice excercise. _____
    d. I am not only delighted about this practice excercise, but I wish all couples who argue could get it. _____

2. How helpful was it to work on this practice excercise? Please check the answer that applies to you.

a.	Not helpful at all	_____	c.	Helpful	_____
b.	Somewhat helpful	_____	d.	Very helpful	_____

3. Which practice exercise did you like best? Rank as No. 1 the one that you liked best, rank as No. 2 the one you liked next best, and so on; mark as N/A the ones you did not like at all or did not apply to you.

Reasons for Arguing		*Your Rank-order*	*Partner's Rank-order*	*Difference Scores*
a.	It's our fault when we do it	________	________	________
b.	One partner wants things one way and the other wants them another way	________	________	________
c.	Work	________	________	________
d.	We do not know how to get along	________	________	________
e.	We do not understand each other	________	________	________
f.	Money	________	________	________
g.	Our children misbehave and do something wrong	________	________	________
h.	One partner is worried about something	________	________	________
i.	Chores or jobs around the house	________	________	________
j.	One partner had a bad day	________	________	________
k.	The other partner had a bad day	________	________	________
l.	People outside the family, relatives/friends	________	________	________
m.	One partner is worried about something	________	________	________
n.	One partner does not feel good	________	________	________
o.	It's our children's fault	________	________	________
p.	One partner does not feel well	________	________	________
q.	The kind of person one partner is	________	________	________
r.	Our children are bad	________	________	________
s.	It's one partner's fault	________	________	________
t.	One partner is the kind of person who likes to argue	________	________	________
u.	The kind of person the partner is	________	________	________
v.	We really do not like each other	________	________	________
w.	It's the other partner's fault	________	________	________
x.	The other partner is the kind of person who likes to argue	________	________	________
y.	State your own reason (________________________)	________	________	________

4. By appointment only, check with your partner and compare, contrast, and discuss your answers to this practice exercise. Write each other's rank orders and subtract them from each other's (even if it results in a minus number). Add all the difference scores and discuss this total score with your professional helper to see how it compares with scores of other couples.

5. Now that you have completed this practice exercise, check which of these answers indicates how you felt about it. There is also space for you to explain further, if you want to:

   a. I did not like it at all, a waste of time. I wish I never worked on this stupid practice exercise. _____
   b. I did not like it very much, but I want to go on with working on practice excercises of this type. _____
   c. I liked it and I want to go on with another practice excercise. _____
   d. I liked it a lot and I wish I had received something like this practice excercise earlier in our life together. ______
   e. I liked it so much that I wish all arguing couples could get something like this to work on. _____

6. How could this practice excercise be improved? Do you have any suggestions? Feel free to write whatever could improve this practice excercise.

____

____

____

____

____

When Parents and Children Argue: From the Eyes of a Child

The purpose of this practice excercise is to help this family have better arguments, that is, instead of arguing, learning how to negotiate by "proacting" with each other rather than reacting to each other. If you all have agreed to work together on this practice excercise, it means that you love each other enough to make things better for yourselves. This practice excercise, however, may be useless unless you set appointments to meet at predetermined, agreed-upon times to discuss your individually completed practice exercises. If, during one of these appointments you find you are getting too angry, call for time out and schedule another appointment at least 24 h ahead. This postponement will allow you to cool off and process what is going on among yourselves.

Practice Exercise 1. What Do You Argue About?

Name_____________________________Sex_______Date__________

The purpose of this practice exercise is to find out how you see the seriousness of your arguments.

1. How often do you have these arguments or fights?

   a. Once a day or more ______
   b. Two or three times a week ______
   c. Once a week ______
   d. Once a month ______
   e. Once every 2 or 3 months ______
   f. Never or hardly ever ______

2. How long do these arguments or fights last?

   a. Sometimes the whole day or more ______
   b. A couple of hours or half a day ______
   c. About an hour ______
   d. Less than 30 minute ______
   e. 1 minute at the most ______

3. How heated, strong, or intense are these arguments or fights?

   a. Very strong to the point of physical violence ______
   b. Very intense but without physical violence ______
   c. Strong and verbally abusive ______
   d. Not very strong ______
   e. We get excited but we calm down soon ______
   f. Usually we keep cool and rational ______
   g. We never lose our cool, we just avoid each other ______
   h. We do not argue or fight, we just bicker ______
   i. Other (explain) ______

4. How do these arguments or fights get started?

   a. I usually start them ______
   b. Another family member usually starts them ______
   c. Sometimes I start them, sometimes someone else starts them ______
   d. I don't know ______
   e. Other (explain) ______

5. How do these arguments or fights end?

   a. We all kiss and make up ______
   b. We stay mad for hours ______
   c. We stay mad for days ______

d. We stay mad for weeks on end ______
e. We stay away from each other until we have another argument or fight ______
f. Other (explain)________________________________ ______

6. Why do you argue or fight? Rank as No. 1 the most troublesome reason for arguing, rank order as No. 2 the second most troublesome reason for arguing, and so on; mark as N/A the reasons that do not apply.

Reasons for Arguing	*Your Rank-order*	*Combined Family Rank-order*
a. Parents want things one way and children want them another way	________	________
b. All of us are at fault	________	________
c. The children do not listen	________	________
d. Parents are worried about something	________	________
e. Chores or jobs around the house	________	________
f. We do not understand each other	________	________
g. Children are upset about something	________	________
h. Children had a bad day	________	________
i. Parents had a bad day	________	________
j. School	________	________
k. One child is mad at another child in the family and is taking it out on the parent	________	________
l. One parent does not feel well	________	________
m. Parents are mad at one child and are taking it out on another child	________	________
n. We do not know how to get along	________	________
o. Money	________	________
p. Parents are mad at each other and one is taking it out on the children	________	________
q. Parents' work	________	________
r. The kind of person the parent is	________	________
s. Parents are unfair	________	________
t. People outside the family, such as relatives and friends	________	________
u. The child is the kind of person who likes to argue	________	________
v. It's the parent's fault	________	________
w. The child does not feel well	________	________
x. The child is a bad child	________	________
y. The parent is the kind of parent who likes to argue	________	________
z. The kind of person the child is	________	________
aa. It's the child's fault	________	________

Reasons for Arguing	*Your Rank-order*	*Combined Family Rank-order*
bb. We really do not like each other	________	________
cc. One parent is a bad parent	________	________
dd. State your own reason (________________)	________	________

7. Now state why you rank-ordered these reasons for arguing the way you did.

____
____
____
____
____

Homework: By preset appointment, compare, contrast, and discuss your answers to this practice exercise. Add up all the family rankings in the last column above. Give copies of your completed practice exercises to whoever is helping you with this practice excercise.

Standard Practice Exercise No.____Title of Practice Exercise_______

Name____________________________Sex______Date___________

The purpose of this practice exercise is to understand more about the reason for arguing listed in the title.

1. How did you start using this reason this way? Please explain in detail:

____
____
____
____
____

2. How often do you use this reason? Check which answer applies to you:

   a. Practically every day ______
   b. Once a week ______
   c. A couple of times a month ______
   d. Once a month ______
   e. Once every 6 months ______
   f. Once a year ______
   g. Once every few years ______

3. Please explain further:

____
____
____
____
____

4. How did this reason come about? Do you remember when you started it? Check which answer fits best:

   a. When I was a child (younger than 5 years of age) ______
   b. In elementary school ______
   c. In middle school ______
   d. In high school ______
   e. Any other time ______

5. Please explain further:

____
____
____
____
____

6. What does this reason get you? Please explain:

____
____
____
____
____

7. Give three specific examples of how using this reason is hurtful to you.

   Example 1:

____
____
____
____
____

Example 2:

Example 3:

8. Give three specific examples of how this reason is hurtful to your family.

Example 1:

Example 2:

Example 3:

Homework: If you want to stop undesirable reasons, learn to start them. Keep in mind that if you learn to start it, you will learn to stop it. Next week plan to repeat this reason at preset times (for instance, at 8 a.m., 12 noon, 4 or 7 p.m.) on at least 3 days (Monday, Wednesday, and Friday, or Tuesday, Thursday, and Saturday).

Write down what happened in detail. For each time make sure to answer in writing the following four questions:

(a) How did you start it?
(b) What followed?
(c) How did it end?
(d) What did this reason get you?

Time 1 (write the time you started__________)

a. ______________________________

b. ______________________________

c. ______________________________

d. ______________________________

Time 2 (write the time you started__________)

a. ______________________________

b. ______________________________

c. ______________________________

d. ______________________________

Time 3 (write the time you started__________)

a. ______________________________

b. ______________________________

c. ____

____

____

d. ____

____

____

Check which of the following shows what you got out of this practice exercise:

a. Completely useless _____
b. Somewhat useless _____
c. So-so _____
d. Somewhat useful _____
e. Extremely useful _____

Now that you have completed this practice exercise, check which of these answers indicates how you feel about it. There is also space for you to explain further, if you want to:

a. I did not like it at all, a waste of time. I want to quit this stupid practice excercise. _____
b. I did not like it very much, but I want to go on with this practice excercise. _____
c. I liked it and I want to go on with this practice excercise. _____
d. I liked it a lot and I wish I had something like this practice excercise earlier. _____
e. I liked it so much that I wish all arguing parents and children could get something like this to work on. _____

Write down how you feel about this homework practice exercise and what you got out of it.

____

____

____

____

____

Concluding Feedback Form

Name______________________________Sex______Date____________

The purpose of this form is to understand what you learned from working on previous practice exercises.

1. Which answer fits how you feel about this practice excercise?

   a. I did not like working on this practice excercise at all. I wish I never saw it. _____

b. I did not like this practice excercise, but I am glad I got to work on it. _____
c. I am happy I got a chance to work on this practice excercise. ____
d. I am not only delighted about this practice excercise, but I wish all couples who argue could get it. _____

2. How helpful was it to work on this practice excercise? Please check the answer that applies to you.

a. Not helpful at all	_____	c. Helpful	_____
b. Somewhat helpful	_____	d. Very helpful	_____

3. Which practice exercise did you like best? Rank as No. 1 the one that you liked best, rank as No. 2 the one you liked next best, and so on; mark as N/A the ones you did not like at all or did not apply to you.

Reasons for Arguing	*Your Rank-order*	*Combined Family Rank-orders*
a. Parents want things one way and children want them another way	______	______
b. All of us are at fault	______	______
c. The children do not listen	______	______
d. Parents are worried about something	______	______
e. Chores or jobs around the house	_______	______
f. We do not understand each other	______	______
g. Children are upset about something	_____	______
h. Children had a bad day	______	______
i. Parents had a bad day	______	______
j. School	_____	______
k. One child is mad at another child in the family and is taking it out on the parent	_____	______
l. One parent does not feel well	_____	______
m. Parents are mad at one child and are taking it out on another child	_____	______
n. We do not know how to get along	______	______
o. Money	______	______
p. Parents are mad at each other and one is taking it out on the children	______	______
q. Parents' work	______	______
r. The kind of person the parent is	______	______
s. Parents are unfair	______	______
t. People outside the family, such as relatives and friends	______	______
u. The child is the kind of person who likes to argue	______	______
v. It's the parent's fault	_____	______
w. The child does not feel well	______	______

Reasons for Arguing	Your Rank-order	Combined Family Rank-orders
x. The child is a bad child	______	______
y. The parent is the kind of parent who likes to argue	______	______
z. The kind of person the child is	______	______
aa. It's the child's fault	______	______
bb. We really do not like each other	______	______
cc. One parent is a bad parent	______	______
dd. State your own reason (__________________)	______	______

4. Compare, contrast, and discuss your answers to this practice exercise with each other (by appointment only). Add all the individual scores and discuss the total rankings you obtained for each practice exercise with your professional helper.

5. Now that you have completed this practice exercise, check which of these answers indicates how you felt about it. Use a separate piece of paper.

   a. I did not like it at all, a waste of time. I wish I never worked on this stupid practice exercise. _____
   b. I did not like it very much, but I want to go on with working on practice exercises of this type. _____
   c. I liked it and I want to go on with another practice exercise. _____
   d. I liked it a lot and I wish I had received something like this practice exercise earlier in our family life. ______
   e. I liked it so much that I wish all arguing parents and children could get something like this to work on. _____

6. How could this practice excercise be improved? Do you have any suggestions? Feel free to write whatever could improve this practice excercise.

____
____
____
____
____

Negotiation

The purpose of this practice excercise is to help couples (and families) learn how to negotiate, problem-solve, and even bargain successfully together. If you have agreed to work on the practice exercises contained in this practice excercise, you must care for each other a great deal. Care and troublesome thought, however, are not enough. Negotiation is also necessary. Many couples and families have not had the experience of knowing how to negotiate because they never saw it take place in their families of origin. Answer all the questions in each practice exercise. Then meet with each other at a time preset at least 24 h in advance. It is very important that you meet by appointment and not discuss your completed individual practice exercises by chance appointments. After you meet, for no more than one hour, read each other's answers and discuss their similarities and differences. Take notes because you may forget what you discussed. If during this meeting either one becomes upset or, worse, angry, interrupt the meeting and set up another appointment for another time 24 h in advance.

Homework Practice Exercise 1. The Goals of Marriage

Name__________________________Sex_________Date__________

The purpose of this homework practice exercise is for you to start thinking about and stating clearly what you want out of this marriage (family).

1. What? Write specific constructive results you want to achieve in this marriage (family).

____
____
____
____
____

2. Why? Write the benefit to each of you from achieving a result.

____
____
____
____
____

3. How? Clarify ways you plan to achieve a result.

____
____
____
____
____

4. When? State clearly frequencies, times, and extent of the ways of achieving a result.

____

____

____

____

____

5. Set goals for tomorrow. Write specifically what you will do tomorrow that you have not done today. Discuss your answers with your partner (family members) for at least 1 h before your meet with your professional helper.
   Results

   Successful (explain why):

____

____

____

____

____

   Unsuccessful (explain why):

____

____

____

____

____

   Canceled (explain why):

____

____

____

____

____

Practice Exercise 2. The Law of Give and Take: The Golden Rule

Name______________________________Sex__________Date___________

The purpose of this practice exercise is for you to practice the Golden Rule. Even though you may know about it, you may not have practiced it in your relationship.

1. Have you ever heard of the Golden Rule? What does the Golden Rule mean to you?

2. How are the Golden Rule and the Law of Give and Take related to each other?

3. Do you agree that the Golden Rule means dealing with others the way we want them to deal with us? Please comment.

4. What happens when we fail to follow this rule in our dealings with others?

5. What happens to your relationship (marriage, family) when you fail to follow this rule?

6. What are the advantages of following the Golden Rule in your relationship?

7. What are the disadvantages?

8. What do you think would happen to your relationship if you were to commit yourself to follow the Golden Rule?

9. What do you think would happen to your relationship if both you and your partner (mate, companion, parent, or child) failed to follow it?

10. How committed are you to following this rule, and why?

11. List specific instances of when and where you failed to follow this rule and the outcome of that failure.

12. List specific instances of when and where you followed this rule and the outcome of having followed it.

13. Discuss your answers with your partner (family members) and discuss similarities and differences in your answers. What did you learn from this discussion?

14. During the next week, concentrate on writing down four specific instances in which you followed the Golden Rule and the outcome.

    Instance 1:

    Outcome:

Instance 2:

Outcome:

Instance 3:

Outcome:

Instance 4:

Outcome:

Practice Exercise 3. "I" Statements

Name____________________________Sex__________Date___________

The purpose of this practice exercise is to help you learn how to speak for yourself and not for your partner or other family members. Some people have trouble starting sentences with the pronoun "I"; instead, they most often use the pronoun "you." Using the "you" pronoun can be very hurtful to marriages and to families. The purpose of this practice exercise is to help you practice making "I" statements. Using sentences that begin with "I" can be especially helpful when trying to express feelings or deal with emotional issues in your relationships.

The following sentence stems have been found helpful in making "I" statements. One blank has been provided under each heading so that you can make up a stem of your own. Write your completions for each of the sentence stems on the lines provided, and start thinking about other possible completions for these sentences. After completing all the responses, discuss your answers with your partner.

1. Self
   I wish ____
   I should ____
   I need ____
   I feel ____
   I ____

2. Marriage/relationship with partner
   It pleases me when _____________________________________
   I fear ____
   I love ____
   I hurt ____
   I ____

3. Children
   I remember ____
   I want ____
   It pleases me when _____________________________________
   It hurts me when ______________________________________
   I ____

4. Parents/in-laws
   I avoid ____
   I understand ____
   I must ____
   I won't ____
   I ____

5. Siblings or relatives
   I feel ____________________
   I ought ____________________
   I avoid ____________________
   I trust ____________________
   I ____________________

6. Work
   Sometimes I ____________________
   I enjoy ____________________
   I dread ____________________
   I'd like ____________________
   I ____________________

7. Friends
   I sense ____________________
   I fear ____________________
   I wonder ____________________
   I enjoy ____________________
   I ____________________

8. Leisure time
   I like ____________________
   If I could ____________________
   I enjoy ____________________
   I don't want ____________________
   I ____________________

Make an appointment with your partner (or family members) to compare and discuss your answers with theirs.

The stimulus sentences listed below represent typical statements made by one partner to another in a relationship. One partner reads the stimulus sentences, one at a time, while the other partner responds in each of the three styles. Blanks have been provided for you to supply your own stimulus sentences unique to your relationship. Write your responses to each stimulus sentence in each of the three styles in the spaces provided. After completion, the partners switch roles.

Don't be overly concerned if a particular style or stimulus sentence does not seem to fit your relationship. Do the best you can in responding to each one. We are interested in your learning the styles at this point and in your being able to note differences between them. Don't be afraid to make mistakes or take risks.

Definitions:

Abusive/apathetic (AA) style: Signs/behaviors of inattentiveness, or using verbal abuse (name-calling, blaming, bringing up the past, blackmailing/bribery, using "you" statements, mind-reading, and ultimatums). Example: Partner: "You're stupid!"

Respondent: “Guess who’s coming over for dinner?” or “I don’t know and I don’t care!”; “It’s all your fault!”

Reactive/repetitive (RR) style: An immediate, impulsive-like statement, often said without thinking, in which you criticize, act defensively, or suggest that you will take care of everything. Example: Partner: “You’re stupid!” Respondent: “What do you think you are?”

Creative/conductive (CC) style: A statement in which you request more information from your partner, rephrase what your partner has said to see if you’ve understood what s/he was trying to say, or otherwise indicate that you are in charge of yourself. Example: Partner: “You’re stupid!” Respondent: “I know that I behave stupidly sometimes. How have I offended you?”

Stimulus sentence 1: Did your mother/father call today?
Styles in responding

AA ____________________
RR ____________________
CC ____________________

Stimulus sentence 2: Did you put the garbage out/do the laundry today as you promised?
Styles in responding

AA ____________________
RR ____________________
CC ____________________

Stimulus sentence 3: The bank called to tell us the last check you wrote bounced.
Styles in responding

AA ____________________
RR ____________________
CC ____________________

Stimulus sentence 4: How late did you get in last night?
Styles in responding

AA ____________________
RR ____________________
CC ____________________

Stimulus sentence 5: How did work/school go today?
Styles in responding

AA ____________________
RR ____________________
CC ____________________

Stimulus sentence 6: I'm going out with the guys/girls Friday night
Styles in responding

AA ______________________________
RR ______________________________
CC ______________________________

Stimulus sentence 7: I'm sorry I wasn't there to pick you up.
Styles in responding

AA ______________________________
RR ______________________________
CC ______________________________

Stimulus sentence 8: What shall we do tonight?
Styles in responding

AA ______________________________
RR ______________________________
CC ______________________________

9. Make up your own stimulus sentences (the more the better):

____
____
____
____
____

Styles in responding

AA ______________________________
RR ______________________________
CC ______________________________

Homework: During the coming week, write down answers that fall in any of the three styles you practiced in this practice exercise. If you do not follow-up by writing them down, chances are you will go back to using AA or RR instead of CC styles.

Practice Exercise 4. Options in Responding: Part 1

Name______________________Sex__________Date__________

The purpose of this task is to identify the first three of five response options – emotional (E), rational (R), and actional (A) – in a relationship and give you and your partner some practice telling them apart. Always using emotional, rational, or actional options in responding often does not result in good outcomes for couples or families when they try to deal with differences or conflicts in their relationship.

The stimulus sentences and situations listed below represent typical statements or typical situations found in relationships. One partner reads the stimulus sentences and situations, one at a time, while the other partner answers in each of the three different response options. Four blanks have been provided for each of you to supply your own stimulus sentences or situations related to your own relationship. Make sure that you write your answers to each of the stimulus sentences and situations in the space provided. After completion, partners must switch roles.

Again, don't be overly concerned if a particular option, stimulus sentence, or stimulus situation does not seem to fit your relationship. Do the best you can in responding to each one. We are interested in your learning the various response options and in your being able to note differences between them. Don't be afraid to make mistakes or take risks.

Definitions:

Emotional response (E): A quick or cutting response given without any thought or awareness. Example: Partner: "That was sure dumb of you!" Respondent: "You're dumb, too!"

Rational response (R): A logical, computer-like, or intellectualized response used in preaching and lecturing, rather than discussing. Example: Partner: "That was sure dumb of you" Respondent: "The word 'dumb' needs to be defined."

Actional response (A): A response including either a nonverbal behavior or a verbal threat involving action. Example: Partner: "That was sure dumb of you!" Respondent: (Slams the door as s/he storms out) or "If you don't take that back, I'm going to________ you!" Actional responses do not need to be acted out. They can be written down as to what one would actually do in response.

Stimulus Sentence 1: I'm very angry at you!
Response Options

Emotional (E) ____
Rational (R) ____
Actional (A) ____

Stimulus Sentence 2: Why are you so late?
Response Options

Emotional (E) ____
Rational (R) ____
Actional (A) ____

Stimulus Sentence 3: You know I love you.
Response Options

Emotional (E)____
Rational (R)____
Actional (A)____

Stimulus Sentence 4: Did you pay the bill?
Response Options

Emotional (E)____
Rational (R)____
Actional (A)____

Stimulus Situation 1: Your partner comes back from the store. You notice s/he didn't get an item you need very badly and that your partner said s/he'd remember to pick up for you.
Response Options

Emotional (E)____
Rational (R)____
Actional (A)____

Stimulus Situation 2: You and your partner both want to take a shower or bath. It's agreed s/he can go first. When it's your turn, you notice that there is no hot water left.
Response Options

Emotional (E)____
Rational (R)____
Actional (A)____

Stimulus Situation 3: You've had a hard day. You go home thinking you will be able to relax. You walk in the door and are immediately reminded by your partner that you promised to go somewhere with him/her right after work.
Response Options

Emotional (E)____
Rational (R)____
Actional (A)____

Stimulus Situation 4: You and your partner have decided to go out this weekend. You think it will be just the two of you. On Friday your partner tells you s/he ran into an old acquaintance who you're not fond of and has invited him/her to join the two of you.

Response Options

Emotional (E)____
Rational (R)____
Actional (A)____

Make up your own stimulus sentences:
Response Options

Emotional (E)____
Rational (R)____
Actional (A)____

Homework: During the coming week, write down answers that fall in any of the three response options you practiced in this practice exercise. If you do not follow-up by writing them down, chances are you will go back to using AA or RR instead of CC styles.

Practice Exercise 5. Options in Responding: Part 2

Name____________________________Sex__________Date___________

The purpose of this practice exercise is to identify two additional response options – awareness and contextual – in a relationship and to give you and your partner practice in telling them apart and in using them. Unlike the first three options covered in Practice Exercise No. 4 (emotional, rational, and actional), both of these response options usually result in good outcomes when partners try to deal with differences or conflicts in their relationship.

The stimulus sentences and situations listed below represent possible statements and situations found in relationships. One partner reads the stimulus sentences and situations one at a time, while the other partner answers using each of the two response options. Blanks have again been provided for each of you to supply stimulus sentences or situations related specifically to your relationship. Write your stimulus sentences or situations along with responses to them and to each of the supplied stimulus sentences and situations using the different options in responding in the spaces provided. When finished, partners change roles.

Again, don't be overly concerned if a particular option, stimulus sentence, or stimulus situation does not seem to fit your relationship. Do the best you can in responding to each one. We are interested in your learning these two additional response options and in your being able to use them. Don't be afraid to make mistakes or take risks.

Definitions:

Awareness response (Aw): A response that starts with the "I" pronoun or an "It," a self statement, indicating an awareness of one's own behavior or internal process.

Example: Partner: "You never listen to me!" Respondent: "I know that I sometimes don't pay attention to you well. I wish we could find a way for me to pay attention to you more often."

Contextual response (C): A response that asks for more information about reasons and background for the other person's statement, which is in the form of a self-statement. Example: Partner: "I don't want to go back to see them again ever!" Respondent: "You seem really upset. Will you tell me what happened? I really need to know more about the situation to understand your response."

Stimulus Sentence 1: You're just like your father/mother!

Response Options

Awareness (Aw) ______________________________
Contextual (C) ______________________________

Stimulus Sentence 2: I can't trust you.
Response Options

Awareness (Aw) ______________________________
Contextual (C) ______________________________

Stimulus Sentence 3: You're really sloppy!
Response Options

Awareness (Aw) ______________________________
Contextual (C) ______________________________

Stimulus Sentence 4: If only you wouldn't do that 20 times a day!
Response Options

Awareness (Aw) ______________________________
Contextual (C) ______________________________

Stimulus situation 1: You and your partner have agreed to go to see a movie that starts at 8 o'clock. Your partner has to work but promises to be home on time to go. By 8:30 s/he's not home and hasn't called. At 8:45 s/he finally walks in the door.
Response Options

Awareness (Aw) ______________________________
Contextual (C) ______________________________

Stimulus situation 2: Your partner appears angry and hasn't said anything to you all day.
Response Options

Awareness (Aw) ______________________________
Contextual (C) ______________________________

Stimulus situation 3: Your partner tells you s/he feels you aren't affectionate or sexy enough toward him/her.
Response Options

Awareness (Aw) ______________________________
Contextual (C) ______________________________

Stimulus situation 4: Your partner teases you about one of your personal or physical characteristics.
Response Options

Awareness (Aw) ______________________________
Contextual (C) ______________________________

Make up your own stimulus sentences:
Stimulus situation:
Response Options

Awareness (Aw) ______________________________
Contextual (C) ______________________________

Homework: During the coming week, write down answers that fall in any of the two response options you practiced in this practice exercise. If you do not follow-up by writing them down, chances are you will go back to using AA or RR instead of CC styles.

Practice Exercise 6. Priorities

Name______________________Sex_________Date__________

The purpose of this homework is to examine important areas of your life and how they relate to your relationship with your partner (and/or family). Listed below are seven stages that represent the development of a family over time. Please circle one stage or category that best fits you currently. If you have been married before, circle the stage or category in which you currently see yourself and your present partner.

Family Life Cycle Stages

1. Unattached young adult
2. Newly married couple
3. Family with young children
4. Family with adolescents
5. Launching children and moving on
6. Family in later life
7. Couple who has decided not to have children

1. Keeping your current family life cycle stage or category in mind, please rank-order in terms of importance the following areas in your life. Use a scale from 1 to 7, with your first ranked area being most important to you down to your seventh ranked area being the least important.

Area	*Rankings of Importance*		
	Now	*Before*	*After*
Selfhood	_____	_____	_____
Marriage/relationship with partner	_____	_____	_____
Children	_____	_____	_____
Parents/in-laws/siblings	_____	_____	_____
Work	_____	_____	_____
Friends	_____	_____	_____
Leisure time	_____	_____	_____

Now rank-order the same areas for both the stage before and the stage following (after) the one you have indicated you are currently in. Example: If you see yourself best fitting into stage 2 now, you would rank-order the areas as you saw them when you were in stage 1 – unattached young adult – and as you expect them to be in the next stage, stage 3 – family with young children. For those of you currently in stage 1, for your previous stage use your late adolescence. For those of you in stage 6 – family in later life – for your next stage use the time when you will be a couple with grandchildren or great-grandchildren. For those of you who chose stage 7 – couple who has decided not to have children – for your previous stage use either stage 1 or 2 – unattached young adult or newly married couple – and for your next stage, use stage 6 – family in later life.

2. The cornerstone of all these priorities is selfhood. How do you define it and what does it mean to you?

____

____

____

____

____

3. Self-fulness. If selfhood is the state of having a self, self-fulness means having a positive sense of self-importance. What does self-fulness mean to you?

____

____

____

____

____

4. How does self-fulness express or manifest itself?

____

____

____

____

____

5. Selfishness: How to you define it and how does it express or manifest itself?

6. How is selfishness different from self-fulness?

7. Selflessness: How do you define it and how does it express or manifest it?

7. How is selfishness different from either self-fulness or selflessness?

8. No-self: How would you define it and how does it express or manifest itself?

9. How does no-self express or manifest itself?

10. Responsibility: What does it mean to you to take responsibility for yourself?

____
____
____
____
____

11. To take responsibility for oneself means to use the personal pronoun "I," instead of the pronoun "You." Give instances where your negative use of the pronoun "You" instead of the pronoun "I," as in blaming, putting down, name-calling, etc., has resulted in negative consequences for your partner and/or your family.

Instance a:

____
____
____
____
____

Instance b:

____
____
____
____
____

Instance c:

____
____
____
____
____

12. Are you convinced that using sentences with the negative "You" produces negative consequences for you and your partner (family)? If you are not yet convinced, go on and use the negative "You." See what happens to you and your partner or family.

13. Perfection: How would you rate yourself as far as having high standards (i.e., perfectionism)? Circle which of these ratings apply to you:

High Medium Low Very Low

If you rate High or Medium, tell what perfectionism does to you and your partner (family).

____
____
____
____
____

14. What are the positive consequences?

____
____
____
____
____

15. What are the negative consequences?

____
____
____
____
____

16. Now briefly describe yourself in four of your major family roles as you were in the past, as you are now in the present, and as you want to be in the future.

Role

a. As a child (son, daughter) to your parents:

Past____________________________________
Present__________________________________
Future__________________________________

b. As a person in your own right:

Past____________________________________
Present__________________________________
Future__________________________________

c. As a partner to your partner:

Past______________________________________
Present____________________________________
Future_____________________________________

d. As a parent to your children:

Past______________________________________
Present____________________________________
Future_____________________________________

e. As a parent to your parents:

Past______________________________________
Present____________________________________
Future_____________________________________

Homework: During the coming week, think about what is important to you in the long run. Answer the following questions in writing and discuss them with your partner or family members by appointment.

1. What will happen to your sense of importance when you retire?

2. What would happen to your sense of importance if you were fired or handicapped by illness?

3. If you do not take good care of yourself, who will?

4. If you do not take care of yourself, how will you be able to take care of those you love and who love you?

____

____

____

____

____

Practice Exercise 7. The Triangle of Living

Name______________________Sex________Date__________

The purpose of this practice exercise is to explain how the three sides of a triangle of living apply to you.

Please answer the following questions to the best of your ability.

A. Having

1. Money

a. What does money mean to you (your partner relationship or family)?

____

____

____

b. What kinds of conflicts are there about money?

____

____

____

2. Goods

a. What do goods (possessions, material things) mean to you (your partner relationship or family)?

____

____

____

b. What kinds of conflicts are there about goods (gifts, things, purchases)?

____

____

____

B. Doing, performance, reading, etc.

1. Services

a. Who performs what chores (or services) in your household?

____
____
____

b. How does this arrangement work for this household?

____
____
____

2. Information: What kind of information is allowed in this home?

a. TV programs (what kind, for how long) and movies:

____
____
____

b. Newspapers and magazines:

____
____
____

c. Books (who reads what?):

____
____
____

d. Relatives, friends and neighbors (get-togethers, frequency of meetings, feelings about visits, etc.):

____
____
____

e. Others (visitors, drop-ins, entertainments, etc.):

____
____
____

f. Which of the preceding are most important?

i. To whom?

___
___
___

ii. How?

___
___
___

iii. Why?

___
___
___

C. Being

1. Love

a. What does love mean to your relationship with your partner or family?

___
___
___

b. How is love shown or demonstrated?

___
___
___

c. Is love used as a commodity to bribe or blackmail family members?

___
___
___

2. Intimacy as defined by the sharing of joys and hurts.

a. How does this definition apply to your intimate relationships?

___
___
___

b. From that definition how intimate is your partner/family?

3. Importance

a. How important are you to yourselves and to others in the family?

b. How is this importance shown or expressed inside the family?

c. How is this importance shown or expressed outside the family?

d. How do you fail to show your individual importance?

D. Balance of having, doing, being

1. Which of these – having, doing, being – is most important to you?

2. Why? (i.e., What does it get you?)

3. Are you satisfied with the way you rank these resources?

____
____
____

4. If you are satisfied, why?

____
____
____

5. If you are not satisfied, why not?

____
____
____

6. How could each of you do better?

____
____
____

Homework: After answering these questions, discuss them with your partner or family by appointment only.

Practice Exercise 8. Guidelines for Negotiation

Name______________________Sex_________Date__________

Dear Partners (or Family Members):
The purpose of these guidelines is to help you learn what most of us do not know how to do, that is, to negotiate important issues and differences with others. These guidelines are based on the assumption that negotiation is the most important factor in most intimate relationships. We cannot promise you happiness. However, we can help you learn this process if each of you is committed to learning. In our experience with countless couples and families, we have found that the major deficit we have is our inability to negotiate creatively and constructively. We hope these guidelines will help you to do so. However, if any one of you is committed to failing and to defeating yourself and the other, there is no question that neither these guidelines nor any other form of service will be helpful to you.

Most of these guidelines are negotiable; that is, if you find that some other approach or deviation from these guidelines is helpful to you, by all means use it. Do let us know what you have found useful so that we can make it part of our experience. There are two guidelines that we feel are not negotiable: (a) negotiating by appointment, and (b) negotiating in writing.

a. Negotiating by appointment: We believe that it is absolutely necessary for a couple or a family to set up 1 h a week in the home to practice and apply the principles and skills we plan to teach you. If you want to save money and time, there is no substitute for your meeting together at a prearranged time, which we consider part of our work. Of course, if you want to defeat us and yourselves, the best way to do it is to avoid setting and keeping these appointments.

b. Negotiating by writing: We believe that it is essential for couples to start keeping a record of what they negotiate about. What you negotiate about is your business, which you may tell us about to the extent that it will help us understand how well you negotiate or fail to negotiate. Each of you should start keeping a notebook in which you jot down issues that arise in your relationship that you feel you need to negotiate with your partner. As you progress, you may be able to develop one notebook for both of you. However, to begin with we would like to see each of you keep separate notes. You may write them before your appointment, during, or after, as you find most comfortable.

Once we have established these two guidelines, we want to let you in on our principle for negotiation, which is at the basis of the next five guidelines to follow: On any issue for couples and family, feelings and emotions must be expressed nonjudgmentally and discussed first, followed by a rational discussion of alternative courses of action (if necessary) and an eventual agreement on which course of action would be mutually satisfactory. Once a course of action is implemented, each of you needs to become more aware of how it is or is not working. You need then to get together to consider how and why this course of action is working (or not working), what changes are necessary, or other action(s) needed to work for both of you.

We have divided this principle into five steps:

Step 1. Emotionality: The function of emotions and feelings in an intimate union is to be discussed to increase intimacy. If there is no intimacy, there is no negotiation possible, since most issues found in couples and families are emotional issues. To deal with emotionality, all of us need to practice "I" statements and avoid making "You" statements. If you want to destroy this marriage and family, continue using "You" statements followed by "never" or "always." We cannot stop you.

Once feelings have been expressed and discussed by both of you (i.e., by using "I" statements) you may be ready to enter the next step. In any of these steps and especially the first step, you may need more than one meeting to conclude matters. The longer it takes to finish each step, the more stressed and troubled the relationship is. If you cannot share your feelings properly, stop! There is no need to go any further.

Step 2. Rationality: At this point, each of you may need to generate as many alternative actions (solutions, possibilities, etc.) that may seem to alleviate or to solve whatever problem you are negotiating. Generate as many alternatives as you can freely, no matter how outlandish they may be. Once each of you has done it, come up with whatever patterns (actions or solutions) may be helpful and satisfactory to you. If you can't and have reached a stalemate or you are becoming emotional, stop, and agree to continue next week at an appointed time to see whether you can come up with a solution to help (re)solve this impasse.

Step 3. Activity: Implement whatever course of action you have agreed upon. However, keep in mind that whatever you have agreed to do or not to do is preliminary and tentative. It does not become set until each of you is able to evaluate its usefulness and you have discussed with the other whatever misgivings (or lack of them) you may have. Give yourself time for this pattern to take place before evaluating its success or failure (up to 3 months if appropriate).

Step 4. Evaluation (awareness and feedback): Is the agreed-upon solution working? How well and at what costs? What rewards? Should you (a) persist with it, (b) change parts of it and improve it, or (c) start using an altogether different solution? At this point (as in Step 1), you need to discuss whatever feelings you may have about what is going on before considering alternatives or changes.

Step 5. Context: It is important that throughout this process (steps 1–4) you become aware of whatever physical and time contexts and constraints you may be negotiating about. Are you negotiating only within your relationship? Or are you negotiating issues or conflicts that include others outside your relationship, such as your children, in-laws, neighbors, or agencies (schools, health care)? Are you dealing with the past, present, or future? You may need to clarify the limits of your negotiation in terms of how and what you control (usually the past and the future are not negotiable).

In spite of these guidelines, we know that you will experience defeats, failures, false starts, wrong turns, detours, and blind alleys. They are all part of the process of trial and error that is necessary to learn to negotiate. To gain some experience in applying these guidelines for negotiation, we have constructed an exercise for you and your partner to do. Please list below five issues, differences, or troublesome aspects of your relationship that you feel you would like to negotiate. Rank-order them from 1 to 5 with your first ranked item being a small difference or issue in your relationship down to your fifth ranked item being one of large conflict size or difficulty. Use all numbers from 1 to 5 only once. Each of you is to make up a list of your own.

After you've made up your list, pick either your number 1 or 2 ranked issue and apply the guidelines for negotiation of this issue with your partner. At this point we want you to tackle only an issue or conflict of low intensity. We suggest you pick an easy issue first because we want you to (a) learn the process of negotiation with a minimum of trouble, and (b) experience some initial success with this new approach. Once you have learned the process, you can use it as an approach to larger and more difficult issues requiring future negotiations in your relationship. Good luck!

Issue/Difference/Conflict	*Rankings*	*Issue/Difference/Conflict*	*Rankings*
1____________________	_______	4____________________	_______
2____________________	_______	5____________________	_______
3____________________	_______		

Feedback Form for Negotiation Practice Exercise

Name__________________________Sex_________Date__________

The purpose of this form is for you to provide feedback to whoever has administered this practice excercise to you about how you feel about completing all the homework practice exercises. Now that you have completed this practice excercise, please respond to the following questions concerning the use of these homework practice exercises.

1. Using a scale of 1–9, rank the homework practice exercises according to their usefulness in developing effective communications for your family. Rank the most useful practice exercise as No. 1, rank the least useful as No. 9. You may use copies of your past practice exercises to reach a decision about these rankings.

Practice Exercise	*Rank-Order*	*Practice Exercise*	*Rank-Order*
The Goals of Marriage or Being a Couple	________	Options in Responding, Part 2	________
The Golden Rule	________	Priorities	________
"I" Statements	________	The Triangle of Living	________
Styles in Intimacy	________	Negotiation Guidelines	________
Options in Responding, Part 1	________		

2. How useful did you find this practice excercise for facilitating/developing more effective negotiation skills in your family?

   a. Very useful ________
   b. Quite useful ________
   c. Somewhat useful ________
   d. Slightly useful ________
   e. Not useful at all ________

3. How helpful would you rate this practice excercise for teaching/developing negotiation skills to other families?

   a. Very helpful ________
   b. Quite helpful ________
   c. Somewhat helpful ________
   d. Slightly helpful ________
   e. Not helpful at all ________

4. How useful would you rate this practice excercise in terms of developing or improving your relationships in general?

a. Very useful ____
b. Quite useful ____
c. Somewhat useful ____
d. Slightly useful ____
e. Not useful at all ____

5. How likely would you be to recommend this practice excercise to other couples you know?

a. Very likely ____
b. Quite likely ____
c. Somewhat likely ____
d. Slightly likely ____
e. Not at all likely ____

6. Using your own words, what did you find useful about this practice exercise?

____
____
____
____
____

7. How could this practice exercise be improved?

____
____
____
____
____

Intimacy

The purpose of this practice excercise is to improve intimacy between partners and among family members. If partners cannot discuss intimacy, it will be very difficult for family members to discuss it as well. Intimacy is the most direct expression of love. Many loving relationships may not discuss intimacy. It is up to you to decide whether you want to become more intimate with your partner and/or family members.

Practice Exercise 1. Loving and Caring

Name______________________Sex_____Date__________

Before we deal with intimacy, however, we need to know more about how you define love. The purpose of this practice exercise is to find out what love means to you.

1. What is love? Please write your own definition.

2. For a moment think about the following definition of love: Love includes at least four separate and distinct parts: (a) caring, (b) seeing the good, (c) forgiveness, and (d) intimacy. Can you improve on these four parts? Feel free to add whatever other part you think is necessary for love.

3. For you, what is caring?

   a. What does it mean to you to show care?

   b. How do you show caring emotionally?

   c. Physically?

d. Mentally?

___

___

___

e. Financially (with money)?

___

___

___

4. How do you take care of yourself?

a. Emotionally

___

___

___

b. Physically

___

___

___

c. Mentally

___

___

___

d. Financially (with money)

___

___

___

5. How do you express your care for people you love and who love you? Please respond in detail.

a. Partner (if any)

___

___

___

b. Children

____
____
____

c. Parents (and in-laws)

____
____
____

d. Other intimates (name them______________________)

____
____
____

6. How could you improve the way you care for yourself? What would you do?

____
____
____
____
____

7. How can you improve caring for those you love and who love you? What exactly would you do?

a. Partner

____
____
____

b. Children

____
____
____

c. Parents

____
____
____

d. In-laws

____
____
____

e. Other intimates. Who are they?____________________

____
____
____

8. How is your caring similar and how is it different from the ways your partner cares for you?

____
____
____
____
____

9. Families differ in the way caring is expressed. For example, different cultures can vary markedly in how they express caring. Does it seem to you that some families you have known are better at showing care than others? Who are they and what did they do?

____
____
____
____
____

Homework: Make an appointment with your partner at least 24 h ahead of time. Compare and contrast your answers with those of your partner. See if you can come up with an agreement about how you both need to care for yourselves and for each other.

____
____
____
____
____

Practice Exercise 2. Seeing the Good

Name________________________________Sex______Date__________

The purpose of this practice exercise is to know more about how you see the good in yourself, your partner, and intimate others.

1. What does "seeing the good" mean to you?

2. What do you see that is good in yourself (explain)?

    a. Is it hard to see the good in yourself? Why?

    b. Write down your positive points or characteristics.

    c. How do you feel when you think of the good in yourself?

3. Why do you have a hard time seeing the good in yourself?

4. Now write down possibly negative points or characteristics about yourself. How does this make you feel?

5. Is it easier/harder to see the bad in yourself? Why?

6. How would we gain by seeing the good in ourselves and in intimate others? Do you see the good in others? Is it easy or hard?

7. Is it easier to see the faults of intimate others? Do you have a reason? What is your reason?

8. Why should we seek the good?

   a. In ourselves?

   b. In our partner?

   c. In intimate others?

9. If we cannot see the good in ourselves, how can we see it in others?

10. Please list your significant others; rate with a checkmark your ability to see the good in each one of them. Who is the easiest/hardest?

Easy Moderate Difficult Impossible Why?

Partner

Mother

Father

Sister(s)

Brother(s)

In-laws

Best friend(s)

Homework: During the next week discuss your answers to these questions with your partner by appointment 24 h ahead and not on impulse.

a. What similarities and differences did you find in each other's answers?

---

b. Can you find a substitute for seeing the good?

---

c. How will you and your partner continue to see the good in yourselves and each other? Make sure that this is a joint decision.

____
____
____
____
____

Practice Exercise 3. Love and Forgiveness

Name______________________________Sex____Date____________

The purpose of this practice exercise is to help you forgive past errors in yourself and in those you love and who love you.

1. What does forgiveness mean to you?

____
____
____
____
____

2. How often do you practice forgiveness? Please check which answer applies to you best:

a. Most of the time	_____	c. Almost never	____
b. Once in a while	_____	d. Never	____

3. Think for a moment about the following definition of forgiveness: Forgiveness is canceling expectations of perfection in ourselves and intimate others. Could you accept this definition? Why yes? Why not?

____
____
____
____
____

4. Expectations could exist in the following ways. Please explain how each way applies to you.

   a. Perfection

   ____
   ____
   ____
   ____
   ____

   b. Performance

      i. At home

      ____
      ____
      ____
      ____
      ____

      ii. At work

      ____
      ____
      ____
      ____
      ____

      iii. In leisure activities

      ____
      ____
      ____
      ____
      ____

   c. Production of:

      i. Money

      ____
      ____
      ____
      ____
      ____

ii. Goods

iii. Services

d. Problem-solving, bargaining, or negotiating

e. Presence, that is, being emotionally available to yourself and to your partner

5. Do you think it is possible to love yourself and others without forgiveness? Explain.

6. What kinds of feeling do you have when you forgive or are forgiven?

a. Is forgiving others the same as forgiving yourself?

b. Can you forgive others if you cannot forgive yourself?

7. Who has been the most forgiving person in your life? What did you learn from him/her?

8. Who has been the least forgiving person in your life? What did you learn from that experience?

9. Often we think that perfection means goodness and imperfection means badness. This is a very destructive match. To be perfect means to be heavenly and to be imperfect means to be human. To be human means to make mistakes. How do you feel about forgiving yourself for being human and for having made mistakes?

10. Why do you not forgive yourself?

    a. Are some things easier to forgive? What are they?

    b. Why some and not others?

11. Do you find it hard to forgive others? If so, why?

12. If you were to forgive yourself or your partner, what would happen to you and to your relationship with your partner?

13. What would you have to give up in order to forgive?

14. Do you think you could use forgiveness to restore or improve love in your life? In what way?

15. List several ways you could use forgiveness to restore a damaged relationship or hurt feelings.

16. What would you give up in the process?

Homework: Discuss your answers to these questions with your partner and/or family members by making an appointment at least 24 h ahead of time. During the next week, list all the instances in which you used forgiveness. Use the rest of this sheet to list all instances of forgiveness during this week. Discuss them with your partner or family members.

Practice Exercise 4. Discussing Hurts: Part 1

Name________________________Sex______Date__________

The purpose of this practice exercise is to help you increase intimacy in your relationship with your partner and/or family members.

1. What does intimacy mean to you?

____

____

____

____

____

2. How intimate are you? Please check which answer applies to you best:

   a. Very intimate ____ c. Not at all intimate ____
   b. Somewhat intimate ____

3. Why are you as intimate as you just checked?

____

____

____

____

____

4. Think for a moment about the following definition of intimacy: Intimacy consists of discussing hurts and fears of being hurt with those we love and who love us.

   a. Does this definition have meaning for you? Yes No

   b. What meaning does this definition have for you?

____

____

____

____

____

c. If you agree, why? If you disagree, why?

5. This definition stresses that love and hurt are intertwined to the extent that we hurt when those we love also hurt. What do you think about this intertwining?

6. If this definition is acceptable to you, we need to define hurt as any action, situation, or event that saddens us, like frustrations, losses, put-downs, rejections, neglect, and humiliations. Facing up to our errors, mistakes, and neediness can also be hurtful. Can you think of other hurts?

7. When was the last time you discussed your hurts with your partner? Do you remember it?

a. How did you feel afterwards?

b. How did your partner feel afterwards?

____
____
____
____
____

c. How often do you and your partner discuss hurts? Check which answer applies to you:

i. Every day ______
ii. Once a week ______
iii. Once a month ______
iv. Once in a while ______
v. Once a year ______
vi. Almost never ______
vii. Never ______

8. Discussing our hurts and our fears of being hurt with those we love and who love us is very hard because:

a. We need to have a sense of self to discuss it with others. How does this point apply to you?

____
____
____
____
____

b. We only hurt the ones we love. How does this point apply to you?

____
____
____
____
____

c. We need to seek comfort from the very ones we have hurt or who have hurt us. How does this point apply to you?

____
____
____
____
____

d. What is your explanation about how hard it is to discuss your hurts and fears with your partner?

____
____
____
____
____

Homework: Make an appointment with your partner and compare your answers to the issues raised in this practice exercise with each other.

1. Think of instances where you were able (or failed) to discuss your hurts with those you love and who love you.
2. Take the risk and tell your partner about a recent failure on your part to discuss your hurts with him/her.
3. Recall instances in which you saw your parents discuss their hurts and fears of being hurt. Perhaps they may have failed in discussing hurts with each other. If that is the case, how could learn how to discuss hurts? Discuss these instances with each other and write them down for future discussions.

Practice Exercise 5. Discussing Hurts: Part 2

Name______________________________Sex______Date__________

The purpose of this practice exercise is to strengthen your intimacy with each other. It is not as easy as you may think.

1. What are some recent instances where you were able to or failed to discuss your hurts with someone you love?

____
____
____
____
____

What happened?

____
____
____
____
____

2. Up till now, how have you dealt with your hurts and fears of being hurt? List these ways and describe how you may have avoided discussing these hurts with someone you love.

3. How did your approach work for you in the past? Did you get what you wanted?

4. How did it work for those who love you?

5. Are you now ready to discuss your hurts with the one you love and who loves you? If yes, why? If no, why not?

6. What are you afraid might happen if you did discuss your hurts with your partner?

7. Discussing hurts is very scary because we are afraid of losing our sense of self, losing our mind, losing control, breaking down, or even losing our lives. What does discussing your hurts mean to you?

____
____
____
____
____

8. If you are not ready to discuss your hurts with your partner, would you be willing to discuss his/her hurts? If yes, why? If no, why not?

____
____
____
____
____

Homework: After you have met by appointment, discuss these issues with your partner and think more about possible reasons why you may not be ready to discuss your hurts with him or her. Write here any added comments you did not have a chance to write above.

____
____
____
____
____

Practice Exercise 6. Discussing Hurts: Part 3

Name______________________Sex______Date__________

The purpose of this practice exercise is to see whether you and your partner can really become intimate with each other, in the sense of discussing hurts and fears of being hurt.

1. What have you concluded about your inability to discuss your hurts with your partner, if that is indeed the case?

____
____
____
____
____

2. Is your not discussing hurts due to unwillingness or to inability?

____
____
____
____
____

3. Where does this inability or unwilling to discuss hurts come from?

____
____
____
____
____

4. Do you think that you could develop this skill of discussing hurts with time?

____
____
____
____
____

5. Are you willing to work on discussing your hurts? If you are not ready, stop here and do not go any further. If you are ready, go on. The two hardest words in the English language are "I hurt." The three hardest words are "It hurts me_" Before discussing with your partner, allow yourself to get in touch with whatever hurts you. Sit close with your partner and join hands with each other. Close your eyes if necessary and concentrate on getting in touch with your hurts. When you are ready, complete the following stems:

   a. I hurt when

   ____
   ____
   ____
   ____
   ____

   b. It hurts me when

   ____
   ____
   ____
   ____
   ____

6. We do not need to find excuses or reasons for our hurts. We hurt because we are human beings, not robots. Do not allow anyone, especially yourself, to belittle your hurts or "reason" yourself out of your hurts. Stay with your hurts and do not try to avoid them. You are entitled to feel hurt. However, we are not entitled to use our hurts to clobber our partners with them. Please comment.

____
____
____
____
____

7. How we feel our hurts is one thing; how we express them is another. We need to feel our hurts but we do not need to hold them inside of us, making ourselves and our partners miserable. Please comment.

____
____
____
____
____

8. Take the risk of discussing your hurts with your partner, as suggested. Then write in the space below what happened.

____
____
____
____
____

Homework: If you still have trouble discussing your hurts with your partner, take 15 minute a day for 4 days to write down all the hurts you received by those you love and all the hurts you have produced in those you love and who love you. After you have finished with this homework, discuss it with your partner by appointment. If this discussing has taken place, did you find it helpful to you? If not, why not? If yes, why?

____
____
____
____
____

Afterwards, review the whole practice excercise practice exercises from the beginning. Write down any comment or reaction that would be useful in improving this practice excercise.

Final Feedback Form for Intimacy

Name______________________________Sex_____Date__________

Now that you have completed this practice excercise, please respond to the following questions concerning the usefulness of these intimacy tasks.

1. On a scale of 1–6, rank-order the six intimacy practice exercises according to their usefulness in improving/developing closeness with your partner. Rank the most useful task as No. 1, rank the least useful task as No. 6.

Task	*Rank-order*	*Task*	*Rank-order*
Loving and Caring	________	Discussing Hurts – Part 1	________
Seeing the good	________	Discussing Hurts – Part 2	________
Love–forgiveness	________	Discussing Hurts – Part 3	________

2. How useful did you find the whole practice excercise for improving/developing greater intimacy between you and your partner or between you and your family members?

a. Very useful	____	d. Slightly useful	____
b. Quite useful	____	e. Not useful at all	____
c. Somewhat useful	____		

3. Please explain why you answered the way you did.

____

____

____

____

____

4. How would you rate this practice excercise's helpfulness for teaching couples and families to develop intimacy?

a. Very helpful	____	d. Slightly helpful	____
b. Quite helpful	____	e. Not helpful at all	____
c. Somewhat helpful	____		

5. Please explain why you answered the way you did.

____

____

____

____

____

6. How likely would you be to recommend this practice excercise to other couples of families you know?

a.	Very likely	____	c.	Somewhat likely	____
b.	Quite likely	____	d.	Not at all likely	____

7. Using your own words, what did you find useful about this practice excercise?

____
____
____
____
____

8. What about this practice excercise did you not find useful? Feel free to express your feelings and opinion.

____
____
____
____
____

9. How could this practice excercise be improved?

____
____
____
____
____

Hurt Feelings

The purpose of these practice exercises is to help you understand and perhaps learn to control and regulate your hurt feelings. You will receive additional practice exercises after completion of this one and after satisfactory completions of others. Make sure that you were given information about the nature of these proactive exercises and that you signed an informed consent form given to you at the beginning.

Practice Exercise 1.

Name____________________________Sex_________Date___________

Step 1. The purpose of this step is to obtain more information about the kind of hurt feelings you have experienced in your life. Rate these hurt feelings on a scale of 10 points, with 0 meaning no hurt feeling was ever experienced, 1 meaning a slightly painful experience, up to 10 meaning extremely and exceedingly painful feeling. Circle the number that best indicates your experience with that particular hurt feeling.

Feeling	*Painfulness*
Anguish	0 1 2 3 4 5 6 7 8 9 10
Bereavement	0 1 2 3 4 5 6 7 8 9 10
Desperation	0 1 2 3 4 5 6 7 8 9 10
Devastation	0 1 2 3 4 5 6 7 8 9 10
Distress	0 1 2 3 4 5 6 7 8 9 10
Grief	0 1 2 3 4 5 6 7 8 9 10
Sorrow	0 1 2 3 4 5 6 7 8 9 10
Suffering	0 1 2 3 4 5 6 7 8 9 10
Trauma	0 1 2 3 4 5 6 7 8 9 10
Upset	0 1 2 3 4 5 6 7 8 9 10

Explain how it felt to complete rating these hurt feelings. Feel free also to explain why you rated the feelings the way you did.

____
____
____
____
____

Could you report on how you feel about answering the above question?

____
____
____
____
____

Step 2. Define the hurt feelings listed below with the help of a dictionary and give two examples of how that particular feeling can be expressed.

1. Anguish

Definition ______________________________

____

Example 1:

____

____

Example 2:

____

____

2. Bereavement

Definition ______________________________

____

Example 1:

____

____

Example 2:

____

____

3. Desperation

Definition ______________________________

____

Example 1:

____

____

Example 2:

____

____

4. Devastation

Definition ______________________________

Example 1:

Example 2:

5. Distress

Definition ______________________________

Example 1:

Example 2:

6. Grief

Definition ______________________________

Example 1:

Example 2:

7. Sorrow

Definition ______________________________

____

Example 1:

____

____

Example 2:

____

____

8. Suffering

Definition ______________________________

____

Example 1:

____

____

Example 2:

____

____

9. Trauma

Definition ______________________________

____

Example 1:

____

____

Example 2:

____

____

10. Upset

Definition ____

____

Example 1:

____

____

Example 2:

____

____

11. A hurt feeling not listed above. Write what it is ______________

Definition ____

____

Example 1:

____

____

Example 2:

____

____

Now that you have defined these feelings according to how painful they are and were to you, please rank-order them according to how much you have experienced these feelings. Rank as No. 1 the feeling that you have experienced the most, rank as No. 2 the feeling that you have experienced next, and so on; mark as N/A the feelings that were not experienced by you, so that you rank only those specific feelings that you have experienced in you life.

Rank-order	*Feeling (Fill in)*	*Rank-order*	*Feeling (Fill in)*
No. 1	____________	No. 6	____________
No. 2	____________	No. 7	____________
No. 3	____________	No. 8	____________
No. 4	____________	No. 9	____________
No. 5	____________	No. 10	____________

Now that you have defined the items in this list and rank-ordered your hurt feelings, please explain how it felt to define and rank-order them. Feel free also to explain why you rank-ordered these feelings the way you did.

____
____
____
____
____

Could you report on how you feel about answering the above question?

____
____
____

After completing this practice exercise you should receive a general form directed to your No. 1 rated hurt feeling.

Practice Exercise No.________Name of Hurt Feeling__________

Name of Participant_______________________Sex_____Date______

The purpose of this practice exercise is to help you improve those hurt feelings that were rated either 10, 9, or 8 or that were ranked from 1 to 6 in your first practice exercise. Usually you should not be working on more than one hurt feeling at a time.

1. How did you experience this hurt feeling? Please explain in detail.

____
____
____
____
____

2. How often do you feel or are you aware of this hurt feeling?

a.	Practically every day	_____	e.	Once every 6 months	_____
b.	Once a week	_____	f.	Once a year	_____
c.	A couple of times a month	_____	g.	Once every few years	_____
d.	Once a month	_____			

3. Please explain further:

____
____
____
____
____

4. How did this hurt feeling come about? Do you remember when you became aware of it? Check which answer fits best:

   a. When I was a child (younger than 5 years of age) ________
   b. When I was in elementary school ________
   c. When I was in middle school ________
   d. When I was in high school ________
   e. After high school ________
   f. Any other time ________

5. Please explain further:

____
____
____

6. Was this hurt feeling acceptable or unacceptable? Why was this hurt feeling acceptable or unacceptable? Please explain:

____
____
____
____
____

7. Give three specific examples of how this hurt feeling affects you in the present

   Example 1:

____
____
____
____
____

Example 2:

___

___

___

___

___

Example 3:

___

___

___

___

___

Homework: Next week, plan to write about this hurt feeling at preset times (for instance, at 8 a.m., 12 noon, 4 or 7 p.m.) on at least 3 days (Monday, Wednesday, and Friday, or Tuesday, Thursday, and Saturday). If you can start thinking about it through writing, you might develop ways to make it stronger than it was in the past. Write down what happened in detail. For each time you start thinking about this hurt feeling, make sure to answer in writing the following four questions:

a. How did you start thinking it?
b. What followed?
c. How did it end?
d. What did this hurt feeling get you?

Time 1 (write the time you started________________)

a. ___

___

___

b. ___

___

___

c ___

___

___

d ___

___

___

Time 2 (write the time you started______________)

a. ______________________________
____
____

b. ______________________________
____
____

c. ______________________________
____
____

d. ______________________________
____
____

Time 3 (write the time you started______________)

a. ______________________________
____
____

b. ______________________________
____
____

c. ______________________________
____
____

d. ______________________________
____
____

Please, check which of the following shows how you feel about this practice exercise:

a. Completely useless _____
b. Somewhat useless _____
c. So-so _____
d. Somewhat useful _____
e. Extremely useful _____

Explain in greater detail how you feel about this practice exercise and what you got out of it if anything.

____
____
____
____
____

(Optional) General Feedback Form for Single Practice Exercises

Name________________________________Sex______Date_______

Practice Exercise No.________

The purpose of this feedback form is to learn how this practice exercise affected you.

Now that you have completed this practice exercise, please respond to the following questions concerning it.

1. How useful did you find this task for understanding the sourcebook topic?

a. Very useful	________	d. Slightly useful	________
b. Quite useful	________	e. Not useful at all	________
c. Somewhat useful	________		

2. How important is the skill or attitude addressed by this practice exercise?

a. Very important	________	d. Slightly important	________
b. Quite important	________	e. Not important at all	________
c. Somewhat important	________		

3. Put into your own words what you got out of doing this practice exercise.

____
____
____
____
____

4. How could this practice exercise be improved or changed?

Causes of Hurt Feelings

The purpose of these practice exercises is to help you understand and perhaps learn more about the causes and sources of hurt feelings in your life. These causes may have produced extremely hurtful feelings that may have affected you all your life.

You will receive one practice exercise after completion of this one and after satisfactory completion of others. Make sure that you were given information about the nature of these practice exercises and that you signed an informed consent form given to you at the beginning of this homework.

Step 1. Define the causes of hurt feelings listed below (with the help of a dictionary if necessary). Give two examples of how that particular cause was hurtful to you. If a cause does not apply to you personally, please define it and give two examples anyway.

1. Abandonment

   Definition

   Example 1:

Example 2:

2. Emotional verbal abuse

Definition

Example 1:

Example 2:

3. Physical abuse

Definition

Example 1:

Example 2:

4. Sexual abuse

Definition

Example 1:

Example 2:

5. Betrayal

Definition

Example 1:

Example 2:

6. Discounting

Definition

Example 1:

Example 2:

7. Frustration

Definition

Example 1:

Example 2:

8. Humiliation

Definition

Example 1:

Example 2:

9. Loss

Definition

Example 1:

Example 2:

10. Neglect

Definition

Example 1:

Example 2:

11. Rejection

Definition

Example 1:

Example 2:

12. Put-downs

Definition

Example 1:

Example 2:

13. A cause not listed above. Write what it is ____________________

Definition

Example 1:

Example 2:

14. A cause not listed above. Write what it is ___________________

Definition

Example 1:

Example 2:

Step 2. The purpose of this step is to obtain more information about present and past causes of hurt feelings you have experienced in your life. Rate these causes hurt feelings on a scale of 10 points, with 0 meaning no hurtfulness was ever experienced, 1 meaning a slightly hurtful experience, up to 10 meaning extremely and exceedingly hurtful feeling. Circle the number that indicates how hurtful that cause was to you and how seriously that cause affected your life.

Causes	*Degree of Hurtfulness*
1. Abandonment	0 1 2 3 4 5 6 7 8 9 10
2. Emotional abuse	0 1 2 3 4 5 6 7 8 9 10
3. Physical abuse	0 1 2 3 4 5 6 7 8 9 10
4. Sexual abuse	0 1 2 3 4 5 6 7 8 9 10
5. Betrayal	0 1 2 3 4 5 6 7 8 9 10
6. Discounting	0 1 2 3 4 5 6 7 8 9 10
7. Frustration	0 1 2 3 4 5 6 7 8 9 10
8. Humiliation	0 1 2 3 4 5 6 7 8 9 10
9. Loss	0 1 2 3 4 5 6 7 8 9 10
10. Neglect	0 1 2 3 4 5 6 7 8 9 10
11. Rejections	0 1 2 3 4 5 6 7 8 9 10
12. Put-down	0 1 2 3 4 5 6 7 8 9 10
13. Your specific cause	0 1 2 3 4 5 6 7 8 9 10
14. Your specific cause	0 1 2 3 4 5 6 7 8 9 10

Now that you have completed this list, please explain how it felt to rate the causes of your hurt feelings. Feel free also to explain why you rated these causes the way you did.

____
____
____
____
____

Could you report on how you feel about answering the above question?

____
____
____
____
____

Step 3. Now that you have defined and rated these causes according to how hurtful they are and were to you, please rank-order them according to how hurtful these causes were to you. Rank as No. 1 the cause that has been the most hurtful, rank as No. 2 the cause that was next in hurtfulness, and so on; mark as N/A the causes that do not apply to you at all.

Rank-order	*Cause (Fill in)*	*Rank-order*	*Cause (Fill in)*
No. 1	______________	No. 8	______________
No. 2	______________	No. 9	______________
No. 3	______________	No. 10	______________
No. 4	______________	No. 11	______________
No. 5	______________	No. 12	______________
No. 6	______________	No. 13	______________
No. 7	______________	No. 14	______________

Now that you have defined, rated, and rank-ordered the causes of your hurt feelings according to how hurtful they were to you, please explain how it felt to define, rate, and rank-order them. Feel free also to explain why you defined, rated, rank-ordered these causes the way you did.

____
____
____
____
____

Could you report on how you feel about answering this practice exercise?

____
____
____
____
____

After completing this practice exercise, you should receive as many general practice exercises as necessary to explain further the nature of the causes you rated on how hurtful they have been to you.

General Practice Exercise No. ________

Name of Hurtful Cause____________________________________

Name of Participant______________________Sex_____Date______

The purpose of this practice exercise is to explain further a cause that produced hurtful feelings that you may suffered all your life.

1. How did you experience this cause? Please explain in detail what happened that hurt your feelings.

____
____
____
____
____

2. How often do you feel or are you aware of this cause?

a.	Practically every day	_____	e.	Once every 6 months	_____
b.	Once a week	_____	f.	Once a year	_____
c.	A couple of times a month	_____	g.	Once every few years	_____
d.	Once a month	_____			

3. Please explain further:

____
____
____
____
____

4. How did this cause come about? Do you remember when you became aware of it? Check which answer fits best:

a. When I was a child (younger than 5 years of age) _____
b. When I was in elementary school _____
c. When I was in middle school _____
d. When I was in high school _____
e. After high school _____
f. Any other time _____

5. Please explain further:

____
____
____
____
____

6. Was this cause acceptable or unacceptable? Why? Please explain:

7. Give three specific examples of how this cause effects you in the present.

Example 1:

Example 2:

Example 3:

Homework: Next week, plan to write about this cause at preset times (for instance, at 8 a.m., 12 noon, 4 or 7 p.m.) on at least 3 days (Monday, Wednesday, and Friday, or Tuesday, Thursday, and Saturday). If you can start thinking about it through writing, you might develop ways to make it weaker than it was in the past. Write down what happened in detail. For each time you start thinking about this cause, make sure to answer in writing the following four questions:

a. How did you start thinking it?
b. What followed?
c. How did it end?
d. What did this hurt feeling get you?

Time 1 (write the time you started__________)

a. ____

____

____

b. ____

____

____

c. ____

____

____

d. ____

____

____

Time 2 (write the time you started__________)

a. ____

____

____

b. ____

____

____

c. ____

____

____

d. ____

____

____

Time 3 (write the time you started__________)

a. ____

____

____

b. ____

____

____

c. ____
____
____

d. ____
____
____

Check which of the following shows how you feel about this practice exercise:

a. Completely useless ______
b. Somewhat useless ______
c. So-so ______
d. Somewhat useful ______
e. Extremely useful ______

Explain in greater detail how you feel about this practice exercise and what you got out of it, if anything:

____
____
____
____
____

(Optional) General Feedback Form for Single Practice Exercises

Name________________________________Sex______Date_______

Practice Exercise No.________

The purpose of this feedback form is to learn how this practice exercise affected you.

Now that you have completed this practice exercise, please respond to the following questions concerning it.

1. How useful did you find this practice exercise for understanding the causes of your hurt feelings?

   a. Very useful ________
   b. Quite useful ________
   c. Somewhat useful ________
   d. Slightly useful ________
   e. Not useful at all ________

2. How important is the way that was used to give you this practice exercise?

a. Very important	________	d. Slightly important	________
b. Quite important	________	e. Not important at all	________
c. Somewhat important	________		

3. In your own words write what you got out of doing this practice exercise.

____
____
____
____
____

4. How could this practice exercise be improved or changed?

____
____
____
____
____

Informed Consent About Hurt Feelings

I______________________________(the undersigned) have been informed about the possible use of written practice exercises about hurt feelings as homework assignments, either by themselves written at a distance (by mail, fax, or Internet), or as additions to other verbal, face-to-face professional approaches, like prevention, psychotherapy, or rehabilitation. I understand that this approach is still experimental and that it needs to be evaluated before being available to everybody. I am aware of the possible dangerous consequences that may be provoked by answering written practice exercises about hurt feelings at a distance. I agree to participate in this type of intervention with the full understanding that it may bring up painful memories in my past and that this approach, at least initially, may produce some upset in me, my partner, or my family. I understand further that all information about me will be considered absolutely confidential because all of my writing will be limited between myself and the professional who is administering these written homework assignments. To maximize this anonymity, I can use the following five-digit number instead of my name in completing practice exercises:

____
____
____
____
____

I can drop out from this type of intervention any time I want without any penalty or consequence and I can only disclose whatever I want at my discretion during the course of these homework assignments. If I were to become upset because of the nature of this approach, it will be up to me to deal with this upset in any way I deem satisfactory to me. First, I should discuss this upset with the professional who is administering this intervention, if I do desire or see fit. Second, I can discuss my upset with whoever I choose. I may keep it to myself or discuss it with my loved ones, friends, clergy, or physician.

I can answer and send my completed homework assignments through the Internet in whatever manner that will guarantee absolute confidentiality, e.g., encryption. I do have the choice of using the Internet to communicate with the professional who is administering these homework assignments.

This professional, after proper evaluation, either through an interview and objective psychological tests, does have the option to inform me whether this approach will or will not be helpful to me. I will be informed of this option verbally and in writing.

I undertake answering in writing homework assignments about hurt feelings at a distance from a professional by my own free will and choice. I will not hold ______ ________________________________ responsible for any possible upset that may result from this intervention. Doctor, Mr., or Ms.___________________________is offering this intervention in good faith, using as many precautions as are humanly and professionally possible. I agree to complete in writing homework assignments given to me until completion of an agreed-upon practice exercise and, if necessary, to be evaluated before administration, after completion of these practice exercises, and even at a given period of time after termination to be agreed with the professional.

Signature of Participant Signature of Professional

___________________ Date_______ ___________Date_________

One copy of this signed informed consent form should be kept by the participant and another copy by the professional.

Note: Do you presently use any antidepressant or mood-changing medication? If so, inform the mental health professional who is offering these practice exercises about this medication. Ask permission and consent from your attending physician to participate in this type of intervention. Make sure you obtain a written consent from your physician that indicates knowledge and consent for you to participate in this type of homework assignments. Give a copy of the physician's consent to the professional. If necessary, have the mental health professional talk with your physician. In this case, you will need to give written permission to this professional to talk with your physician.

Section 3
Self-Help Practice Exercises for Individual Lifelong Learning

Character Strengths

The purpose of this practice exercises is to help you understand your character better You will be asked to complete in writing practice exercises containing a great many questions about the many parts that make up your character. Participation in working on this practice exercises is completely voluntary, and working on these practice exercises will be completely up to you. It is completely up to you whether you want to learn more about yourself and whether you want professionals interested in you to learn more about you. If you complete this practice exercise, it means that you do want to learn more about yourself and that you are interested in improving your condition.

L. L'Abate, *Sourcebook of Interactive Practice Exercises in Mental Health*, DOI 10.1007/978-1-4419-1354-8_13,

Practice Exercise 1. Understanding Your Character

Name________________________Sex_______Date_______________

The purpose of this practice exercise is to understand more about your character. To learn more about yourself, you will need to explain what the words listed below mean to you. Each word indicates a strength. Together with other strengths they make up your character. To understand and define these strengths, you might need the help of a dictionary or of your partner, your relatives, or your friends. In addition to each definition, you need to give two examples of how that strength applies to you or how you understand it in your own words.

Character Strengths	*Definitions and Examples*
a. Creativity ________________	Example 1 ________________
	Example 2 ________________
b. Curiosity ________________	Example 1 ________________
	Example 2 ________________
c. Open-mindedness __________	Example 1 ________________
	Example 2 ________________
d. Love of learning __________	Example 1 ________________
	Example 2 ________________
e. Perspective ______________	Example 1 ________________
	Example 2 ________________
f. Bravery __________________	Example 1 ________________
	Example 2 ________________

g. Persistence ____________________ Example 1 ____________________

____________________ Example 2 ____________________

h. Integrity ____________________ Example 1 ____________________

____________________ Example 2 ____________________

i. Vitality ____________________ Example 1 ____________________

____________________ Example 2 ____________________

j. Love ____________________ Example 1 ____________________

____________________ Example 2 ____________________

k. Kindness ____________________ Example 1 ____________________

____________________ Example 2 ____________________

l. Social intelligence ____________________ Example 1 ____________________

____________________ Example 2 ____________________

m. Citizenship ____________________ Example 1 ____________________

____________________ Example 2 ____________________

n. Fairness ____________________ Example 1 ____________________

____________________ Example 2 ____________________

o. Leadership ____________________ Example 1 ____________________

____________________ Example 2 ____________________

p. Forgiveness ____________________
____
____
____

Example 1 ____________________
____
Example 2 ____________________
____

q. Humility ____________________
____
____
____

Example 1 ____________________
____
Example 2 ____________________
____

r. Prudence ____________________
____
____
____

Example 1 ____________________
____
Example 2 ____________________
____

s. Self-regulation ____________________
____
____
____

Example 1 ____________________
____
Example 2 ____________________
____

t. Appreciation of beauty ____________________
____
____
____

Example 1 ____________________
____
Example 2 ____________________
____

u. Appreciation of excellence ____________________
____
____
____

Example 1 ____________________
____
Example 2 ____________________
____

v. Gratitude ____________________
____
____
____

Example 1 ____________________
____
Example 2 ____________________
____

w. Hope ____________________
____
____
____

Example 1 ____________________
____
Example 2 ____________________
____

x. Humor ____________________
____
____
____

Example 1 ____________________
____
Example 2 ____________________
____

y. Spirituality ____________________ Example 1 ____________________
____________________ ____________________
____________________ Example 2 ____________________
____________________ ____________________

2. Now that you have completed these definitions and examples, it is important to find out how these strengths apply to you. Next to each strength that you have defined, rate it according to how much that particular strength applies to you. Rate with 5 points the strengths that apply to you the most, rate with 4 points the strengths that apply to you next, rate with 3 points the strengths that apply to you next, rate with 2 points the strength that applies to you weakly, and rate with 1 point the strengths that might not apply to you, and rate with 0 the strengths that do not apply to you at all.

Strengths	*Points*	*Strengths*	*Points*
a. Creativity	_______	n. Fairness	_______
b. Curiosity	_______	o. Leadership	_______
c. Open-mindedness	_______	p. Forgiveness	_______
d. Love of learning	_______	q. Humility	_______
e. Perspective	_______	r. Prudence	_______
f. Bravery	_______	s. Self-regulation	_______
g. Persistence	_______	t. Appreciation of beauty	_______
h. Integrity	_______	u. Appreciation of excellence	_______
i. Vitality	_______	v. Gratitude	_______
j. Love	_______	w. Hope	_______
k. Kindness	_______	x. Humor	_______
l. Social intelligence	_______	y. Spirituality	_______
m. Citizenship	_______		

3. Write why you rated your strengths the way you did.

____
____
____
____
____

4. Now that you have completed this practice exercise, check which of these answers indicates how you felt about it. There is also space for you to explain further, if you want to:

   a. I did not like this practice exercise at all. I want to quit this stupid practice exercises. _______
   b. I did not like this practice exercise very much, but I want to go on with this practice exercises. _______

c. I liked this practice exercise and I want to go on with this practice exercises. _______
d. I liked this practice exercise a lot, and I wish I had something like this practice exercises years ago. ______
e. I liked it so much that I wish all my loved ones and friends could get something like this practice exercises to work on. ______

4. Discuss your completed practice exercise with whoever has given it to you.

Homework: During the coming week, think more about the strengths covered by this practice exercise and whether you want to change the ratings of these strengths as listed above, or start working on the next practice exercise.

____
____
____
____
____

Standard Practice Exercise No._____

Title of Strength:______________________________

Name______________________Sex________Date__________

The purpose of this practice exercise is to help you improve those strengths that were rated either 0, 1, 2, or 3 in your first practice exercise. Usually there should not be more than four to five practice exercises of this kind.

1. Why does this strength apply to you so little? Please explain in detail.

____
____
____
____

2. How often do you feel or are you aware of this strength?

a. Practically every day ______
b. Once a week ______
c. A couple of times a month ______
d. Once a month ______
e. Once every 6 months ______
f. Once a year ______
g. Once every few years ______

3. Please explain further:

____
____
____
____
____

4. How did this weak strength come about? Do you remember when you became aware of it? Check which answer fits best:

   a. When I was a child (younger than 5 years of age) ________
   b. When I was in elementary school ________
   c. When I was in middle school ________
   d. When I was in high school ________
   e. After high school ________
   f. Any other time ________

5. Please explain further:

____
____
____
____
____

6. Was this strength acceptable or unacceptable? Why? Please explain:

____
____
____
____
____

7. Give three specific examples of how this weak strength affects you in the present.

   Example 1:

____
____
____
____
____

Example 2:

____
____
____
____
____

Example 3:

____
____
____
____
____

Homework: Next week, plan to write about this weak strength at preset times (for instance, at 8 a.m., 12 noon, 4 or 7 p.m.) on at least 3 days (Monday, Wednesday, and Friday, or Tuesday, Thursday, and Saturday). If you can start thinking about it through writing, you might develop ways to make it stronger than it was in the past. Write down what happened in detail. For each time you start thinking about this strength, make sure to answer in writing the following four questions:

(a) How did you start thinking it?
(b) What followed?
(c) How did it end?
(d) What did this weakness get you?

Time 1 (write the time you started__________)

a. ____
____
____

b. ____
____
____

c. ____
____
____

d. ____
____
____

Time 2 (write the time you started__________)

a. ____

____

____

b. ____

____

____

c. ____

____

____

d. ____

____

____

Time 3 (write the time you started__________)

a. ____

____

____

b. ____

____

____

c. ____

____

____

d. ____

____

____

Check which of the following indicates how you feel about this practice exercise:

a.	Completely useless	______	d.	Somewhat useful	______
b.	Somewhat useless	______	e.	Extremely useful	______
c.	So-so	______			

Explain in greater detail how you feel about this practice exercise and what you got out of it.

____

____

____

____

____

Concluding Feedback Form

Name________________________Sex_________Date____________

The purpose of this form is to review whether this practice exercises was helpful to you or not.

1. Check the answer that best fits how you feel about this practice exercises:
   a. I did not like working on this practice exercises at all. I wish I never saw it. _______
   b. I did not like this practice exercises at all, but I am glad I got to work on it. _______
   c. I am delighted I got a chance to work on this practice exercises. _______
   d. I am not only delighted about working on this practice execises, but I wish all people with anxiety had a chance to work on it. _______

2. How helpful was it to work on this practice exercises? Check the answer that applies to you:

   a. Not helpful at all _______ c. Helpful _______
   b. Somewhat helpful _______ d. Very helpful _______

3. Which practice exercise did you like best? Please rate the practice exercises from the one you liked best (rate No. 5) to the one you liked next best (rate No. 4), and so on, to the one you did not like at all (No. 0); mark as N/A the exercises that did not apply to you.

Strengths	*Points*	*Strengths*	*Points*
a. Creativity	_______	n. Fairness	_______
b. Curiosity	_______	o. Leadership	_______
c. Open-mindedness	_______	p. Forgiveness	_______
d. Love of learning	_______	q. Humility	_______
e. Perspective	_______	r. Prudence	_______
f. Bravery	_______	s. Self-regulation	_______
g. Persistence	_______	t. Appreciation of beauty	_______
h. Integrity	_______	u. Appreciation of excellence	_______
i. Vitality	_______	v. Gratitude	_______
j. Love	_______	w. Hope	_______
k. Kindness	_______	x. Humor	_______
l. Social intelligence	_______	y. Spirituality	_______
m. Citizenship	_______		

4. Please explain why you rated these strengths the way you did.

____

____

____

____

____

5. Sometimes what we like most is not necessarily the most helpful. Which practice exercise was the most helpful to you? Rate the practice exercises according to their helpfulness to you. Rate as No. 5 the most helpful, No. 4 the next most helpful and so on, to the least helpful practice exercise, either 2, 1, or 0 for practice exercises that did help you or did not apply to you.(N/A).

Strengths	*Points*	*Strengths*	*Points*
a. Creativity	_______	n. Fairness	_______
b. Curiosity	_______	o. Leadership	_______
c. Open-mindedness	_______	p. Forgiveness	_______
d. Love of learning	_______	q. Humility	_______
e. Perspective	_______	r. Prudence	_______
f. Bravery	_______	s. Self-regulation	_______
g. Persistence	_______	t. Appreciation of beauty	_______
h. Integrity	_______	u. Appreciation of excellence	_______
i. Vitality	_______	v. Gratitude	_______
j. Love	_______	w. Hope	_______
k. Kindness	_______	x. Humor	_______
l. Social intelligence	_______	y. Spirituality	_______
m. Citizenship	_______		

6. Please explain why you rated these strengths the way you did.

____

____

____

____

____

7. Feel free to write any comments or suggestions that might improve this practice exercises.

____

____

____

____

____

Development of Emotional Competence

The purpose of this practice exercises is to help you improve your emotional competence. The purpose of the first practice exercise is to find how important feelings and emotions (yes, there is a difference between these two!) are for your survival and even your enjoyment of life. Many people do not know how to deal with their feelings and emotions because they have not paid attention to them or have avoided them altogether, for whatever reason. Hence, we will need to find out how important feelings and emotions are to you.

Practice Exercise 1. The Importance of Our Feelings and Emotions

Name________________________Sex__________Date___________

The purpose of this practice exercise is to stress the crucial importance of feelings in our lives and in our relationships.

1. On a scale of 1–10, with 1 meaning complete, absolute control and postpone and procrastinate over your feelings and emotions, and 10 meaning complete, free, and unabashed explosion and discharge of feelings and emotions, regardless of the consequences, circle where you fit most of the time:

   1 2 3 4 5 6 7 8 9 10

2. Check which of these applies to you. For you, feelings and emotions are

a. Completely unimportant	______	d. Important	______
b. Unimportant	______	e. Very important	______
c. Neutral or indifferent	______	f. Extremely important	______

3. Explain how you arrived at this view of feelings and emotions.

____

____

____

____

____

4. List as many feelings and emotions as you are aware of.

____

____

____

____

____

5. From this list of feelings and emotions, which do you experience most often?

6. Why do you experience these particular feelings and emotions?

7. How do you deal with your feelings in most situations?

8. How are these feelings and emotions related to you as a person?

9. How were feelings and emotions dealt with in your family of origin? Explain in detail and give examples of how feelings and emotions were dealt with in your family.

10. In what situations did you experience extreme feelings and how did you express them? Write about three situations where you experienced extreme feelings. Write (a) what happened to you, (b) how you reacted, and (c) what happened to you or others afterwards.

Situation 1:

a. ____

____

____

b. ____

____

____

c. ____

____

____

Situation 2:

a. ____

____

____

b. ____

____

____

c. ____

____

____

Situation 3:

a. ____

____

____

b. ____

____

____

c. ____

____

____

Homework: During the coming week, keep a list of all the feelings or emotional situations that faced you on a daily basis. It is very important for you to keep this daily list if you really want to go on with this practice exercises and understand and improve your emotional competence.

Practice Exercise 2. Awareness of Your Feelings and Emotions

Name__________________________________Sex_____Date______

The purpose of this practice exercise is to help you become more aware of your feelings and emotions because many of us are usually not aware of them. It is hoped that the more aware you become, the better you will be able to express them in a more effective and constructive fashion than you may have done in the past.

1. Is it possible that you may not be aware of certain feelings and emotions? How aware are you?
   Check which applies to you:

a.	Aware all the time	_______	d.	Somewhat aware	_______
b.	Very aware	_______	e.	Not aware at all	_______
c.	Aware	_______			

2. Who is responsible for your feelings and emotions and why?

____
____
____
____
____

3. How do feelings and emotions help you get what you wish for or what you want?

____
____
____
____
____

4. How aware are you of the strength and duration of certain feelings and emotions?

   a. List those feelings and emotions that, in your experience, are not very strong and that do not last very long.

____
____
____
____
____

b. List those feelings and emotions that, in your experience, are very strong and last a long time.

____
____
____
____
____

5. Sometimes, we experience more than one feeling or emotion at the same time. List what feelings or emotions you are aware of that are paired with each other.

____
____
____
____
____

6. How much did your culture, religion, or ethnic group influence you in how aware you are of your own feelings and emotions? Write at will:

____
____
____
____
____

7. How much did your gender influence you in how aware you are of your own feelings and emotions? Write at will:

____
____
____
____
____

8. How much did your social maturity and personality influence you in how aware you are of your own feelings and emotions? Write at will:

____
____
____
____
____

Homework: During the coming week, write whatever feelings come to mind as a result of answering the questions asked in this practice exercise, especially those related to your awareness of your own feelings and emotions.

Practice Exercise 3. Experience of Feelings and of Their Expression

Name________________________________Sex_____Date______

The purpose of this practice exercise is to help you separate what you feel, which belongs to you and you cannot help but feeling, from how you express these feelings. There is a limited number of feelings we can experience. However, there is an almost infinite number of ways in which a feeling can be expressed. One can feel angry and keep this feeling inside, or can say, "I feel angry about...," or, instead of saying anything, hit the one who is the source of that feeling. We have almost no choice about feelings we may experience. However, we have lots of choices on how these feelings can be expressed, shown, and discussed with others.

1. How often do you show and discuss your feelings? Check which applies to you:

a.	Not at all	_______	c.	Most of the time	_______
b.	Sometimes	_______	d.	All the time	_______

2. What kind of taboos and spoken or unspoken rules did your family have about the expression of feelings? Write at will:

____
____
____
____
____

3. Regardless of cultural or family rules about showing and discussing your feelings, what decisions did you personally make about showing and discussing them? Write at will:

____
____
____
____
____

4. Have you ever hidden your feelings and emotions from others? Why? Please explain:

____
____
____
____
____

5. Did you ever deceive others about how you feel? Can you think of any past or present situation when you felt one thing and said another? Try to think of as many situations as you can in how you felt something but said something else.

____
____
____
____
____

6. How much does being a man or a woman have to do with how you did or did not express your feelings openly? Write at will:

____
____
____
____
____

7. There are other factors that may have influenced you in how to show and discuss your feelings in addition to being a man or a woman. These factors are:

   a. Anxiety
   b. Depression or sadness
   c. Having been a latch-key child
   d. Feeling lonely
   e. Isolation
   f. ____________ (write what factor may have influenced you).

Circle which factor or factors may have prevented you from showing and discussing your feelings.

8. Cite some past experiences in which you felt something and you did not express it.

____
____
____
____
____

9. Cite some past experiences when you felt something and you did express it.

____
____
____
____
____

Homework: During the coming week, record what kind of feelings you experienced and how you chose to express them.

Practice Exercise 4. Awareness of Others' Feelings and Emotions

Name________________________Sex_______Date__________

The purpose of this practice exercise is to help you become aware of feelings and emotions in persons that matter to you (partner, children, parents, relatives, friends, coworkers). If we are not aware of our feelings and emotions, how can we be aware of feelings and emotions in those we love and who love us?

1. What kind of clues do you use to understand how others feel? Check all those that apply to you:

a. Face	________	e. Gestures	________
b. Eyes	________	f. Positions	________
c. Mouth	________	g. Movements	________
d. Chin	________	h. Other (explain):	________

2. How much do you rely on facial expressions in understanding other people's emotions and feelings?

a. A great deal	________	c. Not at all	________
b. Somewhat	________		

3. How do you react to feelings and emotions in those you love and who love you?

____
____
____
____
____

4. How do you react when someone you love shows the following feelings toward you? Write about each feeling at will:

a. Anger

b. Anxiety

c. Contempt

d. Disgust

e. Fear

f. Joy

g. Any other feelings you are aware of that are not listed above. Write what kind of feelings and how you react to them.

5. What do you do when someone you love fails to show and discuss feelings that you feel are important? Write at will:

6. Sometimes, whenever we do not receive the information we need about someone else's feelings, we may become judgmental and "mind-read" the other person's feelings. What is your favorite reaction whenever someone fails to tell you how he or she feels? Explain.

7. What kind of excuses do you make whenever you fail to show and discuss your feelings?

8. What kind of excuses do you make whenever someone you love fails to show and discuss his/her feelings with you? For instance, did you use gender? Did you use religion? Did you use culture? Did you use ethnic group? Explain in detail.

Homework: During the coming week, keep a record of situations where you became aware of feelings in intimate others and you checked out that how you saw those feelings was correct.

Practice Exercise 5. Using Words for Emotional Experience and Expression

Name____________________________________Sex____Date______

The purpose of this practice exercise is to help you expand your vocabulary about feelings and emotions. However, there are some individuals who are completely unable to talk about their feelings and emotions. Are you one of those individuals? If you are, or if you feel limited about how you feel and how you show and discuss your feelings, perhaps this practice exercise may help.

1. List as many feelings as you are aware of that you experience but do not express.

____
____
____
____
____

2. Among all the feelings you have listed above, pick at least three feelings that you experience most often. For each feeling, write the situations that provoked or aroused them.

   Feeling 1:

____
____
____
____
____

   Feeling 2:

____
____
____
____
____

Feeling 3:

3. List as many feelings as you can think of and show how you express them. For instance, we may feel very sad. However, we can express this feeling through criticism of self or others, or we may show and discuss anger. Whatever we may feel does not necessarily match what we may express. If necessary, use a dictionary and start listing all the emotions we can express. List as many as you can find.

4. From this list of emotions, pick three emotions that are most common to you and explain how you expressed them in at least three situations:

Emotion 1 .... (fill in)

Situation a:

Situation b:

Situation c:

Emotion 2 .... (fill in)

Situation a:

Situation b:

Situation c:

Emotion 3 .... (fill in)

Situation a:

Situation b:

Situation c:

5. Now complete the following sentence stems:

   a. When someone I love is angry at me I …

   b. When someone I love is frustrated with me I …

   c. When someone I love is disappointed in me I …

   d. When someone I love is…………………….. (write in the emotion) at me, I …

6. Complete the following sentence stems:

   a. When I am angry at someone I love, I …

   b. When I am frustrated with someone I love, I …

   c. When I am disappointed with someone I love, I

   d. When I feel…………………….. (write in the feeling) with someone I love, I …

7. Write what other feelings you would like to experience and express better.

8. Why? Explain your reasons for wanting to experience and express the feelings you have listed in the previous item, No. 7.

Homework: During the coming week, record all instances of how you reacted to the feelings and emotions of those who matter to you, as well as of those who may not matter.

Practice Exercise 6. Capacity for Putting oneself into another's shoes

Name___________________________________Sex____Date______

The purpose of this practice exercise is to help you become more aware of and understand others' feelings, especially of those you love and who love you, and to help you communicate that you care about their feelings.

1. How aware and sympathetic are you of others' feelings? Check which answer applies to you:

   a. Very sympathetic _____
   b. Sympathetic enough _____
   c. Somewhat sympathetic _____
   d. Not very sympathetic _____
   e. Not at all sympathetic _____

2. Would you like to become more sympathetic or are you satisfied that you are sympathetic enough and you do not need to complete this practice exercise? Check which answer applies to you:

   a. I am sympathetic enough and I do not need to complete this practice exercise. ________
   b. I am somewhat sympathetic but I still would like to improve my care for others' feelings. ________
   c. I really need to become more sympathetic and I very much want to complete this practice exercise and the whole practice exercises. ________

3. Write about three instances when you did show your care for others' feelings. Write (a) who the person was, (b) what feelings were expressed, (c) how you reacted to these feelings, and (d) how you felt afterwards.

   Instance 1:

a. ____

b. ____

c. ____

d. ____

Instance 2:

a. ____
____
____

b. ____
____
____

c. ____
____
____

d. ____
____
____

Instance 3:

a. ____
____
____

b. ____
____
____

c. ____
____
____

d. ____
____
____

4. Now write about three instances when you failed to care for someone else's feelings, following the same outline given above: (a) who was the person. (b) what feelings were expressed, (c) how you reacted, and (d) how you felt afterwards.

Instance 1:

a. ____
____
____

b. ______

c. ______

d. ______

Instance 2:

a. ______

b. ______

c. ______

d. ______

Instance 3:

a. ______

b. ______

c. ______

d. ______

5. How do you explain your caring or not caring about others' feelings? Trace the development of your sympathy or lack of it since you can remember.

____
____
____
____
____

6. What special experiences or events do you remember that relate to your being sympathetic or not sympathetic of others' feelings? Try to remember as many as you can and write about them.

____
____
____
____
____

Homework: During the coming week record as many instances in which you were sympathetic or not sympathetic of the feelings of those you care about and who care for you.

Practice Exercise 7. Coping with Painful Feelings and Distressful Situations

Name______________________Sex_____Date______

The purpose of this practice exercise is to help you control, regulate, and express constructively and positively painful feelings in distressful situations.

1. List as many painful and distressful situations as you have experienced in the past and that you may have not discussed with anyone until now. Write for 15 minute a day for four consecutive days. Make sure that you do not spend more than 15 minute a day by using an alarm clock or a kitchen timer to remind you to stop after 15 minute. If possible, try to write always at the same time of day.

   Day 1:

____
____
____
____
____

Day 2:

Day 3:

Day 4:

2. From this list, pick three experiences that were the most painful and distressful to you and write about them in greater detail.

Experience a:

Experience b:

Experience c:

____
____
____
____
____

3. What effects or influence have these painful experiences had on you? Please explain in detail.

____
____
____
____
____

4. What have you done to deal with, cope with, and control your past or present painful or stressful experiences? Below are listed a variety of helpful steps that can be taken. Which one did you use and how useful was it to you? Circle all that apply to you.

   a. Problem solving as a rational and reasonable way to cope
      i. Used ______ Not used ______
      ii. Useful _____ Not useful _____
   b. Seeking support from others
      i. Used ______ Not used ______
      ii. Useful _____ Not useful _____
   c. Seeking help from close ones (parents, partner, relatives, and friends)
      i. Used ______ Not used ______
      ii. Useful _____ Not useful _____
   d. Seeking help from professionals (physician, therapist, counselor, clergy, others)
      i. Used ______ Not used ______
      ii. Useful _____ Not useful _____
   e. Distancing or avoiding painful/distressful situation
      i. Used ______ Not used ______
      ii. Useful _____ Not useful _____
   f. Keeping inside and not discussing with anyone
      i. Used ______ Not used ______
      ii. Useful _____ Not useful _____
   g. Getting it out and acting it out verbally or physically
      i. Used ______ Not used ______
      ii. Useful _____ Not useful _____

h. Emotion focused on, that is, discussing your feelings with someone who cares about you
   i. Used ______ Not used ______
   ii. Useful _____ Not useful _____
i. Any other direction not listed above. Write what it was:
   i. Used ______ Not used ______
   ii. Useful _____ Not useful _____

5. Pick the step that was most useful to you and write about it in detail.

____
____
____
____
____

6. What could you do in the future that you have not done in the past to cope with painful/stressful experiences? Develop a plan consisting of how you would handle a painful/stressful experience in a more positive and constructive fashion than you have done in the past.

____
____
____
____
____

7. Discuss this plan with someone you trust and ask him or her to help you make it more specific and more detailed to help you cope with future painful/stressful experiences in better ways than you have done in the past.

8. Make whatever changes are necessary in your plan after you receive helpful feedback from someone you trust. Make sure that these changes are put in writing.

Homework: In the coming week, apply your plan to possibly painful/stressful experiences and see how it works. Make whatever corrections in your plan will be more helpful to you.

Practice Exercise 8. Awareness of Emotional Communications in Intimate Relationships

Name____________________________________Sex____Date______

The purpose of this practice exercise is to help you handle potentially painful experiences in the future in better ways than you may have done in the past.

1. List as many conflict situations as you can remember that have provoked anger or other extreme feelings in you. Write (1) that the situation was, (2) who provoked it, (3) how you reacted, and (4) how you felt afterwards.

Situation a:

a. ______________________________

b. ______________________________

c. ______________________________

d. ______________________________

Situation b:

a. ______________________________

b. ______________________________

c. ______________________________

d. ______________________________

Situation c:

a. ______________________________

b. ____

____

____

c. ____

____

____

d. ____

____

____

2. Make up at least three possible or pretend situations that might confront you in the future that you want to handle in more creative ways than you might have done in the past. List (1) the possible situation, (2) whom the situation involves, (3) how you would react, and (4) how you would feel afterwards.

Situation a:

a. ____

____

____

b. ____

____

____

c. ____

____

____

d. ____

____

____

Situation b:

a. ____

____

____

b. ____

____

____

c. ____
____
____

d. ____
____
____

Situation c:

a. ____
____
____

b. ____
____
____

c. ____
____
____

d. ____
____
____

3. How fast or how slow are you in reacting to emotional situations? Check which applies to you the most:

a. Very, very fast ______
b. Very fast ______
c. Fast enough ______
d. Not very fast ______
e. Not fast at all ______
f. Very slow ______
g. Very, very slow ______

4. Explain why you react the way you checked in No. 3.

____
____
____
____
____

5. What are the advantages of reacting slowly to emotional situations? Please explain.

____
____
____
____
____

6. What are the disadvantages of reacting very fast to emotional situations? Please explain.

____
____
____
____
____

7. What emotional situations require fast reactions? List as many situations you can think of.

____
____
____
____

8. What emotional situations require fast reactions? List as many situations that you can think of.

____
____
____
____
____

Homework: During the coming week, try to implement, apply, or actually start a painful/stressful situation to see how you would handle it. If possible, start more than one situation. Remember that if you can start it, you can stop it!

Practice Exercise 9. Capacity for Emotional Self-Effectiveness

Name______________________________Sex____Date______

The purpose of this practice exercise is to help you improve your emotional effectiveness.

1. One way to improve self-effectiveness is to accept your own feelings and your own sense of well-being. How much are you able to accept both feelings and well-being?

    a. A great deal ______
    b. Somewhat ______
    c. Not yet, but I am working at it ______
    d. Not at all, I need further help with my feelings and emotions ______

2. How could you improve your acceptance of your feelings and how you express them? Write about possible ways in which you can improve your acceptance.

____
____
____
____
____

3. There are some ways in which self-effectiveness can be improved. In order to achieve this goal, you may need to become aware of possible conflicts within yourself:

    Conflict a: Your feelings are weaker than how you have expressed them. Give three examples of how this conflict applies to you.

    Example 1:

____
____
____
____
____

    Example 2:

____
____
____
____
____

    Example 3:

____
____
____
____
____

Conflict b: You feelings are stronger and may overpower how you express them. Give three examples of how this conflict applies to you.

Example 1:

Example 2:

Example 3:

Conflict c: How you express your feelings, that is, your emotions, is not equal to how you feel. Give three examples of how this conflict applies to you.

Example 1:

Example 2:

Example 3:

4. Another source of conflict may result from you feeling one way and presenting it another way. For instance, you may be very angry at your boss, but you cannot express your feelings unless you want to jeopardize your job. Give three instances when you had to act in different ways from what you felt.

Example 1:

Example 2:

Example 3:

5. Another source of conflict may relate to a comparison of your feelings with the feelings of another person who is important to you, Write about three situations when your feelings were different from the feelings of someone else.

Situation a. Your feelings were stronger than the feelings of another:

Situation b. Your feelings were weaker than the feelings of another:

Situation c. Your feelings were as strong or the same as the feelings of another:

6. Knowing what you know now, how would you handle a conflict situation where your feelings were quite different from the feelings of another?

7. An important part of owing one's feelings is to talk about them using the personal pronoun "I." Start as many sentences with "I" to practice owning your feelings.

8. Now you need to practice recognition and affirmation of someone else's feelings. Restate or rephrase but do not repeat the feelings expressed in No. 7 as if someone else said them to you. It is important to convey to the other person that you have understood and value their feelings.

Homework: During the coming week, record instances where you reacted too fast or to slow to an emotional situation. If possible, report where you failed to express your feelings using the personal pronoun, and failed to indicate to another how you cared for their feelings. If you did not fail, record any possible success you may have achieved.

Practice Exercise 10. Emotional Incompetence and Deviancy

Name_________________________________Sex_____Date______

The purpose of this final practice exercise is to make you aware of any possible emotional incompetence or deviancy that may slow down your progress toward an improvement of your emotional effectiveness. In order to complete this practice exercise answer all the following questions to the best of your abilities.

1. What happens if awareness of one's feelings and emotions is inadequate?

____

____

____

____

____

2. What happens if understanding others' emotional experience is limited?

____

____

____

____

____

3. What happens if there is a limited emotional vocabulary?

____

____

____

____

____

4. What happens if one is either overwhelmed by others' emotional experience, or, at the other extreme, one is unable to respond appropriately to another's feelings?

____

____

____

____

____

5. What happens if one cannot separate feelings, on one hand, and emotions, on the other hand, in most emotional situations?

6. What happens if one's ability to handle emotional situations is limited and one is defective in the ability to control one's feelings and emotions?

7. What happens when emotional communication in relationships is impaired or distorted?

8. What happens when emotional effectiveness is seldom experienced?

Homework: During the coming week, you need to reflect on, think about, and consider whether working on these practice exercises was helpful to you. It is important for you to think about it because in the follow-up practice exercise you will be asked to answer which practice exercise was most helpful to you and which was not.

Final Follow-Up Form

Name__________________________________Sex______Date_______

The purpose of this follow-up practice exercise is to find what you have learned from completing the practice exercises in this practice exercises. Congratulations to you for reaching this point!

1. Check which answer applies to you best:

   a. I wish I never saw any practice exercise in this practice exercises. It was a complete waste of my time. ________
   b. These practice exercises were hard to complete and I did not get out of them what I wished I should have gotten. ________
   c. These practice exercises were okay. I really do not know whether I learned anything new or not. ________
   d. I enjoyed working on these practice exercises and I am delighted I was able to complete them. ________
   e. I cannot think of anything better in my life. These practice exercises gave me a completely different perspective on myself and my life. ________
   f. I cannot think of where I would be if I did not have these practice exercises to work on. I wish everybody were able to work on them. ________
   g. I cannot begin to tell you how much these practice exercises meant to me. They saved my life. ________

2. Which practice exercise was the most helpful to you? Rank-order them from most useful to least useful. Rank as No. 1 the most useful, rank as No. 2 the second most useful, and so on until the very last one, which should be ranked No. 9.

Practice Exercises	*Rank-order*
a. The Importance of Our Feelings and Emotions	________
b. Awareness of Your Feelings and Emotions	________
c. The Experience of Feelings and the Expression of Emotions	________
d. Awareness of Others' Feelings and Emotions	________
e. Using the Vocabulary of Emotional Experience and Expression	________
f. Capacity for Empathic Involvement	________
g. Coping with Painful Feelings and Distressful Situations	________
h. Awareness of Emotional Communication within Relationships	________
i. Capacity for Emotional Self-Effectiveness	________

3. Explain why you rank-ordered the practice exercises the way you did. Why did you rank one practice exercise as the most useful and why did you rank another as the least useful?

____
____
____
____
____

4. Do you have any suggestions to improve these practice exercises? We would appreciate any kind of critical and constructive feedback that would allow an improvement in these practice exercises.

____
____
____
____
____

Self-Importance

This practice exercises is to be administered after determining objectively whether importance is attributed to self more than to significant others or whether others are attributed more importance than self. The purpose of this practice exercises is to help you improve your sense of self-importance.

Practice Exercise 1. How Important Am I?

Name________________________Sex______Date______

The purpose of this practice exercise is to understand how the characteristics listed below are related to your sense of self-importance.

1. Rate from 0 to 10 how each characteristic listed below is related to your sense of self-importance: 0 means absolutely no importance, 10 means a great deal of importance. Circle the number that indicates how important each characteristic is for you.

a. Intelligence	0	1	2	3	4	5	6	7	8	9	10
b. Physical attractiveness	0	1	2	3	4	5	6	7	8	9	10
c. Sports success	0	1	2	3	4	5	6	7	8	9	10
d. Sense of humor	0	1	2	3	4	5	6	7	8	9	10
e. School/job competence	0	1	2	3	4	5	6	7	8	9	10

f.	Sociability/popularity	0	1	2	3	4	5	6	7	8	9	10
g.	Morality	0	1	2	3	4	5	6	7	8	9	10
h.	Self-worth or self-esteem	0	1	2	3	4	5	6	7	8	9	10
i.	Any other characteristic not listed above (______________)	0	1	2	3	4	5	6	7	8	9	10

2. Rank-order the characteristics listed above by how much they contribute to your sense of self-importance. Rank as No. 1 the characteristic that contributes the most to your sense of self-importance, rank as No. 2 the characteristic that contributes second to your sense of self-importance, and so on, until the characteristic that does not contribute at all is ranked 8 or 9, based on whether you have filled in another characteristic (item i).

Characteristic	*Rank-order*
a. Intelligence	________
b. Physical attractiveness	________
c. Sports success	________
d. Sense of humor	________
e. School/job competence	________
f. Sociability/popularity	________
g. Morality	________
h. Self-worth or self-esteem	________
i. Any other characteristic not listed above (______________________)	________

3. What guided your thinking as you rank-ordered these characteristics?

____
____
____
____
____

Homework: During the coming week, think how each characteristic could affect your sense of importance in a positive way. Write down what you come up with and discuss it with whoever is giving you these assignments.

Standard Practice Exercise for Self-Importance

Practice Exercise No.___Characteristic______________________________

Name____Sex_____Date______

The purpose of this practice exercise is to understand in greater detail how the characteristic listed above is linked to your sense of self-importance.

1. How does this characteristic influence your sense of importance?

____

____

____

____

____

2. When did you become aware of this characteristic? Check which age applies:

a.	Preschool	______	d.	High school	______
b.	Elementary school	______	e.	College	______
c.	Middle school	______	f.	Graduate school	______

3. How did you become aware of this characteristic? Write as much as you possibly can.

____

____

____

____

____

4. How has this characteristic handicapped your sense of self-importance in the past?

____

____

____

____

____

5. How does this characteristic handicap your sense of self-importance in the present?

____

____

____

____

____

6. How much do you want this characteristic to handicap your sense of self-importance in the future?

____

____

____

____

____

7. How often did this characteristic affect your sense of self-importance? Check which answer applies to you:

a.	Practically every day	______	e.	Once every 6 months	______
b.	Once a week	______	f.	Once a year	______
c.	A couple of times a month	______	g.	Once every few years	______
d.	Once a month	______			

8. Please explain further:

____
____
____
____
____

9. Give three specific examples of how this characteristic handicaps your sense of self-importance.

Example 1:

____
____
____
____
____

Example 2:

____
____
____
____
____

Example 3:

____
____
____
____
____

Homework: During the next few days think of how you could either give up this characteristic if it handicaps you, or change it so that it has a positive effect on you.

1. Write down what you want to do about this characteristic.

____
____
____
____
____

2. Do you want this characteristic to control you or do you want to control it?

____
____
____
____
____

Concluding Feedback Form

Name_______________________Sex_______Date________

The purpose of this form is to find out what you have learned from this practice exercises.

1. How was this practice exercises helpful to you?

   a. Very little _______ c. A great deal _______
   b. Somewhat _______

2. In your own words, write how this practice exercises was helpful to you (if at all).

____
____
____
____
____

3. Rank-order the practice exercises listed below according to helpful they were to you. Rank as No. 1 the practice exercise that was most helpful, rank as No. 2 the practice exercise that was helpful next, and so on, down to a practice exercise that was not helpful to you at all.

Characteristic	*Rank-order*
a. Intelligence	_________
b. Physical attractiveness	_________

c. Sports success ________
d. Sense of humor ________
e. School/job competence ________
f. Sociability/popularity ________
g. Morality ________
h. Self-worth or self-esteem ________
i. Any other characteristic not listed above ________
(____________________)

4. Write in greater detail how the first three ranked practice exercises were helpful to you.

____
____
____
____
____

5. Write in greater detail why the least ranked practice exercises was not helpful to you.

____
____
____
____
____

6. Why was this practice exercise not helpful to you?

____
____
____
____
____

7. How would you improve this practice exercises?

____
____
____
____
____

Others' Importance

The purpose of this practice exercises is to help you develop a better understanding of people who in one way or another, positively or negatively, have affected your sense of self- importance.

Practice Exercise 1. Who Are the Others?

Name__________________________________Sex_____Date_______

The purpose of this practice exercise is to understand better who are the people who affected your sense of self-importance.

1. Explain in great detail who these people are by giving their names and more information about the nature of their relationship with you.

   a. Close friends

   ____

   b. Boy/girlfriend or partner/mate/spouse

   ____

   c. Children (if any)

   ____

   d. Mother or mother substitute[1]

   ____

   e. Father or father substitute[2]

   ____

   f. Brothers/sisters (list all of them by name and age)

   ____

   g. Coworkers or fellow students

   ____

[1]Female caregiver could be biological, stepmother, or other institutional caregiver of feminine gender (check which).

[2]Male caregiver could be biological, stepfather, or other institutional caregiver of masculine gender (check which).

h. Neighbors

____

i. Other relatives (list only those who were close to you)

____

j. Teachers/mentors

____

k. Write the name of anybody else who affected your sense of importance: (______________________)

____

2. Now that you have identified further those people who in one way or another affected your sense of self-importance, rank-order these people according to how they compare in how they affected your sense of self-importance. Rank as No. 1 the person who had the greatest effect on your sense of self-importance, rank as No. 2 the person who had the next greatest effect on your sense of self-importance, and so on, until the person who ranked the lowest among these people in affecting your sense of self-importance.

Person	*Rank-order*
a. Close friends	________
b. Boy/girlfriend or partner/mate/spouse	________
c. Children (if applicable)	________
d. Mother or mother substitute	________
e. Father or father substitute	________
f. Brothers/sisters	________
g. Coworkers	________
h. Neighbors	________
i. Other relatives (as listed above)	________
j. Teachers/mentors	________
k. Anybody else (______________________):	________

3. Now that you have rank-ordered all these people according to how much they affected your sense of self-importance, explain why you ranked them in the way you did.

____
____
____
____
____

Homework: During the next week, start thinking whether there are other people who affected your sense of self-importance. Write down whatever new information about others comes to your mind and discuss with whoever is giving you these assignments.

Standard Practice Exercises for Others' Importance

Practice Exercise No.___Person described (write name)___________

Name____________________________Sex_____Date____________

The purpose of this practice exercise and of all other practice exercises is to tell more about the particular person (whose name is listed above) who affected your sense of self-importance.

1. What kind of relationship did you have with this person? Write about it for as long as it is necessary.

   ____
   ____
   ____
   ____
   ____

2. How did this person affect your sense of self-importance?

   ____
   ____
   ____
   ____
   ____

3. How often did this person affect your sense of self-importance? Check which answer applies to you:

a.	Practically every day	_____	e.	Once every 6 months	_____
b.	Once a week	_____	f.	Once a year	_____
c.	A couple of times a month	_____	g.	Once every few years	_____
d.	Once a month	_____			

4. Please explain further:

____
____
____
____
____

4. When did this person start to influence your sense of self-importance? Check which answer fits best:

   a. When I was a child (younger than 5 years of age) ________
   b. When I was in elementary school ________
   c. When I was in middle school ________
   d. When I was in high school ________
   e. After high school ________
   f. Any other time ________

5. Please explain further:

____
____
____
____
____

6. Give three specific examples of how this person affected your sense of self-importance.

   Example 1:

____
____
____
____
____

   Example 2:

____
____
____
____
____

Example 3:

7. How did you feel and react to this person? Write in detail.

8. What is the nature of you relationship with this person now?

9. If you could say something to this person, what would you say to her or him?

10. How do you want to relate to this person in the future (provided this person is still alive)?

11. If you could change your behavior toward this person, how would you change it?

12. If you could say something positive to this person, what would you say?

____
____
____
____
____

Homework: During the coming week, write down how you could undo whatever damage has been done to your sense of self-importance by this person. Discuss your writing with whoever is helping you with this practice exercises.

Concluding Feedback Form

Name_________________________Sex_____Date________

The purpose of this form is to find out what you have learned from this practice exercise.

1. Was this practice exercise helpful to you?

   a. Very little _______ c. A great deal _______
   b. Somewhat _______

2. In your own words, write how this practice exercises was helpful to you.

____
____
____
____
____

3. Rank-order the practice exercises listed below according to helpful they were to you. Rank as No. 1 the practice exercise that was most helpful, rank as No. 2 the practice exercise that was helpful next, and so on, down to a practice exercise was not helpful to you at all.

Practice Exercise	*Rank-order*
a. Close friends	_________
b. Boy/girlfriend or partner/mate/spouse	_________
c. Children (if applicable)	_________
d. Mother or mother substitute	_________
e. Father or father substitute	_________
f. Brothers/sisters	_________
g. Coworkers	_________

h. Neighbors ________
i. Other relatives (as listed above) ________
j. Teachers/mentors ________
k. Anybody else (________________________): ________

4. Write in greater detail how the first three ranked practice exercises were helpful to you.

____
____
____
____
____

5. Write in greater detail why the least ranked practice exercise was not helpful to you.

____
____
____
____
____

6. How would you improve this practice exercises?

____
____
____
____
____

Emotional Expression

The purpose of this practice exercises is to help you become more aware of your feelings and, perhaps, learn how to express them in a more helpful and constructive fashion than you may have done in the past.

Practice Exercise 1. Becoming Aware of Feelings

Name________________________________Sex____Date________

The purpose of this practice exercise is to list some of the most common feelings that take place within individuals, between couples, and among family members. The remainder of this practice exercises consists of feelings drawn from this list.

1. Please define what you understand about the meaning of each feeling listed below, and give two examples of how each feeling is used. Use a dictionary or online information if you need help in defining these feelings.

Emotion and Definitions	*Examples*
a. Amusement __________	Example 1 __________
__________	Example 2 __________
b. Anger __________	Example 1 __________
__________	Example 2 __________
c. Contempt __________	Example 1 __________
__________	Example 2 __________
d. Disgust __________	Example 1 __________
__________	Example 2 __________
e. Distress __________	Example 1 __________
__________	Example 2 __________
f. Enjoyment __________	Example 1 __________
__________	Example 2 __________
g. Fear __________	Example 1 __________
__________	Example 2 __________
h. Guilt __________	Example 1 __________
__________	Example 2 __________

i. Interest ______________________	Example 1 ______________________
______________________	______________________
______________________	Example 2 ______________________
______________________	______________________
j. Sadness ______________________	Example 1 ______________________
______________________	______________________
______________________	Example 2 ______________________
______________________	______________________
k. Surprise______________________	Example 1 ______________________
______________________	______________________
______________________	Example 2 ______________________
______________________	______________________
l. Any other feeling not listed above. Please fill in the feeling before defining it (______________) and giving two examples.	Example 1 ______________________ ______________________ Example 2 ______________________ ______________________
______________________	______________________
m. Same as above (______________)	Example 1 ______________________
______________________	______________________
______________________	Example 2 ______________________
______________________	______________________
n. Same as above (______________)	Example 1 ______________________
______________________	______________________
______________________	Example 2 ______________________
______________________	______________________

2. Now you need to rank-order this list of feelings according to how much each feeling is used by you and according to its strength in comparison to other feelings. Rank as No. 1 the strongest feeling among all the feelings listed above, rank as No. 2 the next second strongest feeling, and so on, until the last one is numbered from 11 to 14, based on how many feelings you have defined above.

Feelings	*Rank-order*	*Feelings*	*Rank-order*
a. Amusement	________	h. Guilt	________
b. Anger	________	i. Interest	________
c. Contempt	________	j. Sadness	________
d. Disgust	________	k. Surprise	________
e. Distress	________	l. (______)	________
f. Enjoyment	________	m. (______)	________
g. Fear	________	n. (______)	________

3. (For partners only; single individuals skip to Practice Exercise No. 4.) If you are married or living with someone in a committed relationship, rank-order this list of feelings according to how strong they are in your partner. Rank as No. 1 the strongest feeling, rank as No. 2 the second strongest feeling, and so on, until the last one ranked is the weakest feeling that is not present or evident in your relationship.

Feelings	*Rank-order*	*Feelings*	*Rank-order*
a. Amusement	________	h. Guilt	________
b. Anger	________	i. Interest	________
c. Contempt	________	j. Sadness	________
d. Disgust	________	k. Surprise	________
e. Distress	________	l. (______________)	________
f. Enjoyment	________	m. (______________)	________
g. Fear	________	n. (______________)	________

4. Rank-order these feelings according to how strong they are or were among members of your family of origin. Rank as No. 1 the strongest feeling, rank as No. 2 the second strongest feeling, and so on, until the last one ranked is the weakest feeling that is or was not present or evident in your mother (stepmother, female caregiver, or mother substitute; circle which is relevant), your father (stepfather, male caregiver, or father substitute, circle which is relevant), and your brothers or sisters (state their age and gender).

Feelings	*Rank-orders*				
	Mother	*Father*	*Sibling*	*Sibling*	*Sibling*
Age	_____	_____	_____	_____	_____
Gender	_____	_____	_____	_____	_____
a. Amusement	_____	_____	_____	_____	_____
b. Anger	_____	_____	_____	_____	_____
c. Contempt	_____	_____	_____	_____	_____
d. Disgust	_____	_____	_____	_____	_____
e. Distress	_____	_____	_____	_____	_____
f. Enjoyment	_____	_____	_____	_____	_____
g. Fear	_____	_____	_____	_____	_____
h. Guilt	_____	_____	_____	_____	_____
i. Interest	_____	_____	_____	_____	_____
j. Sadness	_____	_____	_____	_____	_____
k. Surprise	_____	_____	_____	_____	_____
l. (____________)	_____	_____	_____	_____	_____
m. (____________)	_____	_____	_____	_____	_____
n. (____________)	_____	_____	_____	_____	_____

Homework: During the coming week, think about the list of feelings given in the first practice exercise and assess them according to how constructive (helpful) or destructive they are for you, for your partner (if you have one), and for members of your family. Write them down according to how helpful or hurtful these feelings are for you.

Standard Practice Exercises

Practice Exercise No.______________Title of Feeling:____________

Name___________________________Sex________Date_________

The purpose of this practice exercise is to understand more about the feeling listed in the title.

1. How is this emotion expressed by you? Please explain in detail.

____

____

____

____

____

2. How often do you express this feeling? Check which answer applies to you:

a. Practically every day	_____	e. Once every 6 months	_____
b. Once a week	_____	f. Once a year	_____
c. A couple of times a month	_____	g. Once every few years	_____
d. Once a month	_____	h. Please explain further:	

____

____

____

____

____

3. How often is this feeling expressed by your partner (if your have one, otherwise skip this question)? Check which answer applies to your partner:

a. Practically every day	_____	e. Once every 6 months	_____
b. Once a week	_____	f. Once a year	_____
c. A couple of times a month	_____	g. Once every few years	_____
d. Once a month	_____	h. Please explain further:	

____
____
____
____
____

4. How often is (was) this feeling expressed by your mother or mother substitute? Check which answer applies to her:

a.	Practically every day	_____	e.	Once every 6 months	_____
b.	Once a week	_____	f.	Once a year	_____
c.	A couple of times a month	_____	g.	Once every few years	_____
d.	Once a month	_____	h.	Please explain further:	

____
____
____
____
____

5. How often is (was) this feeling expressed by your father or father substitute? Check which answer applies to him:

a.	Practically every day	_____	e.	Once every 6 months	_____
b.	Once a week	_____	f.	Once a year	_____
c.	A couple of times a month	_____	g.	Once every few years	_____
d.	Once a month	_____	h.	Please explain further:	

____
____
____
____
____

6. Pick one sibling (brother or sister) whose emotional expression matters or mattered to you a great deal, more than any other sibling, and check which answer applies to her or him:

a.	Practically every day	_____	e.	Once every 6 months	_____
b.	Once a week	_____	f.	Once a year	_____
c.	A couple of times a month	_____	g.	Once every few years	_____
d.	Once a month	_____	h.	Please explain further:	

____
____
____
____
____

7. Can you remember how this feeling came about? Do you remember when you started it? Check which answer fits best:

   a. When I was a child (younger than 5 years of age) ______
   b. When I was in elementary school ______
   c. When I was in middle school ______
   d. When I was in high school ______
   e. After high school ______
   f. Any other time ______
   g. Please explain further: ______

____
____
____
____
____

8. Did expressing this feeling ever get you in trouble? Please explain:

____
____
____
____

9. Give three specific examples of how this feeling got you in trouble.

   Example 1:

____
____
____
____
____

   Example 2:

____
____
____
____
____

Example 3:

____

10. Can you make any connection or link between how you express your feelings now and how they were expressed by your mother, father, or siblings?

Homework: Next week, in order for you to learn to express this feeling in more helpful ways ("Start it if you want to stop it!"), plan, recall, or pretend to repeat this feeling at preset times (for instance, at 8 a.m., 12 noon, 4 or 7 p.m.), at least three times. Write down what happened in detail. For each time make sure to answer in writing the following four questions:

(a) How did you start this feeling?
(b) What followed your expression?
(c) How did it end?
(d) What did expressing this feeling get you?

Time 1 (write the time you started__________)

a.

b.

c.

d.

Time 2 (write the time you started__________)

a. ____
____
____

b. ____
____
____

c. ____
____
____

d. ____
____
____

Time 3 (write the time you started__________)

a. ____
____
____

b. ____
____
____

c. ____
____
____

d ____
____
____

Check which of the following indicates what you got out of this practice exercise:

a. Completely useless	_______	d. Somewhat useful	_______
b. Somewhat useless	_______	e. Extremely useful	_______
c. So-so	_______		

Feel free to explain how you feel about the homework practice exercise and what you got out of it.

____
____
____
____
____
____
____
____

Concluding Feedback Form

Name______________________________Sex__________Date____________

The purpose of this form is to review whether this practice exercises was helpful to you or not.

1. Check the answer that best fits how you feel about this practice exercises:

   a. I did not like working on this practice exercises at all. I wish I never saw it. ________
   b. I did not like this practice exercises at all, but I am glad I got to work on it. ________
   c. I am delighted I got a chance to work on this practice exercises. ________
   d. I am not only delighted about this practice exercises, but I wish all people in my situation had a chance to work on it ________

2. How helpful was it to work on this practice exercises? Check the answer that applies to you:

   a. Not helpful at all ________ c. Helpful ________
   b. Somewhat helpful ________ d. Very helpful ________

3. Which practice exercise did you like best? Please rank-order the practice exercises from the one that you liked best (rank as No. 1), to the one you liked next best (rank as No. 2), down to the one you did not like at all (No. 11–14).

Feelings	*Rank-order*	*Feelings*	*Rank-order*
a. Amusement	________	h. Guilt	________
b. Anger	________	i. Interest	________
c. Contempt	________	j. Sadness	________
d. Disgust	________	k. Surprise	________
e. Distress	________	l. (________________)	________
f. Enjoyment	________	m. (________________)	________
g. Fear	________	n. (________________)	________

4. Why did you rank-order the practice exercises the way you did?

____

____

____

____

____

5. Which practice exercise was the most helpful to you? Sometimes what we like most is not necessarily the most helpful. Consequently, rank the practice exercises according to their helpfulness to you. Rank as No. 1 the most helpful, rank as No. 2 the next most helpful, and so on, until the least helpful (No. 11–14):

Feelings	*Rank-order*	*Feelings*	*Rank-order*
a. Amusement	________	h. Guilt	________
b. Anger	________	i. Interest	________
c. Contempt	________	j. Sadness	________
d. Disgust	________	k. Surprise	________
e. Distress	________	l. (______________)	________
f. Enjoyment	________	m. (______________)	________
g. Fear	________	n. (______________)	________

6. Why did you rank-order the practice exercises the way you did?

____
____
____
____
____

7. Feel free to write any comments that might improve this practice exercises.

____
____
____
____
____
____
____
____

Emotional Intelligence

The purpose of this practice exercises is to help you become more aware of your emotional behaviors and perhaps learn ho.w to express them in a more helpful and constructive fashion than you may have in the past.

Practice Exercise 1. Becoming Aware of Emotional Behaviors

Name______________________________Sex__________Date_____________

The purpose of this practice exercise is to list the most common emotional behaviors that take place within individuals, between couples, and among family members. If necessary, use a dictionary or ask your partner (if you have one), family members, relatives, or friends to help you define these behaviors. The remainder of this practice exercises consists of practice exercises about emotional behaviors drawn from this list.

1. Define what you understand about the meaning of each emotional behavior listed below. Give two examples of a situation where that emotional behavior would be appropriate.

Emotional Behaviors and Definitions	*Examples*
a. Emotional self-awareness ________	Example 1 ____________
______________________	______________________
______________________	Example 2 ____________
______________________	______________________
b. Assertiveness ____________	Example 1 ____________
______________________	______________________
______________________	Example 2 ____________
______________________	______________________
c. Self-regard ____________	Example 1 ____________
______________________	______________________
______________________	Example 2 ____________
______________________	______________________
d. Self-actualization ________	Example 1 ____________
______________________	______________________
______________________	Example 2 ____________
______________________	______________________
e. Independence ____________	Example 1: ____________
______________________	______________________
______________________	Example 2: ____________
______________________	______________________
f. Empathy ____________	Example 1: ____________
______________________	______________________
______________________	Example 2: ____________
______________________	______________________

g. Close relationships with loved ones ______ Example 1: ______ Example 2: ______

h. Social responsibility ______ Example 1: ______ Example 2: ______

i. Problem solving ______ Example 1: ______ Example 2: ______

j. Reality testing ______ Example 1: ______ Example 2: ______

k. Flexibility ______ Example 1: ______ Example 2: ______

l. Stress tolerance ______ Example 1: ______ Example 2: ______

m. Impulse control ______ Example 1: ______ Example 2: ______

n. Happiness ______ Example 1: ______ Example 2: ______

o. Optimism ______ Example 1: ______ Example 2: ______

p. Positive impression ______________ Example 1: ______________________
______________________________________ ______________________________
______________________________________ Example 2: ______________________
______________________________________ ______________________________

q. Negative impression ______________ Example 1: ______________________
______________________________________ ______________________________
______________________________________ Example 2: ______________________
______________________________________ ______________________________

2. Now rank-order this list of emotional behaviors according to how much you want to use each behavior in more helpful ways than you may have done in the past. Rank as No. 1 the emotional behavior you want to use the most in comparison to the other emotional behaviors, rank as No. 2 the emotional behavior you want to use second most, and so on, until you reach emotional behaviors that are either not applicable to you (N/A) or that you do not want or need to learn at all (No. 17).

Emotional Behaviors	*Rank-orders*	*Emotional Behaviors*	*Rank-orders*
a. Emotional self-awareness	________	j. Reality testing	________
b. Assertiveness	________	k. Flexibility	________
c. Self-regard	________	l. Stress tolerance	________
d. Self-actualization	________	m. Impulse control	________
e. Independence	________	n. Happiness	________
f. Empathy	________	o. Optimism	________
g. Interpersonal relationships	________	p. Positive impression	________
h. Social responsibility	________	q. Negative impression	________
i. Problem solving	________		

4. Explain why you rank-ordered the emotional behaviors the way you did.

____
____
____
____
____

Homework: During the coming week, think about the list of feelings given in the first practice exercise and assess them according to how constructive (helpful) or destructive they are for your, for your partner (if you have one), and for members of your family. Write them down according to how helpful or hurtful these feelings are for you.

Standard Practice Exercise

Practice Exercise No.____Title of Emotional Behavior:____________

Name____________________________Sex______Date___________

The purpose of this practice exercise is to understand more about the emotional behavior listed in the title.

1. How do you express this emotional behavior? Please explain in detail.

____
____
____
____
____
____

2. How often do you express this emotional behavior? Check which answer applies to you:

   a. Practically every day _____ e. Once every 6 months _____
   b. Once a week _____ f. Once a year _____
   c. A couple of times a month _____ g. Once every few years _____
   d. Once a month _____ h. Please explain further:

____
____
____
____
____

3. How often is this emotional behavior expressed by your partner (if your have one, otherwise skip this question)? Check which answer applies to your partner:

   a. Practically every day _____ e. Once every 6 months _____
   b. Once a week _____ f. Once a year _____
   c. A couple of times a month _____ g. Once every few years _____
   d. Once a month _____ h. Please explain further:

____
____
____
____
____

4. How often is (was) this emotional behavior expressed by your mother or mother substitute? Check which answer applies to her:

a. Practically every day	_____	e. Once every 6 months	_____
b. Once a week	_____	f. Once a year	_____
c. A couple of times a month	_____	g. Once every few years	_____
d. Once a month	_____	h. Please explain further:	

____

____

____

____

____

5. How often is (was) this emotional behavior expressed by your father or father substitute? Check only if you did have one. Check which answer applies to him:

a. Practically every day	_____	e. Once every 6 months	_____
b. Once a week	_____	f. Once a year	_____
c. A couple of times a month	_____	g. Once every few years	_____
d. Once a month	_____	h. Please explain further:	

____

____

____

____

____

6. Pick one sibling (brother or sister, if you have one) whose emotional behavior matters or mattered to you a great deal, more than any other sibling. Check which answer applies to her or him. How often did this sibling behaved emotionally in this way?

a. Practically every day	_____	e. Once every 6 months	_____
b. Once a week	_____	f. Once a year	_____
c. A couple of times a month	_____	g. Once every few years	_____
d. Once a month	_____	h. Please explain further:	

____

____

____

____

____

7. Can you remember how this emotional behavior came about? Do you remember when you started it? Check which answer fits best:

   a. When I was a child (younger than 5 years of age) ______
   b. When I was in elementary school ______
   c. When I was in middle school ______
   d. When I was in high school ______
   e. After high school ______
   f. Any other time ______
   g. Please explain further:

____
____
____
____
____

8. Did this emotional behavior ever get you in trouble? Please explain.

____
____
____
____
____

9. Give three specific examples of how this emotional behavior got you in trouble.

   Example 1:

____
____
____
____
____

   Example 2:

____
____
____
____
____

Example 3:

____
____
____
____
____

10. Can you make any connection or link between how you express your feelings and emotions now and how they were expressed by your mother, father, or sibling?

____
____
____
____
____

Homework: Next week, in order for you to learn to express this emotional behavior in more helpful ways ("Start it if you want to stop it!") than you did in the past, plan, recall, or pretend to repeat it at preset times (for instance, at 8 a.m., 12 noon, 4 or 7 p.m.), at least three times. Write down what happened in detail. For each time make sure to answer in writing the following four questions:

(a) How did you start this emotional behavior?
(b) What followed your expression?
(c) How did it end?
(d) What did this behavior get you?

Time 1 (write the time you started__________)

a. ____
____
____

b. ____
____
____

c. ____
____
____

d. ____
____
____

Time 2 (write the time you started__________)

a. ____
____
____

b. ____
____
____

c. ____
____
____

d. ____
____
____

Time 3 (write the time you started__________)

a. ____
____
____

b. ____
____
____

c. ____
____
____

d. ____
____
____

Check which of the following indicates what you got out of this practice exercise:

a. Completely useless _____
b. Somewhat useless _____
c. So-so _____
d. Somewhat useful _____
e. Extremely useful _____

Feel free to explain how you feel about the homework practice exercise and what you got out of it.

____
____
____
____
____

Concluding Feedback Form

Name____________________________Sex__________Date___________

The purpose of this form is to review whether this practice exercises was helpful to you or not.

1. Check the answer that best fits how you feel about this practice exercises:

   a. I did not like working on this practice exercises at all. I wish I never saw it. _______
   b. I did not like this practice exercises at all, but I am glad I got to work on it. _______
   c. I am delighted I got a chance to work on this practice exercise. _______
   d. I am not only delighted about this practice exercises but I wish all people in trouble or distress had a chance to work on it. _______

2. How helpful was it to work on this practice exercise? Check the answer that applies to you:

   a. Not helpful at all _____
   b. Somewhat helpful _____
   c. Helpful _____
   d. Very helpful _____

3. Which practice exercise did you like best? Rank as No. 1 the one that you liked best, rank as No. 2 the one you liked next best, and so on; mark as N/A the ones you did not like at all or did not apply to you.

Emotional Behaviors	*Rank-orders*	*Emotional Behaviors*	*Rank-orders*
a. Emotional self-awareness	_________	j. Reality testing	_________
b. Assertiveness	_________	k. Flexibility	_________
c. Self-regard	_________	l. Stress tolerance	_________
d. Self-actualization	_________	m. Impulse control	_________
e. Independence	_________	n. Happiness	_________
f. Empathy	_________	o. Optimism	_________
g. Interpersonal relationships	_________	p. Positive impression	_________
h. Social responsibility	_________	q. Negative impression	_________
i. Problem solving	_________		

4. Explain why you rank-ordered the practice exercises the way you did.

____
____
____
____
____

5. Which practice exercise was the most helpful to you? Sometimes what we like most is not necessarily the most helpful. Consequently, rank the practice exercises according to their helpfulness to you. Rank as No. 1 the most helpful, rank as No. 2 the next most helpful, and so on, until the least helpful (No. 11–14):

Emotional Behaviors	*Rank-orders*	*Emotional Behaviors*	*Rank-orders*
a. Emotional self-awareness	________	j. Reality testing	________
b. Assertiveness	________	k. Flexibility	________
c. Self-regard	________	l. Stress tolerance	________
d. Self-actualization	________	m. Impulse control	________
e. Independence	________	n. Happiness	________
f. Empathy	________	o. Optimism	________
g. Interpersonal relationships	________	p. Positive impression	________
h. Social responsibility	________	q. Negative impression	________
i. Problem solving	________		

6. Explain why you rank-ordered the practice exercises the way you did.

____
____
____
____
____

7. Feel free to write any comments that might improve this practice exercises.

____
____
____
____
____

Social Skills

The purpose of this practice exercises is to help you understand the importance of social skills in how we all function in the real world. The purpose of this first practice exercise is to find out what skills you want to work on and, possibly, improve.

Practice Exercise 1. What Are My Social Skills?

Name____________________Sex________Date__________

The purpose of this practice exercise is to find what your social skills are.

1. Below there is a list of social skills. Please define each skill according to how you understand it. You may use a dictionary or ask close friends about the meaning of each skill. Give two examples of how each skill is applied in your experience.

Skill and Definitions Examples

a. Approval from others ________	Example 1 ________
________	________
________	Example 2 ________
________	________
b. Assertiveness ________	Example 1 ________
________	________
________	Example 2 ________
________	________
c. Confidence ________	Example 1 ________
________	________
________	Example 2 ________
________	________
d. Control (social) ________	Example 1 ________
________	________
________	Example 2 ________
________	________
e. Defense of (own) rights ________	Example 1 ________
________	________
________	Example 2 ________
________	________
f. Being direct ________	Example 1 ________
________	________
________	Example 2 ________
________	________
g. Emotional control ________	Example 1 ________
________	________
________	Example 2 ________
________	________
h. Emotional expression ________	Example 1 ________
________	________
________	Example 2 ________
________	________

i. Empathy ______________________ Example 1 ______________________

______________________ ______________________

______________________ Example 2 ______________________

______________________ ______________________

j. Expression (social) ______________ Example 1 ______________________

______________________ ______________________

______________________ Example 2 ______________________

______________________ ______________________

k. Expression of positive feelings ___ Example 1 ______________________

______________________ ______________________

______________________ Example 2 ______________________

______________________ ______________________

l. Need for approval ______________ Example 1 ______________________

______________________ ______________________

______________________ Example 2 ______________________

______________________ ______________________

m. Sensitivity ______________ Example 1 ______________________

______________________ ______________________

______________________ Example 2 ______________________

______________________ ______________________

n. Any other skill (fill in) Example 1 ______________________

(______________) and define it: ______________________

______________________ Example 2 ______________________

______________________ ______________________

______________________ ______________________

2. Now rank-order these skills according to how frequent, serious, or strong they are in you. Rank as No. 1 the skill that is the strongest or most frequent, rank as No. 2 the skill that is second strongest or most frequent; mark as N/A the skills that do not apply to you.

Skills	*Rank-orders* *Self*	*Mother*	*Father*	*Siblings*
a. Approval from others	_____	_____	_____	_____
b. Assertiveness	_____	_____	_____	_____
c. Confidence	_____	_____	_____	_____
d. Control (social)	_____	_____	_____	_____
e. Defense of (own) rights	_____	_____	_____	_____
f. Directiveness	_____	_____	_____	_____

g.	Emotional control	______	______	______	______
h.	Emotional expression	______	______	______	______
i.	Empathy	______	______	______	______
j.	Expression (social)	______	______	______	______
k.	Expression of positive feelings	______	______	______	______
l.	Need for approval	______	______	______	______
m.	Sensitivity	______	______	______	______
n.	Any other skill (____________)	______	______	______	______

3. Which of these skills were present in your family of origin? Check whether they applied to your mother (or mother substitute), father (or father substitute), or brothers or sisters. Check all that apply.

Homework: During the next few days write down all of the advantages and disadvantages you get from using self-defeating behaviors.

Standard Practice Exercise for Social Skills

Practice Exercise No.____Name of Skill:______________________________

Name______________________________Sex__________Date____________

The purpose of this practice exercise is to understand more about the skill named above:

1. What does this skill mean to you? Please explain in detail.

____
____
____
____
____

2. How often do you use this skill? Check which answer applies to you:

a.	Practically every day	_____	e.	Once every 6 months	_____
b.	Once a week	_____	f.	Once a year	_____
c.	A couple of times a month	_____	g.	Once every few years	_____
d.	Once a month	_____			

Please explain further:

3. How did this skill (or lack of it) come about? Do you remember when you started using it? Check which answer fits best:

   a. When I was a child (younger than 5 years of age) ______
   b. In elementary school ______
   c. In middle school ______
   d. In high school ______
   e. Any other time ______

   Please explain further:

4. What does this skill get you or fails to get you? Please explain:

5. Give three specific examples of how this skill or lack of it was hurtful to you.

   Example 1:

Example 2:

Example 3:

6. Give three specific examples of how this skill was hurtful to those you love and who love you.

Example 1:

Example 2:

Example 3:

7. Now that you have completed this practice exercise, check which of these answers indicates how you feel about it. There is also space for you to explain further, if you want to.

   a. I did not like it at all, a waste of time. I want to quit this stupid practice exercises. ______
   b. I did not like it very much, but I want to go on with this practice exercises. ______
   c. I liked it and I want to go on with this practice exercises. ______
   d. I liked it a lot and I wish I had something like this practice exercises earlier. ______
   e. I liked it so much that I wish all people with limited social skills could get something like this practice exercises to work on. ______

Homework: Next week, plan to repeat this skill at preset times (for instance, at 8 a.m., 12 noon, 4 or 7 p.m.), at least three times. Write down what happened in detail. For each time make sure to answer in writing the following four questions:

(a) How did you start it?
(b) What followed?
(c) How did it end?
(d) What did this behavior get you?

Time 1 (write the time you started__________)

a. ____
____
____

b. ____
____
____

c. ____
____
____

d. ____
____
____

Time 2 (write the time you started__________)

a. ____
____
____

b. ____
____
____

c. ____
____
____

d. ____
____
____

Time 3 (write the time you started__________)

a. ____
____
____

b. ____
____
____

c. ____
____
____

d. ____
____
____

Check which of the following indicates what you got out of this practice exercise:

a. Completely useless _____
b. Somewhat useless _____
c. So-so _____
d. Somewhat useful _____
e. Extremely useful _____

Write down how you feel about this homework practice exercise and what you got out of it.

____
____
____
____
____

Concluding Feedback Form

Name________________________________Sex_______Date______

The purpose of this form is to review whether practice exercises in this practice exercises were helpful to you.

1. Which answer fits how you feel about this practice exercises?

   a. I did not like working on this practice exercises at all. I wish I never saw it. ________
   b. I did not like this practice exercises, but I am glad I got to work on it. ________
   c. I am happy I got a chance to work on this. ________
   d. I am not only delighted about this practice exercises, but I wish all people with limited social skills could get it. ________

2. How helpful was it to work on this practice exercises? Check the answer that applies to you.

   a. Not helpful at all ________ c. Helpful ________
   b. Somewhat helpful ________ d. Very helpful ________

3. Which practice exercise did you like best? Rank as No. 1 the one that you liked best, rank as No. 2 the one you liked next best, and so on; mark as N/A the ones you did not like at all or did not apply to you.

Skill	*Rank-order*
a. Approval from others	________
b. Assertiveness	________
c. Confidence	________
d. Control (social)	________
e. Defense of (own) rights	________
f. Directiveness	________
g. Emotional control	________
h. Emotional expression	________
i. Empathy	________
j. Expression (social)	________
k. Expression of positive feelings	________
l. Need for approval	________
m. Sensitivity	________
n. Any other skill (__________________________)	________

4. Now that you have completed this practice exercise, check which of these answers indicates how you felt about it. There is also space for you to explain further, if you want to.

   a. I did not like it at all, a waste of time. I wish I never worked on this stupid practice exercises. _______
   b. I did not like it very much, but I want to go on with working on practice exercisess of this type. _______
   c. I liked it and I want to go on with another practice exercises. _______
   d. I liked it a lot and I wish I had received something like this practice exercises earlier in my life. _______
   e. I liked it so much that I wish all individuals with limited social skills could get something like this practice exercises to work on. _______

5. How could this practice exercises be improved? Do you have any suggestions? Feel free to write whatever could improve this practice exercises.

____
____
____
____
____

Basic Abilities

The purpose of this practice exercises is to help you understand more about your basic abilities and learn how it might be possible for you to improve the abilities you want to improve.

Practice Exercise 1. Basic Definitions and Ordering

Name______________________________________Sex_____Date____

The purpose of this practice exercise is to help you define these abilities and order them according to how you want to improve those that need improvement.

1. Here are brief definitions of 15 abilities that cover most of if not all the range of human abilities. In addition to these definitions, give two examples for each definition of how it applies to your experience, how you use or have used that specific ability in your life, if at all. Try to answer all these definitions. However, if you do not understand it or are not interested in it, leave it blank.

a. Language: reading a book or writing a poem ________________

Example 1 ________________

Example 2 ________________

b. Logical–mathematical: deriving a logical proof or solving a mathematical problem ________________

Example 1 ________________

Example 2 ________________

c. Spatial: fitting suitcases in the trunk of a car or finding ones way when driving ________________

Example 1 ________________

Example 2 ________________

d. Musical: singing a song, playing an instrument, or composing a symphony ________________

Example 1 ________________

Example 2 ________________

e. Bodily-kinesthetic: dancing or playing football or other sports ________________

Example 1 ________________

Example 2 ________________

f. Interpersonal: understanding and interacting with other people ________________

Example 1 ________________

Example 2 ________________

g. Intrapersonal: understanding oneself ________________

Example 1 ________________

Example 2 ________________

h. Naturalistic: discerning patterns in nature ____________________

Example 1 ____________________

Example 2 ____________________

i. Spiritual: troublesome thoughts with cosmic achievement of a state of being ____________________

Example 1 ____________________

Example 2 ____________________

j. Existential: troublesome thoughts with ultimate issues of life ____________________

Example 1 ____________________

Example 2 ____________________

k. Emotional: ability to access and/or generate feelings and emotions ____________________

Example 1 ____________________

Example 2 ____________________

l. Practical: ability to deal with real, concrete world situations not covered by other abilities ____________________

Example 1 ____________________

Example 2 ____________________

m. Analytical: evaluation of choices and options available to oneself in life ____________________

Example 1 ____________________

Example 2 ____________________

n. Creative: required to generate unusual problem-solving choices and options ____________________

Example 1 ____________________

Example 2 ____________________

o. Sexual: interest and concentration on body-skin pleasure ____________ Example 1 ____________

____________ Example 2 ____________

____________ ____________

____________ ____________

2. Now that you have defined these abilities, you need to rank-order them according to how they describe you (perceived ability). Rank as No. 1 the ability you feel describes you the most, rank as No. 2 the ability that describes you next, and so on; mark as N/A the abilities that describe you little or not at all.

Abilities	*Rank-orders Perceived Ability*	*Rank Desired Ability*	*Average*
a. Language	______	______	______
b. Logical–mathematical	______	______	______
c. Spatial	______	______	______
d. Musical	______	______	______
e. Bodily-kinesthetic	______	______	______
f. Interpersonal	______	______	______
g. Intrapersonal	______	______	______
h. Naturalistic	______	______	______
i. Spiritual	______	______	______
j. Existential	______	______	______
k. Emotional	______	______	______
l. Practical	______	______	______
m. Analytical	______	______	______
n. Creative	______	______	______
o. Sexual	______	______	______

3. Explain why you have rank-ordered these abilities the way you did.

____

____

____

____

____

4. Now rank these abilities according to your desire to excel or improve that ability (desired ability). Rank as No. 1 the ability that you want to improve the most, rank as No 2 the ability you want to improve second most, and so on, down to the abilities you do not want or need to improve. Rank-order all the abilities even though you may not want to improve them.

5. Explain why you ranked these abilities the way you did.

____
____
____
____
____

6. Calculate the average in the third column by adding the two ranks, your perceived ability and your desired ability, and dividing by 2. The reason for averaging lies in the possibility that your perceived abilities may not agree with your desired abilities. Consequently, we need to find a compromise between the two views of your abilities. Furthermore, the averaged rank-order will serve as the basis for the order of administration of practice exercises for each of the abilities listed above.

Homework: During the coming week, think more about your perceived and desired abilities and whether you are comfortable with how you rank-ordered them. There is still time to change how you have ranked perceived and desired abilities.

Practice Exercise 2. Goals, Plans, and Priorities (to be administered after the first practice exercise for a specific ability)

Title of Ability__________________

Name__________________________________Sex_____Date_____

The purpose of this practice exercise is to follow-up on the previous practice exercise about increasing your mastery in one particular ability. To achieve your goal, there are certain steps that must be taken, regardless of the ability involved.

1. What direction toward your goal do you want to take? State clearly what steps you need to take to achieve your goal. For instance, you could describe

   a. Daily goals
   b. Weekly goals
   c. Monthly goals
   d. Yearly goals
   e. Where to you want to be with this ability 5 years from now?

____
____
____
____
____

f. Where do you want to be with this ability 10 years from now?

g. Why do you want to reach these goals? Write down your answer.

Note: It is very important to check on whether you have achieved your goals or not. Are you just spinning your wheels? If you are not able to complete your daily goals, how are you going to complete your weekly goals? Only by starting small, that is, every day, can you achieve big. If you want to climb the Himalayas without way-stations, you will never reach the desired peak. If you do not check on whether you have achieved even the smallest goal, there is no sense making any goal.

2. What are your priorities? You need to think through what is most important to you, what is next most important, and what is least important. Write down everything you can think of, separating persons, things or possessions, activities, into at least three or more different lists. Then, within each list, rank items in order of importance.

After you have listed them by order of importance, rank them in order of urgency. What person, possession, or activity needs your most urgent attention, which needs some attention, and which needs the least attention. In order to think through what is important and what is urgent, you may need to follow guidelines that may become part of your priorities:

a. *Flexibility versus rigidity*: You can try to reach your goals leisurely, in a relaxed fashion, or you can try to reach them rigorously, in a driven, rigid fashion. Somewhere in between these two extremes there is a happy medium for you. What is this happy medium? Write down *how* you are going to achieve your goals, flexibly or rigidly? However, whatever way you choose, you must explain *why* you followed it.

b. *Speed in the service of direction:* How fast or how slow do you want to reach your goals? Again, between the two extremes of very fast and very slow there must be a happy medium for you. What is it, and why do you want to follow it?
c. *Overcoming obstacles*: What barriers, events, or other possibilities may take place in your life that will slow down your progress? Write down all the possible future obstacles that may come between you and reaching your final goal.
d. *Long-term perspective*: There are life-cycle stages in your future goals that may need to be recognized. For instance, you may have to leave home and get a job, or you may want to get married and raise children, you may want to take early retirement, etc. What stages of your life cycle do you suppose may either hinder or help the progress toward your final goal with this ability? Answer in writing.

3. *Skills*: To achieve your goal of mastery of the ability considered in this practice exercise, there are at least four necessary skills that need to be considered:
   a. *Resilience:* What do you understand by this word? Define it (look it up in the dictionary, if necessary) and then rate yourself on this skill on a scale from 1 to 10, with 1 being not having any resilience at all and 10 being extremely resilient. After you have rated yourself, explain why you rated yourself the way you did. Give at least two examples that show how resilient you are. How is this skill related to your ultimate goal? Answer in writing.
   b. *Relentlessness:* What do you understand by this word? Define it (look it up in the dictionary, if necessary) and then rate yourself on this skill on a scale from 1 to 10, with 1 being not relentless at all and 10 being extremely relentless. After you have rated yourself, explain why have you rated yourself the way you did. Give at least two examples that show how relentless you are. How is this skill related to your ultimate goal? Answer in writing.
   c. *Restlessness:* What do you understand by this word? Define it (look it up in the dictionary, if necessary) and then rate yourself on this skill on a scale from 1 to 10, with 1 being not restless at all and 10 being extremely restless. After you have rated yourself explain why you rated yourself the way you did. Give at least two examples that show how restless you are. How is this skill related to your ultimate goal? Answer in writing.
   d. *Risk taking:* What do you understand by this word? Define it (look it up in the dictionary, if necessary) and then rate yourself on this skill on a scale from 1 to 10, with 1 being not a risk taker at all and 10 being an extreme risk taker. After you have rated yourself explain why you rated yourself the way you did. Give at least two examples that show what a risk taker you are. How is this skill related to your ultimate goal? Answer in writing.

4. *Planning*: Without planning there is no sense pursuing any goal. If you have answered all the previous items, you may be on the way to reaching your goal. However, it is important to plan beforehand to avoid making hasty decisions that in the long run may interfere with your goal. Outline in writing a general plan of action that you are going to follow in order to reach your goal.
5. *Wisdom*: One may be very wise in one aspect of life, for instance, work, and be very unwise in one's home life. Some of us may be wise in fixing an electric short while unable to write a personal letter. Some others may be very wise in shopping but not in making money to support the shopping. In what areas of your life do you show wisdom, and in what areas do you show less than wisdom? It is important to separate the two sides to link your wisdom to the ability you want to master. Answer in writing.
6. *Motivation:* It is important for you to rate your motivation or desire necessary to achieve your goal, ranging from 1 for no motivation at all to 10 for extreme desire and motivation. Write in detail how desirous and motivated you are to reach your goal, giving at least two examples that show your motivation.
7. *Competence:* Perhaps this item may have been answered by the four skills listed above. On the other hand, it is important for you to rate your competence. Write down at least two examples that show how competent you are in dealing with this ability. You may be highly motivated and incompetent at the same time (back to the wisdom item). On the other hand, you may be very unmotivated and still highly competent. How are these two qualities related to your final goal to master this ability? Answer in writing.
8 *Personality*: What kind of personality do you have that would fit into your goal? Are you introverted but want to work with people? Are you extroverted and want to become a computer scientist? Are you more interested in people or in things? Are you tense and driven or relaxed and at ease? What personality traits do you see yourself as having that may help or hinder your final goal with this ability? Answer in detail and in writing.

Homework: During the coming week, keep thinking about your goals and plans. If you change your mind, do so in writing; change whatever your have already written in this practice exercise.

Follow-Through Practice Exercise

Practice Exercise No._____Title of Ability__________________

Name____________________________________Sex_____Date_________

The purpose of this practice exercise is to follow through with the previous practice exercise about goals, plans, and priorities.

1. Are your satisfied about what you wrote in the previous practice exercise? If you are not, write why and how you have changed your goals.

2. Are you clear about how you are going to reach your goals? If you are not, write whatever changes you need to make to reach your stated goals.

3. Did you check on your daily goals? Did you accomplish them? If not, write why you did not.

4. Are you satisfied with your priorities? If you are not, write why and how you have changed them.

5. Are you clear about your priorities? If you are not, write how you would like to change them.

6. Are you satisfied with your plans to reach your goals? If you are not, write why and how you want to change your plans.

____
____
____
____
____

7. Are you clear about your plans? If you are not, write how you need to change them.

____
____
____
____
____

Homework: Give yourself some time (1–3 months, or even more) to see whether your goals, priorities, and plans have been reached. If they have not been reached, what changes do you need to make to facilitate accomplishing your goals. Were the goals too unrealistic? Were you confused about them? Were they impossible to reach? Write down whatever realistic, clear, and possible changes you need to make to reach your goals.

Spatial Ability

This ability is used by people who have a strong sense of color, line, texture, and style. They like to draw or paint, use maps well, understand directions, learn visually, draw or highlight or underline when taking notes, and cluster notes in boxes or sections on the page to give the visual cues helpful for study. Books with charts, diagrams, or pictures are helpful to them in synthesizing the information in the text. The way places look matters to these people. They learn better in pleasant or soothing surroundings. They may want to clean up the room or the desk before they sit down to work. They like to be shown and then try things themselves.

Practice Exercise 1. Spatial Ability

Name_________________________Sex______Date____

The purpose of this practice exercise is to understand in greater detail the nature of this ability. How did it develop? How have you used it in the past? How can you use it in the present and future?

1. Why is this ability important to you? Give as many reasons as you can think of.

____
____
____
____

2. How does this ability apply to you?

   a. A great deal _____ c. Not at all _____
   b. Somewhat _____

3. Explain in detail how this ability applies to you.

____
____
____
____
____

4. How did this ability develop in you? Explain in detail.

____
____
____
____
____

5. When did you find out that you had this ability?

   a. In prekindergarten _____ e. In high school _____
   b. In kindergarten _____ f. In college _____
   c. In elementary school _____ g. After college _____
   d. In middle school _____

6. Explain in greater detail how you found out about this ability.

____
____
____
____
____

7. How have you used this ability in the past? Explain in detail.

____
____
____
____
____

8. How are you using this ability in the present? Explain in detail.

____
____
____
____
____

9. How are you planning to use this ability in the future? Explain in detail.

____
____
____
____
____

10. How do you feel about having this ability? Explain through your feelings rather than through your thinking.

____
____
____
____
____

Homework: During the coming week, think more about how you could develop this ability. Jot down anything that comes to mind about this ability during the course of this week. At the end of the week, see whether you can put all these thoughts into one single plan to develop this ability even more than you have done in the past.

Body-Kinesthetic Ability

This ability describes people who relax with movement and remember by moving. Some pace back and forth when memorizing something, some tap a pencil or jiggle a foot, some need to rock in a chair in order to read or study. They express emotions through movement as well. They may throw things, hit the table, hug and kiss a lot, physically back away from tasks, or dance when happy or excited. As children they could not sit still in class. They also invent or create through movement; they do a lot of trial-and-error testing (by climbing, jumping, hanging from trees or poles). They take in information about what's possible by moving their bodies through space.

Practice Exercise 1. Body-Kinesthetic Ability

Name________________________________Sex______Date____

The purpose of this practice exercise is to understand in greater detail the nature of this ability. How did it develop? How have you used it in the past? How can you use it in the present and future?

1. Why is this ability important to you? Give as many reasons as you can think of.

____

____

____

____

____

2. How does this ability apply to you?

   a. A great deal _____ c. Not at all _____
   b. Somewhat _____

3. Explain in detail how this ability applies to you.

____

____

____

____

____

4. How did this ability develop in you? Explain in detail.

____

____

____

____

____

5. When did you find out that you had this ability?

a. In prekindergarten	_______	e. In high school	_______
b. In kindergarten	_______	f. In college	_______
c. In elementary school	_______	g. After college	_______
d. In middle school	_______		

6. Explain in greater detail how you found out about this ability.

____

____

____

____

____

7. How have you used this ability in the past? Explain in detail.

____

____

____

____

____

8. How are you using this ability in the present? Explain in detail.

____

____

____

____

____

9. How are you planning to use this ability in the future? Explain in detail.

____

____

____

____

____

10. How do you feel about having this ability? Explain through your feelings rather than through your thinking.

____

____

____

____

____

Homework: During the coming week, think more about how you could develop this ability. Jot down anything that comes to mind about this ability during the course of this week. At the end of the week, see whether you can put all these thoughts into one single plan to develop this ability even more than you have done in the past.

Musical Ability

People may love music but don't have to be musicians. They are acutely aware of rhythms. They hear the rhythms in nature; they're acutely aware of how random sounds form harmonic or rhythmic patterns (water, birds, crickets, wind in trees, etc.). They learn auditorily and can mimic sounds, such as voices and accents. When they learn a song, they learn not just the words but the total sound: the beat the rhythms in the instruments and the inflection in the singer's voice and even nonsense sounds.

Practice Exercise 1. Musical Ability

Name________________________________Sex______Date____

The purpose of this practice exercise is to understand in greater detail the nature of this ability. How did it develop? How have you used it in the past? How can you use it in the present and future?

1. Why is this ability important to you? Give as many reasons as you can think of.

____
____
____
____
____

2. How does this ability apply to you?

   a. A great deal ________ c. Not at all ________
   b. Somewhat ________

3. Explain in detail how this ability applies to you.

____
____
____
____
____

4. How did this ability develop in you? Explain in detail.

____
____
____
____
____

5. When did you find out that you had this ability?

a.	In prekindergarten	______	e.	In high school	______
b.	In kindergarten	______	f.	In college	______
c.	In elementary school	______	g.	After college	______
d.	In middle school	______			

6. Explain in greater detail how you found out about this ability.

____
____
____
____
____

7. How have you used this ability in the past? Explain in detail.

____
____
____
____
____

8. How are you using this ability in the present? Explain in detail.

____
____
____
____
____

9. How are you planning to use this ability in the future? Explain in detail.

____
____
____
____
____

10. How do you feel about having this ability? Explain through your feelings rather than through your thinking.

____
____
____
____
____

Homework: During the coming week, think more about how you could develop this ability. Jot down anything that comes to mind about this ability during the course of this week. At the end of the week, see whether you can put all these thoughts into one single plan to develop this ability even more than you have done in the past.

Linguistic Ability

People endowed with this ability enjoy words and language. They like to write stories or poems and they communicate easily with words. They are in tune with the nuances of language and can sense shades of meaning. They are aware of meaning in a person's tone of voice. They remember using words ("That's not what I said; what I said was...") and can replay conversations – even lengthy ones – almost verbatim. They have an awareness of the possibilities with words (puns, made-up words, sounds that words make when said aloud). These people learn auditorily because they can easily remember much of what was said; they can also remember the atmosphere the words created when they were said. They easily link words to emotions.

Practice Exercise 1. Linguistic Ability

Name______________________Sex______Date_____

The purpose of this practice exercise is to understand in greater detail the nature of this ability. How did it develop? How have you used it in the past? How can you use it in the present and future?

1. Why is this ability important to you? Give as many reasons as you can think of.

____
____
____
____
____

2. How does this ability apply to you?

   a. A great deal _______ c. Not at all _______
   b. Somewhat _______

3. Explain in detail how this ability applies to you.

____
____
____
____
____

4. How did this ability develop in you? Explain in detail.

____
____
____
____
____

5. When did you find out that you had this ability?

   a. In prekindergarten ______ e. In high school ______
   b. In kindergarten ______ f. In college ______
   c. In elementary school ______ g. After college ______
   d. In middle school ______

6. Explain in greater detail how you found out about this ability.

____
____
____
____
____

7. How have you used this ability in the past? Explain in detail.

____
____
____
____
____

8. How are you using this ability in the present? Explain in detail.

____
____
____
____
____

9. How are you planning to use this ability in the future? Explain in detail.

____
____
____
____
____

10. How do you feel about having this ability? Explain through your feelings rather than through your thinking.

____
____
____
____
____

Homework: During the coming week, think more about how you could develop this ability. Jot down anything that comes to mind about this ability during the course of this week. At the end of the week, see whether you can put all these thoughts into one single plan to develop this ability even more than you have done in the past.

Logical/Mathematical Ability

People endowed with this ability are organized. They enjoy numbers and use numbers to remember. They think sequentially. They're the ones who always say, "Well first, …, and second, …" Numbers take on the same function for them as size does for spatially intelligent people. People who sew or knit or make furniture have to use math (often geometry) but they work with shape and space as well as numbers. The logical function can work with words as well as with numbers too.

Practice Exercise 1. Logical/Mathematical Ability

Name__________________________________Sex______Date____

The purpose of this practice exercise is to understand in greater detail the nature of this ability. How did it develop? How have you used it in the past? How can you use it in the present and future?

1. Why is this ability important to you? Give as many reasons as you can think of.

____
____
____
____
____

2. How does this ability apply to you?

   a. A great deal _______ c. Not at all _______
   b. Somewhat _______

3. Explain in detail how this ability applies to you.

____
____
____
____
____

4. How did this ability develop in you? Explain in detail.

____
____
____
____
____

5. When did you find out that you had this ability?

   a. In prekindergarten ______ e. In high school ______
   b. In kindergarten ______ f. In college ______
   c. In elementary school ______ g. After college ______
   d. In middle school ______

6. Explain in greater detail how you found out about this ability.

____
____
____
____
____

7. How have you used this ability in the past? Explain in detail.

____
____
____
____
____

8. How are you using this ability in the present? Explain in detail.

____
____
____
____
____

9. How are you planning to use this ability in the future? Explain in detail.

____
____
____
____
____

10. How do you feel about having this ability? Explain through your feelings rather than through your thinking.

____
____
____
____
____

Homework: During the coming week, think more about how you could develop this ability. Jot down anything that comes to mind about this ability during the course of this week. At the end of the week, see whether you can put all these thoughts into one single plan to develop this ability even more than you have done in the past.

Interpersonal Ability

People endowed with this ability enjoy other people, empathize easily, and mediate well when situations get difficult. They have a strong social sense because they can understand the sense of things from someone else's point of view and imagine what that person is feeling. They like social situations; they study best with others even if they're all studying different subjects. For these people, the relationship they have with the teacher can affect how well they learn the material or try to learn; the social makeup of the class matters, too. They listen well, hearing not just the sense of what is said, but the subtle messages encoded in the discussion. (This ability often dovetails with musical and linguistic abilities.) These people can easily motivate others because they understand what makes people tick. Actors depend heavily on this intelligence when they work on character. Feelings surface easily and strongly for these people. Their biggest task is to control feelings so that they can use them in a positive way. Feelings can block their ability to remember or listen openly. Out-of-control feelings can sap the energy they need to learn.

Practice Exercise 1. Interpersonal Ability

Name________________________________Sex______Date____

The purpose of this practice exercise is to understand in greater detail the nature of this ability. How did it develop? How have you used it in the past? How can you use it in the present and future?

1. Why is this ability important to you? Give as many reasons as you can think of.

____

____

____

____

____

2. How does this ability apply to you?

a.	A great deal	_____	c.	Not at all	_____
b.	Somewhat	_____			

3. Explain in detail how this ability applies to you.

____

____

____

____

____

4. How did this ability develop in you? Explain in detail.

____
____
____
____
____

5. When did you find out that you had this ability?

a. In prekindergarten ______
b. In kindergarten ______
c. In elementary school ______
d. In middle school ______
e. In high school ______
f. In college ______
g. After college ______

6. Explain in greater detail how you found out about this ability.

____
____
____
____
____

7. How have you used this ability in the past? Explain in detail.

____
____
____
____

8. How are you using this ability in the present? Explain in detail.

____
____
____
____
____

9. How are you planning to use this ability in the future? Explain in detail.

____
____
____
____
____

10. How do you feel about having this ability? Explain through your feelings rather than through your thinking.

____
____
____
____
____

Homework: During the coming week, think more about how you could develop this ability. Jot down anything that comes to mind about this ability during the course of this week. At the end of the week, see whether you can put all these thoughts into one single plan to develop this ability even more than you have done in the past.

Intrapersonal Ability

This ability depends upon a highly developed sensitivity, as does the interpersonal ability, but this time the sensitivity is internal. These people enjoy their own company, feel very comfortable with themselves and who they are. They understand their own motivation and can examine their own reactions (analysis that combines interpersonal with logical abilities to understand why they react to certain things the way they do). They can be objective while examining very emotional feelings. They can also connect what they have learned about themselves to help them understand others.

Practice Exercise 1. Intrapersonal Ability

Name____________________________________Sex______Date____

The purpose of this practice exercise is to understand in greater detail the nature of this ability. How did it develop? How have you used it in the past? How can you use it in the present and future?

1. Why is this ability important to you? Give as many reasons as you can think of.

____
____
____
____
____

2. How does this ability apply to you?

a. A great deal _____ c. Not at all _____
b. Somewhat _____

3. Explain in detail how this ability applies to you.

____
____
____
____
____

4. How did this ability develop in you? Explain in detail.

____
____
____
____
____

5. When did you find out that you had this ability?

a.	In prekindergarten	______	e.	In high school	______
b.	In kindergarten	______	f.	In college	______
c.	In elementary school	______	g.	After college	______
d.	In middle school	______			

6. Explain in greater detail how you found out about this ability.

____
____
____
____
____

7. How have you used this ability in the past? Explain in detail.

____
____
____
____
____

8. How are you using this ability in the present? Explain in detail.

____
____
____
____
____

9. How are you planning to use this ability in the future? Explain in detail.

____
____
____
____
____

10. How do you feel about having this ability? Explain through your feelings rather than through your thinking.

____
____
____
____
____

Homework: During the coming week, think more about how you could develop this ability. Jot down anything that comes to mind about this ability during the course of this week. At the end of the week, see whether you can put all these thoughts into one single plan to develop this ability even more than you have done in the past.

Naturalistic Ability

This ability means being interested in and curious about nature in all its various forms: plants, herbs, flower, animals, and country, sea, and mountains. It implies wanting to know more about how things in nature develop and what functions they perform in the environment. It may mean being aware and protective of how the environment is maintained, wanting to make sure that products do not endanger the environment. It may mean an interest in biology, zoology, and astronomy.

Practice Exercise 1. Naturalistic Ability

Name________________________Sex______Date____

The purpose of this practice exercise is to understand in greater detail the nature of this ability. How did it develop? How have you used it in the past? How can you use it in the present and future?

1. Why is this ability important to you? Give as many reasons as you can think of.

____
____
____
____
____

2. How does this ability apply to you?

   a. A great deal _____
   b. Somewhat _____
   c. Not at all _____

3. Explain in detail how this ability applies to you.

____
____
____
____
____

4. How did this ability develop in you? Explain in detail.

____
____
____
____
____

5. When did you find out that you had this ability?

   a. In prekindergarten _____
   b. In kindergarten _____
   c. In elementary school _____
   d. In middle school _____
   e. In high school _____
   f. In college _____
   g. After college _____

6. Explain in greater detail how you found out about this ability.

____
____
____
____
____

7. How have you used this ability in the past? Explain in detail.

____
____
____
____
____

8. How are you using this ability in the present? Explain in detail.

____
____
____
____
____

9. How are you planning to use this ability in the future? Explain in detail.

____
____
____
____
____

10. How do you feel about having this ability? Explain through your feelings rather than through your thinking.

____
____
____
____
____

Homework: During the coming week, think more about how you could develop this ability. Jot down anything that comes to mind about this ability during the course of this week. At the end of the week, see whether you can put all these thoughts into one single plan to develop this ability even more than you have done in the past.

Spiritual Ability

This ability implies troublesome thoughts with cosmic achievement and its relationship to a higher power or powers. It may involve a deep, personal interest in religious matters and activities, including membership in organized religion, belonging to a church, praying, and believing in the importance of spiritual activities as being foremost in one's life, including faith in what is not known and accepting faith as being more important than scientific evidence or facts.

Practice Exercise 1. Spiritual Ability

Name____________________________________Sex______Date____

The purpose of this practice exercise is to understand in greater detail the nature of this ability. How did it develop? How have you used it in the past? How can you use it in the present and future?

1. Why is this ability important to you? Give as many reasons as you can think of.

____

____

____

____

____

2. How does this ability apply to you?

   a. A great deal _________
   b. Somewhat _________
   c. Not at all _________

3. Explain in detail how this ability applies to you.

____

____

____

____

____

4. How did this ability develop in you? Explain in detail.

____

____

____

____

____

5. When did you find out that you had this ability?

   a. In prekindergarten _______
   b. In kindergarten _______
   c. In elementary school _______
   d. In middle school _______
   e. In high school _______
   f. In college _______
   g. After college _______

6. Explain in greater detail how you found out about this ability.

7. How have you used this ability in the past? Explain in detail.

8. How are you using this ability in the present? Explain in detail.

9. How are you planning to use this ability in the future? Explain in detail.

10. How do you feel about having this ability? Explain through your feelings rather than through your thinking.

Homework: During the coming week, think more about how you could develop this ability. Jot down anything that comes to mind about this ability during the course of this week. At the end of the week, see whether you can put all these thoughts into one single plan to develop this ability even more than you have done in the past.

Existential Ability

This ability involves interest in the meaning of life and the purpose of one's being within a larger historical and contextual framework. It may mean and it may be related to spiritual and emotional interests, but in itself it includes valuing life as the main reason for living, and enjoying the subjective experience rather than an objective reality. It may mean interest in philosophical pursuits, either formally or informally, that give more information about this subject.

Practice Exercise 1. Existential Ability

Name________________________________Sex______Date_____

The purpose of this practice exercise is to understand in greater detail the nature of this ability. How did it develop? How have you used it in the past? How can you use it in the present and future?

1. Why is this ability important to you? Give as many reasons as you can think of.

____

____

____

____

____

2. How does this ability apply to you?

   a. A great deal ________ c. Not at all ________
   b. Somewhat ________

3. Explain in detail how this ability applies to you.

____

____

____

____

____

4. How did this ability develop in you? Explain in detail.

____

____

____

____

____

5. When did you find out that you had this ability?

a.	In prekindergarten	______	e.	In high school	______
b.	In kindergarten	______	f.	In college	______
c.	In elementary school	______	g.	After college	______
d.	In middle school	______			

6. Explain in greater detail how you found out about this ability.

____
____
____
____
____

7. How have you used this ability in the past? Explain in detail.

____
____
____
____
____

8. How are you using this ability in the present? Explain in detail.

____
____
____
____

9. How are you planning to use this ability in the future? Explain in detail.

____
____
____
____
____

10. How do you feel about having this ability? Explain through your feelings rather than through your thinking.

____
____
____
____
____

Homework: During the coming week, think more about how you could develop this ability. Jot down anything that comes to mind about this ability during the course of this week. At the end of the week, see whether you can put all these thoughts into one single plan to develop this ability even more than you have done in the past.

Emotional Ability

This ability consists of being aware of and accessible to one's feelings and emotions, as shown by crying appropriately, speaking about one's feelings using the personal pronoun "I," valuing feelings and emotions over reason and thinking or even behavior. It implies being emphatic and sympathetic about how others feel, valuing their feelings and not allowing reason and thinking to distract from one's emotional state. It implies also consideration of feelings as the bottom line of one's existence.

Practice Exercise 1. Emotional Ability

Name____________________________Sex__________Date___________

The purpose of this practice exercise is to understand in greater detail the nature of this ability. How did it develop? How have you used it in the past? How can you use it in the present and future?

1. Why is this ability important to you? Give as many reasons as you can think of.

____
____
____
____
____

2. How does this ability apply to you?

   a. A great deal _________
   b. Somewhat _________
   c. Not at all _________

3. Explain in detail how this ability applies to you.

____
____
____
____
____

4. How did this ability develop in you? Explain in detail.

____
____
____
____
____

5. When did you find out that you had this ability?

a. In prekindergarten ______
b. In kindergarten ______
c. In elementary school ______
d. In middle school ______
e. In high school ______
f. In college ______
g. After college ______

6. Explain in greater detail how you found out about this ability.

____
____
____
____
____

7. How have you used this ability in the past? Explain in detail.

____
____
____
____
____

8. How are you using this ability in the present? Explain in detail.

____
____
____
____
____

9. How are you planning to use this ability in the future? Explain in detail.

____
____
____
____
____

10. How do you feel about having this ability? Explain through your feelings rather than through your thinking.

____
____
____
____
____

Homework: During the coming week, think more about how you could develop this ability. Jot down anything that comes to mind about this ability during the course of this week. At the end of the week, see whether you can put all these thoughts into one single plan to develop this ability even more than you have done in the past.

Practical Ability

This ability deals with interest in solving problems, ranging from simple decision making, to choosing one option over other options, to being able to explain the pros and cons of making choices. It involves finding appropriate solutions to a variety of problems, including manual, rational, or even irrational or verbal complexities. It may mean bringing down to earth issues and ideas that seem at first blush too abstract and complex to be solved.

Practice Exercise 1. Practical Ability

Name______________________________Sex__________Date__________

The purpose of this practice exercise is to understand in greater detail the nature of this ability. How did it develop? How have you used it in the past? How can you use it in the present and future?

1. Why is this ability important to you? Give as many reasons as you can think of.

____
____
____
____
____

2. How does this ability apply to you?

a. A great deal ________ c. Not at all ________
b. Somewhat ________

3. Explain in detail how this ability applies to you.

____
____
____
____
____

4. How did this ability develop in you? Explain in detail.

____
____
____
____

5. When did you find out that you had this ability?

a.	In prekindergarten	_______	e.	In high school	_______
b.	In kindergarten	_______	f.	In college	_______
c.	In elementary school	_______	g.	After college	_______
d.	In middle school	_______			

6. Explain in greater detail how you found out about this ability.

____
____
____
____
____

7. How have you used this ability in the past? Explain in detail.

____
____
____
____
____

8. How are you using this ability in the present? Explain in detail.

____
____
____
____
____

9. How are you planning to use this ability in the future? Explain in detail.

____
____
____
____
____

10. How do you feel about having this ability? Explain through your feelings rather than through your thinking.

____
____
____
____
____

Homework: During the coming week, think more about how you could develop this ability. Jot down anything that comes to mind about this ability during the course of this week. At the end of the week, see whether you can put all these thoughts into one single plan to develop this ability even more than you have done in the past.

Analytical Ability

This ability involves a critical evaluation of an issue, idea, problem, or confrontation, being able to break down the various components of a situation into their relationship within themselves as well as with external or historical determinants. Its content may be political, academic, philosophical, or even mechanical. However, the major aspect that distinguishes this ability from the practical relies on criticalness, being aware of the various pros and cons of many ideological situations, and being able to get down to the core issue of many situations.

Practice Exercise 1. Analytical Ability

Name____________________________Sex_________Date____________

The purpose of this practice exercise is to understand in greater detail the nature of this ability. How did it develop? How have you used it in the past? How can you use it in the present and future?

1. Why is this ability important to you? Give as many reasons as you can think of.

____
____
____
____
____

2. How does this ability apply to you?

a. A great deal ________
b. Somewhat ________
c. Not at all ________

3. Explain in detail how this ability applies to you.

____
____
____
____
____

4. How did this ability develop in you? Explain in detail.

____
____
____
____
____

5. When did you find out that you had this ability?

a. In prekindergarten ______
b. In kindergarten ______
c. In elementary school ______
d. In middle school ______
e. In high school ______
f. In college ______
g. After college ______

6. Explain in greater detail how you found out about this ability.

____
____
____
____
____

7. How have you used this ability in the past? Explain in detail.

____
____
____
____
____

8. How are you using this ability in the present? Explain in detail.

____

____

____

____

____

9. How are you planning to use this ability in the future? Explain in detail.

____

____

____

____

____

10. How do you feel about having this ability? Explain through your feelings rather than through your thinking.

____

____

____

____

____

Homework: During the coming week, think more about how you could develop this ability. Jot down anything that comes to mind about this ability during the course of this week. At the end of the week, see whether you can put all these thoughts into one single plan to develop this ability even more than you have done in the past.

Creative Ability

This ability implies being able to generate unusual problem-solving choices, plans, and options, whether in the arts, sciences, or any other human endeavor. It involves being able to come up with a solution, idea, product, or composition that no one else ever thought of before. It may refer to physical patterns, literary compositions, visual assignments, or mechanical solutions.

Practice Exercise 1. Creative Ability

Name_______________________Sex_________Date____________

The purpose of this practice exercise is to understand in greater detail the nature of this ability. How did it develop? How have you used it in the past? How can you use it in the present and future?

1. Why is this ability important to you? Give as many reasons as you can think of.

____
____
____
____
____

2. How does this ability apply to you?

a.	A great deal	______	c.	Not at all	______
b.	Somewhat	______			

3. Explain in detail how this ability applies to you.

____
____
____
____
____

4. How did this ability develop in you? Explain in detail.

____
____
____
____

5. When did you find out that you had this ability?

a.	In prekindergarten	______	e.	In high school	______
b.	In kindergarten	______	f.	In college	______
c.	In elementary school	______	g.	After college	______
d.	In middle school	______			

6. Explain in greater detail how you found out about this ability.

____
____
____
____
____

7. How have you used this ability in the past? Explain in detail.

8. How are you using this ability in the present? Explain in detail.

9. How are you planning to use this ability in the future? Explain in detail.

10. How do you feel about having this ability? Explain through your feelings rather than through your thinking.

Homework: During the coming week, think more about how you could develop this ability. Jot down anything that comes to mind about this ability during the course of this week. At the end of the week, see whether you can put all these thoughts into one single plan to develop this ability even more than you have done in the past.

Sexual Ability

This ability involves being very interested in sensual and sexual pleasures, involving skin and body sensations obtained through masturbation or sexual intercourse, but also caressing, massaging, or touching one's or someone else's body. It may involve thinking and fantasizing about body pleasures, wanting to be with someone to discuss these pleasures, and even buying books, videotapes, and paraphernalia relating to sex and sexual activities, or watching so-called pornographic movies or videotapes.

Practice Exercise 1. Sexual Ability

Name______________________________Sex_________Date__________

The purpose of this practice exercise is to understand in greater detail the nature of this ability. How did it develop? How have you used it in the past? How can you use it in the present and future?

1. Why is this ability important to you? Give as many reasons as you can think of.

____
____
____
____
____

2. How does this ability apply to you?

   a. A great deal ________
   b. Somewhat ________
   c. Not at all ________

3. Explain in detail how this ability applies to you.

____
____
____
____
____

4. How did this ability develop in you? Explain in detail.

____
____
____
____
____

5. When did you find out that you had this ability?

   a. In prekindergarten ______
   b. In kindergarten ______
   c. In elementary school ______
   d. In middle school ______
   e. In high school ______
   f. In college ______
   g. After college ______

6. Explain in greater detail how you found out about this ability.

7. How have you used this ability in the past? Explain in detail.

8. How are you using this ability in the present? Explain in detail.

9. How are you planning to use this ability in the future? Explain in detail.

10. How do you feel about having this ability? Explain through your feelings rather than through your thinking.

Homework: During the coming week, think more about how you could develop this ability. Jot down anything that comes to mind about this ability during the course of this week. At the end of the week, see whether you can put all these thoughts into one single plan to develop this ability even more than you have done in the past.

Concluding Feedback Form

Name___________________________Sex__________Date____________

The purpose of this practice exercise is to review what you learned from working on selected practice exercises in this practice exercises.

1. Below are listed all the abilities that are included in the practice exercises. Some of these abilities may not have been included in your practice exercises because you listed them as not being interesting to you. Perhaps you may have changed your mind. If so, feel free to rank-order them according to how important they are to you now. Rank as No. 1 the ability that you think is the most important to you, rank as No. 2 the ability that is second in importance to you, and so on, until you reach abilities that are not important to you, for which you can either write N/A or give a rank number if you think you can rank-order the abilities that do not apply to you.

Ability	*Rank-order*	*Ability*	*Rank-order*
a. Language	________	i. Spiritual	________
b. Logical–mathematical	________	j. Existential	________
c. Spatial	________	k. Emotional	________
d. Musical	________	l. Practical	________
e. Bodily-kinesthetic	________	m. Analytical	________
f. Interpersonal	________	n. Creative	________
g. Intrapersonal	________	o. Sexual	________
h. Naturalistic	________		

2. What did you learn from working on the practice exercises given to you? Please explain freely.

____

____

____

____

____

3. What did you like best about working on these practice exercises?

____

____

____

____

____

4. What did you like the least about these practice exercise?

____
____
____
____
____

5. How did this practice exercises help in reaching your goals? Check which answer applied to you:

a. A lot _______ c. Not at all _______
b. Somewhat _______

6. What suggestions could you make to improve this practice exercises?

____
____
____
____
____

Normative Experiences: Form AB5C

The purpose of this practice exercises is to help you understand the nature of your normal experiences. You will be asked to answer in writing many practice exercises containing a great many questions about the experiences that make up your normality. Participation in working on this practice exercises is completely voluntary, and you do not have to answer any questions or complete any practice exercise if you do not want to do it. It is completely up to you whether you want to learn more about yourself and whether you want professionals interested in your welfare to learn more about you. If you complete this practice exercise, it means that you do want to learn more about yourself and that you are interested in improving your condition.

Practice Exercise 1. Understanding Your Normality

Name______________________________Sex_______Date_________

The purpose of this first practice exercise is to understand more about your normality and determine the best course of action to deal with it. To learn more about yourself, you will need to explain what the behaviors listed below mean to you. Each behavior, together with other behaviors, very likely makes up your personality.

Some behaviors may be hard for you to know or understand. Use a dictionary or ask relatives or friends for the meaning of behaviors you do not know or do not understand. Make sure to explain what each behavior means to you. For each behavior, give two concrete examples to make sure you understand what that behavior means.

Behaviors and Definitions	*Examples*
a. Dutifulness ________	Example 1 ________
________	________
________	Example 2 ________
________	________
b. Moderation ________	Example 1 ________
________	________
________	Example 2 ________
________	________
c. Morality ________	Example 1 ________
________	________
________	Example 2 ________
________	________
d. Impulse control ________	Example 1 ________
________	________
________	Example 2 ________
________	________
e. Happiness ________	Example 1 ________
________	________
________	Example 2 ________
________	________
f. Calmness ________	Example 1 ________
________	________
________	Example 2 ________
________	________
g. Cautiousness ________	Example 1 ________
________	________
________	Example 2 ________
________	________

h. Purposefulness ______________ Example 1 ______________
______________ ______________
______________ Example 2 ______________
______________ ______________

i. Cooperation ______________ Example 1 ______________
______________ ______________
______________ Example 2 ______________
______________ ______________

j. Tranquility ______________ Example 1 ______________
______________ ______________
______________ Example 2 ______________
______________ ______________

k. Leadership ______________ Example 1 ______________
______________ ______________
______________ Example 2 ______________
______________ ______________

l. Orderliness ______________ Example 1 ______________
______________ ______________
______________ Example 2 ______________
______________ ______________

m. Stability ______________ Example 1 ______________
______________ ______________
______________ Example 2 ______________
______________ ______________

n. Efficiency ______________ Example 1 ______________
______________ ______________
______________ Example 2 ______________
______________ ______________

o. Imperturbability ______________ Example 1 ______________
______________ ______________
______________ Example 2 ______________
______________ ______________

p. Nurturance ______________ Example 1 ______________
______________ ______________
______________ Example 2 ______________
______________ ______________

q. Conscientiousness ____________	Example 1 ____________
____________	____________
____________	Example 2 ____________
____________	____________
r. Depth ____________	Example 1 ____________
____________	____________
____________	Example 2 ____________
____________	____________
s. Talkativeness ____________	Example 1 ____________
____________	____________
____________	Example 2 ____________
____________	____________

2. Now that you have explained the meaning of these behaviors, it is important to find out which behaviors you want to improve. Each behavior that you have just explained needs to be rank-ordered according to how much you want to improve that particular behavior. Rank as No. 1 the behavior that you want to improve the most, rank as No. 2 the behavior that you want to improve next, and so on; mark as N/A the behaviors that do not need any improvement.

Behaviors	*Rank-order*	*Behaviors*	*Rank-order*
a. Dutifulness	________	k. Leadership	________
b. Moderation	________	l. Orderliness	________
c. Morality	________	m. Stability	________
d. Impulse control	________	n. Efficiency	________
e. Happiness	________	o. Imperturbability	________
f. Calmness	________	p. Nurturance	________
g. Cautiousness	________	q. Conscientiousness	________
h. Purposefulness	________	r. Depth	________
i. Cooperation	________	s. Talkativeness	________
j. Tranquility	________		

3. Write why you ranked these behaviors the way you did.

____

____

____

____

____

4. Now that you have completed this practice exercise, check which of these answers indicates how you felt about it. There is also space for you to explain further, if you want to.

   a. I did not like this practice exercise at all. I want to quit this stupid practice exercises. ______
   b. I did not like this practice exercise very much, but I want to go on with this practice exercises. ______
   c. I liked this practice exercise and I want to go on with this practice exercises. ______
   d. I liked this practice exercise a lot and I wish I had something like this practice exercises years ago. ______
   e. I liked it so much that I wish all people with the same condition I have could get something like this practice exercises to work on. ______

Homework: During the next week, think more about the behaviors you rank-ordered and whether you want to change their rank-order.

Concluding Follow-Up Form

Name______________________________Sex__________Date____________

The purpose of this form is to review whether this practice exercises was helpful to you or not.

1. Check the answer that best fits how you feel about this practice exercises:

   a. I did not like working on this practice exercises at all. I wish I never saw it. ______
   b. I did not like this practice exercises at all, but I am glad I got to work on it. ______
   c. I am delighted I got a chance to work on this practice exercises. ______
   d. I am not only delighted about working on this practice exercises, but I wish everybody had a chance to work on it. ______

2. How helpful was it to work on this practice exercises? Check the answer that applies to you.

   a. Not helpful at all ______ c. Helpful ______
   b. Somewhat helpful ______ d. Very helpful ______

3. Which practice exercise did you like best? Rank as No. 1 the one that you liked best, rank as No. 2 the one you liked next best, and so on; mark as N/A the ones you did not like at all or did not apply to you.

Behaviors	*Rank-order*	*Behaviors*	*Rank-order*
a. Dutifulness	________	k. Leadership	________
b. Moderation	________	l. Orderliness	________
c. Morality	________	m. Stability	________
d. Impulse control	________	n. Efficiency	________
e. Happiness	________	o. Imperturbability	________
f. Calmness	________	p. Nurturance	________
g. Cautiousness	________	q. Conscientiousness	________
h. Purposefulness	________	r. Depth	________
i. Cooperation	________	s. Talkativeness	________
j. Tranquility	________		

4. Explain why you rank-ordered these behaviors the way you did.

____
____
____
____
____

5. Sometimes what we like most is not necessarily the most helpful. Which practice exercise was the most helpful to you? Rank the practice exercises according to their helpfulness to you. Rank as No. 1 the most helpful, rank as No. 2 the next most helpful, and so on, down to the least helpful practice exercise; mark as N/A the practice exercises that did not apply to you.

Behaviors	*Rank-order*	*Behaviors*	*Rank-order*
a. Dutifulness	________	k. Leadership	________
b. Moderation	________	l. Orderliness	________
c. Morality	________	m. Stability	________
d. Impulse control	________	n. Efficiency	________
e. Happiness	________	o. Imperturbability	________
f. Calmness	________	p. Nurturance	________
g. Cautiousness	________	q. Conscientiousness	________
h. Purposefulness	________	r. Depth	________
i. Cooperation	________	s. Talkativeness	________
j. Tranquility	________		

6. Explain why you rank-ordered these behaviors the way you did.

____
____
____
____
____

7. Feel free to write any comments that might improve this practice exercises.

____
____
____
____
____
____

Normative Experiences: Form IPIP

The purpose of this practice exercise is to help you understand the nature of your normal experiences. You will be asked to answer in writing many practice exercises containing a great many questions about the many experiences that make up your personality. Of course, you do not have to answer any question or complete any practice exercise if you do not want to. Participation in working on this practice exercises is completely voluntary. It is completely up to you whether you want to learn more about yourself and whether you want professionals interested in your welfare to learn more about you. If you complete this practice exercise, it means that you do want to learn more about yourself and that you are interested in improving your condition.

Practice Exercise 1. Understanding Your Normality

Name______________________________Sex_______Date_________

The purpose of this first practice exercise is to understand more about your normality and to determine the best course of action to deal with it. To learn more about yourself, explain what the behaviors listed below mean to you. Each behavior, together with other ones, very likely makes up your personality. To understand how each behavior applies to you, define each behavior and give two examples. Make sure to explain what each behavior means to you. Use a dictionary if you need one.

Behavior and Definitions	*Examples*
a. Stability ________________	Example 1 ________________
________________	________________
________________	Example 2 ________________
________________	________________
b. Cooperation ________________	Example 1 ________________
________________	________________
________________	Example 2 ________________
________________	________________
c. Temperance ________________	Example 1 ________________
________________	________________
________________	Example 2 ________________
________________	________________
d. Dutifulness ________________	Example 1 ________________
________________	________________
________________	Example 2 ________________
________________	________________
e. Self-control ________________	Example 1 ________________
________________	________________
________________	Example 2 ________________
________________	________________
f. Calmness ________________	Example 1 ________________
________________	________________
________________	Example 2 ________________
________________	________________
g. Happiness ________________	Example 1 ________________
________________	________________
________________	Example 2 ________________
________________	________________
h. Satisfaction ________________	Example 1 ________________
________________	________________
________________	Example 2 ________________
________________	________________
i. Impulse control ________________	Example 1 ________________
________________	________________
________________	Example 2 ________________
________________	________________

j. Imagination ____________________ Example 1 ____________________
____________________ ____________________
____________________ Example 2 ____________________
____________________ ____________________

k. Immoderation ____________________ Example 1 ____________________
____________________ ____________________
____________________ Example 2 ____________________
____________________ ____________________

2. Now that you have explained the meaning of all these behaviors, it is important to find out how they apply to you. Each behavior that you have just explained needs to be rank-ordered according to how much that particular behavior applies to you. Rank as No. 1 the behavior that applies to you the most, rank as No. 2 the behavior that applies to you next, and so on; mark as N/A the behaviors that do not apply to you at all.

Behaviors	*Rank-order*	*Behaviors*	*Rank-order*
a. Stability	________	g. Happiness	________
b. Cooperation	________	h. Satisfaction	________
c. Temperance	________	i. Impulse control	________
d. Dutifulness	________	j. Imagination	________
e. Self-control	________	k. Immoderation	________
f. Calmness	________		

3. Write why you ranked these behaviors the way you did.

____
____
____
____

4. Now that you have completed this practice exercise, check which of these answers indicates how you felt about it. There is also space for you to explain further, if you want to.

   a. I did not like this practice exercise at all. I want to quit this stupid practice exercises. ______
   b. I did not like this practice exercise very much, but I want to go on with this practice exercises. ______
   c. I liked this practice exercise and I want to go on with this practice exercises. ______
   d. I liked this practice exercise a lot and I wish I had something like this practice exercises years ago. ______
   e. I liked it so much that I wish all people with the same condition I have could get something like this practice exercises to work on. ______

Homework: During the coming week, think more about the behaviors you ranked.

Concluding Follow-Up Form

Name____________________________Sex________Date____________

The purpose of this form is to review whether this practice exercises was helpful to you or not.

1. Check the answer that best fits how you feel about this practice exercises:

   a. I did not like working on this practice exercises at all. I wish I never saw it. _______
   b. I did not like this practice exercises at all, but I am glad I got to work on it. _______
   c. I am delighted I got a chance to work on this practice exercises. _______
   d. I am not only delighted about working on this practice exercises, but I wish everybody had a chance to work on it. _______

2. How helpful was it to work on this practice exercises? Check the answer that applies to you.

   a. Not helpful at all _______ c. Helpful _______
   b. Somewhat helpful _______ d. Very helpful _______

3. Which practice exercise did you like best? Rank as No. 1 the one that you liked best, rank as No. 2 the one you liked next best, and so on; mark as N/A the ones you did not like at all or did not apply to you.

Behaviors	*Rank-order*	*Behaviors*	*Rank-order*
a. Stability	________	g. Happiness	________
b. Cooperation	________	h. Satisfaction	________
c. Temperance	________	i. Impulse control	________
d. Dutifulness	________	j. Imagination	________
e. Self-control	________	k. Immoderation	________
f. Calmness	________		

4. Sometimes what we like most is not necessarily the most helpful. Which practice exercise was the most helpful to you? Rank the practice exercises according to their helpfulness to you. Rank as No. 1 the most helpful, rank as No. 2 the next most helpful, and so on, down to the least helpful practice exercise; mark as N/A the practice exercises that did not apply to you.

Behaviors	*Rank-order*	*Behaviors*	*Rank-order*
a. Stability	________	g. Happiness	________
b. Cooperation	________	h. Satisfaction	________
c. Temperance	________	i. Impulse control	________
d. Dutifulness	________	j. Imagination	________
e. Self-control	________	k. Immoderation	________
f. Calmness	________		

5. Explain why you rank-ordered these behaviors the way you did.

____
____
____
____
____

6. Feel free to write any comments that might improve this practice exercises.

____
____
____
____
____

Normative Experiences: Form PSC

The purpose of this practice exercises is to help you understand the nature of your normal experiences. You will be asked to answer in writing many practice exercises containing a great many questions about the many experiences that make up your condition. Of course, you do not have to answer any question or complete any practice exercise. It is completely up to you whether you want to learn more about yourself and whether you want professionals interested in your welfare to learn more about you. If you complete this practice exercise, it means that you do want to learn more about yourself and that you are interested in improving your condition.

Practice Exercise 1. Understanding Your Normality

Name________________________________Sex___Date_____

The purpose of this first practice exercise is to understand more about your normality and to determine the best course of action to deal with it. To learn more about yourself, you will need to explain what the behaviors listed below mean to you. Each behavior, together with other behaviors, very likely makes up your personality. To understand how each behavior applies to you, define each behavior and give two examples. Make sure to explain what each behavior means to you. Use a dictionary if you need one.

Behaviors and Definitions	*Examples*
a. Socialization ________________	Example 1 ________________
________________	________________
________________	Example 2 ________________
________________	________________
b. Reliability ________________	Example 1 ________________
________________	________________
________________	Example 2 ________________
________________	________________
c. Good impression ________________	Example 1 ________________
________________	________________
________________	Example 2 ________________
________________	________________
d. Prudence ________________	Example 1 ________________
________________	________________
________________	Example 2 ________________
________________	________________
e. Dutifulness________________	Example 1 ________________
________________	________________
________________	Example 2 ________________
________________	________________
f. Self-control ________________	Example 1 ________________
________________	________________
________________	Example 2 ________________
________________	________________
g. Work orientation ________________	Example 1 ________________
________________	________________
________________	Example 2 ________________
________________	________________
h. Managerial potential ________________	Example 1 ________________
________________	________________
________________	Example 2 ________________
________________	________________

i. Responsibility ______________ Example 1 ______________

______________ ______________

______________ Example 2 ______________

______________ ______________

j. Enlightened second nature ______ Example 1 ______________

______________ ______________

______________ Example 2 ______________

______________ ______________

k. Abstractness ______________ Example 1 ______________

______________ ______________

______________ Example 2 ______________

______________ ______________

l. Forgetfulness ______________ Example 1 ______________

______________ ______________

______________ Example 2 ______________

______________ ______________

m. Impulsiveness ______________ Example 1 ______________

______________ ______________

______________ Example 2 ______________

______________ ______________

2. Now that you have explained the meaning of all these behaviors, it is important to find out how they apply to you. Each behavior that you have just explained needs to be rank-ordered according to how much that particular behavior applies to you. Rank as No. 1 the behavior that applies to you the most, rank as No. 2 the behavior that applies to you next, and so on; mark as N/A the behaviors that do not apply to you at all.

Behaviors	*Rank-order*	*Behaviors*	*Rank-order*
a. Socialization	________	h. Managerial potential	________
b. Reliability	________	i. Responsibility	________
c. Good impression	________	j. Enlightened second nature	________
d. Prudence	________	k. Abstractness	________
e. Dutifulness	________	l. Forgetfulness	________
f. Self-control	________	m. Impulsiveness	________
g. Work orientation	________		

3. Write why you ranked these items the way you did.

____
____
____
____
____

4. Now that you have completed this practice exercise, check which of these answers indicates how you felt about it. There is also space for you to explain further, if you want to.

   a. I did not like this practice exercise at all. I want to quit this stupid practice exercises. _____
   b. I did not like this practice exercise very much, but I want to go on with this practice exercises. _____
   c. I liked this practice exercise and I want to go on with this practice exercises. _____
   d. I liked this practice exercise a lot and I wish I had something like this practice exercises years ago. _____
   e. I liked it so much that I wish all people with the same condition I have could get something like this practice exercises to work on. _____

Homework: During the coming week, think more about the items you rank-ordered and whether you want to change their rank-order.

Concluding Follow-Up Form

Name_________________________Sex____Date______

The purpose of this form is to review whether this practice exercises was helpful to you or not.

1. Check the answer that best fits how you feel about this practice exercises:

   a. I did not like working on this practice exercises at all. I wish I never saw it. _____
   b. I did not like this practice exercises at all, but I am glad I got to work on it. _____
   c. I am delighted I got a chance to work on this practice exercises. _____
   d. I am not only delighted about working on this practice exercises, but I wish everybody had a chance to work on it. _____

2. How helpful was it to work on this practice exercises? Check the answer that applies to you:

a. Not helpful at all	_____	c. Helpful	_____
b. Somewhat helpful	_____	d. Very helpful	_____

3. Which practice exercise did you like best? Rank as No. 1 the one that you liked best, rank as No. 2 the one you liked next best, and so on; mark as N/A the ones you did not like at all or did not apply to you.

Behaviors	*Rank-order*	*Behaviors*	*Rank-order*
a. Socialization	_________	h. Managerial potential	_________
b. Reliability	_________	i. Responsibility	_________
c. Good impression	_________	j. Enlightened second nature	_________
d. Prudence	_________	k. Abstractness	_________
e. Dutifulness	_________	l. Forgetfulness	_________
f. Self-control	_________	m. Impulsiveness	_________
g. Work orientation	_________		

4. Sometimes what we like most is not necessarily the most helpful. Which practice exercise was the most helpful to you? Rank the practice exercises according to their helpfulness to you. Rank as No. 1 the most helpful, rank as No. 2 the next most helpful, and so on, down to the least helpful practice exercise; mark as N/A the practice exercises that did not apply to you.

Behaviors	*Rank-order*	*Behaviors*	*Rank-order*
a. Socialization	_________	h. Managerial potential	_________
b. Reliability	_________	i. Responsibility	_________
c. Good impression	_________	j. Enlightened second nature	_________
d. Prudence	_________	k. Abstractness	_________
e. Dutifulness	_________	l. Forgetfulness	_________
f. Self-control	_________	m. Impulsiveness	_________
g. Work orientation	_________		

5. Explain why you rank-ordered these item the way you did.

____

____

____

____

____

6. Feel free to write any comments that might improve this practice exercises.

____

____

____

____

____

Priorities

The purpose of these practice exercises is to help participants become more aware of their priorities, that is, goals that in some way or another determine how one behaves and self-regulates in relationship with oneself and with important others. Priorities are goals that have been ranked according to a specific stage of the life cycle, as well as their importance, urgency, temporal perspective, and reality

There are three types of priorities considered in these practice exercisess: (1) self-oriented; (2) others oriented; and (3) general, abstract or concrete ones. These priorities change developmentally from one stage of the life cycle to another. That is the reason for having different practice exercisess for different stages of the life cycle.

Elementary-School Age

The purpose of this practice exercises is to help you become more aware of your priorities. Priorities are goals that in some way or another determine how you behave in relationship to yourself and to important others. There are three types of priorities (1) self-oriented, (2) others oriented, and (3) general.

Practice Exercise 1. Priorities

Name__________________Sex_______Age_________Date_______

Please rank-order the self-priorities from the most important (1) to the least important (10), according to how important these priorities are to you.

Self-Oriented	*Rank-order*	*Self-Oriented*	*Rank-order*
a. School grades	_________	f. Sense of humor	_________
b. Physical	_________	g. Intelligence	_________
c. Attractiveness	_________	h. Self-worth	_________
d. Sports success	_________	i. Other characteristic that is important to you: write it down: (_____________)	_________
e. School conduct	_________		

Please rank-order the others-oriented priorities from the most important (1) to the least important (8), according to how important these priorities are to you.

Others Oriented	*Rank-order*
a. Close friends	________
b. Boy/girlfriend	________
c. Mother or mother substitute (see Footnote 1)	________
d. Father or father substitute (see Footnote 2)	________
e. Brothers/sisters	________
f. Other relatives	________
g. Teachers	________
h. Write the name of anybody else who makes you feel important (____________________)	________

Please rank-order the general priorities listed below according to how important they are to you. Rank as No. 1 the most important priority, rank as No. 2 the second most important, and so on, until you have ranked all the priorities in this list.

General Priorities	*Rank-order*
a. Being sociable	________
b. Being smart	________
c. Talking with others	________
d. Being close to others	________
e. Being physically strong	________
f. Being clean	________
g. Being in good health	________
h. Being attractive	________
i. Having lots of things	________
j. Being happy	________
k. Being honest	________
l. Being independent	________
m. Having lots of money	________
n. Being popular	________
o. Feeling important	________
p. Having many friends	________
q. Becoming a champion in sports	________
r. Becoming a great scientist	________
s. Make up your own priority: what is it? (................)	________
t. Make up your own priority: what is it? (..................)	________

Explain why you ordered the priorities listed above in the way that you did.

____

____

____

____

____

Middle-School Age

The purpose of this practice exercises is to help you become more aware of your priorities, that is, goals that in some way or another determine how you behave in relationship to yourself and to others.

Practice Exercise 1. Priorities

Name____________________Sex_____Age_____Date_______

Please rank-order the self-priorities from the most important (1) to the least important (9), according to how important these priorities are to you.

Self-Oriented	*Rank-order*
a. School grades	_______
b. Physical attractiveness	_______
c. Sports	_______
d. School conduct	_______
e. Sense of humor	_______
f. Intelligence	_______
g. Self-worth	_______
h. Write any other self characteristic that makes you feel important: (______________)	_______
i. Write any other self characteristic that makes you feel important: (______________)	_______

Please rank-order these others-oriented priorities from the most important (1) to the least important (8), according to how important these persons are to you.

Others Oriented	*Rank-order*
a. Close friend	_______
b. Boy/girlfriend	_______
c. Mother or mother substitute (see Footnote 1)	_______
d. Father or father substitute (see Footnote 2)	_______
e. Brothers/sisters	_______
f. Other relatives	_______
g. Teachers	_______
h. Write the name of anybody else who makes you feel important (________)	_______

Please rank-order the priorities listed below according to how important they are to you. Start with the most important priority as No. 1, then to the second most important No. 2, and so on until you have ranked all the priorities in this list.

General Priorities	*Rank-order*
a. Being sociable	________
b. Being smart	________
c. Sharing with others	________
d. Being close to others	________
e. Being physically strong	________
f. Being clean	________
g. Being in good health	________
h. Being attractive	________
i. Having lots of things	________
j. Being happy	________
k. Being honest	________
l. Being independent	________
m. Having lots of money	________
n. Being popular	________
o. Feeling important	________
p. Having many friends	________
q. Becoming a champion in sports	________
r. Becoming a great scientist	________
s. Make up your own priority: what is it? (............................)	________
t. Make up your own priority: what is it? (........................)	________

Explain why you ranked-ordered the general priorities as you did.

High-School Age

The purpose of this practice exercises is to help you become more aware of your priorities, that is, goals that in some way or another determine how you behave in relationship to yourself and to others. There are three types of priorities: (1) self-priorities, (2) others priorities, and (3) general priorities.

Practice Exercise 1. Priorities

Name__________________________Sex____Age______Date_______

Please rank-order the self-oriented priorities from the most important (1) to the least important (10), according to how important these priorities are to you.

Self-Oriented	*Rank-order*
a. School grades	________
b. Physical attractiveness	________
c. Sports success	________
d. School conduct	________

e. Popularity with peers	________
f. Sense of humor	________
g. Intelligence	________
h. Job or work competence	________
i. Self-worth	________
j. Write any other self characteristic that makes you feel important: (__________________)	________

Please rank-order the others-oriented priorities from the most important (1) to the least important (8), according to how important these persons are to you.

Others Oriented	*Rank-order*
a. Close friends	________
b. Boy/girlfriend	________
c. Mother or mother substitute (see Footnote 1)	________
d. Father or father substitute (see Footnote 2)	________
e. Brothers/sisters	________
f. Other relatives	________
g. Teachers	________
h. Write the name of anybody else who makes you feel important: (__________________)	________

Please rank-order the general priorities listed below according to how important they are to you. Start with the most important priority as No. 1, then to the second most important No. 2, and so on until you have ranked all the priorities in this list.

General Priorities	*Rank-order*
a. Being sociable	________
b. Being smart	________
c. Sharing with others	________
d. Being close to others	________
e. Being physically strong	________
f. Being clean	________
g. Being in good health	________
h. Being attractive	________
i. Having lots of things	________
j. Being happy	________
k. Being honest	________
l. Being independent	________
m. Having lots of money	________
n. Being popular	________
o. Feeling important	________
p. Having many friends	________
q. Becoming a champion in sports	________

r. Becoming a great scientist ________
s. Make up your own priority: what is it? (......................) ________
t. Make up your own priority: what is it? (.........…….....…..) ________

Explain why you ranked-ordered the general priorities as you did.

College Age

The purpose of this practice exercises is to help you become more aware of your priorities, that is, goals that in some way or another determine how you behave in relationship to yourself and others. There are three types of priorities (1) self-priorities, (2) others-priorities, and (3) general.

Practice Exercise 1. Priorities

Name__________________________Sex____Age_____Date________

Please rank-order the self-priorities from the most important (1) to the least important (10), according to how important these priorities are to you.

Self-Oriented *Rank-order*
a. School achievement ________
b. Physical attractiveness ________
c. Sports success ________
d. Intelligence ________
e. Creativity ________
f. Sense of humor ________
g. Popularity ________
h. Morality ________
i. Self-worth or self-esteem ________
j. Any other characteristic that makes you feel important: (_______) ________

Please rank-order the others-oriented priorities listed below from the most important (1) to the least important (9), according to how important these priorities are to you.

Others Oriented *Rank-order*
a. Close friendships ________
b. Romantic relationships ________
c. School/job/career ________
d. Mother or mother substitute (see Footnote 1) ________
e. Father or father substitute (see Footnote 2) ________
f. Siblings ________

g. Relatives ________
h. Teachers/mentors ________
i. Other person that makes you feel important (................) ________

Please rank-order the general priorities listed below according to how important they are to you. Start with the most important priority as No. 1, then to the second most important as No. 2, and so on until you have ranked all the priorities in this list.

General Priorities	*Rank-order*
a. Being sociable	________
b. Being smart	________
c. Sharing with others	________
d. Being close to others	________
e. Being physically strong	________
f. Being clean	________
g. Being in good health	________
h. Being attractive	________
i. Having lots of things	________
j. Being happy	________
k. Being honest	________
l. Being independent	________
m. Having lots of money	________
n. Being popular	________
o. Feeling important	________
p. Having many friends	________
q. Becoming a champion in sports	________
r. Becoming a great scientist	________
s. Make up your own priority: what is it? (......................)	________
t. Make up your own priority: what is it? (.....................)	________

Explain why you ranked-ordered the general priorities as you did.

____
____
____
____
____

Adulthood

The purpose of this practice exercises is to help you become more aware of your priorities, that is, goals that in some way or another determine how you behave in relationship to yourself and to others. There are at least three types of priorities (1) self-priorities, (2) others priorities, and (3) general priorities.

Practice Exercise 1. Priorities

Name________________________Age_____Sex_____Date________

Please rank-order the self-priorities from the most important (1) to the least important (9), according to how important these priorities are to you.

Self-Oriented	*Rank-order*
a. Intelligence	________
b. Physical attractiveness	________
c. Sports success	________
d. Sense of humor	________
e. Job competence	________
f. Sociability	________
g. Morality	________
h. Self-worth or self-esteem	________
i. Any other self-oriented priority not listed above (______________)	________

Please rank-order the others-oriented priorities listed below from the most important (1) to the least important (12), according to how important these priorities are to you.

Others Oriented	*Rank-order*
a. Partner/mate or boy/girlfriend	________
b. Children (if applicable)	________
c. Mother or mother substitute (see Footnote 1)	________
d. Father or father substitute (see Footnote 2)	________
e. In-laws (if applicable)	________
f. Siblings	________
g. Friends	________
h. Coworkers	________
i. Neighbors	________
j. Relatives	________
k. Teachers/mentors	________
l. Any other others-oriented priority not listed above (______)	________

Please rank-order the priorities listed below according to how important they are to you. Start with the most important priority as No. 1, then the second most important as No. 2, and so on until you have ranked all the priorities in this list.

General Priorities	*Rank-order*
a. Being sociable	________
b. Being smart	________
c. Sharing with others	________
d. Being close to others	________
e. Being physically strong	________

f. Being clean ________
g. Being in good health ________
h. Being attractive ________
i. Having lots of things ________
j. Being happy ________
k. Being honest ________
l. Being independent ________
m. Having lots of money ________
n. Being popular ________
o. Feeling important ________
p. Having many friends ________
q. Becoming a champion in sports ________
r. Becoming a great scientist ________
s. Make up your own priority: what is it? (............................) ________
t. Make up your own priority: what is it? (........................) ________

Explain why you rank-ordered the general priorities as you did.

Instructions to the Professional Administrator for Standard Practice Exercises for Priorities practice exercise

From the rank-orders given in the first practice exercise, administer standard practice exercises for priorities according to the rank-orders given there. The priority given first place should be numbered and written down for self-oriented, others-oriented, and general priorities. After this practice exercise is completed, just follow the rank-orders given in the first practice exercise – No. 2, No. 3, and so on – until the agreed-upon number of standard practice exercises that was decided beforehand is completed.

Standard Practice Exercise for Priorities

Self-Priority No.___ Title of Priority______________________________

Name______________________________Age______Sex_____Date_____

The purpose of this practice exercise is to understand more about the self-priority listed above in the title.

1. How does this priority apply to you? Please explain in detail.

____
____
____
____
____

2. How often do you think about this priority?

a.	Practically every day	______	e.	Once every 6 months	______
b.	Once a week	______	f.	Once a year	______
c.	A couple of times a month	______	g.	Once every few years	______
d.	Once a month	______			

3. Please explain further:

____

____

____

____

____

4. How did this priority come about? Do you remember when you started to think about it? Check which answer fits best:

a. When I was a child (younger than 5 years of age) ______
b. When I was in elementary school ______
c. When I was in middle school ______
d. When I was in high school ______
e. Any other time ______

5. Please explain further:

____

____

____

____

____

6. How acceptable or unacceptable is this priority to your family?

a. Why was it acceptable? Please explain.

____

____

____

____

____

b. Why was it unacceptable? Please explain.

7. Give three specific examples of how this priority affects you.

Example 1:

Example 2:

Example 3:

8. Give three specific examples of how this priority affects others.

Example 1:

Example 2:

____

Example 3:

Others-Priority No.___Name of Other Person__________________

The purpose of this practice exercise is to understand more about the person listed above as being important to you.

1. How does this person relate to you? Please explain in detail.

2. How often do you see this person?

   a. Practically every day ______
   b. Once a week ______
   c. A couple of times a month ______
   d. Once a month ______
   e. Once every 6 months ______
   f. Once a year ______
   g. Once every few years ______

3. Please explain further:

4. Do you remember when you started to consider this person as being important to you? Check which answer fits best:

   a. When I was a child (younger than 5 years of age) ______
   b. When I was in elementary school ______
   c. When I was in middle school ______
   d. When I was in high school ______
   e. Any other time ______

5. Please explain further:

____
____
____
____
____

6. Give three specific examples of how this person affects you.

   Example 1:

____
____
____
____
____

   Example 2:

____
____
____
____
____

   Example 3:

____
____
____
____
____

7. Give three specific examples of how this person affects others.

Example 1:

____
____
____
____
____

Example 2:

____
____
____
____
____

Example 3:

____
____
____
____
____

General Priority No.____Title of Priority______________________

The purpose of this practice exercise is to understand more about the general priority listed above.

1. How does this general priority apply to you? Please explain in detail.

____
____
____
____
____

2. How often do you think about this priority?

a. Practically every day _____
b. Once a week _____
c. A couple of times a month _____
d. Once a month _____
e. Once every 6 months _____
f. Once a year _____
g. Once every few years _____

3. Please explain further:

____
____
____
____
____

4. How did this priority come about? Do you remember when you started thinking about it? Check which answer fits best:

   a. When I was a child (younger than 5 years of age) ________
   b. When I was in elementary school ________
   c. When I was in middle school ________
   d. When I was in high school ________
   e. Any other time ________

5. Please explain further:

____
____
____
____
____

6. Is this priority acceptable or unacceptable to your family?

   a. Why was it acceptable? Please explain.

____
____
____
____
____

   b. Why was it unacceptable? Please explain.

____
____
____
____
____

7. Give three specific examples of how this priority affects you.

Example 1:

Example 2:

Example 3:

8. Give three specific examples of how this priority affects others.

Example 1:

Example 2:

Example 3:

____
____
____
____
____

Check which of the following indicates how you feel about this practice exercise:

a. Completely useless _____
b. Somewhat useless _____
c. So-so _____
d. Somewhat useful _____
e. Extremely useful _____

Explain in greater detail how you feel about this practice exercise and what you got out of it.

____
____
____
____
____

Concluding Feedback Form for Priorities Practice exercisess

Name__________________________Sex______Age_____Date______

The purpose of this form is to review whether this practice exercises was helpful to you or not.

1. Check the answer that best fits how you feel about this practice exercises:

   a. I did not like working on this practice exercises at all. I wish I never saw it. _______
   b. I did not like this practice exercises at all, but I am glad I got to work on it. _______
   c. I am delighted I got a chance to work on this practice exercises. _______
   d. I am not only delighted about working on this practice exercises, but I wish everybody had a chance to work on it. _______

2. How helpful was it to work on this practice exercises? Check the answer that applies to you:

   a. Not helpful at all _______
   b. Somewhat helpful _______
   c. Helpful _______
   d. Very helpful _______

3. Which practice exercise did you like best? Rank as No. 1 the one that you liked best, rank as No. 2 the one you liked next best, and so on; mark as N/A the ones you did not like at all or did not apply to you.

General Priorities	*Rank-order*
a. Being sociable	________
b. Being smart	________
c. Sharing with others	________
d. Being close to others	________
e. Being physically strong	________
f. Being clean	________
g. Being in good health	________
h. Being attractive	________
i. Having lots of things	________
j. Being happy	________
k. Being honest	________
l. Being independent	________
m. Having lots of money	________
n. Being popular	________
o. Feeling important	________
p. Having many friends	________
q. Becoming a champion in sports	________
r. Becoming a great scientist	________
s. Make up your own priority: what is it? (............)	________
t. Make up your own priority: What is it? (............)	________

3. Sometimes what we like most is not necessarily the most helpful. Rank the practice exercises according to their helpfulness to you. Rank as No. 1 the most helpful, rank as No. 2 the next most helpful, and so on, down to the least helpful practice exercise; mark as N/A the practice exercises that did not apply to you.

General Priorities	*Rank-order*
a. Being sociable	________
b. Being smart	________
c. Sharing with others	________
d. Being close to others	________
e. Being physically strong	________
f. Being clean	________
g. Being in good health	________
h. Being attractive	________
i. Having lots of things	________
j. Being happy	________
k. Being honest	________
l. Being independent	________

m. Having lots of money ________
n. Being popular ________
o. Feeling important ________
p. Having many friends ________
q. Becoming a champion in sports ________
r. Becoming a great scientist ________
s. Make up your own priority: what is it? (......................) ________
t. Make up your own priority: what is it? (........................) ________

5. Please explain why you rank-ordered the practice exercises the way you did.

____
____
____
____
____

6. Feel free to write any comments that might improve this practice exercises.

____
____
____
____
____

Enhancing Self-Awareness

The purpose of this practice exercise is to improve mental and emotional functioning and one's self-awareness. The practice exercises must be followed to the letter. Think of the mind as a never-ending tape that is continuously running, made up of various thoughts, one running into another, such as sad and happy thoughts. These thoughts can consist of experiences that range from happy, enjoyable comedies to very sad, painful tragedies. If there are pleasant and happy thoughts, the tape keeps on running. If there are unhappy and painful thoughts, the tape slows downs and may even stop running, as in the case of limited self-awareness. Hence, this practice exercises was designed to help the tape of your mind to run more smoothly than has been the case in the past.

This practice exercises consists of 12 homework practice exercises. The first practice exercise consists of an introduction to this practice exercises, setting up appointment times for when you want to work on it, and choosing how you want to work on it. You may have a choice about the order in which to work on the practice exercises; ask the mental health professional that is helping you. However, all of the practice exercises should be completed to fulfill the purpose of this practice exercises. A 12th practice exercise seeks your feedback about this practice exercises.

Practice Exercise 1. Setting Appointment Times and Choosing the Order of Administration

Name__________________Sex_____Date__________Time__________

The purpose of this practice exercise is to set times and choose the order of administration for all future practice exercises.

1. Set appointments first: Before you start working on this practice exercises, you must decide on a work schedule. This schedule will consist of prearranged, predetermined appointment times when you will be working on this practice exercises for no longer than 1 h at one time. These appointments could take place once, twice, or three times a day, or once, two, or three times a week, unless the mental health professional who is administering this practice exercises suggests a different schedule. You must sign an informed consent form before starting the practice exercises.

   It is important that you choose the specific times on which you are going to work on this practice exercises beforehand (e.g., Monday at 9 a.m.), and that you stick to those preset times no matter what. If, for whatever reason, you are unable to work at the time you have chosen beforehand, make an appointment with yourself at least 24 h ahead. Never work on this practice exercises on the spur of the moment, but work on it always by appointment at least 24 h ahead of time.

2. Defining the contents of your thoughts: These practice exercises are composed of at least ten types of thoughts:

   (T1) Extremely painful tragedies are extremely sad experiences and events of great intensity to you that did not allow any escape or solution, such as great losses, terrible traumas, and major hurts and defeats. These experiences may have produced and provoked intense feelings of shame and guilt in you, and may have taught you to become aware of errors and mistakes in your life, influencing your mood very negatively.

   (T2) Very painful tragedies are experiences or events whose intensity is minor compared to the intensity of extremely painful experiences (T1). You were not dealing with total darkness here; there was a light at the end of the tunnel. The themes may be the same, that is, errors, painful experiences, humiliations, losses, defeats, etc. However, these experiences or events were of lesser importance to you than extremely painful tragedies. Nonetheless, these tragedies did influence your mood negatively.

   (T3) Somewhat painful tragedies were experiences that, although of lesser importance to you than extremely painful and very painful ones, are still somewhat vivid in your mind, including minor losses, small errors, slights and humiliations of lower intensity than the two previous types of tragedies, having little if any effect on your mood.

(C1) Extremely enjoyable comedies were extremely funny experiences and events in your life that can still make you laugh uproariously and keep you always in a very good mood.

(C2) Very enjoyable comedies are different from extremely funny experiences because, even though they may keep you in a good mood, they do not make you laugh.

(C3) Somewhat enjoyable comedies consist of enjoyable experiences or events that were pleasant, but did not make you laugh or kept you in a good mood.

(TD) Things you need to do, such as going to the grocery store, calling a friend, or paying an overdue bill, to deal with practical matters that are necessary for daily living.

(TT) Thoughts about triumphs relate to events or experiences in which you felt victorious and proud of your achievement; you felt indestructible, invincible, and positively full of yourself, making you feel on top of the world.

(MP) Memories from the past that do not fit into the previous categories of thoughts or memories that are neither tragic nor comedic but that, nevertheless, represent simple memories of rather simple events or experiences in your life.

(DF) Dreams about the future consist of daydreams, fantasies, aspirations, and hopes for the future, such as what you would like to see happen in your life to make you feel happier and in a better mood.

3. Choosing the order of practice exercises: Now choose in which order you want to work on the homework practice exercises defined above. Below, rank-order which practice exercise you want to work on first by writing 1 for the rank-order, which practice exercise you want to work on second by writing 2 for the rank-order, and so on, until the last practice exercise is ranked 10.

Title of Practice Exercise	*Rank-order*
(T1) Extremely painful tragedies	________
(T2) Very painful tragedies	________
(T3) Somewhat painful tragedies	________
(C1) Extremely enjoyable comedies	________
(C2) Very enjoyable comedies	________
(C3) Somewhat enjoyable comedies	________
(TD) Things you need to do	________
(TT) Thoughts about triumphs	________
(MP) Memories from the past	________
(DF) Dreams about the future	________

Practice Exercise (T1). Extremely Painful Tragedies

Name______________________Sex______Date_______Time______

These tragedies are made up of extremely sad and painful experiences and events of great intensity to you that did not allow any escape or solution, such as great losses, terrible traumas, and major hurts and defeats. These experiences may have produced and provoked intense feelings of shame and guilt in you, and may have taught you to become aware of errors and mistakes in your life, influencing your mood very negatively.

Write in great detail about experiences and events in your life that fit into the definition given above. Write about these experiences even if you have not discussed them with anybody, for whatever reason.

____

____

____

____

____

Practice Exercise (T2). Very Painful Tragedies

Name_________________________Sex______Date_______Time___

This type of experiences or events is of lesser intensity than extremely painful experiences or events. You are not dealing with complete darkness here. There was a light at the end of the tunnel. The themes may be the same, that is, errors, painful experiences, humiliations, losses, defeats, etc. However, these experiences or events were of lesser importance to you than extremely painful tragedies, but, nonetheless, these tragedies did influence your mood negatively.

Write in great detail about experiences and events in your life that fit into the definition given above. Write about these experiences even if you have not discussed them with anybody, for whatever reason.

____

____

____

____

____

Practice Exercise (T3). Somewhat Painful Tragedies

Name_____________________Sex_______Date______Time______

These are experiences that, although of lesser importance to you than extremely painful and very painful ones, are still somewhat vivid in your mind, including minor losses, small errors, slights and humiliations of lower intensity than the two previous types of tragedies, having little if any effect on your mood.

Write in great detail about experiences and events in your life that fit into the definition given above. Write about these experiences even if you have not discussed them with anybody, for whatever reason.

____
____
____
____
____

Practice Exercise (C1). Extremely Enjoyable Comedies

Name______________________Sex______Date______Time______

These are very funny experiences and events in your life that can still make you laugh uproariously and keep you always in a good mood.

Write in great detail about experiences and events in your life that fit into the definition given above. Write about these experiences even if you have not discussed them with anybody, for whatever reason.

____
____
____
____

Practice Exercise (C2). Very Enjoyable Comedies

Name____________________Sex______Date________Time_____

These are funny experiences or events that are different from extremely enjoyable experiences because, even though they may keep you in a good mood, they do not make you laugh.

Write in great detail about experiences and events in your life that fit into the definition given above. Write about these experiences even if you have not discussed them with anybody, for whatever reason.

____
____
____
____
____

Practice Exercise (C3). Somewhat Enjoyable Comedies

Name____________________Sex_____Date_________Time_____

These comedies consist of experiences or events that were enjoyable and pleasant, but did not make you laugh or kept you in a good mood.

Write in great detail about experiences and events in your life that fit into the definition given above. Write about these experiences even if you have not discussed them with anybody, for whatever reason.

____
____
____
____
____

Practice Exercise (TD). Things You Need to Do

Name______________________Sex______Date______Time_____

These are thoughts about what you need to do, including chores and "to-do" list items, such as going to the grocery store, calling a friend, or paying an overdue bill, to deal with practical matters that are necessary for daily living.

Write in great detail about experiences and events in your life that fit into the definition given above. Write about these experiences even if you have not discussed them with anybody, for whatever reason.

____
____
____
____
____

Practice Exercise (TT). Thoughts About Triumphs

Name______________________Sex_______Date______Time______

Triumphs are events or experiences in which you felt victorious and proud of your achievement, when you felt indestructible, invincible, and positively full of yourself, making you feel on top of the world.

Write in great detail about experiences and events in your life that fit into the definition given above. Write about these experiences even if you have not discussed them with anybody, for whatever reason.

Practice Exercise (MP). Memories from the Past

Name______________________Sex______Date______Time_______

These memories from the past may not fit into of the previous categories of thoughts. They may be memories that are neither tragic nor comedic but that, nevertheless, represent simple memories of rather simple events or experiences in your life that do not affect your mood.

Write in great detail about experiences and events in your life that fit into the definition given above. Write about these experiences even if you have not discussed them with anybody, for whatever reason.

Practice Exercise (DF). Dreams About the Future

Name______________________Sex_______Date______Time______

This practice exercise consists of daydreams, fantasies, aspirations, and hopes for the future, about what you would like to see happen in your life to make you feel happier and keep you in a better mood.

Write in great detail about experiences and events in your life that fit into the definition given above. Write about these experiences even if you have not discussed them with anybody, for whatever reason.

____

____

____

____

____

Feedback Practice Exercise About Self-Awareness

Name_________________________Sex____Date______Time______

During this appointment time, it is important to write about what you think or feel about this practice exercises. Please rank the practice exercises of this practice exercises according to how much you liked them and how useful and helpful they were to you. Write 1 for the one you liked best and also for the one that was the most useful; these can be different practice exercises. Write 2 for the one you liked next and for the one that was the next most useful, and so on, until you reach the last practice exercises, which are ranked 10 for liking and 10 for usefulness to you.

Title of Practice Exercises		*Rank-orders Liking*	*Usefulness*
(T1)	Extremely painful tragedies	________	______
(T2)	Very painful tragedies	________	______
(T3)	Somewhat painful tragedies	________	______
(C1)	Extremely enjoyable comedies	________	______
(C2)	Very enjoyable comedies	________	______
(C3)	Somewhat enjoyable comedies	________	______
(TD)	Things you need to do	________	______
(TT)	Thoughts about triumphs	________	______
(MP)	Memories from the past	________	______
(DF)	Dreams about the future	________	______

Your feedback about this practice exercises is very important to us. Please write your reactions about it as directly and honestly as you can. Write as much and as long as you want. We need your honest opinion in order to improve this practice exercises. Do not hold back any negative reactions that you may have about it. How could we change it? How could we improve it?

____

____

____

____

____

Who Am I? Aspects of Identity Formation

This practice exercises aims at identifying which aspects of your identity are more important to you than other aspects.

Practice Exercise 1. Aspects of Identity Formation

Name__________________________Sex____________Date__________

We are all the products of many identities acquired since and before birth. The purpose of this practice exercise is to expand on various aspects of these many identities.

1. Below you will find many aspects of identity. For each aspect explain what it is and what it means to you is. Define each aspect and give two examples of how that identity is applied either in your life experience or in general.

Aspects of Identity and Definitions	*Examples*
a. Gender ______________	Example 1 ______________
______________	______________
______________	Example 2 ______________
______________	______________
b. Sexual orientation/preference	Example 1 ______________
______________	______________
______________	Example 2 ______________
______________	______________
c. Body: no examples necessary; just supply this information:	Shape______ Size_____ Height____ Weight ______________
______________	
______________	Any other body characteristics?
______________	______________
d. Geographical (where you were born) ______________	Example 1 ______________
	______________
______________	Example 2 ______________
______________	______________
e. Geographical (where you have lived the longest)	Example 1 ______________
	______________
______________	Example 2 ______________
______________	______________
f. Geographical (where your heart is)	Example 1 ______________
______________	______________
______________	Example 2 ______________
______________	______________
g. Son/daughter	Example 1 ______________
______________	______________
______________	Example 2 ______________
______________	______________
h. Brother/sister	Example 1 ______________
______________	______________
______________	Example 2 ______________
______________	______________

i. Partner ______________________ Example 1 ______________________
______________________ Example 2 ______________________

j. Parent ______________________ Example 1 ______________________
______________________ Example 2 ______________________

k. Caregiver ______________________ Example 1 ______________________
______________________ Example 2 ______________________

l. Homemaker ______________________ Example 1 ______________________
______________________ Example 2 ______________________

m. Provider ______________________ Example 1 ______________________
______________________ Example 2 ______________________

n. Grandparent ______________________ Example 1 ______________________
______________________ Example 2 ______________________

o. Ethnic/cultural ______________________ Example 1 ______________________
______________________ Example 2 ______________________

p. Religion/spirituality ______________________ Example 1 ______________________
______________________ Example 2 ______________________

q. Educational ______________________ Example 1 ______________________
______________________ Example 2 ______________________

r. Occupational/work/job ____________ ____________ ____________	Example 1 ____________ ____________ Example 2 ____________ ____________
s. Political affiliation or ideology ____________ ____________ ____________	Example 1 ____________ ____________ Example 2 ____________ ____________
t. Leisure time activities ____________ ____________ ____________	Example 1 ____________ ____________ Example 2 ____________ ____________
u. Sports fan ____________ ____________ ____________	Example 1 ____________ ____________ Example 2 ____________ ____________
v. Sports activities ____________ ____________ ____________	Example 1 ____________ ____________ Example 2 ____________ ____________
w. Military experience and identity ____________ ____________ ____________	Example 1 ____________ ____________ Example 2 ____________ ____________
x. Membership in fraternal/social or similar organizations (Elks, Rotary, Masons, etc.) ____________	Example 1 ____________ ____________ Example 2 ____________ ____________
y. Any other identity not mentioned above that is important to you. Write what it is ____________	Example 1 ____________ ____________ Example 2 ____________ ____________
z. Any other identity not mentioned above that is important to you. Write what it is. ____________	Example 1 ____________ ____________ Example 2 ____________ ____________

2. Now that you have defined various aspects of your identity, rank them according to how much each aspect is important to you. Rank as No. 1 the most important aspect, rank as No. 2 the next most important aspect, and so on, giving a rank-order to each aspect; mark as N/A the aspects that do not apply to you at all.

Aspects of Identity	*Rank-order*
a. Gender	________
b. Sexual orientation/preference	________
c. Body	________
d. Geographical (where you were born)	________
e. Geographical (where you have lived the longest)	________
f. Geographical (where your heart is)	________
g. Son/daughter	________
h. Brother/sister	________
i. Partner	________
j. Parent	________
k. Caregiver	________
l. Homemaker	________
m. Provider	________
n. Grandparent	________
o. Ethnic/cultural	________
p. Religion/spirituality	________
q. Educational	________
r. Occupational/work/job	________
s. Political affiliation or ideology	________
t. Leisure time activities	________
u. Sports fan	________
v. Sports activities	________
w. Military	________
x. Fraternal organizations	________
y. Any other identity not mentioned above that is important to you: write what it is	________
z. Any other identity not mentioned above that is important to you; write what it is	________

Homework: During the next week, think about how you have rank-ordered your many identities and whether your need to change the rank-order you have completed. Feel free to make whatever changes you want to make to the rank-order.

Standard Practice Exercise No.____

Aspect of Identity____

Name_______________________________Sex_________Date_________

The purpose of this and future practice exercises is to expand on aspects of your identity that are most important to you. Above write the aspect of your identity that you have ranked as No.____

1. How does this aspect apply to you? Please explain in detail.

____
____
____
____
____

2. How often do you identify yourself in this way?

   a. Practically every day _____
   b. Once a week _____
   c. A couple of times a month _____
   d. Once a month _____
   e. Once every 6 months _____
   f. Once a year _____
   g. Once every few years _____

3. Please explain further:

____
____
____
____
____

4. How did this aspect of your identity come about? Do you remember when you started to identify yourself in this way? Check which answer best fits this aspect of your identity:

   a. When I was a child (younger than 5 years of age) ________
   b. When I was in elementary school ________
   c. When I was in middle school ________
   d. When I was in high school ________
   e. After high school ________
   f. Any other time ________

5. Please explain further:

6. Was this aspect of your identity acceptable or unacceptable? Why? Please explain.

7. Give three specific examples of how this aspect affects you.

Example 1:

Example 2:

Example 3:

Homework: The purpose of this homework is to help you achieve greater control over the aspect of your identity completed in this practice exercise. Next week, plan to focus on this aspect at preset times (for instance, at 8 a.m., 12 noon, 4 or 7 p.m.) on at least 3 days (Monday, Wednesday, and Friday, or Tuesday, Thursday, and Saturday). During this focus time, answer in writing the following questions:

a. How much does this aspect of identity mean to you?
b. Why does it mean so much to you?
c. What would you do if you did not have it?
d. Do you want to keep it or abandon it?
e. Why do you want to keep it or abandon it?

Time 1 (write the time you started__________)

a. ____
____
____

b. ____
____
____

c. ____
____
____

d. ____
____
____

e. ____
____
____

Time 2 (write the time you started__________)

a. ____
____
____

b. ____
____
____

c. ____
____
____

d. ____
____
____

e. ______________________________
____
____

Time 3 (write the time you started__________)

a. ______________________________
____
____

b. ______________________________
____
____

c. ______________________________
____
____

d. ______________________________
____
____

e. ______________________________
____
____

Check which of the following indicates how you feel about this practice exercise:

a.	Completely useless	_______	d.	Somewhat useful	_______
b.	Somewhat useless	_______	e.	Extremely useful	_______
c.	So-so	_______			

Explain in greater detail how you feel about this practice exercise and what you got out of it.

____
____
____
____
____

Note: Use the same format of this practice exercise for all future practice exercises that cover aspects of your identity according to the rank-order given in the first practice exercise.

Concluding Follow-Up Form

Name______________________________Sex______Date______

The purpose of this form is to review whether this practice exercises was helpful to you or not.

1. Check the answer that best fits how you feel about this practice exercises:

   a. I did not like working on this practice exercises at all. I wish I never saw it. _______
   b. I did not like this practice exercises at all, but I am glad I got to work on it. _______
   c. I am delighted I got a chance to work on this practice exercises. _______
   d. I am not only delighted about working on this practice exercises, but I wish all people had a chance to work on it. _______

2. How helpful was it to work on this practice exercises? Check the answer that applies to you:

   a. Not helpful at all _______
   b. Somewhat helpful _______
   c. Helpful _______
   d. Very helpful _______

3. Which practice exercise did you like best? Rank as No. 1 the one that you liked best, rank as No. 2 the one you liked next best, and so on; mark as N/A the ones you did not like at all or did not apply to you.

Aspects of Identities	*Rank-order*
a. Gender	________
b. Sexual orientation/preference	________
c. Body	________
d. Geographical (where you were born)	________
e. Geographical (where you have lived the longest)	________
f. Geographical (where your heart is)	________
g. Son/daughter	________
h. Brother/sister	________
i. Partner	________
j. Parent	________
k. Caregiver	________
l. Homemaker	________
m. Provider	________
n. Grandparent	________
o. Ethnic/cultural	________
p. Religion/spirituality	________
q. Educational	________

r. Occupational/work/job ________
s. Political affiliation or ideology ________
t. Leisure time activities ________
u. Sports fan ________
v. Sports activities ________
w. Military ________
x. Fraternal organizations ________
y. Any other identity not mentioned above that is important to you; write what it is ________
z. Any other identity not mentioned above that is important to you; write what it is ________

4. Please explain why you rank-ordered aspects of your identity the way you did.

____
____
____
____
____

5. Sometimes what we like most is not necessarily the most helpful. Which practice exercise was the most helpful to you? Rank the practice exercises according to their helpfulness to you. Rank as No. 1 the most helpful, rank as No. 2 the next most helpful, and so on, until the least helpful practice exercise; mark as N/A the practice exercises that did not apply to you.

Aspects of Your Identity *Rank-order*

a. Gender ________
b. Sexual orientation/preference ________
c. Body ________
d. Geographical (where you were born) ________
e. Geographical (where you have lived the longest) ________
f. Geographical (where your heart is) ________
g. Son/daughter ________
h. Brother/sister ________
i. Partner ________
j. Parent ________
k. Caregiver ________
l. Homemaker ________
m. Provider ________
n. Grandparent ________
o. Ethnic/cultural ________
p. Religion/spirituality ________
q. Educational ________
r. Occupational/work/job ________

s. Political affiliation or ideology ________
t. Leisure time activities ________
u. Sports fan ________
v. Sports activities ________
w. Military ________
x. Fraternal organizations ________
y. Any other identity not mentioned above that is important to you; write what it is ________
z. Any other identity not mentioned above that is important to you; write what it is ________

6. Explain why you rank-ordered these behaviors the way you did.

____
____
____
____
____

7. Feel free to write any comments that might improve this practice exercises.

____
____
____
____
____

Speak Up for Yourself!

The purpose of this practice exercises is to help you learn how to speak up for yourself instead of speaking down to yourself or to others. To communicate helpfully, we need to become more aware of the errors (and horrors!) of hurtful, abusive communication by increasing our sensitivity to these errors and leaving them behind. When we become fully aware of how painful and hurtful these errors are, we will be better able to give them up. These errors should be replaced by the secrets of successful, helpful communication, by being proactive rather than behaving reactively.

To communicate better, we need to become aware of all the hurts we have accumulated in our lives and discuss them, reciprocally, with those we love and who love us. Discussing hurts is another skill that can facilitate successful communication and emotional intimacy. Couples or families may meet at home at a prearranged, preset times to exchange and discuss their practice exercises. If we do not discuss hurts, there cannot be full discussing of joys. Once they become aware of these hurts and are able to discuss them, partners can learn to communicate in helpful ways and give up hurtful, defensive patterns.

Helpful and successful communication is based on the use of three small core words that are critical to speaking up for oneself: "I," "It," and "We."

"I" Statements

Many people are trained to avoid speaking up for themselves. As a result, they grow up without any awareness of their own selves and with an inadequate, incomplete sense of self-importance. If we do not speak up for ourselves, who will? If not now, when?

"It" Statements

When it is necessary to address a negative behavior (after use of the "You" pronoun is given up), we need to speak about the noxious or unpleasant behavior ("It") rather than about the person. We must learn to speak in a nonjudgmental, impersonal (rather than personal) manner. This is a much more difficult undertaking. It requires that one learn to discriminate between what we do (performance) and what we are (person). Sometimes even perfectly wonderful people make errors of omission and commission that impact others unpleasantly or even hurtfully. We need to learn to speak about this (mis)behavior in a way that enhances both ourselves and the other. Rather than debasing self and other, using "It" statements makes the process less threatening and more constructive.

We need to address the behavior that upsets us in ways that eliminate blame, judgment, and punishment. "I feel very bad about forgetting to check the answering machine before attacking you. I should have known better. You are very good about letting me know when you are late. From now on I will check the answering machine before I jump the gun. Please forgive me." Exercise No. 3 deals with this issue.

"We" Statements

If you live with others, whatever affects one person will affect everybody else who lives under the same roof. If this relationship is important, we learn to assert the importance of the relationship by speaking about "Us" rather than "Them," and "We" rather than "You." For instance, "I thought we agreed together that we would always check our answering machines before calling. Isn't that right?" By jumping from the specific behavior itself to the overall issues of whether agreements should be honored, and whether further consideration of an agreement is in order, puts the whole situation in a different perspective. Hence, the unpleasant or obnoxious behavior is put within the greater context of honoring agreements and possibly renegotiating agreements, rather that just being on time.

Practice Exercise 1. Practicing "I" Statements

Name______________________Sex______Date_______Time_____

The purpose of this practice exercise is to learn to speak up for yourself. Learning to speak up for oneself begins with speaking about how one feels, thinks, and acts. Many people think that using the personal pronoun "I" indicates selfishness. Nothing could be further from the truth. Speaking and standing up for one self shows that we are admitting and acknowledging personal responsibility rather than blaming the other (partner, mate, parent, friend). Taking personal responsibility and speaking for oneself is shown by the pronoun "I" and using "I" statements. The sentence completions in the following three practice exercises show how to speak up for oneself rather than speaking about another person. It is easier to speak about the shortcomings of others than about one's shortcomings.

Complete the following sentences ten times. Complete them with different persons and/or objects.

a. "I like":

1. I ______________________________
2. I ______________________________
3. I ______________________________
4. I ______________________________
5. I ______________________________
6. I ______________________________
7. I ______________________________
8. I ______________________________
9. I like ______________________________
10. I like ______________________________

B. "I want":

1. I want______________________________
2. I want______________________________
3. I want______________________________
4. I want______________________________
5. I want______________________________
6. I want______________________________
7. I want______________________________
8. I want______________________________
9. I want______________________________
10. I want______________________________

C. "I need":

1. I need______________________________
2. I ______________________________
3. I ______________________________
4. I ______________________________
5. I ______________________________

6. I ______________________________
7. I ______________________________
8. I need______________________________
9. I need______________________________
10. I need______________________________

D. "I am":
1. I am ______________________________
2. I am ______________________________
3. I am ______________________________
4. I am ______________________________
5. I am ______________________________
6. I am ______________________________
7. I am ______________________________
8. I am ______________________________
9. I am ______________________________
10. I am ______________________________

Homework: During the next week, become aware of how you feel when you speak about yourself and when you speak about another. Write down in great detail whatever you feel and experience during this week.

Practice Exercise 2. Practicing Feelings Statements

Name______________________Sex_______Date_______Time_____

The purpose of this practice exercise is to become aware of one's feelings and especially hurts that have been kept hidden from yourself and from those you love and who love you.

Complete the following sentence stems in writing. Repeat each stem ten times with different completions for each time.

Note: It may take more than 1 day to complete all these stems. Therefore, it is okay to complete this practice exercise over a period of time.

I hurt when …	I fear …
1. ______________	1. ______________
2. ______________	2. ______________
3. ______________	3. ______________
4. ______________	4. ______________
5. ______________	5. ______________
6. ______________	6. ______________
7. ______________	7. ______________
8. ______________	8. ______________
9. ______________	9. ______________
10. ______________	10. ______________

I am disappointed …
1. ______________
2. ______________
3. ______________
4. ______________
5. ______________
6. ______________
7. ______________
8. ______________
9. ______________
10. ______________

I feel bad when …
1. ______________
2. ______________
3. ______________
4. ______________
5. ______________
6. ______________
7. ______________
8. ______________
9. ______________
10. ______________

I feel sad when …
1. ______________
2. ______________
3. ______________
4. ______________
5. ______________
6. ______________
7. ______________
8. ______________
9. ______________
10. ______________

I feel frustrated when …
1. ______________
2. ______________
3. ______________
4. ______________
5. ______________
6. ______________
7. ______________
8. ______________
9. ______________
10. ______________

I feel scared when …
1. ______________
2. ______________
3. ______________
4. ______________
5. ______________
6. ______________
7. ______________
8. ______________
9. ______________
10. ______________

I feel angry when …
1. ______________
2. ______________
3. ______________
4. ______________
5. ______________
6. ______________
7. ______________
8. ______________
9. ______________
10. ______________

I feel disappointed when …
1. ______________
2. ______________
3. ______________
4. ______________
5. ______________
6. ______________
7. ______________
8. ______________
9. ______________
10. ______________

Homework: For four consecutive days, write for 15–20 minute about all the hurts that you have experienced in your life. Make appointments with yourself to write at preset, predetermined times (e.g., 8 a.m., 1 p.m., and 7 p.m.). If you have an appointment book, write down the times you will use to complete this homework practice exercise. Include also hurts that you have not discussed with anyone until now. If possible discuss these hurts with your partner or family members, provided they have completed the same lessons and are willing to discuss them with you.

After you have finished writing about your hurts, practice expressing them in a positive way with those you love and who love you. Do not allow anyone to put down your hurts. You hurts are yours and they are important. If anyone puts your feelings down, they are putting you down. Do not allow it under any conditions. Love means accepting one's feelings. Your feelings are very important because they are yours, and you are very important. If we do not assert our importance through our feelings, no one is going to assert it for us.

Practice Exercise 3. Discussing Hurts

Name________________________Sex______Date_______Time_____

The purpose of this practice exercise is to learn to discuss your hurts with those who discuss their hurts with you. Discuss your hurts only with those who discuss theirs with you. This is one way to find out whether we love them and whether they love us. Even though this may be a brief practice exercise, it is an important one.

Instructions: Complete the following sentences ten times:

I hurt when ...

1. ______________
2. ______________
3. ______________
4. ______________
5. ______________
6. ______________
7. ______________
8. ______________
9. ______________
10. ______________

It hurts me when ...

1. ______________
2. ______________
3. ______________
4. ______________
5. ______________
6. ______________
7. ______________
8. ______________
9. ______________
10. ______________

It is very hurtful for me to ...

1. ______________
2. ______________
3. ______________
4. ______________
5. ______________
6. ______________
7. ______________
8. ______________
9. ______________
10. ______________

Homework: During the next week, make sure to complete all the sentences that you have not yet completed.

Practice Exercise 4. Practicing "It" Statements

Name________________________Sex______Date_______Time_____

The purpose of this practice exercise is for you to learn to talk about a person's (mis)behavior in an impersonal rather than personal fashion. Instead of speaking about the person, speak about the behavior, as in: "I cannot accept cigarette smoke because smoking is bad for everybody. I know smoking is extremely dangerous and I am extremely uncomfortable about it. I would appreciate it if you smoked outside the home. I do not appreciate being the victim of second-hand smoke."

Think of at least ten offending behaviors that affect you and write about these behaviors using the personal pronoun "I." Write how the offending behavior makes you feel. Remember that "It" is the offending behavior.

Hint: Use "I appreciate" and "I do not appreciate" to begin your sentences. Write down what you want to say before saying it. Discuss these statements with your partner or family member after they have completed the same practice exercise.

Practice Exercise 5. Practicing "We" Statements

Name________________________Sex______Date_______Time_____

The purpose of this practice exercise is to learn to speak about the relationship ("We") rather than the person or personality of another one ("You").

1. Write down at least ten issues or problem situations between you and your partner (or intimate other) in which you both were equally involved. For instance: "We will need to talk about the checkbook because we need to record exactly what we spend in order to keep track of whether we are within our budget or not." Write down these statements before saying them. After each partner has written down these statements, discuss them with each other and talk about them.
2. Write about the following statements by giving at least two examples of how they apply to you and your relationship. Discuss your examples with your partner, family members, or friend. Make sure you write down what everybody says during these discussions.

"One of us cannot win at the expense of the other."

Example 1:

Example 2:

"We both win, or if one of us loses we both lose."

Example 1:

Example 2:

"I cannot win at your expense and neither can you."

Example 1:

Example 2:

"We either hang together or we hang."

Example 1:

Example 2:

"If we both win, we will go forward in our relationship."

Example 1:

Example 2:

"If we both lose, we will stay put or go back, but we will not go forward in our relationship."

Example 1:

Example 2:

Homework: If you have trouble standing up for yourself, you may need personal, face-to-face help from a professional. Remember, that it takes a lot of strength to ask for help. Very weak people are unable to ask for it. Asking for help is another way of standing up for oneself.

Section 4
Relational Self-Help Practice Exercises for Lifelong Learning of Couples and Families

Couples

Premarital Preparation

We prepare for life through education. We even prepare for a driving license through education. Yet we often assume that being married or entering a relationship will take place naturally, without preparation. Marriage is one of the most responsible roles of our lives, but getting married and becoming a partner is expected to happen without any effort on our part. The purpose of this practice exercises is to help you learn more about why you want to get married or become a couple at this time. It is hoped that identifying these reasons will allow you to have a better relationship.

Practice Exercise 1. Reason for Marriage (or Living Together)

Name________________________________Sex_____Date______

The purpose of this practice exercise is to explore the reasons why you want to get married or live together now. Question No. 1 should be completed by each partner independently of the other. It would be extremely self-defeating if the couple worked together on answering this question. After you have completed answering it, get together with your partner to discuss how each of you has answered it.

L. L'Abate, *Sourcebook of Interactive Practice Exercises in Mental Health*, DOI 10.1007/978-1-4419-1354-8_14,

1. Why do you want to get married? Rank-order the goals listed below according to your reasons for getting married. Rank as No. 1 the most important reason for marrying your partner now, rank as No. 2 the second most important reason, and so on; mark as N/A (not applicable) the reasons tat may not apply to you at all. Try to rank-order at least ten reasons. Make an appointment with your partner at least 24 h in advance to compare, contrast, and spend your answers. Make sure to keep notes of your meeting.

Reasons	*Rank-orders*		
	Yours	*Partner's*	*Combined*
a. I want to make my partner happy	______	______	______
b. I want to make myself happy	______	______	______
c. I cannot think of life without my partner	______	______	______
d. I love my partner and I cannot think of spending my life with anybody else	______	______	______
e. He or she is the most wonderful person in the world	______	______	______
f. Isn't "being in love" a good reason?	______	______	______
g. I love having sex with my partner	______	______	______
h. I need the love I get from my partner	______	______	______
i. I want to discuss the rest of my life with my partner	______	______	______
j. I love my partner for the security that this relationship gives me	______	______	______
k. To escape painful family relationships	______	______	______
l. This seems the right time	______	______	______
m. We have to marry because we are expecting a child	______	______	______
n. Our families arranged it	______	______	______
o. To fulfill a promise	______	______	______
p. All our friends are getting married	______	______	______
q. My biological clock is ticking and I need to have a child	______	______	______
r. My religion requires marriage for sex	______	______	______
s. My father caught us having sex and now he wants us to get married	______	______	______
t. I caught a sexually transmitted disease from my partner and it would be hard to find other partners	______	______	______
u. My horoscope said that this time is right	______	______	______

Reasons	*Rank-orders* *Yours*	*Partner's*	*Combined*
v. Our children wanted us to get married	________	________	________
w. My partner is terminally ill and wants to provide for me after death	________	________	________
x. My parents will disown me if I do not provide them with a legal grandchild	________	________	________
y. I want to marry an American citizen to become an American myself	________	________	________
z. Write your own reason for marrying: (________________)	________	________	________

2. Now that you have finished with the rank-order, explain why you ranked the reasons for marrying the way you did.

____
____
____
____
____

3. Compare and contrast your rank-order with the rank-order of your partner. Add both rank-orders in the middle column and give your combined rankings to whoever is helping you with this practice exercises.

Homework: During the coming week, think about the rank-order you have completed, the rank-order completed by your partner, and whether the combined rank-order obtained from you both represents a useful way to proceed with this practice exercises. If you have any misgivings about your and your partner's rank-orders, or your combined rank-order, discuss them with your partner and with the professional who is helping you with this practice exercises.

Standard Practice Exercise for Marital Preparation

Practice Exercise No.______Reason________________________

Name______________________________Sex__________Date______

The purpose of this practice exercise is to understand in greater detail how the reason listed above is linked to your wanting to get married now.

1. When did you become aware of this reason? Check which age applies:

a.	In preschool	______	d.	In high school	______
b.	In elementary school	______	e.	In college	______
c.	In middle school	______	f.	In graduate school	______

2. How did you become aware of this reason? Tell as much as you possibly can:

____
____
____
____
____

3. How has this reason helped you in the present?

____
____
____
____
____

4. How much do you want this reason to help you in the future?

____
____
____
____
____

5. Now that you have completed this practice exercise, check which of these answers indicates how you felt about it. There is also space for you to explain further, if you want to:

   a. I did not like it at all. I want to quit this practice exercises. ______
   b. I did not like it very much, but I want to go on with this practice exercises. ______
   c. I liked it and I want to go on with this practice exercises. ______
   d. I liked it a lot and I wish I had something like this practice exercises years ago. ______
   e. I liked it so much that I wish all couples planning to get married could get a practice exercises like this to work on before they get married. ______

6. Discuss your answers with whoever has given you this practice exercises.

Homework: During the next few days, think of how you could either give up this reason if it is negative for you and your partner, or change it to have a positive effect on you and your partner. Write down what you want to do about this reason.

____
____
____
____
____

Concluding Follow-Up Form for Marital Preparation

Name______________________________ Sex__________ Date_______

The purpose of this form is to review whether this practice exercises was helpful to you.

1. Please select the answer that fits how you feel about this practice exercises:

   a. I did not like working on this practice exercises at all. I wish I never saw it. _________
   b. I did not like this practice exercises at all, but I am glad I got to work on it. _________
   c. I am delighted I got a chance to work on this practice exercises. _________
   d. I am not only delighted about this practice exercises, but I wish all premarital couples had a chance to work on it. _________

2. How helpful was it to work on this practice exercises? Please check the answer that applies to you:

   a. Not helpful at all _____ c. Helpful _____
   b. Somewhat helpful _____ d. Very helpful _____

3. Which practice exercise did you like best? Rank as No. 1 the one that you liked best, rank as No. 2 the one you liked next best, and so on; mark as N/A the ones you did not like at all or did not apply to you.

Reasons	*Rank-orders*		
	Yours	*Partner's*	*Subtracted*
a. I want to make my partner happy	________	________	________
b. I want to make myself happy	________	________	________
c. I cannot think of life without my partner	________	________	________
d. I love my partner and I cannot think of spending my life with anybody else	________	________	________

Reasons	*Rank-orders* *Yours*	*Partner's*	*Subtracted*
e. He or she is the most wonderful person in the world	________	________	________
f. Isn't "being in love" a good reason?	________	________	________
g. I love having sex with my partner	________	________	________
h. I need the love I get from my partner	________	________	________
i. I want to discuss the rest of my life with my partner	________	________	________
j. For the security that this relationship gives me	________	________	________
k. To escape painful family relationships	________	________	________
l. This seems the right time	________	________	________
m. We have to marry because we are expecting a child	________	________	________
n. Our families arranged it	________	________	________
o. To fulfill a promise	________	________	________
p. All our friends are getting married	________	________	________
q. My biological clock is ticking and I need to have a child	________	________	________
r. My religion requires marriage for sex	________	________	________
s. My father caught us having sex and now he wants us to get married	________	________	________
t. I caught a sexually transmitted disease from my partner and it would be hard to find other partners	________	________	________
u. My horoscope said that this time is right	________	________	________
v. Our children wanted us to get married	________	________	________
w. My partner is terminally ill and wants to provide for me after death	________	________	________
x. My parents will disown me if I do not provide them with a legal grandchild	________	________	________
y. I want to marry an American citizen to become an American myself	________	________	________
z. Write your own reason for wanting to marry now rather than later: (______________________________)	________	________	________
Total discrepancy score	________	________	________

4. Write why you ranked the practice exercises the way you did.

___

___

___

___

___

5. After completing item 4, discuss your rank-orders with your partner and write them in the column next to your rank-orders. Discuss similarities and differences in your rank-orders. In this case, however, instead of adding your scores, you will need to subtract your rank-order from the rank-orders of your partner, even if a minus number results. Add all these scores at the bottom of the table and discuss with each other the meaning of this total discrepancy score. You can use differences between yourselves to enhance the relationship or you can use the same differences to sabotage it. The choice is yours.

6. Please write any comments that might improve this practice exercises.

___

___

___

___

___

Sexual Motivation

The purpose of this practice exercises is to help you understand your motivations about sex and sexuality and possibly improve your sexual relationship with your partner, either in marriage or in a committed couple relationship.

Answer each practice exercise individually and get together with your partner at preset, predetermined times (at least 24 h ahead) to discuss your completed practice exercises for no longer than 1 h. If you get upset during this time, end the discussion and make another appointment for another time at least 24 h ahead.

Practice Exercise 1. Defining Sexual Motives

Name________________________Sex_______Date________

The purpose of this practice exercise is to help you define more clearly your motivation for sex and sexuality. Most couples need to know and discuss this motivation about their relationships. Make sure that you understand and discuss with each other the meaning of each item that makes up this practice exercise.

1. Below are listed various sexual motives that cover a range of possibilities. If you have a motive not found in this list, add it at the end (there is room for additional features). Define each motive, and give two examples of how that motive is shown concretely in your relationship. Feel free to use a dictionary; it may help you in the process of defining these motives.

Motives and Definitions	*Examples*
a. Affirmation ________	Example 1 ________
________	________
________	Example 2 ________
________	________
b. Intimacy ________	Example 1 ________
________	________
________	Example 2 ________
________	________
c. Pleasure ________	Example 1 ________
________	________
________	Example 2 ________
________	________
d. Peer influence ________	Example 1 ________
________	________
________	Example 2 ________
________	________
e. Insecurity ________	Example 1 ________
________	________
________	Example 2 ________
________	________
f. Coping ________	Example 1 ________
________	________
________	Example 2 ________
________	________
g. Partner's power ________	Example 1 ________
________	________
________	Example 2 ________
________	________
h. Expression of worth ________	Example 1 ________
________	________
________	Example 2 ________
________	________

i. Relief from stress ______________ Example 1 ______________
______________ ______________
______________ Example 2 ______________
______________ ______________

j. Procreation ______________ Example 1 ______________
______________ ______________
______________ Example 2 ______________
______________ ______________

k. Enhance power ______________ Example 1 ______________
______________ ______________
______________ Example 2 ______________
______________ ______________

l. To feel valued ______________ Example 1 ______________
______________ ______________
______________ Example 2 ______________
______________ ______________

m. Nurturance ______________ Example 1 ______________
______________ ______________
______________ Example 2 ______________
______________ ______________

n. Lust ______________ Example 1 ______________
______________ ______________
______________ Example 2 ______________
______________ ______________

o. To say you have done it ______________ Example 1 ______________
______________ ______________
______________ Example 2 ______________
______________ ______________

p. To fit in better ______________ Example 1 ______________
______________ ______________
______________ Example 2 ______________
______________ ______________

q. To make partner love you more ______________ Example 1 ______________
______________ ______________
______________ Example 2 ______________
______________ ______________

r. Short-term avoidance of emotions ______ Example 1 ______
______ Example 2 ______
______

s. To brag about it ______ Example 1 ______
______ Example 2 ______
______

t. Curiosity ______ Example 1 ______
______ Example 2 ______
______

u. A motive not listed above (specify) Example 1 ______
______ Example 2 ______
______

v. A motive not listed above (specify) Example 1 ______
______ Example 2 ______
______

w. A motive not listed above (specify) Example 1 ______
______ Example 2 ______
______

2. Now that you have defined the meaning of each motive, you need to rank-order them according to how important they are to you in this relationship under the column "Yours." Rank as No. 1 the motive that is most important to you, rank as No. 2 the motive that is next in importance, and so on; mark as N/A the motives that may not be important to you at all or do not apply to this relationship.

Motive	*Rank-orders* *Yours*	*Partner's*	*Joint*
a. Affirmation	______	______	______
b. Intimacy	______	______	______
c. Pleasure	______	______	______
d. Peer influence	______	______	______
e. Insecurity	______	______	______
f. Coping	______	______	______

Motive	*Rank-orders* *Yours*	*Partner's*	*Joint*
g. Partner's power	________	________	________
h. Expression of worth	________	________	________
i. Relief from stress	________	________	________
j. Procreation	________	________	________
k. Enhance power	________	________	________
l. To feel valued	________	________	________
m. Nurturance	________	________	________
n. Lust	________	________	________
o. To say you have done	________	________	________
p. To fit in better	________	________	________
q. To make partner love you more	________	________	________
r. Short-term avoidance of emotions	________	________	________
s. To brag about it	________	________	________
t. Curiosity	________	________	________
u. A motive not listed above	________	________	________
v. A motive not listed above	________	________	________
w. A motive not listed above	________	________	________

3. Why did you rank-order these motives the way you did?

____

____

____

____

____

Homework: During the coming week, make an appointment with your partner and go over your definitions and your rank-orders. Record your partner's rank-orders in the appropriate column and add both to achieve a joint rank-order. Take notes of your discussion while you are discussing (comparing and contrasting) your answers. Give your completed practice exercises and your notes to the professional who is assisting you with this practice exercises. If you are completing these practice exercises on your own, without professional help, make sure to keep your notes for future reference.

Whatever joint rank-order you agree on will determine the order of future practice exercises. The next practice exercise should be given the title of the motive that has been rated jointly as No. 1. After that practice exercise, the other practice exercises should follow the joint rank-order given above.

Standard Practice Exercise for Sexual Motivation

Practice Exercise No.____Title:________________________________

Name____________________________Sex__________Date__________

The purpose of this practice exercise is to understand more about the sexual motive listed in the title:

1. How did this motive start? Please explain in detail.

____
____
____
____
____

2. How often does this sexual motive take place? Check which answer applies to you:

a.	Practically every day	_____	e.	Once every 6 months	_____
b.	Once a week	_____	f.	Once a year	_____
c.	A couple of times a month	_____	g.	Once every few years	_____
d.	Once a month	_____			

3. Please explain further:

____
____
____
____
____

4. How did this sexual motive come about? Do you remember how it started? Check which answer fits best:

a. As we met for the first time ______
b. During courtship or while dating ______
c. Before marriage or before we started living together ______
d. During the honeymoon or as we were moving in together ______
e. Right after the honeymoon or right after we moved in together ______
f. A few months after the marriage or after we moved in together ______
g. 1 year after the marriage or when we moved in together ______
h. Years after marriage or when we moved in together ______

5. Please explain further:

6. What does this sexual motive get you? Please explain:

7. Give three specific examples of how this sexual motive might be helpful to you.

   Example 1:

   Example 2:

   Example 3:

8. Give three specific examples of how this sexual motive might be hurtful to you.

   Example 1:

   Example 2:

   Example 3:

9. Give three specific examples of how this sexual motive might be helpful to those you love and who love you.

   Example 1:

   Example 2:

Example 3:

10. Give three specific examples of how this sexual motive might be hurtful to those you love and who love you.

Example 1:

Example 2:

Example 3:

Homework: Next week, plan to think about this motive, whether it belongs to you or not, or remind your partner to think about it if it belongs to him or her. Make sure this thinking is repeated at preset times (for instance, at 8 a.m., 12 noon, 4 or 7 p.m.), at least three times. Write down what happened in detail.

In case you wonder why this motive should be thought about, keep in mind that if you or your partner think about it, whoever thinks about it will acquire the power to end it, if you want to.

For each time you think about this motive, make sure to answer in writing the following four questions:

a. How did your thinking about this motive start?

b. What followed?
c. How did it end?
d. What did this thinking get you or your partner?

Time 1 (write the time you started__________)

a. ______________________________
____
____

b. ______________________________
____
____

c. ______________________________
____
____

d. ______________________________
____
____

Time 2 (write the time you started__________)

a. ______________________________
____
____

b. ______________________________
____
____

c. ______________________________
____
____

d. ______________________________
____
____

Time 3 (write the time you started__________)

a. ______________________________
____
____

b. ______________________________
____
____

c. ______________________________
____
____

d. ____

____

____

Check which of the following shows what you got out of this practice exercise:

a. Completely useless _____
b. Somewhat useless _____
c. So-so _____
d. Somewhat useful _____
e. Extremely useful _____

Write down how you feel about this homework practice exercise and what you got out of it.

____

____

____

____

____

Final Follow-Up Form for Sexual Motivation

Name__________________________Sex____________Date________

The purpose of this form is to review whether the practice exercises in this practice exercises were helpful to you.

1. Which answer best fits how you feel about this practice exercises?

   a. I did not like working on this practice exercises at all. I wish I never saw it. _________
   b. I did not like this practice exercises, but I am glad I got to work on. _________
   c. I am happy I got a chance to work on it. _________
   d. I am not only delighted about this practice exercises, but I wish all partners could discuss their sexual motivation. _________

2. How helpful was it to work on this practice exercises? Please check the answer that applies to you:

   a. Not helpful at all _____
   b. Somewhat helpful _____
   c. Helpful _____
   d. Very helpful _____

3. Which practice exercise did you like best that was the most helpful to you? Rank as No. 1 the one that you liked best, rank as No. 2 the one you liked next best, and so on; mark as N/A the ones you did not like at all or did not apply to you.

Motives	*Rank-orders* *Yours*	*Partner's*	*Joint*
a. Affirmation	________	________	________
b. Intimacy	________	________	________
c. Pleasure	________	________	________
d. Peer influence	________	________	________
e. Insecurity	________	________	________
f. Coping	________	________	________
g. Partner's power	________	________	________
h. Expression of worth	________	________	________
i. Relief from stress	________	________	________
j. Procreation	________	________	________
k. Enhance power	________	________	________
l. To feel valued	________	________	________
m. Nurturance	________	________	________
n. Lust	________	________	________
o. To say you have done it	________	________	________
p. To fit in better	________	________	________
q. To make partner love you more	________	________	________
r. Short-term avoidance of emotions	________	________	________
s. To brag about it	________	________	________
t. Curiosity	________	________	________
u. A motive not listed above	________	________	________
v. A motive not listed above	________	________	________
w. A motive not listed above	________	________	________

4. Explain why you rank-ordered the practice exercises the way you did.

____

____

____

____

____

5. Make an appointment with your partner and write down in the appropriate column your partner's rank-orders. Discuss (compare and contrast) whatever differences you may find in your individual rank-orders.

6. After completion of this practice exercise, check which of these answers indicates how you felt about it. There is also space for you to explain further, if you want to:
   a. I did not like it at all, a waste of time. I wish I never saw this stupid practice exercises. ________
   b. I did not like it very much, but I want to go on with another practice exercises. ________

c. I liked it and I want to go on with another practice exercises. ________
d. I liked it a lot and I wish I had something like this practice exercises earlier. ______
e. I liked it so much that I wish all couples could get something like this practice exercises to work on. ________

7. How could this practice exercises be improved? Do you have any suggestions? Feel free to write whatever could improve this practice exercises.

____
____
____
____
____

Relational Quality: Part 1

The purpose of this practice exercises is to improve your relationship with your partner, either in marriage or in a committed couple relationship. Answer each practice exercise individually and get together with your partner at preset, predetermined times (at least 24 h ahead) to discuss your completed practice exercises for no longer than 1 h. If you get upset during this time, end the discussion and make another appointment for another time at least 24 h ahead.

Practice Exercise 1. Defining Relational Quality

Name______________________________Sex__________Date_______

The purpose of this practice exercise is to help you define more clearly the nature and quality of your relationship with your partner. Make sure that you understand and discuss with each other the meaning of each feature that is included in this practice exercise.

1. Below are listed various features that cover a range of possibilities in a relationship. If you have a feature not found in this list, add it at the end (there is room for additional features). Define each feature and give two examples of how that feature is shown concretely in your relationship.

Features and Definitions	*Examples*
a. Taking time for each other ______	Example 1 ____________
______________________	______________________
______________________	Example 2 ____________
______________________	______________________

b. Talking with each other __________ Example 1 __________

__________ __________

__________ Example 2 __________

__________ __________

c. Empathy __________ Example 1 __________

__________ __________

__________ Example 2 __________

__________ __________

d. Listening to each other __________ Example 1 __________

__________ __________

__________ Example 2 __________

__________ __________

e. Taking an interest in partner __________ Example 1 __________

__________ __________

__________ Example 2 __________

__________ __________

f. Consideration __________ Example 1 __________

__________ __________

__________ Example 2 __________

__________ __________

g. Openness __________ Example 1 __________

__________ __________

__________ Example 2 __________

__________ __________

h. Affection __________ Example 1 __________

__________ __________

__________ Example 2 __________

__________ __________

i. Paying attention to partner Example 1 __________

__________ __________

__________ Example 2 __________

__________ __________

j. Understanding __________ Example 1 __________

__________ __________

__________ Example 2 __________

__________ __________

k. Safety ____________________ Example 1 ____________________
____________________ Example 2 ____________________

l. Honesty ____________________ Example 1 ____________________
____________________ Example 2 ____________________

m. Being there for each other ________ Example 1 ____________________
____________________ Example 2 ____________________

n. Mutual respect ____________________ Example 1 ____________________
____________________ Example 2 ____________________

o. Trust ____________________ Example 1 ____________________
____________________ Example 2 ____________________

p. Discussing everything ____________ Example 1 ____________________
____________________ Example 2 ____________________

q. Love ____________________ Example 1 ____________________
____________________ Example 2 ____________________

r. Displaying emotions ____________ Example 1 ____________________
____________________ Example 2 ____________________

s. Tenderness ____________________ Example 1 ____________________
____________________ Example 2 ____________________

t. Accepting partner ______ Example 1 ______
______ ______
______ Example 2 ______
______ ______

u. Fidelity ______ Example 1 ______
______ ______
______ Example 2 ______
______ ______

v. Looking forward to seeing each other ______ Example 1 ______
______ ______
______ Example 2 ______
______ ______

w. Longing for each other ______ Example 1 ______
______ ______
______ Example 2 ______
______ ______

x. Dependability ______ Example 1 ______
______ ______
______ Example 2 ______
______ ______

y. Forgiveness ______ Example 1 ______
______ ______
______ Example 2 ______
______ ______

z. A feature not listed above (specify) Example 1 ______
______ ______
______ Example 2 ______
______ ______

aa. A feature not listed above (specify) Example 1 ______
______ ______
______ Example 2 ______
______ ______

2. Now that you have defined the meaning of each feature, you need to rank-order those features according to how important they are to you in this relationship in the column "Yours." Rank as No 1 the feature that is the most important to you, rank as No. 2 the feature that is next in importance, and so on; mark as 0 the

features that are not important to you at all, and mark as N/A the features that do not apply to your relationship.

Features	*Rank-orders* *Yours*	*Partner's*	*Joint*
a. Taking time for each other	______	______	______
b. Talking with each other	______	______	______
c. Empathy	______	______	______
d. Listening to each other	______	______	______
e. Taking an interest in partner	______	______	______
f. Consideration	______	______	______
g. Openness	______	______	______
h. Affection	______	______	______
i. Paying attention to partner	______	______	______
j. Understanding	______	______	______
k. Safety	______	______	______
l. Honesty	______	______	______
m. Being there for each other	______	______	______
n. Mutual respect	______	______	______
o. Trust	______	______	______
p. Discussing everything	______	______	______
q. Love	______	______	______
r. Displaying emotions	______	______	______
s. Tenderness	______	______	______
t. Accepting partner	______	______	______
u. Fidelity	______	______	______
v. Looking forward to seeing each other	______	______	______
w. Longing for each other	______	______	______
x. Dependability	______	______	______
y. Forgiveness	______	______	______
z. A feature not listed above	______	______	______
aa. A feature not listed above	______	______	______

3. Why did you rank-order these features the way you did?

____

____

____

____

____

Homework: During the coming week, make an appointment with your partner and go over your definitions and your rank-orders. Record your partner's rank-orders in the appropriate column and add both to achieve a joint rank-order.

Take notes of your discussion while you are comparing and contrasting your answers. Keep your completed practice exercises and, if you work with a professional who is assisting you with this practice exercises, discuss these notes with her or him in addition to discussing copies of your completed practice exercises.

Note: Whatever joint rank-order you agree on will determine the order of future practice exercises. However, you need to decide whether you want to work on practice exercises where there are the greatest discrepancies in your rankings or whether you want to work on practice exercises where there is the least discrepancy.

Consequently, based on your decision, the next practice exercise should be given the title of the joint feature that has been rated either as No. 1 or as one lower in your joint rank-order. After that practice exercise, all other practice exercises should follow the joint rank-order you have agreed on, either from the top or from the bottom of your rank-orders.

Standard Practice Exercise for Features of Relational Quality (Parts One, Two, and Three)

Practice Exercise No.____Feature:____________________

Name________________________Sex__________Date_______

The purpose of this practice exercise is to understand more about the feature listed in the title.

1. How did this feature start? Please explain in detail.

____
____
____
____
____

2. How often does this feature take place in your relationship? Check which answer applies to you:

a.	Practically every day	_____	e.	Once every 6 months	_____
b.	Once a week	_____	f.	Once a year	_____
c.	A couple of times a month	_____	g.	Once every few years	_____
d.	Once a month	_____			

3. Please explain further:

____
____
____
____
____

4. How did this feature come about? Do you remember when it started? Check which answer fits best:

   a. As we met for the first time ______
   b. During courtship or while dating ______
   c. Before marriage or before we started living together ______
   d. During the honeymoon or as we were moving in together ______
   e. Right after the honeymoon or right after we moved in together ______
   f. A few months after the marriage or after we moved in together ______
   g. 1 year after the marriage or when we moved in together ______
   h. Years after marriage or when we moved in together ______

5. Please explain further:

____
____
____
____
____

6. What does this feature get you? Please explain.

____
____
____
____
____

7. Give three specific examples of how this feature is helpful to you.

   Example 1:

____
____
____
____
____

   Example 2:

____
____
____
____
____

Example 3:

8. Give three specific examples of how this feature is helpful to your partner.

Example 1:

Example 2:

Example 3:

Homework: Next week, plan to repeat this feature, if it belongs to you, or remind your partner to repeat it if it belongs to him or her. Make sure it is repeated at preset times (for instance, at 8 a.m., 12 noon, 4 or 7 p.m.), at least three times. Write down what happened in detail. In case you wonder why this feature should be started, keep in mind that if you or your partner start it, whoever starts it will acquire the power to end it. This power should strengthen your relationship.

For each time make sure to answer in writing the following four questions:

a. How did it start?
b. What followed?
c. How did it end?
d. What did this behavior get you or your partner?

Time 1 (write the time you started__________)

a. ______________________________

____

____

b. ______________________________

____

____

c. ______________________________

____

____

d. ______________________________

____

____

Time 2 (write the time you started__________)

a. ______________________________

____

____

b. ______________________________

____

____

c. ______________________________

____

____

d. ______________________________

____

____

Time 3 (write the time you started__________)

a. ______________________________

____

____

b. ______________________________

____

____

c. ______________________________

____

____

d. ______________________________

____

____

Check which of the following shows what you got out of this practice exercise:

a.	Completely useless	_______	d.	Somewhat useful	_______
b.	Somewhat useless	_______	e.	Extremely useful	_______
c.	So-so	_______			

Write down how you feel about this homework practice exercise and what you got out of it.

____
____
____
____
____

Final Follow-Up Form for Relational Quality (Parts 1–3)

Name_______________________Sex__________Date________

The purpose of this form is to review whether the practice exercises in this practice exercises were helpful to you.

1. Which answer best fits how you feel about this practice exercises?

   a. I did not like working on this practice exercises at all. I wish I never saw it. _________
   b. I did not like this practice exercises, but I am glad I got to work on. _________
   c. I am happy I got a chance to work on this. _________
   d. I am not only delighted about this practice exercises, but I wish all couples could get it. _________

2. How helpful was it to work on this practice exercises? Please check the answer that applies to you:

a.	Not helpful at all	_____	c.	Helpful	_____
b.	Somewhat helpful	_____	d.	Very helpful	_____

3. Which practice exercise did you like best and that was the most helpful to you? Rank as No. 1 the one that you liked best, rank as No. 2 the one you liked next best, and so on; mark as 0 the ones you did not like at all, and mark as N/A the ones that did not apply to you.

Features	*Rank-orders*		
	Yours	*Partner's*	*Joint*
a. Taking time for each other	_________	_________	_________
b. Talking with each other	_________	_________	_________
c. Empathy	_________	_________	_________
d. Listening to each other	_________	_________	_________

Features	*Rank-orders*		
	Yours	*Partner's*	*Joint*
e. Taking an interest in partner	________	________	________
f. Consideration	________	________	________
g. Openness	________	________	________
h. Affection	________	________	________
i. Paying attention to partner	________	________	________
j. Understanding	________	________	________
k. Safety	________	________	________
l. Honesty	________	________	________
m. Being there for each other	________	________	________
n. Mutual respect	________	________	________
o. Trust	________	________	________
p. Discussing everything	________	________	________
q. Love	________	________	________
r. Displaying emotions	________	________	________
s. Tenderness	________	________	________
t. Accepting partner	________	________	________
u. Fidelity	________	________	________
v. Looking forward to seeing each other	________	________	________
w. Longing for each other	________	________	________
x. Dependability	________	________	________
y. Forgiveness	________	________	________
z. A feature not listed above	________	________	________
aa. A feature not listed above	________	________	________

4. Explain why you rank-ordered the practice exercises the way you did.

____

____

____

____

____

5. Make an appointment with your partner and write down in the appropriate column your partner's rank-orders. Discuss (compare and contrast) whatever differences you may find in your individual rank-orders. Add both columns and compare your joint rank-orders with the rank-orders given in your first practice exercise. Are there any changes in your rank-orders, and if there are, why? If there are no changes, why? Please explain.

____

____

____

____

____

6. After completion of this practice exercise, check which of these answers indicates how you felt about it. There is also space for you to explain further, if you want to:

   a. I did not like it at all, a waste of time. I wish I never saw this stupid practice exercises. _________
   b. I did not like it very much, but I want to go on with another practice exercises. _________
   c. I liked it and I want to go on with another practice exercises. _________
   d. I liked it a lot and I wish I had something like this practice exercises earlier. _________
   e. I liked it so much that I wish all couples could get something like this practice exercises to work on. _________

7. How could this practice exercises be improved? Do you have any suggestions? Feel free to write whatever could improve this practice exercises.

____
____
____
____
____

Relational Quality: Part 2

The purpose of this practice exercises is to improve your relationship with your partner, either in marriage or in a committed couple relationship. Answer each practice exercise individually and get together with your partner at preset, predetermined times (at least 24 h ahead) to discuss your completed practice exercises for no longer than 1 h. If you get upset during this time, end the discussion and make another appointment for another time at least 24 h ahead.

Practice Exercise 1. Defining Relational Quality

Name__________________________Sex______Date________

The purpose of this practice exercise is to help you define more clearly the nature and quality of your relationship. Make sure that you understand and discuss with each other the meaning of each feature that is included in this practice exercise.

1. Below are listed various features that cover a range of possibilities in a relationship. If you have a feature not found in this list, add it at the end (there is room for additional features). Define each feature and give two examples of how that feature is shown concretely in your relationship.

Features and Definitions	*Examples*
a. Support ________________	Example 1 ________________
________________	________________
________________	Example 2 ________________
________________	________________
b. Knowing partner ________________	Example 1 ________________
________________	________________
________________	Example 2 ________________
________________	________________
c. Friendship ________________	Example 1 ________________
________________	________________
________________	Example 2 ________________
________________	________________
d. Running the household together	Example 1 ________________
________________	________________
________________	Example 2 ________________
________________	________________
e. Similarities ________________	Example 1 ________________
________________	________________
________________	Example 2 ________________
________________	________________
f. Mutual goals ________________	Example 1 ________________
________________	________________
________________	Example 2 ________________
________________	________________
g. Similar interests ________________	Example 1 ________________
________________	________________
________________	Example 2 ________________
________________	________________
h. Only a few quarrels ________________	Example 1 ________________
________________	________________
________________	Example 2 ________________
________________	________________
i. Mutual friends ________________	Example 1 ________________
________________	________________
________________	Example 2 ________________
________________	________________

j. Common activities ____________ Example 1 ____________
Example 2 ____________

k. Harmony ____________ Example 1 ____________
Example 2 ____________

l. Security ____________ Example 1 ____________
Example 2 ____________

m. Similar beliefs ____________ Example 1 ____________
Example 2 ____________

n. Deferring to partner's wishes ____ Example 1 ____________
Example 2 ____________

o. Helping one another ____________ Example 1 ____________
Example 2 ____________

p. Spending as much time together as possible ____________ Example 1 ____________
Example 2 ____________

q. Solving problems together ______ Example 1 ____________
Example 2 ____________

r. Willingness to compromise ______ Example 1 ____________
Example 2 ____________

s. Autonomy ______ Example 1 ______ Example 2 ______

t. Maintaining individuality ______ Example 1 ______ Example 2 ______

u. Independence ______ Example 1 ______ Example 2 ______

v. Having and allowing for freedom Example 1 ______ Example 2 ______

w. A feature not listed above (specify) Example 1 ______ Example 2 ______

x. A feature not listed above (specify) Example 1 ______ Example 2 ______

2. Now that you have defined the meaning of each feature, rank-order these features according to how important they are to you in this relationship in the column "Yours." Rank as No 1 the feature that is the most important to you, rank as No. 2 the feature that is next in importance, and so on; mark as 0 the features that may not be important to you at all, and mark as N/A the features that do not apply to your relationship.

Features	*Rank-orders*		
	Yours	*Partner's*	*Joint*
a. Support	______	______	______
b. Knowing partner	______	______	______
c. Friendship	______	______	______
d. Running the household together	______	______	______
e. Similarities	______	______	______

Features	*Rank-orders* *Yours*	*Partner's*	*Joint*
f. Mutual goals	________	________	________
g. Similar interests	________	________	________
h. Only a few quarrels	________	________	________
i. Mutual friends	________	________	________
j. Common activities	________	________	________
k. Harmony	________	________	________
l. Security	________	________	________
m. Similar beliefs	________	________	________
n. Deferring to partner's wishes	________	________	________
o. Helping one another	________	________	________
p. Spending as much time together as possible	________	________	________
q. Solving problems together	________	________	________
r. Willingness to compromise	________	________	________
s. Autonomy	________	________	________
t. Maintaining individuality	________	________	________
u. Independence	________	________	________
v. Having and allowing for freedom	________	________	________
w. A feature not listed above(____________________)	________	________	________
x. A feature not listed above (____________________)	________	________	________

3. Why did you rank-order these features the way you did?

Homework: During the coming week, make an appointment with your partner at least 24 h in advance and go over your definitions and your rank-orders. Record your partner's rank-orders in the appropriate column and add both to achieve a Joint rank-order.

Take notes of your discussion while you are comparing and contrasting your answers. Keep your completed practice exercises and, if you work with a professional who is assisting you with this practice exercises, discuss those notes with her or him in addition to discussing your completed practice exercises.

Note: Whatever joint rank-order you agree on will determine the order of future practice exercises. However, you need to decide whether you want to work on practice exercises where there are the greatest discrepancies in your rankings or whether you want to work on practice exercises where there is the least discrepancy.

Consequently, based on your decision, the next practice exercise should be given the title of the joint feature that has been rated either as No. 1 or as one lower in your joint rank-order. After that practice exercise, all other practice exercises should follow the joint rank-order you have agreed on, either from the top or from the bottom of your rank-orders.

Concluding Follow-Up Form for Relational Quality

Name__________________________________Sex_____Date______

The purpose of this form is to review whether the practice exercises in this practice exercises were helpful to you.

1. Which answer best fits how you feel about this practice exercises?

   a. I did not like working on this practice exercises at all. I wish I never saw it. ________
   b. I did not like this practice exercises, but I am glad I got to work on. ________
   c. I am happy I got a chance to work on this. ________
   d. I am not only delighted about this practice exercises, but I wish all couples could use it. ________

2. How helpful was it to work on this practice exercises? Please check the answer that applies to you:

   a. Not helpful at all _______ c. Helpful _______
   b. Somewhat helpful _______ d. Very helpful _______

3. Which practice exercise did you like best and that was the most helpful to you? Rank as No. 1 the one that you liked best, rank as No. 2 the one you liked next best, and so on; mark as 0 the ones you did not like at all, and mark as N/A the ones that did not apply to you.

Features	*Rank-Orders*		
	Yours	*Partner's*	*Joint*
a. Support	______	______	______
b. Knowing partner	______	______	______
c. Friendship	______	______	______
d. Running the household together	______	______	______
e. Similarities	______	______	______
f. Mutual goals	______	______	______
g. Similar interests	______	______	______
h. Only a few quarrels	______	______	______
i. Mutual friends	______	______	______
j. Common activities	______	______	______
k. Harmony	______	______	______
l. Security	______	______	______
m. Similar beliefs	______	______	______
n. Deferring to partner's wishes	______	______	______
o. Helping one another	______	______	______
p. Spending as much time together as possible	______	______	______

Features	*Rank-Orders* *Yours*	*Partner's*	*Joint*
q. Solving problems together	______	______	______
r. Willingness to compromise	______	______	______
s. Autonomy	______	______	______
t. Maintaining individuality	______	______	______
u. Independence	______	______	______
v. Having and allowing for freedom	______	______	______
w. A feature not listed above (______________)	______	______	______
x. A feature not listed above (______________)	______	______	______

4. Explain why you rank-ordered the practice exercises the way you did.

____

____

____

____

____

5. Make an appointment with your partner and write down in the appropriate column your partner's rank-orders. Discuss (compare and contrast) whatever differences you may find in your individual rank-orders. Add both columns and compare your joint rank-orders from the rank-orders made in your first-practice exercise. Are there any changes in your rank-orders, and if there are, why? If there are no changes, why? Please explain.

____

____

____

____

____

6. After completion of this practice exercise, check which of these answers indicates how you felt about it. There is also space for you to explain further, if you want to:

   a. I did not like it at all, a waste of time. I wish I never saw this stupid practice exercises. ______
   b. I did not like it very much, but I want to go on with another practice exercises. ______
   c. I liked it and I want to go on with another pr actice exercises. ______
   d. I liked it a lot and I wish I had something like this practice exercises earlier. ______

e. I liked it so much that I wish all couples could get something like this practice exercises to work on. ________

7. How could this practice exercises be improved? Do you have any suggestions? Feel free to write whatever could improve this practice exercises.

____
____
____
____
____

Relational Quality: Part 3

The purpose of this practice exercises is to improve your relationship with your partner, either in marriage or in a committed couple relationship. Answer each practice exercise individually and get together with your partner at preset, predetermined times (at least 24 h ahead) to discuss your completed practice exercises for no longer than 1 h. If you get upset during this time, end the discussion and make another appointment for another time at least 24 h ahead.

Practice Exercise 1. Defining Relational Quality

Name__________________________Sex___________Date________

The purpose of this practice exercise is to help you define more clearly the nature and quality of your relationship. Make sure that you understand and discuss with each other the meaning of each feature that is included in this practice exercise.

1. Below are listed various features that cover a range of possibilities in a relationship. If you have a feature not found in this list, add it at the end (there is room for additional features). Define each feature and give two examples of how that feature is shown concretely in your relationship.

Features and Definitions *Examples*

a. One's own friends ____________ Example 1 ____________________
______________________ ____________________
______________________ Example 2 ____________________
______________________ ____________________

b. Willingness to discuss friends ____ Example 1 ____________________
______________________ ____________________
______________________ Example 2 ____________________
______________________ ____________________

c. Willingness to argue when necessary ______ Example 1 ______

______ Example 2 ______

d. Tolerance ______ Example 1 ______

______ Example 2 ______

e. Equality ______ Example 1 ______

______ Example 2 ______

f. Flexibility ______ Example 1 ______

______ Example 2 ______

g. Different interests ______ Example 1 ______

______ Example 2 ______

h. Humor ______ Example 1 ______

______ Example 2 ______

i. No dominance ______ Example 1 ______

______ Example 2 ______

j. Arguments ______ Example 1 ______

______ Example 2 ______

k. Responsibility ______ Example 1 ______

______ Example 2 ______

l. Not taking each other for granted ______ Example 1 ______

______ Example 2 ______

m. Sexuality ______ Example 1 ______

______ Example 2 ______

n. Sexual harmony ______ Example 1 ______

______ Example 2 ______

o. Sexual satisfaction ______ Example 1 ______

______ Example 2 ______

p. Physical contact ______ Example 1 ______

______ Example 2 ______

q. Having fun ______ Example 1 ______

______ Example 2 ______

r. A feature not listed above (specify) Example 1 ______

______ Example 2 ______

s. A feature not listed above (specify) Example 1 ______

______ Example 2 ______

2. Now that you have defined the meaning of each feature, rank-order these features according to how important they are to you in this relationship in the column "Yours." Rank as No 1 the feature that is the most important to you, rank as No. 2 the feature that is next in importance, and so on; mark as 0 the features that are not important to you at all, and mark as N/A the features that do not apply to your relationship.

Features	*Rank-orders* *Yours*	*Partner's*	*Joint*
a. One's own friends	________	________	________
b. Willingness to discuss friends	________	________	________
c. Willingness to argue when necessary	________	________	________
d. Tolerance	________	________	________
e. Equality	________	________	________
f. Flexibility	________	________	________
g. Different interests	________	________	________
h. Humor	________	________	________
i. No dominance	________	________	________
j. Arguments	________	________	________
k. Responsibility	________	________	________
l. Not taking each other for granted	________	________	________
m. Sexuality	________	________	________
n Sexual harmony	________	________	________
o. Sexual satisfaction	________	________	________
p. Physical contact	________	________	________
q. Having fun	________	________	________
r. A feature not listed above (______________)	________	________	________
s. A feature not listed above (______________)	________	________	________

3. Why did you rank-order these features the way you did?

Homework: During the coming week, make an appointment with your partner and go over your definitions and your rank-orders. Record your partner's rank-orders in the appropriate column and add both to achieve a joint rank-order.

Take notes of your discussion while you are comparing and contrasting your answers. Keep your completed practice exercises and, if you work with a professional who is assisting you with this practice exercises, discuss these notes with her or him in addition to discussing copies of your completed practice exercises.

Note: Whatever joint rank-order you agree on will determine the order of future practice exercises. However, you need to decide whether you want to work on practice exercises where there are the greatest discrepancies in your rankings or whether you want to work on practice exercises where there is the least discrepancy.

Consequently, based on your decision, the next practice exercise should be given the title of the joint feature that has been rated either as No. 1 or as one lower in your joint rank-order. After that practice exercise, all other practice exercises should follow the joint rank-order you have agreed on, either from the top or from the bottom of your rank-orders.

Concluding Follow-Up Form for Relational Quality

Name_____________________________Sex_________Date_________

The purpose of this form is to review whether the practice exercises in this practice exercises were helpful to you.

1. Which answer fits how you feel about this practice exercises?

   a. I did not like working on this practice exercises at all. I wish I never saw it. _________
   b. I did not like this practice exercises, but I am glad I got to work on. _________
   c. I am happy I got a chance to work on this. _________
   d. I am not only delighted about this practice exercises, but I wish all husbands who use abusive or violent thinking could get it. _________

2. How helpful was it to work on this practice exercises? Please check the answer that applies to you:

   a. Not helpful at all _____ c. Helpful _____
   b. Somewhat helpful _____ d. Very helpful _____

3. Which practice exercise did you like best and that was the most helpful to you? Rank as No. 1 the one that you liked best, rank as No. 2 the one you liked next best, and so on; mark as 0 the ones you did not like at all, and mark as N/A the ones that did not apply to you.

Features	*Rank-orders*		
	Yours	*Partner's*	*Joint*
a. One's own friends	_____	_____	_____
b. Willingness to discuss friends	_____	_____	_____
c. Willingness to argue when necessary	_____	_____	_____
d. Tolerance	_____	_____	_____
e. Equality	_____	_____	_____
f. Flexibility	_____	_____	_____
g. Different interests	_____	_____	_____
h. Humor	_____	_____	_____
i. No dominance	_____	_____	_____
j. Arguments	_____	_____	_____
k. Responsibility	_____	_____	_____
l. Not taking each other for granted	_____	_____	_____
m. Sexuality	_____	_____	_____
n. Sexual harmony	_____	_____	_____
o. Sexual satisfaction	_____	_____	_____
p. Physical contact	_____	_____	_____
q. Having fun	_____	_____	_____

Features	*Rank-orders* *Yours*	*Partner's*	*Joint*
r. A feature not listed above (____________)	________	________	________
s. A feature not listed above (____________)	________	________	________

4. Explain why you rank-ordered the practice exercises the way you did.

____

____

____

____

____

5. Make an appointment with your partner and write down in the appropriate column your partner's rank-orders. Discuss (compare and contrast) whatever differences you may find in your individual rank-orders. Add both columns and compare your joint rank-orders with the rank-orders made in your first practice exercise. Are there any changes in your rank-orders, and if there are, why? If there are no changes, why? Please explain.

____

____

____

____

____

6. After completion of this practice exercise, check which of these answers indicates how you felt about it. There is also space for you to explain further, if you want to:

   a. I did not like it at all, a waste of time. I wish I never saw this stupid practice exercises. ________
   b. I did not like it very much, but I want to go on with another practice exercises. ________
   c. I liked it and I want to go on with another practice exercises. ________
   d. I liked it a lot and I wish I had something like this practice exercises earlier. ________
   e. I liked it so much that I wish all couples could get something like this practice exercises to work on. ________

7. How could this practice exercises be improved? Do you have any suggestions? Feel free to write whatever could improve this practice exercises.

____

____

____

____

____

Relationship Styles

The purpose of this practice exercises is to help you become more aware of the many styles that are found in intimate relationships.

Practice Exercise 1. Understanding Relationship Styles

Name______________________________Sex___________Date_________

The purpose of this practice exercise is to help you understand various types of relationship styles.

1. There are 16 types of styles in intimate relationships. Define each pair of words according to what it means to you; you can use a dictionary or consult your partner, a relative, a friend, or a mental health professional. Please add two examples of your own to make sure that you understood these definitions.

Definitions of Relationship Styles	*Examples*
a. Empty/absent ________________	Example 1 ________________
______________________________	______________________________
______________________________	Example 2 ________________
______________________________	______________________________
b. Participant/sharing____________	Example 1 ________________
______________________________	______________________________
______________________________	Example 2 ________________
______________________________	______________________________
c. Solitary/reserved______________	Example 1 ________________
______________________________	______________________________
______________________________	Example 2 ________________
______________________________	______________________________

d. Tenacious/egocentric ____________ Example 1 ____________

e. Docile/surrendering ____________ Example 1 ____________ Example 2 ____________

Example 2 ____________

f. Altruist/involved ____________ Example 1 ____________ Example 2 ____________

g. Mysterious/ambiguous ____________ Example 1 ____________ Example 2 ____________

h. Collaborative/mediator ____________ Example 1 ____________ Example 2 ____________

i. Abstract/unpredictable ____________ Example 1 ____________ Example 2 ____________

j. Sharing/innovative ____________ Example 1 ____________ Example 2 ____________

k. Rebel/antagonist ____________ Example 1 ____________ Example 2 ____________

l. Dominant/dictatorial ____________ Example 1 ____________ Example 2 ____________

m. Two-faced/false-altruist ________	Example 1 ________
________	________
________	Example 2 ________
________	________
n. Unpredictable/altruist ________	Example 1 ________
________	________
________	Example 2 ________
________	________
o. Inconclusive/disorganized ________	Example 1 ________
________	________
________	Example 2 ________
________	________
p. Confused/chaotic ________	Example 1 ________
________	________
________	Example 2 ________
________	________

2. Now that you understand various types of relationship styles, it is important to find out how they apply to you. Rank-order them according to how much they apply to you. Rank as No. 1 the style that applies to you the most, rank as No. 2 the style that applies to you next, and so on; mark as N/A the styles that do not apply to you. If you have trouble ranking these styles, ask your partner to help you, and make yourself available to help your partner with his or her rankings. Often, others can see us more accurately than we can.

Styles	*Rank-orders*			
	First	*Partner*[1]	*Other*[2]	*Final*
a. Empty/absent	____	____	____	____
b. Participant/sharing	____	____	____	____
c. Solitary/reserved	____	____	____	____
d. Tenacious/egocentric	____	____	____	____
e. Docile/surrendering	____	____	____	____
f. Altruist/involved	____	____	____	____
g. Mysterious/ambiguous	____	____	____	____
h. Collaborative/mediator	____	____	____	____
i. Abstract/unpredictable	____	____	____	____
j. Sharing/innovative	____	____	____	____
k. Rebel/antagonist	____	____	____	____
l. Dominant/dictatorial	____	____	____	____
m. Two-faced/false-altruist	____	____	____	____

[1]Indicate here who your partner (or relative) is:________________.

[2]Indicate here who "other" is:______________________________.

Styles	*Rank-orders*			
	First	*Partner*[1]	*Other*[2]	*Final*
o. Unpredictable/altruist	_______	_______	_______	_______
p. Inconclusive/ disorganized	_______	_______	_______	_______
r. Confused/chaotic	_______	_______	_______	_______

3. Write or type this list on a separate sheet of paper and give it to your partner, relative, or friend, without their seeing your rank-orders. Ask your partner, relative, or friend to rank-order how these styles apply to you.

4. Now you need to ask another person who knows you very well (parents, siblings, relatives, close friends) to rank-order these styles as they apply to you, using the column "Other." To make sure that this rank-order is independent of yours, type or write this list on a separate sheet of paper.

Homework: During the next week, compare and contrast your rank-order with the other two rank-orders and write down (under "Final") how you would re-rank these styles on the basis of the feedback you received from your partner and from the other person.

Standard Practice Exercise for Relational Styles

Practice Exercise No.____Adjectives:__________________

Name______________________________Sex_________Date_______

The purpose of this practice exercise is to understand more about the relationship style described by the two adjectives listed in the title above.

1. How does the style described by these adjectives apply to you? Please explain in detail.

____
____
____
____
____

2. How often do you feel like the style described by the adjectives listed above?

a. Practically every day	_____	e. Once every 6 months	_____
b. Once a week	_____	f. Once a year	_____
c. A couple of times a month	_____	g. Once every few years	_____
d. Once a month	_____		

3. Please explain further:

____
____
____
____
____

4. How did the style described by these adjectives come about? Do you remember when you started it? Check which answer fits best:

   a. When I was a child (younger than 5 years of age) ______
   b. When I was in elementary school ______
   c. When I was in middle school ______
   d. When I was in high school ______
   e. After high school ______
   f. Any other time ______

5. Please explain further:

____
____
____
____
____

6. Was the style described by these adjectives acceptable or unacceptable? Why? Please explain.

____
____
____
____
____

7. Give three specific examples of how the style described by these adjectives affects you.

   Example 1:

____
____
____
____
____

Example 2:

____
____
____
____
____

Example 3:

____
____
____
____
____

Homework: Next week, plan to repeat the style described by these adjectives at preset times (for instance, at 8 a.m., 12 noon, 4 or 7 p.m.) on at least 3 days (Monday, Wednesday, and Friday, or Tuesday, Thursday, and Saturday). If you can start it, you can stop it. Write down what happened in detail. For each time you start this style, make sure to answer in writing the following four questions:

(a) How did you start it?
(b) What followed?
(c) How did it end?
(d) What did the style described by these adjectives get you?

Time 1 (write the time you started__________)

a. ____
____
____

b. ____
____
____

c. ____
____
____

d. ____
____
____

Time 2 (write the time you started__________)

a. ____
____
____

b. ____
____
____

c. ____
____
____

d. ____
____
____

Time 3 (write the time you started__________)

a. ____
____
____

b. ____
____
____

c. ____
____
____

d. ____
____
____

Please check which of the following shows how you feel about this practice exercise:

a. Completely useless _____
b. Somewhat useless _____
c. So-so _____
d. Somewhat useful _____
e. Extremely useful _____

Explain in greater detail how you feel about this practice exercise and what you got out of it.

____
____
____
____
____

Concluding Feedback Form for Relational Styles

Name____________________________Sex__________Date_________

The purpose of this form is to review whether this practice exercises was helpful to you or not.

1. Please check the answer that best fits how you feel about this practice exercises:

   a. I did not like working on this practice exercises at all. I wish I never saw it. ______
   b. I did not like this practice exercises at all, but I am glad I got to work on it. ______
   c. I am delighted I got a chance to work on this practice exercises. ______
   d. I am not only delighted about working on this practice exercises, but I wish all people with relational problems had a chance to work on it. ______

2. How helpful was it to work on this practice exercises? Please check the answer that applies to you:

   a. Not helpful at all ______ c. Helpful ______
   b. Somewhat helpful ______ d. Very helpful ______

3. Which practice exercise did you like best? Please rank-order the practice exercises. Rank as No. 1 the one you liked best, rank as No. 2 the one you liked next best, and so on; mark as N/A the ones you did not like at all or that did not apply to you.

Styles	*Rank-orders*			
	First	*Partner*	*Other*	*Final*
a. Empty/absent	____	____	____	____
b. Participant/sharing	____	____	____	____
c. Solitary/reserved	____	____	____	____
d. Tenacious/egocentric	____	____	____	____
e. Docile/surrendering	____	____	____	____
f. Altruist/involved	____	____	____	____
g. Mysterious/ambiguous	____	____	____	____
h. Collaborative/mediator	____	____	____	____
i. Abstract/unpredictable	____	____	____	____
j. Sharing/innovative	____	____	____	____
k. Rebel/antagonist	____	____	____	____
l. Dominant/dictatorial	____	____	____	____

Styles	*Rank-orders*			
	First	*Partner*	*Other*	*Final*
m. Two-faced/false-altruist	____	____	____	____
o. Unpredictable/altruist	____	____	____	____
p. Inconclusive/disorganized	____	____	____	____
r. Confused/chaotic	____	____	____	____

4. Now ask your partner, relative, or friend (Partner) as well as another person (Other) to rank-order these styles. Write down their rank-orders and then calculate the final rank-order that represents whether you paid attention to these other opinions.
5. Sometimes what we like most is not necessarily the most helpful. Rank the practice exercises according to their helpfulness to you. Rank as No. 1 the most helpful, rank as No. 2 the next most helpful, and so on, down to the least helpful practice exercise; mark as N/A the practice exercises that did not apply to you.

Styles	*Rank-order*	*Styles*	*Rank-order*
a. Empty/absent	________	i. Abstract/unpredictable	________
b. Participant/sharing	________	j. Sharing/innovative	________
c. Solitary/reserved	________	k. Rebel/antagonist	________
d. Tenacious/egocentric	________	l. Dominant/dictatorial	________
e. Docile/surrendering	________	m. Two-faced/false-altruist	________
f. Altruist/involved	________	o. Unpredictable/altruist	________
g. Mysterious/ambiguous	________	p. Inconclusive/disorganized	________
h. Collaborative/mediator	________	r. Confused/chaotic	________

6. Please feel free to write any comments that might improve this practice exercises.

____
____
____
____
____
____

Families

Foster/Adoptive Care

The purpose of this practice exercises is to help potential foster/adoptive parents prepare for caring for their foster or adoptive child(ren).

Practice Exercise 1. Learning to Think Like a Foster/Adoptive Parent

Name________________________________Sex_____Date_________

The purpose of this practice exercise is to help you think like an adoptive/foster parent.

Be sure that the numbers and letters in your answer sheets match those in these practice exercises.

1. This is a list of the most commonly asked questions about foster or adoptive care. Answer these questions to the best of your ability even if you have to guess. After you have completed your answers, discuss them and their implications with your partner.

   a. Question for the natural family:

      i. Why did we lose our child?

____
____
____

      ii. Will they give him/her back?

____
____
____

      iii. Could we keep in touch with him/her?

____
____
____

      iv. Would foster/adoptive care help us too?

____
____
____

   b. Question for the foster/adoptive child:

      i. Who are these foster people?

____
____
____

ii. What can I do now?

iii. What can I not do?

iv. What do they expect from me?

v. What do they think about me?

vi. Who can I rely on?

vii. What will my family think about me?

viii. Will they accept me or reject?

ix. What have I done to deserve this?

c. Question for the foster or adoptive parents:

i. Are we fit for this experience?

ii. Have we got enough strength?

iii. How can we get to know him/her, his/her habits, and his/her difficulties?

iv. How can we raise him/her?

v. What will our natural children say about the ways the foster child is different? Will they become friends with the foster child?

vi. What will happen if we become too fond of him/her?

vii. What will we do if his/her family pesters or bothers us?

d. Questions for the natural children of foster or adoptive parents:

i. Is s/he taking my space away?

ii. What will s/he demand from us?

iii. Is s/he being a pest?

iv. Can we live now as before?

v. Will my parents love me as much as before?

e. Questions for the extended family of foster/adoptive parents:

i. Have they got enough strength to deal with this child?

ii. Will this child turn out to be as rejected as he or she may seem?

iii. What will happen when the child goes back to his/her family, will s/he be worse off?

f. Questions for social workers:

i. Is this experience worth the trouble?

ii. Is this family right for this child?

iii. How long will the child stay in this house?

iv. How will the natural parents behave?

v. In which way can we help all of them?

2. In your opinion, are there other important questions? Write as many questions you can think of that were not contained in the above list.

3. Go back to the list above and reread carefully all the questions most asked by foster/adoptive parents.

   a. What questions did you ask yourself before reading these questions? Write out at least three new ones:

      i. Question 1

      ____
      ____
      ____

      ii. Question 2

      ____
      ____
      ____

      iii. Question 3

      ____
      ____
      ____

   b. What questions are new to you, questions that you wonder about?

   ____
   ____
   ____

   c. Are there other questions that would be worth asking?

   ____
   ____
   ____

4. After your have discussed your answers with those of your partner, answer the following questions:

   a. Did you answer all the questions listed above?

   ____
   ____
   ____

b. Which questions did your partner answer differently from you?

____

____

____

c. What questions did you answer that your partner did not? (Put a question mark beside them.)

____

____

____

d. What question are not yet answered? (Put an asterisk beside them.)

____

____

____

e. Summarize in a few words what you feel about the prospect of becoming foster/adoptive parents.

____

____

____

5. Which people do you think are most troublesome in facing a foster/adoptive situation? Rank them from the most troublesome (No. 1) to the least troublesome (No. 7 or 8):

People	*Rank-order*
Natural family	________
Foster child	________
Our children	________
Our extended family	________
Neighbors	________
Friends	________
Social workers	________
Other (specify________)	________

6. Where would you put yourselves in the above ranking?

____

____

____

____

____

7. What could you say or give to people who are in more trouble than you?

____
____
____
____
____

8. What do you wish to receive from people who are in less trouble than you?

____
____
____
____
____

Homework:

1. Who would you like to talk about foster/adoptive care with:

   a. Your children
   b. Your parents
   c. Your relatives
   d. Your neighbors
   e. Your friends
   f. Your coworkers
   g. Other (specify____________)

2. Schedule a meeting with as many people listed above as possible. Set the specific time (date and hour) and arrange the proper accommodations. Open the discussion in this way: "Both my partner and I would like to hear your views about foster/adoptive care. Before embarking on such a difficult responsibility we would like to hear from all of you because, without your support, we may not want to start on this journey."

3. Keep notes on the discussion. Bring these notes to the next training session.

Practice Exercise 2. Foster or Adoptive Child Checkup

Name________________________________Sex_____Date_________

The purpose of this practice exercise is to help foster/adoptive children to connect effectively with their foster or adoptive parents. The child is the main subject of this experience. The natural parents, if they are effective parents, know their children well; they saw them from birth, they named them, they have watched them day by day, they saw them through highs and lows. They love them as much as anyone can love. However, they may not be able to take care of them as well as you might. Foster/adoptive parents need to acquire their information, if at all possible, so that they can enter into the relationship with the child by knowing beforehand his/her situation, in order to show their love to this child. Since this is an important part of the process, we need to work on a "foster/adoptive child checkup."

1. What do you wish to know about a child before she/he comes into your home? We need to consider first the age of the child.

   a. Family relationships with preschool children: Think about a daily family situation, for example, suppertime. What would a child do in this situation? There are many possibilities, but choose three typical ones. Cite the child's age or age range _________. Write down some typical child's behaviors for the age stated above.

____

____

____

      i. How would his/her parents react?

____

____

____

      ii. Now place the same child into another family (i.e., in the family of the parents' friends, but not the child's friends). How would s/he behave?

____

____

____

      iii. How would the adults react or exert parental responsibilities?

____

____

____

   b. Family relationships with elementary school children. Think about the same situation, but with an elementary school child. Cite the child's age or age range _________.

      i. Some typical child's behaviors:

____

____

____

ii. How would his/her parents react?

____
____
____

iii. Some behaviors of the same child in a different family:

____
____
____

iv. The response of the adults with parental duties:

____
____
____

c. Family relationships with teenagers
Apply the same situation to a teenager. Cite the teenager's age or age range __________.

i. Some typical teenager's behaviors:

____
____
____

ii. How would his/her parents react?

____
____
____

iii. Some behaviors of the same teenager in a different family:

____
____
____

iv. The response of the adults with parental duties:

____
____
____

d. Child's behavior in an unknown family

____
____
____

2. Think again about the child's behavior and the parents'/adults' response. Specify the age and sex of the child____________.

   i. Some typical child's behaviors:

____
____
____

   ii. How would his/her parents react?

____
____
____

   iii. Some behaviors of the same child in a different family:

____
____
____

3. Questions for adults with parental duties: A foster or adoptive child, coming into a family, behaves as any child would who is put into a strange situation, at least until s/he becomes accustomed to living in that family without anxieties and fears.

   a. What would you feel if you were in the same situation?

____
____
____

   b. What would you think if you were in the same situation?

____
____
____

c. What would you do if you were in the same situation?

4. Foster/adoptive child's behaviors

There is no such thing as a "normal" child. Children have different personalities, feelings, and habits, resulting from their past experiences. A foster/adoptive child usually has had a more difficult past than most other children. His/her natural family has had more troubles than most other families. The child may have lived apart from his/her natural family for a long time.

a. Maybe s/he has not acquired habits that, for most children of the same age, we consider important. Considering the child's age and sex, write your thoughts about the habits listed below:

i. Body care

ii. Eating and drinking

iii. Playing/leisure time

iv. School/work

v. Relating to others

vi. Other (specify)________________________

____
____
____

b. The child may have acquired some negative habits. Consider those listed below and add others, if necessary. Rank them from the most troublesome (No. 1) to the least troublesome (No. 6).

Negative Habits	*Rank-order*
i. Temper tantrum	________
ii. Stealing	________
iii. Smoking	________
iv. Fighting	________
v. Lying	________
vi. Other (specify)	________

c. She could have: such as the following:

	Rank-order
i. Bad eyesight	________
ii. Faulty hearing	________
iii. Stuttering	________
iv. Emotional or mental troubles	________
v. Learning disabilities	________
vi. Poor memory	________
vii. Lack of concentration/attention	________
viii. Hyperactivity	________
List other possible handicaps:	________
ix. ______________________	________
x. ______________________	________

d. Write your reasons for ranking the negative habits and handicaps they way you did.

____
____
____

5. Consider gender differences: Specify the child's age and sex ______. Suppose the child demonstrates some behaviors among those listed in item 4.

a. Make up a worst-case scenario for what your reactions would be to it.

____
____
____

b. Do you feel you could accept a child with these qualities? Is there full agreement between you and your partner?

c. How would you try to find a solution to any problem arising with the child?

6. The meaning of behavior

In dealing with relationships between the foster/adoptive child and foster/adoptive parents, we have to consider the following possibilities

a. The child behaves in certain ways because

i. S/he does not know how to behave differently
ii. S/he does not want to behave differently
iii. S/he wants the opposite from what you want

b. Why do these behaviors take place? Discuss these possibilities and others, and write down your conclusions.

7. Any parent, whether natural, adoptive, or foster, has to keep in mind positive rather than negative reactions to the child's behavior or misbehavior:

a. A constant positive feeling: the child must have the experience of feeling wanted and loved
b. A realistic view of the level of skill necessary for the child's age, that is, what he/she can have, make, hold, spend, etc.
c. What do you think about these issues?

Homework: What will you do to cope with potential problems? Will you two parent the child as individuals or will you parent as a couple? This is a very important issue that needs a great deal of thought and discussion because foster/adoptive care requires much more energy and thought than caring for natural children. In what ways is it possible to cope with potential difficulties? Keep notes of your discussion. Bring these notes to the next training session.

Practice Exercise 3. Foster/Adoptive Care: Needs and Demands

Name_____________________________________Sex____Date______

The purpose of this practice exercise is to review some aspects of foster or adoptive care in order to increase your effectiveness as parents. The foster/adoptive child is not responsible for the foster/adoptive family's satisfaction. This child needs a positive family experience.

1. It is necessary to combine the child's needs with the emotional availability of his/her caregivers.

   a. What do the words "emotional availability" mean to you?

____
____
____

   b. Are you able to be emotionally available to each other? How?

____
____
____

   c. Are you able to be emotionally available to others? List as many people as you can think of with whom you have been emotionally available in the past, including your natural children (if any).

____
____
____

   d. If you are unable to be emotionally available to yourselves as individuals and to each other as a couple, you may need to reconsider undergoing the experience of foster/adoption care. If there is a problem here, discuss it with your trainer or professional helper.

____
____
____

2. In addition to emotional availability, there are a host of other issues you need to become aware of. Here is a range of possibilities in foster/adoptive care:

   a. Temporary custodianship for just some weeks or months because of serious emergencies in the child's natural family.
   b. Foster care experience after the child has grown in an institution or in another foster family, and a positive family experience is important before facing life without such an experience.
   c. Foster care before a reintroduction to his/her natural family. This reintroduction depends on the nature of the disturbance in the natural family, such as: physical, psychiatric, financial, legal, etc.
   d. Foster care awaiting court decision for adoption. Adoption is not a prospect for the foster family.
   f. Foster care as preadoptive step. This represents the first step toward adoption after all legal formalities and court decision have been taken into consideration.
   g. Discuss the implications of these possibilities with your partner, close friend, or professional helper.
   h. Consider any other possibility not listed above.

____

____

____

3. Which of these foster/adoptive care possibilities are you considering and why?

____

____

____

____

____

4. Which of these possibilities are you excluding and why?

____

____

____

____

____

5. Write down the advantages and disadvantages of each age range for a foster/adoptive child:

   a. Toddler to nursery school

____

____

____

b. Kindergarten

c. Elementary school

d. Middle school

e. High school

f. Which age do you consider suitable for a foster child in your home and why?

g. Which age do you exclude and why?

h. How did you decide on a suitable age?

7. Do you prefer a boy or a girl?

a. What are the reasons for your preference?

b. Which disadvantages do you think you could handle with a child of the other sex?

---

c. What do your children (if your have any) think about the foster child's sex and why?

---

d. What do your relatives/friends/neighbors think about this issue?

---

8. What do you think about the child's race or ethnic origin?

   a. What do you prefer and what do you exclude? Why?

---

   b. What do think your children, relatives, or neighbors may feel about this issue and why?

---

9. Which health conditions in the foster/adoptive child's do you exclude and why?

---

10. Which psychological and emotional troubles (in the foster child) you do not want or feel able to face and why?

____

____

____

____

____

11. Foster/adoptive care is not a bank transaction; nevertheless, this service is expensive and requires money. Which of the following financial conditions do you think is the most appropriate, keeping in mind your financial situation?

    a. No financial reward ________
    b. Money needed for hospital treatment ________
    c. Money needed for school assistance ________
    d. Money needed for board and room ________
    e. Money needed for college education ________
    f. The money provided by welfare will be sufficient to cover our expenses for this child ________
    g. Explain your choices:

____

____

____

    h. Write down what you will need in terms of future expenses for this child until s/he reaches 18 years of age.

____

____

____

12. Family foster/adoptive care is a service connected with social services. Below are some possible relationships with these services:

    a. A mental health helper will visit you every week ________
    b. A mental health helper will visit you every month ________
    c. A mental health helper will be at your disposal every time you need help ________
    d. A mental health helper will participate to your family conference ________
    e. A mental health helper will communicate all information, even if not in person ________
    f. What other type of relationship with the mental health helper would you like? Why?

____

g. Which would be your preference and why?

h. Which of these possibilities do you think are most suitable to your situation and why?

Homework: Family foster/adoptive care represents a complex endeavor, with many requirements and responsibilities. It may or it may not offer many nourishing advantages to the family. Plan a family meeting to discuss issues presented in this or previous practice exercises. Keep notes of the discussion. Bring these notes to the next training session.

Practice Exercise 4. The Skills of Adoptive/Foster Parents

Name______________________________Sex_____Date_________

The purpose of this practice exercise is to stress that adoptive/foster children require an extra dose of understanding, patience, and forbearance.

1. As we have stressed, the child is the main subject of the foster/adoptive care experience. Of course, foster parents are just as important! Their skills are not so different from those of natural parents' skills. Nevertheless, it is important to stress some specific aspects of the foster/adoptive care experience. Write down some skills you think are important in parenting children.

2. Now that you have listed these skills rank them in terms of their importance to you and to the child. Rank the most important as No. 1, rank the next most important as No. 2, and so on, until you have ranked all these skills in order of importance.

3. Explain the reasons for your ranking order.

4. If you have natural children, you know some of their friends.

   a. Do you use the same skills with them that you use with your children?

   b. What is the difference between skills used with your children and the skills you use with their friends?

5. How about the foster/adoptive child?

   a. Are the skills needed for your children the same as the skills needed for a foster/adoptive child? Why?

b. How are the skills necessary for your children different from skills necessary for the foster/adoptive child?

____
____
____

c. What skills are they?

____
____
____

6. A good foster parent should able to:

   a. Put him/herself in the child's shoes ________
   b. Understand the child's needs ________
   c. Stress the child's positive aspects ________
   d. Respect the child's individuality ________

7. Are these skills in your list?

   a. Which of these skills do you feel you have? Why?

____
____
____

   b. Which of these skills do you not have? Why?

____
____
____

   c. Do you agree about the importance of these skills? Why?

____
____
____

8. When foster/adoptive parents have to manage their natural children and their foster child together, the situation can become difficult. Paying attention to the natural children can be seen as preference by the foster/adoptive child and vice versa.

a. What do you think about this possibility?

b. How do you plan to deal with this possibility?

9. Below is a list of suggestions to avoid possible preferences or conflicts about problem behaviors:

   a. Consider the age of each child.
   b. Explain your position in advance and give some reasons for it.
   c. Clarify the relationship between the specific situation or context and how adults as well as children need to behave accordingly.
   d. Pay attention to sex differences.
   e. Forbid any criticism about the topic of parental preference.
   f. Debrief the children periodically by arranging regular family conferences.

10. Rebut and respond to any verbal expression of preference or any other complaint by writing the complaint down and informing the child(ren) that this topic will be dealt with in a family meeting after discussion with your partner.
11. Do what you said you will do and after discussion with your partner develop a plan of how to deal with the issue after negotiation with family members in a preset family meeting.
12. There will be moments of stress from the beginning. The foster/adoptive child can provoke serious problems because she:

   a. Is depressed
   b. May want to be sent home
   c. Feels uneasy and unhappy
   d. May test the limits of your acceptance capacity by wanting to see whether you can express unconditional love
   e. May feel rejected by your children and may want to test whether there are parental preferences
   f. Needs to be asked for reasons why s/he behaved the way s/he did; very likely s/he will not know or will make up an excuse that many or may not be relevant to the situation at hand

13. Regardless of the child's behavior, it is your choice whether you want to react immediately to the child's (mis)behavior or whether you can keep your council, avoid reacting, and remain in charge. Reacting may mean exploding in the face of an unusual or deviant situation. It is more conducive to keep cool and ask for information before responding. Extreme reacting may border on child abuse, which should be avoided at all costs. Conducive behavior means taking stock of the situation, obtaining all the possible information, and processing it with your partner and/or trainer or professional helper before responding to the child.

    a. Give as many examples of reactive behavior as you can.

____

____

____

    b. Give as many examples of conducive behavior as you can.

____

____

____

    c. Which behavior offers more positive solutions? Why?

____

____

____

____

14. To help you reach a conducive rather than reactive level of parenting, consider the following suggestions for increasing skills in stress management. This is a partial list, and you and your partner need to develop a plan on how to deal with various situations that will come up (see Homework).

    a. Minimize disruptive behaviors (if they do not require the immediate intervention of social services or the police) by giving the child alternative and more positive ways of responding.
    b. Distinguish actions from feelings.
    c. Do not put down or ridicule inappropriate behaviors.
    d. Debrief the initial or previous agreement by asking for further information and whether the child has understood what was expected of him or her.
    e. Do not threaten corporal punishment.
    f. Do not threaten moral punishment or rejection.
    g. Do not preach to the child.

h. Distinguish what is relevant from what is not; discuss these possibilities at length.
i. Schedule a family meeting at least 24 h in advance. The planned-parenting practice exercises shown below may be helpful in this regard.
j. Write down other types of management that have helped lower the stress in your family.

Homework: Review the parenting skills listed above and choose the three or four you think are the most important for the child's sake. With your partner's help, develop a detailed plan for parenting the child in for the next few weeks.

Practice Exercise 5. The Foster/Adoptive Child Is Not an Orphan

Name__________________________________Sex____Date__________

The purpose of this practice exercise is to stress that the adoptive/foster child comes into the new family with baggage from past relationships that is going to impinge on and affect new relationships.

1. The child does not came alone into a foster/adoptive family. S/he brings complex relationships with other people. Consider the relationships that have been important in determining the foster/adoptive child's life. These relationships are the basis for the child's personal identity, even though there might have been difficulties, tensions, and pain. If foster/adoptive parents do not consider these relationships, they risk repeating the same kind of relationship problems with the child.

2. Get information about his or her natural family. The child may still be a member of that family, if not legally, then emotionally This family has affected most of the (positive or negative) development of this child. To know more about the child's natural family is a consistent part of knowing more about the child. If you have obtained this information, what are the chances of:

   a. Success?
   b. Failure?
   c. Be realistic in writing down what these chances will be.

____
____
____

3. If the child was removed from his/her natural home, very likely it was due to problems. Consider what these problems could have been:

   a. Chronic poverty, with an event that put the family in an emergency situation
   b. Alcohol or drug addiction
   c. Physical abuse

i. Beatings
ii. Scolding
iii. Burning
iv. Wounds

d. Sexual abuse or molestation

i. Oral intercourse
ii. Anal intercourse

e. A neglectful situation in fundamental life needs

f. Verbal abuse

i. Blaming
ii. Put-downs
iii. Criticisms
iv. Scolding
v. Name calling

4. Did you know other families in similar situations?

a. What reactions did you have to these abusive behaviors?

____
____
____

b. Is there something about these behaviors to understand before condemning them?

____
____
____

c. Write down some positive aspects of families like these.

____
____
____

5. Is separation from the family worse than abuse? The child may have gotten used to negative behaviors! Maybe s/he feels more pain about the separation than about abusive treatment.

a. Most likely, his/her feelings are despair and abandonment.

i. Did you ever feel something similar? Describe the situation.

____
____
____

ii. In what way did you overcome the situation?

____
____
____

b. A child can feel angry about being abandoned.

i. Did you feel abandoned in the presence of your children or relatives?

____
____
____

ii. How long did you feel this way?

____
____
____

iii. Could you control and bear it?

____
____
____

c. If a child sees a new environment that contrasts drastically from the former, the child may feel loyalty conflict: "If I do this, will I receive love from my family? If I behave in different way, what will the foster family say?" This loyalty conflict may lead to passivity, indecision, and an incapacity to do anything.

i. Did you ever experience such a feeling?

____
____
____

ii. How long did you feel this way?

____
____
____

iii. How is it possible to overcome it?

____
____
____

6. Write down your possible solutions for overcoming a loyalty conflict.

____
____
____
____
____

7. Continuity of intimate relationships is very important. Foster/adoptive families must learn to respect the history and origins of foster children and love them without owning them.

   a. Do you agree?

____
____
____

   b. How is it possible to do this?

____
____
____

8. The relationships between foster/adoptive and natural families need to be viewed as a possible reality. The child's natural family may want to visit the child's foster home. They may want to arrange visit with their child outside of the foster home. One needs to consider the circumstances, and foster/adoptive parents may need to consult with appropriate authorities or social services. These visits may represent the key element in bringing together the families as well as in terminating the parental rights. These visits may be the main tool for overcoming many issues already considered in previous sessions. If they are possible, plans should be prepared to deal with them.

a. Preparation of the natural parents: They need to complete a training program appropriate to their needs and level of functioning. This training could be found in the planned-parenting practice exercises that follows this one.
b. Foster parents will need to:
a. Talk with the foster child concerning the meaning of these visits
b. Talk with their own children and relatives
c. Set up a time and place for the visit, and arrange any legal forms required
d. Manage these visits in a way that will be positive for all, especially for the child

9. What strategies could you use to deal with these visits?

a. After the visit of the natural parents, discuss it with the child or a social worker; focus on the behaviors and attitudes of:
a. The foster/adoptive parents
b. The natural children and relatives
c. The foster child
d. The natural parents of the child

10. To put home visits in perspective, the discussion should ask:

a. What did we learn, so that the next visit can be more positive than this one?

____
____
____

b. Is the discussion compatible with our lifestyle?

____
____
____

c. What can we do differently next time?

____
____
____

11. The Achilles' heel of a visit from the natural parents can found in behaviors to which the child may react with negative feelings. For example, talking to the natural parents about the child's arrival in the foster family, you can say: "Our children welcomed him/her with open arms! We hope they will became good friends." But the natural mother may hear that you are criticizing her, and proclaim in response: "But we always loved him/her!" Thus, the foster/adoptive parents must be careful not to say anything that will sound critical of the natural parents or suggest that they do not love the child. Thus, any possibly invidious comparison needs to be avoided.

12. Foster/adoptive parents can intervene in different ways. Prepare a variety of worst-case scenarios and consider how to respond to them if they arise. Think of at least one scenario for each of the following possibilities:

    a. Jealousy
    b. Hostility or aggressiveness
    c. Exploitation
    d. Indifference

Homework: Review the natural parents' attitudes and possible behaviors and then answer this question: If these attitudes and behaviors were ours, what would happen? Keep notes on the discussion. Bring these notes to the next training session.

Practice Exercise 6. The Foster/Adoptive Child vs. Your Own Children

Name________________________________Sex____Date_________

The purpose of this practice exercise is to understand the inevitable conflicts that may arise between natural and adoptive/foster children.

1. The foster/adoptive child faces new parents as well as new children, both in your home and in school.

    a. Discuss with your natural children the possible availability of your family for foster children. Write down your children's reactions, positive and negative, and discuss them with the children and in another meeting with your partner or professional trainer or helper.

____
____
____

    b. You need to explore your natural children's feelings about the foster/adoptive child. Below are reactions that your children may have toward receiving in your home a foster/adoptive child:

        i. S/he is a stranger. S/he is not a member of our family.

____
____
____

        ii. S/he does not have our habits.

____
____
____

iii. We don't know him/her and we do not want to.

iv. S/he is the enemy; s/he is too big, too little, bad, a bully, etc.

v. S/he does not talk much or do things like we do.

vi. S/he is a rival for our parents' love; s/he stole our parents from us.

vii. S/he demands too much attention from our parents that we need and want for ourselves.

viii. S/he is a pest; s/he occupies our room, breaks our toys, plays with our things.

ix. S/he is a sponger; s/he eats up all the food that belongs to us.

x. S/he is our little slave; s/he should do what we want; s/he must do what we tell her/him.

2. Discuss all of your children's stated objections, as well as others that they may not express directly in words.

   a. Ask yourself why do they have these feelings?

   b. Whatever their feelings may be, assume that your children feel insecure about your loving them.

   c. You need to ask yourself what behavior on your part has rendered your children so insecure.

   d. You need to answer this question before you are able to consider foster/adoptive care, since the foster/adoptive child will need a double dose of security because, chances are, s/he will be an even more insecure child than your own children.

   e. Discuss the issue of security-insecurity with your partner. How secure or insecure were you about your parents' love?

f. If either one of you was insecure, how do you expect to give security either to your children or to a foster/adoptive child?

____

____

____

3. After this discussion, practice finding positive aspects in:

a. Your partner/friend

____

____

____

b. Your own children

____

____

____

c. The foster/adoptive child

____

____

____

3. Complaints may be voiced not only from your children about the foster/adoptive child, but also from either parent because you both might be worried about the influence of this child on your children. Rank-order the behaviors that may become sources of conflict between you and the foster/adoptive child. Rank as No. 1 the greatest potential source of conflict that worries you the most, rank as No. 2 the next potential source of conflict, and so on, until you have ranked all potential sources of conflict.

Behavior	*Rank-order*
a. Inappropriate habits in general (does not bathe or does not practice personal hygiene)	________
b. Does not brush his/her teeth	________
c. Eats with hands	________
d. Throws temper tantrums	________
e. Disobeys requests	________
f. Inclined to steal	________
g. Smokes	________
h. Has had premature sexual experiences	________
i. Tells lies	________

Behavior	*Rank-order*
j. Uses foul language	_________
k. Is aggressive and hostile	_________
l. Other worrisome behavior (specify)	_________
m. Other worrisome behavior (specify)	_________

4. In trying to help the child, below are some choices that might help you deal with undesirable behaviors:

   a. Speak to your own children about these behaviors.
   b. Explain to the foster child that these behaviors are unacceptable, giving the reason for their unacceptability.
   c. Tell the child what consequences may follow unacceptable behavior.
   d. Make sure that these consequences have been thought through and are not made up on the spur of the moment or out of anger or frustration. Discuss these consequences with your partner before discussing them with the children, both your own and the foster/adoptive child. Discuss the pros and cons for each choice with your partner, writing them down.
   e. Make sure that these consequences follow naturally from the unacceptable behavior. Discuss them also with your trainer or professional helper.
   f. Make sure that these consequences are applied with care, troublesome thoughts, consideration, and compassional, and that they apply to your own children as much as to the foster/adoptive child.

5. What are some opportunities for increasing the pros and reducing the cons of the child's behavior?

   a. If have no plan, develop one. (See the planned-parenting practice exercises.)
   b. A poor plan can be improved.

6. Another aspect of foster/adoptive family care to take into account troublesome thoughts the possible impact (influence) that this child might have on your children. Write down all the possible influences that this child could have on your own children. Compare and contrast your list with the list made up by your partner. Make up a master list from both. For each troublesome thoughts write one or two ways of dealing with it.

Homework: Decide whether you want to parent with a plan or without a plan. If you have no plan, you do not need to parent anybody. (See the planned-parenting practice exercises.)

1. If you have no plan but want to develop one, do so with the help of your partner, other parents, friends, or a professional helper. Part of this plan would contain troublesome thoughts written in response to item 6.

2. Review the main point of this lesson and then write down some notes for a possible discussion with all the children in a preset family meeting.

3. If at all possible, hold this family meeting and write down a detailed summary of what occurred, keeping notes of what went on. Bring these notes to the next training session.

Practice Exercise 7. A Welcome Plan

Name________________________________Sex____Date_________

The purpose of this practice exercise is to help to prepare a plan to welcome to your home the new adoptive/foster child.

1. This practice exercise puts together various ideas that have emerged during this training program. Structure a possible plan to receive the foster/adaptive child in your home. Let us suppose that your preparation is completed. Your availability as foster/adoptive parents has been positively evaluated by social services. There are no formal or legal obstacles or unforeseen events. Consider this situation:

   a. It is Monday afternoon. You receive a call from a social worker whom you know, who says. "There is a child who needs to be received in a family, because his father, an alcoholic, is in jail and his mother has been hospitalized in an emergency this morning for an contagious illness. He does not have any relatives locally. He does not present any particular problems, but he does not do too well in school. This emergency could last up to 6 months. We think that your family could be a good placement for this child. What do you think? If you are favorably disposed, this child could visit with you as early as Wednesday evening. I will give you more details if you accept. We would like, if possible, for the child to be received by next weekend." Given the sex, age, and ethnic origin of the child, draw up a plan for receiving the child:

   a. People to meet:

      i. Social worker
      ii. The child
      iii. The lawyer
      iv. Ask if there other people who will be present (i.e., newspaper, police, etc.)

   b. Information to ask about

   c. Agreements to sign

d. Preparation of family members

   i. What to say
   ii. What to ask
   iii. What not to say
   iv. What not to ask
   v. What to do
   vi. What not to do

e. Preparation of people outside the immediate family (relatives, in-laws, siblings, extended family members, neighbors, friends, clergyman)

   i. What to say
   ii. What to ask
   iii. What not to say
   iv. What not to ask
   v. What to do
   vi. What not to do

2. Things to prepare:

   a. Bed and space for belongings
   b. Schedule for driving the child to the doctor, social services, school, etc.
   c. Extra food
   d. Extra clothing if necessary

3. Plan for the weekend by considering some possibilities for receiving the child:

   a. Where to pick him up
   b. Will the social worker brings him to your home?
   c. Prepare a party with neighbor children of the same age
   d. Ask neighbors to come to welcome the child
   e. Structure the weekend with activities as well as rest periods
   f. Invite friends who are involved in your support group
   g. Invite relatives who are part of your support group

4. Review these possibilities and then choose which of them seem attractive to you. Consider the possibility that the child may be very shy, very fearful, or very tired and upset. Consequently, discuss your plans with the social worker who is acquainted with the natural family and the child.
5. In considering all the possibilities listed above, talk with your partner about the pros and cons of each possibility, considering the information about the child given to you by the social worker.
6. Which possibility is the most advantageous?

7. Unforeseen events can arise. To prepare yourself for them, suppose that you receive a call from the social worker, who says, "There are some unforeseen circumstances that will make it impossible for the child to be placed in your home. Tomorrow evening I'll explain more."

   a. What will be your reaction? Why? To whom will your express it and how?

____
____
____

   b. What will you say to your family?

____
____
____

   c. What will you say to your neighbors and friends?

____
____
____

   d. Will you express your disappointment to the social worker?

____
____
____

   e. Will you be available as foster/adoptive parent in the future?

____
____
____

Homework: During the coming week, discuss with your partner whether you still want to consider becoming foster/adoptive parents or not. What are the pros and cons of becoming one? Bring your conclusions to the training session.

Concluding Feedback Form

Name________________________________Sex____Date_________

The purpose of this form is to review what has been learned from this series of homework practice exercises. Now that you have completed this practice exercises, please respond to the following questions concerning the use of written homework practice exercises.

1. Rank-order the homework practice exercises according to their usefulness in developing an effective introduction to foster/adoptive family care. Rank the most useful practice exercise as No. 1, rank the next most useful as No. 2, and so on, ranking the least useful as 7.

Practice Exercises	*Rank-order*
a. Learning to think like a foster/adoptive parent	______
b. Foster/adoptive child checkup	______
c. Foster/adoptive care: needs and demands	______
d. Foster/adoptive parenting skills	______
e. The foster/adoptive child is not an orphan	______
f. Foster/adoptive child vs. one's own children?	______
g. A welcome plan	______

2. How useful was this practice exercises to help you prepare as a foster/adoptive parent?

a. Very useful	______	d. Slightly useful	______
b. Quite useful	______	e. Not useful at all	______
c. Somewhat useful	______		

3. How useful did you find this practice exercises in improving your relationship with your partner?

a. Very useful	______	d. Slightly useful	______
b. Quite useful	______	e. Not useful at all	______
c. Somewhat useful	______		

4. How useful was this practice exercises in increasing your potential for foster/adoptive care?

a. Very useful	______	d. Slightly useful	______
b. Quite useful	______	e. Not useful at all	______
c. Somewhat useful	______		

5. How useful was this practice exercises in helping you decide whether you want to be considered for foster/adoptive care?

a. Very useful	______	d. Slightly useful	______
b. Quite useful	______	e. Not useful at all	______
c. Somewhat useful	______		

6. Using your own words, what did you find useful about this practice exercises?

____
____
____
____
____

7. How could this practice exercises be improved? Your suggestions will be welcome and appreciated.

____
____
____
____
____

Planning Parenthood

Note to professional helpers: The purpose of this practice exercises is to reduce cumbersome and abstract models, derived from a developmental, contextual competence theory (L'Abate, 2005, 2006), to concrete and specific practice exercises to be used as homework to evaluate interactively, rather than statically, as in test instruments, models, and the theory behind them. As most sources have demonstrated, parenting and parenting preparation are crucial to personality development of the child. These skills have become even more crucial given the increase of nontraditional family structures, which, no matter their composition or level of functioning, will need to have parents exercising these skills. Note that there are other theory-derived practice exercises that deal with parts of the theory, such as (1) depression, (2) negotiation, (3) intimacy, (4) selfhood, and (5) identity. The depression practice exercises (L'Abate, 1986) contains the drama triangle, the distance regulation triangle, and the paradoxical prescription of depression positively reframed as a "friend." The negotiation practice exercises (1986) was patterned after the ERAAwC (Emotionality, Rationality, Activity, Awareness, and Context) model, and contains practice exercises about the ARC (Abusive/Apathetic, Reactive/Repetitive Conductive/Creative) and resources exchanged models. The intimacy practice exercises (1986) contains practice exercises about seeing the good in self and intimate others, caring, forgiveness, and three practice exercises about sharing of hurts. The identity practice exercises, located in (section 3) contains about a variety of self-definitions that are not contained in the selfhood model. The selfhood model is represented in two separate practice exercises about receiving importance from self-attributes and from intimate others.

By the same token, there are theory-related and theory-independent practice exercises that are, however, in some way or another conceptually related to the models of the theory. They could be compared with this one and other practice exercises, or other parenting skills programs. What would happen when a parenting program taking place face to face through talk between parents and professionals is compared with this practice exercises administered at a distance through the Internet, with a minimum of face-to-face talk between parents and professionals?

Responsible professionals should be aware of and follow the ethical and professional guidelines of their respective national and state organizations, and should obtain from participants a signed informed consent form. Also, they should conduct a structured or unstructured screening interview and administer a battery of tests relating to the level of individual, couple, or multirelational functioning, as well as a baseline parenting inventory to evaluate the level of parenting skills present in prospective or actual parent(s) before administering this practice exercises. These tests and parenting inventories should be readministered after completion of the practice exercises, and, ideally, 6 months or even 1 year after completion.

Make sure that partners, parents, caregivers, and single parents complete these practice exercises at specific, preset, predetermined times, ideally always in the same place. The purpose of stressing the same place and time in practice exercises is to teach parents to become regular and predictable in how they are going to complete the practice exercises in this practice exercises. Perhaps this regularity may generalize to other parts of their parenting and of their relationships. It would help the process of homework practice exercises if families were taught from the outset how to be together, how to say how much they love each other, and how to communicate nonverbally through hugging, holding, and cuddling.

Practice Exercise 1. The Purpose of This Practice exercises

Name______________________________________Sex_____Date_____

A practice exercises consists of written homework practice exercises to be completed by partners, parents, or single parents who want to improve their parenting skills according to a positive plan. Rather than reacting to your children immediately and with no forethought, without thinking about the consequences of your or your children's actions, the purpose of this practice exercises is to make you think about what you are doing as an individual, as a partner, and as a parent. If you do not have a partner, perhaps you can enlist the help of a caring friend, or use the professional who is administering this practice exercises to you as a sounding board and a source of support and feedback.

The reason for calling this practice exercises "planned parenting" stems from the fact that responsible and responsive parenting does not come about automatically in a vacuum. Parenting is too serious, important, and responsible an activity to assume that we can parent our children without learning any skills. The only parenting skills we know usually are those we learned from our parents. If our parents' skills were in some ways defective or incomplete, we are doomed to repeat their mistakes. Parenting, to be effective, needs to be planned carefully and sensitively.

1. What do you want to get from working on the practice exercises of this practice exercises? Check all that apply:

    a. I want to improve my skills as a parent. ________
    b. I would like to plan what I do with my children, rather than simply respond or react to them. ________
    c. I am so limited in my parenting skills that I can use any help I can get. ________
    d. My parents were not models of parenting skills, and I hope I can improve on what they did. ________
    e. My parenting background was so erratic and unplanned that I need to become more consistent and more positive in my parenting skills. ________
    f. I have read many books on parenting, but none gave me a hands-on experience of really working interactively with down-to-earth practice exercises. ________
    g. My parents were so abusive that I need to make sure I do not repeat the mistakes they made. ________
    h. Parenting is too important to think that one can learn it without thinking and learning more about it. ________
    i. Parenting is the most important skill one needs to learn in life. ________
    j. My parenting skills definitely need improvement. ________
    k. Any other reason not listed above (state what it is) ________

2. In your own words, write what you plan to get out of working on the practice exercises of this practice exercises.

____
____
____
____
____

3. What kind of parenting experience have you had so far? Please describe in detail, from your past family of origin to the present family of procreation.

____
____
____
____
____

Homework: During the coming week, write down all the hurts that you experienced as a child that were related to your parents' parenting mistakes. Write only for exactly 15 minute a day for 4 days in a row. Make sure to write always at the same preset times and predetermined place.

After you have finished, discuss these hurts with your partner by setting an appointment at least 24 h in advance. Take notes during your discussion. If you do not have either a partner or a friend to discuss your notes with, discuss them with the professional who is administering these practice exercises.

Practice Exercise 2. The Ability to Love and to Parent

Name________________________________Sex______Date______

Parenting skills do not grow in a vacuum automatically. They develop from how love and responsibility are experienced and expressed in one's family of origin and in one's family of procreation, your family now.

The purpose of this practice exercise is to make you aware of how love is shown through different types of parenting, allowing you then to choose how to show and discuss love with your children and what kind of parenting you want to learn and practice. By improving your parenting skills, you will also be able to show your love for your children in more constructive and positive ways than you might have followed heretofore.

1. Answer the following questions in detail.

   a. Describe the love and parenting in your family of origin.

      i. How was love shown in your family of origin?

____
____
____

      ii. How was affection shown in your family of origin?

____
____
____

      iii. How do you show love in your family now?

____
____
____

      iv. How do you show affection in your family now?

____
____
____

v. How do you feel about love and parenting being part of the same process?

b. There are three major types of parenting that will be explained below:

i. Abusive–apathetic or neglectful (AA)
ii. Reactive–repetitive (RR)
iii. Creative–conductive (CC)

2. Characteristics of abusive–apathetic (AA, neglectful) parenting: an abusive or neglectful parent usually denies being abusive or neglectful:

a. Using immediate physical punishment, like hitting, yelling, spanking with a switch or belt, throwing things, sexual abuse, or kicking
b. Using verbal punishment, like name calling, screaming, raging, etc.
c. Specific examples of verbal AA parenting:

i. Bringing up past errors or misdeeds on the part of the child: "I remember what you did (or did not do) 2 years ago."
ii. Blackmail: "If you don't do this or that, I will do this or that to you."
iii. Bribery: "I will give you something if you do or do not do something."
iv. Blaming: "It's all your fault."
v. Reading someone else's mind: "I know what you want to do and I know how and why you want to do it."
vi. Ultimatums: "If you do not do this right away, I will do this to you!"
vii. Avoidance of any consequences for the child's behavior, or the consequences are angrily (through tantrums) or extremely enforced in an inconsistent fashion.
viii. Going from one extreme of abuse to another extreme of making up for the abuse, as in asking for forgiveness, promising to change what the parent has said or done, buying gifts to make up, or allowing the child to do or have whatever the child wants, sometimes going from one extreme of punishment to another extreme of letting the child do or get what he or she wants.
ix. Setting no limits on the child and letting the child do whatever he or she wants.
x. Favoring one child over another.
xi. Denial of the abuse or belittling the strength or the damage of abusive or neglectful parenting on the child, let alone the parent.
xii. Being addicted to alcohol, drugs, food, or medication.

xiii. Repeating without stop the deadly triangle composed of three parts – victim, rescuer or savior, and persecutor – in which each member of the family plays three parts or roles well.

(a) The victim is usually the one who feels tormented, put upon, or blamed, collecting all the real, perceived, or imagined hurts that have been received from another intimate, who is perceived as the persecutor. The victim feels innocent of any blamed misdeed or feels that the persecutor is unfair or not justified in punishing and abusing.
(b) The persecutor is the one who blames, hits, yells, and abuses another intimate, the victim, without regard to the consequences of his or her actions.
(c) The savior or rescuer is the one who comes in between, intervenes, and supposedly protects the victim from the cruel persecutor. Since most intimates play these parts well, this deadly triangle tends to repeat itself from one generation to another. Children repeat the same roles/parts that were played by their parents. Most mental illness develops from this triangle. This is why this triangle is deadly.
(d) How does this triangle apply to your experience? Check a choice that applies to you:

(i) A great deal ________
(ii) Somewhat ________
(iii) Not at all ________

3. Characteristics of reactive-repetitive (RR) parenting: A reactive parent repeats himself or herself without getting the desired behavior from the child.

a. Immediacy, that is, doing quickly whatever seems to be in the best, immediate interest of the child or of the parent, without thinking about possible consequences of what has been done or said. As a result the undesirable behavior on the child's part keeps on repeating itself without a stop.
b. Acting right away to deal with the child without consulting the partner or anybody else.
c. Not setting any limits on the child, by letting the child do whatever he or she wants to do or giving the child whatever he or she wants.
d. Protecting and shielding the child from experiencing the natural consequences of his or her actions.
e. Trusting the child's word rather than the word of authorities (police, teachers, doctors).
f. Rescuing the child from whatever trouble the child may have created.
g. Thinking that "unconditional love" without any limits will make the child happier, more self-reliant, or more independent.
h. Exaggerating the good in the child and ignoring potentially negative aspects of the child's behavior.

i. Giving the child toys, money, and clothes without limit, rather than giving affection with firm, consistent limits to the child's behavior.
j. Putting responsibility for the child's behavior on others (teachers, peers, doctors, friends, neighbors) rather than on the child.
k. Taking on too much responsibility and faulting oneself for the child's behavior rather than faulting the child.
l. Making the child dependent on the parent by taking away the child's initiative except through short-cuts, such as giving into the child's immediate wishes.
m. Wanting to become the child's best friend, and allowing the child to become the parent's confidant. These positions leads to role confusion and identity conflicts in the child.
n. Playing the distance–resolution triangle, consisting of pursuer, distancer, and regulator parts or roles, where intimates play all three parts in different areas of their lives. For instance, one could be a sexual pursuer but an emotional distancer. By the same token, a regulator in one area could play the other parts in another area.

    i. The pursuer seeks, approaches, and wants to get close physically and emotionally to another intimate.
    ii. The distancer avoids getting close and wants to be left alone, rejecting the advances of the pursuer.
    iii. The regulator switches from one part to another. For instance, "I want (need, like) your helpGo away, your help did not do me any good."

    How does this triangle apply to your experience? Check a choice that applies to you:

    (a) A great deal ________
    (b) Somewhat ________
    (c) Not at all ________

4. Characteristics of creative–conductive, planned parenting:
A caring, creative, and conductive[3] parent

    a. Thinks before he or she acts or reacts with the child.
    b. Discuss any parenting problem with one's partner, parent, close friend, or professional before taking action.
    c. Plans ahead what to do or say before doing it or saying it.
    d. Does not confuse or become confused by mixing "unconditional love" with "planned parenting."
    e. Takes time and makes time to spend time with the child at every opportunity.
    f. Stresses what it is rather than what "should," "could," or "must" be.

[3]A conductor is a leader who does not get angry during confrontations but who follows an orchestrated score or a thought-out plan rather than acting and reacting, at the spur of the moment, to the child's behavior haphazardly and inconsistently. A conductor thinks before acting. A conductor leads rather than reacts.

g. Stresses the child's strengths rather than the child's weaknesses.
h. Does not use the child to satisfy his or her own self-centered needs or wants.
i. Models how to express and discuss painful and pleasurable emotions in a nonjudgmental way.
j. Models how to delay immediate gratification for more important, future goals.
k. Helps the child distinguish between immediate needs, desires, and delayed wants and goals.
l. Lives and helps the child live in the present and not in the past.
m. Knows one's self limits and helps the child discover his or her own strengths and become aware of his or her limits.
n. Helps the child become aware of and respect differences in self and others, not allowing scapegoating on others but assuming responsibility for his or her behavior.
o. Is consistent in saying what he or she means and what he or she does.
p. Allows the child to grow up and be autonomous according to his or her rights.

Homework: During this coming week, review the characteristics of parenting listed above. Pick those that are familiar to you and that are part of your past and present experience, and write about them in great detail, 15 minute a day, for 4 days in a row.

If your pick either the drama or distance triangles, or both, write about how they have affected your life and your parenting skills.

After the 4 days of writing, discuss your writing with your partner at a preset time and place, planned at least 24 h ahead. Make sure you take notes of your discussion. If you do not have a partner, discuss your writing with a friend. Whether you have a partner or not, discuss your writing and discussion notes with a professional helper.

Practice Exercise 3. Who Am I? Who Do I Want to Be?

Name__________________________________Sex______Date______

The purpose of this practice exercise is to help you clarify who you are as an individual, as a partner, as a parent, and as a child of a parent; how you developed into the person you are now; and whether you want to improve on who you are now.

1. Write about how you feel about yourself and how you developed these feelings.

____

____

____

____

____

2. Write about how close you were to those who took care of you as you grew up.

____
____
____
____
____

3. There are at least six ways we develop as we grow up:

   a. Symbiotically means that you lived to satisfy your parents' needs and not your own: "I cannot live without you!" This way produces extreme dependency on the child, to the point that the child cannot separate from the caregiver. In extremes, this way produces either complete dependence or complete alienation (or both) in the child.
   b. Sameness means that your parents required blind and uncritical conformity to their wishes and behaviors: "Be exactly like me and do exactly what I want you to do and you will be all right." This way is bound to produce either dependency, on one hand, or rebellion and oppositeness, on the other.
   c. Similarity means that your parents did not demand conformity to their behaviors but modeled for you desirable and positive behavior worthy of being followed. This way gives enough room to the child to grow in his or her ways without constraints from the parents.
   d. Differentness means that your parents gave you the freedom to be different from them and from others without going to extremes of nonconformity or rebellion. This way allows the child to be creative and free to develop his or her best abilities.
   e. Oppositeness means that you chose to be the opposite of what your parents required of you, and in so doing, by rebelling, you likely chose to conform to the rules and behavior of another group that similarly rebelled against the norms of their parents and of society. This way can produce extremely rebellious children who are also very conforming to the rules and guidelines of a fringe or borderline group.
   f. Alienation means that you grew up completely separated from your parents as well as from society. This way produces the highest probability of criminal or severely problematic behavior.

4. Rate yourself on a three-point scale in how you define yourself according to the six ways defined above with persons listed below:

   Symbiosis = 3
   Sameness = 2
   Similarity = 1

Differentness = 1
Oppositeness = 2
Alienated = 3

a. With your mother _______
b. With your father _______
c. With your siblings _______
d. With your peers _______
e. With your friends _______
f. With your present partner _______
g. With your past partners _______
h. With your teacher(s) _______
i. With anybody else who is not listed above: identify () _______

6. Why did you rate yourself the way you did? Please explain.

Homework: In the coming week, write how you grew up according to the six ways that make us develop into who we are. Write 15 minute a day for 4 days in a row and meet by appointment with your partner, a friend, or a professional to discuss your writing. Keep notes on your discussion.

Practice Exercise 4. Me as Parent to My Child

Name________________________________Sex______Date_______

The purpose of this practice exercise is to explore how you define yourself with your child according to the six ways you developed as an individual, as a partner, and as a parent. Please answer all these questions:

1. Symbiosis:

   a. Are you raising your child as a symbiotic expression of your needs? If yes, why? If no, why not?
   b. Is the child fulfilling your unrequited dreams or wishes? For instance, do you want the child to be a movie star or performer because you wanted (and failed) to be a movie star or a performer?
   c. Will you be able to live without the child, once your child is grown up and leaves your home?
   d. Are you letting this child become independent or do you want for the child to always be dependent on you?

2. Sameness:

   a. Do you want your child to follow your rules and requests blindly without discussion, without allowing him or her to make up his or her mind about anything?

b. Do you require uncritical conformity to your wishes and rules, as it was perhaps required during your growing up?
c. Do you want your child to be a carbon copy of you?
d. What makes you think that your way of thinking and behaving is correct or constructive? How do you know you are "right?"
e. Is more important to you to be "right" or to be close to your child (or to your partner for this matter)?

3. Similarity:

   a. Do you model desirable behavior for your child in ways that allow him or her to follow your example rather than always being told what to do?
   b. Do you give your child enough leeway to follow your example rather than to do or say what you do or say?
   c. Do you show the child what to do or say rather than telling him or her what to do or say?

4. Differentness:

   a. Do you allow your child the freedom to be different without being considered weird or inappropriate?
   b. Do you strengthen his or her creativity by encouraging it directly or indirectly?
   c. What are you doing to encourage his or her creativity?

5. Oppositeness:

   a. How did your child's rebellion and oppositeness come about?
   b. What did you do that forced your child to do the opposite of what you do or say?
   c. How do you know he or she is oppositional to you?

6. Alienation:

   a. What is it about your parenting practices as parents and as partners that brought about this complete separation from you (and your partner)?
   b. Why do you think your child is now alienated from you?

Homework: Answer in writing each set of questions one at a time, perhaps one a day for 1 day in a row. If you have a partner, discuss each other's answers, keeping notes of what you have talked about. If you do not have a partner, discuss your answers with the professional who administering these practice exercises.

Practice Exercise 5. Selfhood

Name________________________________Sex______Date______

The purpose of this practice exercise is to help you define yourself even further by learning about how importance was expressed and discussed in your family of origin, as well as how importance is expressed and discussed now in your present family. Importance means showing troublesome thoughts and care toward both self and intimate others, such as parents, partner, child, siblings, teachers, or friends.

1. There are four major ways in which importance can be expressed toward self and intimate others:

   a. Importance, troublesome thoughts, and care are expressed positively toward self and others: "We are both important. We both must win." This way leads to a position called self-fulness. Parenting here means working things out with your child in ways in which you both win. You as a parent are authoritative (firm and consistent) in your parenting stance. This is one way to create a responsible, creative child.
   b. Importance is expressed positively toward self but negatively toward others: "I am important but you are not. I win, you lose." This way leads to a position called selfishness. Parenting here means you put on your child the weight of your authority and demand blind and uncritical conformity and obedience from the child without any backtalk or disobedience. This is one way to create either a bully and a rebel or a very dependent and fearful individual.
   c. Importance is expressed negatively toward self but positively toward others: "I am not important and you are more important than I am. You win, I lose." This way leads to a position called selflessness. Parenting here means that you let the child permissively win at your expense, and you are unable to set clear and firm limits to the child's behavior. This is one way to create a spoiled, pampered child.
   d. Importance is expressed negatively toward both self and others: "Neither one of us is important. Neither one of us is going to win." This way leads to a position called no-self. Parenting here means that neither you nor the child will win, without limits but with inconsistent and contradictory extremes from one destructive behavior to another, or from one permissive behavior to another, leading to eventual alienation and separation from each other. This is the way to create a confused, mixed up, and alienated child.

2. Family of origin. Answer the following questions about your family of origin:

   a. How did your mother express or deny her importance to herself and others?

   ____
   ____
   ____

   b. How did your father express or deny his importance to himself and others?

   ____
   ____
   ____

   c. How did any of your siblings express or deny their importance to themselves and others?

   ____
   ____
   ____

   d. How did anybody else in your family of origin express or deny importance to oneself and others?

   ____
   ____
   ____

   e. How do you express your importance with your parents?

   ____
   ____
   ____

   f. How do you express your importance with your siblings?

   ____
   ____
   ____

   g. How do you express your importance with other family members, such as in- laws and extended family members?

   ____
   ____
   ____

3. Present family:

    a. How do you express your importance with your partner?

    ____
    ____
    ____

    b. How do you express your importance with your child?

    ____
    ____
    ____

    c. How do you express your importance with your friends?

    ____
    ____
    ____

    d. How do you express your importance with anybody else?

    ____
    ____
    ____

4. Your children:

    a. How did you teach your children that they are important without putting anybody else down, or winning at someone else's expense?
    b. What do you need to do to teach your children that they are important but do not need to do it at anybody else's expense?

5. Yourself:

    a. How did you acquire a sense of self-importance, if any?

    ____
    ____
    ____

    b. What qualities in yourself make you feel important?

    ____
    ____
    ____

c. Who, among all the people mentioned above, helped you gain a sense of self-importance?

____

____

____

d. What qualities in yourself make you feel unimportant, if any?

____

____

____

e. Who, among all the people mentioned above, did not help and, indeed, tried to make you feel unimportant?

____

____

____

Homework: In the coming week, spend at least 20 minute a day answering the questions asked in this practice exercise. Compare and discuss your answers with your partner at a preset time and place, keeping notes on what you discussed. If you do not have a partner, discuss your answers with a professional helper.

Practice Exercise 6. Priorities

Name________________________Sex______Date______

The purpose of this practice exercise is to learn more about your priorities, that is, what is most important to you and to those who love you.

1. Rank-order the importance to you of the persons listed below. Rank as No. 1 the person who is most important to you, rank as No. 2 the person who is next in importance, and so on, down to the person who might not be as important to you as the others.

People Important to You	*Rank-order*
a. Grandparent	________
b. Mother	________
c. Father	________
d. Siblings	________
e. Self	________
f. Partner	________
g. Child(ren)	________

h. Relative (specify______) ________
i. Friend ________
j. Coworker ________
k. Classmate ________
l. Any other person (specify______) ________

2. Why did you rank-order these persons the way you did?

____
____
____
____
____

3. Rank-order the following roles according to their importance to you:

a. Bread winner ________
b. Homemaker ________
c. Supporter ________
d. Rule maker ________
e. Parent ________
f. Partner ________
g. Employer ________
h. Employee ________

4. Why did you rank-ordered these roles the way you did?

____
____
____
____
____

5. On a scale of 1–5, where 1 is extremely unimportant and 5 is extremely important, rate the following resources available to you on how important they are to you:

Resource	*Rank-order*
a. Being and feeling important	________
b. Being intimate emotionally	________
c. Performing	________
d. Being informed	________
e. Money	________
f. Goods/possessions	________

6. Why did you rate these resources the way you did?

____
____
____
____
____

7. The triangle of living: What we exchange in life – presence, performance, production.

   a. Importance together with intimacy constitute presence, being emotionally available to those you love and who love you. This is the base of the triangle. If this base is narrow, the other two sides of the triangle tend to become longer and larger. Too long or too large a base of presence is another extreme that leads to passivity and neglect of self and intimate others. Finding a balance among the three sides of the triangle is the most difficult task of our lives.
   b. Services together with information constitute performance, doing something to survive/enjoy. If and when performance is greater than presence, as in perfectionism, workholism, or drivenness, then presence suffers and problems develop.
   c. Money together with goods and possessions constitute production, having the wherewithal to survive financially and enjoy life. However, if production becomes exaggerated, as in hoarding, being a packrat, or developing an obsession with making money or accumulating things, then presence is decreased and problems develop.

8. Write how you feel about each of these modalities of exchange and how important they are to you.

____
____
____
____
____

9. On a scale of 1–5, where 1 is extremely unimportant and 5 is extremely important, rate the following channels of communication within yourself and with other resources available to you on how important they are to you:

   a. Feelings and emotions, leading to whom one gets close to or distant from, that is, presence ______
   b. Reason and logic, leading to how fast or slow one will behave ______
   c. Activities and actions, leading to stress on performance/production with lessened consideration about being together with loved ones ______

d. Awareness and reflection, that is, thinking about the consequences of one's actions or activities that provide feedback to your feelings and thinking, changing the whole process ______
e. Context and surroundings, being aware of one's feelings, thinking, and actions, and the behavior of loved ones and nonintimates ______

10. Why did you rate these channels of communication in the way you did? Please explain.

____
____
____
____
____

Homework: During the coming week, spend at least 20 minute a day answering the questions in this practice exercise. Compare and discuss your answers with your partner and with a professional helper. Make sure you keep notes on all your discussions.

Practice Exercise 7. Sharing Hurts and Achieving Closeness

Name________________________Sex______Date______

The purpose of this practice exercise is to help you get closer to the people who love you and whom you love.

Answer all these questions.

1. Crying: Go back to Practice Exercise No. 1, and recall what you wrote about whatever past hurts you may have received as a result of parenting.

   a. Were you able to cry about these past hurts?

____
____
____

   b. Why were you able to cry and, if not, why were you not able to cry?

____
____
____

c. Did you ever see your parents cry together?

d. What happened when one parent cried? What did the other parent do?

e. Have you and your partner cried together? When and why?

f. When is the last time you cried?

g. What reactions did you get from others when you cried?

2. Affection:

   a. How affectionate were your parents and how did they show their affection?

   b. How affectionate are you with your partner and vice versa?

c. How affectionate are your with your children?

3. Sharing hurts and fears of being hurt:

a. How did your family of origin discuss its hurts?

b. How does your present family discuss its hurts?

c. If hurts are not discussed constructively, how is happiness going to be discussed?

4. Forgiveness of errors

a. How was forgiveness expressed in your family of origin?

b. Who forgave whom and what was forgiven?

c. How is forgiveness expressed now in your present family?

d. Who forgives whom and for what?

____
____
____

e. Are you able to forgive yourself, or do you need to be perfect?

____
____
____

f. Can you accept being imperfect, or do you need to perform and produce to consider yourself perfect?

____
____
____

g. How about the members of your family? Do they need to perform and produce to be accepted?

____
____
____

Homework: During the coming week, take about 15–20 minute a day to answer all the questions asked above. Once you have finished, discuss your answers with your partner at a preset time and place. Keep notes on your discussion, and discuss them with the professional helper who is administering these practice exercises to you. If you are a single parent, discuss your answer with a trusted friend who is willing and able to work with you on these practice exercises, as well as with your professional helper.

Practice Exercise 8. Setting Boundaries/Limits

Name________________________________Sex________Date______

The purpose of this practice exercise is to help you set limits and boundaries for yourself and your children.

1. What do limits and boundaries mean to you? Please give a definition of limits and boundaries and give two examples of what these terms mean to you.

   Definition

____
____
____
____

Example 1:

Example 2:

2. Why are limits and boundaries important?

3. How were limits and boundaries set for you as you were growing up?

4. Are you able to set limits and boundaries for yourself? How? In what areas of your life?

5. Are you able to set limits and boundaries for your partner? If yes, why? If no, why not?

6. How do you set limits for your child?

   a. Are you successful? If yes, why? If no, why not?

   b. Are you able to say no to you child clearly and firmly, sticking to it without feeling guilty?

7. Do you set limits for the child by yourself or with the help of your partner? How?

8. Have you and your partner discussed how you are going to set limits for your child together?

9. If you do not have a partner, have you enlisted someone else to help you set limits for your child?

10. If you are not successful in setting limits for your child now, how successful will you be in the future?

11. If and when your child pushes the limits, how does he or she do it?

12. What can you and your partner do to set realistic, consistent, firm, and positive limits for your child?

13. Agree with your partner beforehand (if you have one) that from now on any request made at the last minute by your children is met by an automatic no. Any request made of one parent, when the other parent is absent, is met by a qualified no, adding, "Your [father, mother] and I will discuss it and we will let you know." If the child persists with the request, say, without anger or feelings, "The more you repeat this request, the longer it will take for your [father, mother] and I to make a decision about it." Give two examples of how you dealt with immediate requests from your child in the past and how you are handling them now.

Example 1:

Example 2:

14. If you are a single parent, any last minute request should be met with an automatic no, adding: "I will think about it and I will let you know when and what I decide about this request." If the child persists with the request, say, without anger or feelings, "The more you repeat this request,. the longer it will take me to make a decision about it." Give two examples of how you have handled this problem in the past and how you are handling it now.

Example 1:

Example 2:

15. What are the long-term consequences to the child of satisfying his or her immediate requests and decreasing the joint power and decision making of the parents by separating them in the process? What about a single parent's authority and decision making? The child will learn to think that the parent will always satisfy all his or her needs without thinking about the long-term outcome of this process.

Please comment:

____
____
____
____
____

Homework: After you have completed your answers to the questions raised in this practice exercise, discuss them with your partner by setting an appointment 24 h ahead in the same place you usually meet. An exception to this homework are points 13 and 14. Give at least two examples of how your child tries to have his or her own way to making requests at the last minute and from one parent alone when the other parent is absent. Keep in mind that your child will test the limits of your resolve, especially if past requests were immediately satisfied.

Practice Exercise 9. Solving Problems Together

Name________________________________Sex_____Date_______

The purpose of this practice exercise is to learn to solve problems with your partner, if you have one, and your child. Solving problems is a skill that needs to be practiced continually, lest you forget how important this skill is to help you, your child, and your family.

1. "Problems in the family are not solved on the spur of the moment." Please comment on this statement. Why is it correct or incorrect?

____
____
____
____
____

2. "Problems in the family are not solved when anyone in the family is upset, depressed, or angry." Please comment on this statement. Why is it correct or incorrect?

____
____
____
____
____

3. "Problems in the family are solved by appointment, by making time to sit down face to face and talk about what the problem is and how it can be solved and resolved responsibly and sensitively by planned problem solving." Please comment on this statement. Why is it correct or incorrect?

____
____
____
____
____

4. How to solve problems in the family:

   a. Make an appointment for the whole family at least 24 h ahead at a time that is agreeable to every one. Do not make more than one appointment a week. Ideally, once-a-month family meetings would be appropriate.
   b. Make sure that the meeting does not last longer than 1 h. Set a timer or alarm clock. If the meeting risks going over the 1 h limit, set the time for another appointment 24 h ahead. By the same token, if tempers are too strong and nothing is being accomplished, set the time for another appointment, if and when tempers cool down.
   c. Decide who should be in charge of the meeting and who should keep notes on what is being discussed at each meeting, including the date of the meeting. If you or your partner are in charge of the meeting, make sure that you alternate being in charge from one meeting to another. If you are a single parent, then you are in charge. The child must not be in charge under any condition; you, the parent, are in charge, but the child can take the notes if he or she wants to. The child, however, does have one vote if he or she contributes to the process of problem solving.
   d. You may get resistance to the idea of a meeting at an appointed time. The one in the family who feels a possible loss of power may want to sabotage the process. This resistance will need to be met in terms of what other choices are available to the family. How can the family solve its problems otherwise? Can anyone come up with a better choice? Then the choice for the resistant family members is whether he or she wants to solve family problems or not. This resistance also says something about how this family member was allowed to be powerful without taking responsibility for the family's welfare.
   e. To break the ice, it would help the whole family climate if some levity were added, not during family meetings but during the main evening meal. For instance, you could ask family members, including yourself, to tell a joke or relate a funny incident or story. A quarter could be painted red and given to whoever, by consensus, told the funniest joke, story, or event. This quarter would circulate around as funny stories, jokes, or events are brought to the table. If there are disagreements about who should get the quarter, use this disagreement to call for a family meeting.

f. Even though family meetings should not take place more often that once a month, family members should be allowed to call a family meeting for special emergencies or important issues that cannot wait until the next family meeting. Even emergency or special meetings should be scheduled 24 h ahead, unless it is a matter of life or death.
g. Once these prerequisites have been taken care of and the meeting has started, begin by asking everyone to raise any troublesome thoughts or worries. Start to model how an issue or problem should be addressed.
h. Make a list of all these troublesome thoughts and talk about how they should be ranked in terms of importance to each family member If one troublesome thoughts, issue, or problem raised by one family member is ranked first, then other issues raised by another member should be ranked second and third, and so on, to make sure that everyone is heard. Then another troublesome thoughts by the same family member who raised issue No. 1 is rated fourth, and so on. Make sure that all this information is recorded for future meetings.
i. Make sure that everyone is allowed to talk without interruption. If a family member keeps interrupting and cannot be silent, that problem must be ranked as No. 1 over the other problems.
j. Allow everyone to speak in a sequence that is reversed from one time to another. For instance, if the parents speak first, then the sequence should follow the ages of the children. Once this sequence is followed, the next discussion should start with youngest member speaking first and the parents speaking last.
k. Start a sequence by expressing your feelings about the problem, using the personal pronoun "I" and starting a sentence with: "I feel (am concerned, worried, etc.)about this problem." Make sure you say how you feel and not how you think about solving the problem. Allow everyone else to do the same. Feelings first, no thinking and no actions at this point.
l. Once a troublesome thoughts, issue, or problem is agreed upon and rank-ordered by everyone in the family, allow everyone to suggest possible solutions, making sure that all the pros and cons about each suggestions are fully expressed: thinking only at this point. Record all suggestions with the name of the one who made them.
m. After a full discussion of the pros and cons is completed, select which course of action seems the most feasible and agreeable to all the members of the family. If necessary and agreeable to all family members, have each member sign this document.
n. Suggest that this course of action will be followed for a predetermined period of time (e.g., 4 weeks, 3 months) and monitored, by keeping notes week by week, and future once-a-month family meetings will be held to see that the plan is fully implemented and that the desired results were obtained. Feedback and reflection at this point are important.
o. If the process does not seem to work within 4 weeks, discuss why it did not work, and what needs to be corrected, or consider an alternative course of action. Still feedback and reflection are offered with an awareness of the context of the problem solving.

p. At the end of each meeting, make sure to hug each family member, and, looking members of the family in the eyes, tell them how much you love them. If appropriate, thank them for their contribution to the family meeting. However, do not play favorites. You either praise everybody or do not praise at all: "I really appreciate how all of us worked together to solve our problems."

Homework: Make sure that the meaning and implications of the foregoing statements are discussed thoroughly over a period of weeks.

Concluding Follow-Up Feedback Form

Name________________________________Sex______Date________

The purpose of this form is to evaluate the usefulness of all the work you have been doing in the last several weeks.

1. What are your reactions to the whole practice exercises. Choose which answer best reflects how you feel about the whole process:

   a. This practice exercises was a complete waste of my time and energy. I could have gotten more information from the Internet or from my neighbor. ______
   b. The practice exercises was okay, but no big deal. ______
   c. I liked working on the practice exercises but it was a lot of work. ______
   d. I enjoyed working on the practice exercises of this practice e xercises and I learned a great deal from them. ______
   e. Not only did I enjoy working on the practice exercises of this practice exercises, but I think that all parents should learn all the many skills necessary to parent through planning. ______

2. Below there is a list of all the practice exercises in this practice exercises. Rank-order them according to how useful they were to you. Rank as No. 1 the most useful practice exercise, rank as No. 2 the second most useful practice exercise, and so on, until all practice exercises have been ranked.

Titles of Practice Exercises	*Rank-order*
1. Purpose of this practice exercises	________
2. The ability to love and to parent	________
3. Who am I? Who do I want to be	________
4. Me as parent to my child	________
5. Selfhood	________
6. Priorities	________
7. Sharing hurts and achieving closeness	________
8. Setting boundaries	________
9. Solving problems together	________

3. Why did you rank-order the practice exercises the way you did?

4. Feel free to comment and give whatever suggestions you have to improve this practice exercises.

Section 5
Self-Help Practice Exercises from Lists and Single- and Multiple-Score Tests

Children: Mixed Internalizing and Externalizing Disorders

School Conduct Problems
School Social Skills
Unusual or Troublesome Behavior

Adults
Butcher Treatment Planning Inventory (BTPI)

Single-Score Tests

Axis II Cluster C Internalizing Disorders
Beck Depression Inventory
Beck Anxiety Inventory
Hamilton Anxiety Inventory
Hamilton Depression Inventory
Other Troublesome thoughts

Axis II Cluster B Externalizing Personalities
Anger Expression
Self-Suffering (Masochism)
Help-Seeking (Dependent)
Serious (Depressed)

Selected Cluster B Personality Disorders
Self-Interested (Narcissistic)
Nonconformist (Negativistic)
Compelling (Compulsive)
Unusual (Sadistic)
Unpopular (Antisocial)
Exciting (Histrionic)
Private (Avoidant)
Distinct (Schizoid)

Mixed Internalizing and Externalizing Disorders
Personality Disorders: Form 1992
Personality Disorders: Form 1989
Personality Disorders: Form 1990

Multiple Score Tests
Personality Dimensions from the Minnesota Multiphasic Personality Inventory-2
Personality Dimensions from the Five-Factor Model of Personality (Neuroticism Extraversion Openness [NEO] Inventory)
Personality Dimensions from the Personality Assessment Inventory (PAI)

L. L'Abate, *Sourcebook of Interactive Practice Exercises in Mental Health*, DOI 10.1007/978-1-4419-1354-8_15,

Couples
Improving Relationships
Relationship Conflict
Couple Satisfaction

Families
Family Profile Form (FPF)
Family Functioning

Children: Mixed Internalizing and Externalizing Disorders

School Conduct Problems

The purpose of this practice exercise is to help you deal with behaviors that get you into trouble in school, outside school, and perhaps at home.

Practice Exercise 1. Definitions

This practice exercise may be difficult for some children to answer in just one sessions. In such cases, allow the child to work on the first part of this practice exercise.

Name ______________________________ Sex ____ Date _____

This beginning practice exercise helps you learn more about the behaviors that get you into trouble in school.

1. Define what each behavior listed below means to you. Use a dictionary or the Internet if you need information. Give two examples to make sure you understand the definition. It might take you more than a day to write down all these definitions. Take your time. After you have completed this list, go to item No. 2.

Behaviors	*Definitions and Examples*
a. Disruptive in class ____________	Example 1 ____________
______________________	______________________
______________________	Example 2 ____________
______________________	______________________
b. Disrespectful and discourteous to others ____________	Example 1 ____________
______________________	______________________
______________________	Example 2 ____________
______________________	______________________

c. Stealing or destroying others' property ________________________________	Example 1 ________________________
________________________________	Example 2 ________________________
d. Using excessive profanity (bad words) or verbal aggression ______	Example 1 ________________________
________________________________	Example 2 ________________________
e. Uncooperative in school-related group activities ____________	Example 1 ________________________
________________________________	Example 2 ________________________
f. Not obeying commands from authority figures ____________	Example 1 ________________________
________________________________	Example 2 ________________________
g. Fighting others without provocation ____________	Example 1 ________________________
________________________________	Example 2 ________________________
h. Intimidating, bullying, or victimizing other students ____________	Example 1 ________________________
________________________________	Example 2 ________________________
i. Expressing extremely negative feelings about school ____________	Example 1 ________________________
________________________________	Example 2 ________________________
j. Testing classroom and school rules to extreme limits ____________	Example 1 ________________________
________________________________	Example 2 ________________________

2. Rank-order the behaviors defined above according to how hurtful they are to you, that is, according to how much they get you into trouble now. Rank as No. 1 the most hurtful behavior, rank as No. 2 the next most hurtful behavior, and so on; mark as N/A (not applicable) the behaviors that do not get you into trouble.

Behaviors	*Rank-order*
a. Disruptive in class	________
b. Disrespectful and discourteous to others	________
c. Stealing or destroying others' property	________
d. Using excessive profanity (bad words) or verbal aggression	________
e. Uncooperative in school-related group activities	________
f. Not obeying commands from authority figures	________
g. Fighting others without provocation	________
h. Intimidating, bullying, or victimizing other students	________
i. Expressing extremely negative feelings about school	________
j. Testing classroom and school rules to extreme limits	________

3. Why did you rank-order these behaviors the way you did?

____

____

____

____

____

Homework: During the coming week, think about these behaviors and how you rank-ordered them. Perhaps the more you face these behaviors instead of avoiding them, the easier it will be for you to forget about them and for them to have no effect on your behavior. Before going on with the next practice exercise, answer these two questions in writing:

1. What w ill happen to you if you go on with the same hurtful and troublesome behaviors?

____

____

____

____

____

2. What would happen to you if you were to change these behaviors from hurtful to helpful and from troublesome to trouble free?

____
____
____
____
____

Standard Practice Exercise for School Conduct Problems

Practice Exercise No. ____ Title of Behavior ____________________

Name ____________________ Sex ________ Date ________

The purpose of this practice exercise is to understand more about the behavior listed in the title above.

1. How does this behavior apply to you?

   Please explain in detail.

____
____
____
____
____

a. Practically every day ________
b. Once a week ________
c. A couple of times a month ________
d. Once a month ________
e. Once every 6 months ________
f. Once a year ________
g. Once every few years ________

2. How often do you behave this way?

   Please explain further:

____
____
____
____
____

3. How did this behavior come about? Do you remember when it started? Check which answer fits best:

   a. When I was a child (younger than 5 years of age) ________
   b. When I was in elementary school ________
   c. When I was in middle school ________
   d. When I was in high school ________
   e. Any other time ________

   Please explain further:

____
____
____
____
____

4. Is this behavior acceptable (cool, OK) or unacceptable (not cool, not OK) to you? Why is this behavior acceptable (OK) to you?
   Please explain:

____
____
____
____
____

5. Give three specific examples of how this behavior got you into trouble in the past.

   Example 1:

____
____
____
____
____

   Example 2:

____
____
____
____
____

Example 3:

6. Give three specific examples of how this behavior gets you into trouble now.

Example 1:

Example 2:

Example 3:

7. Give three specific examples of how this behavior will get you into trouble in the future.

Example 1:

Example 2:

____

Example 3:

____

Homework: Next week, pretend doing this behavior by writing it on paper at preset times (for instance, at 8 a.m., 12 noon, 4 or 7 p.m.) on at least 3 days (Monday, Wednesday, and Friday, or Tuesday, Thursday, and Saturday). It may sound strange to you to be asked to repeat this behavior, especially when it is so hurtful and troublesome to you. However, keep in mind that if you can start it, you can learn to control it. If you can learn to control it, you may be able to let go of it. Otherwise, this behavior may come back when you will be the one who is hurt. Each time you pretend doing this behavior, write down what you thought would happen in detail. Make sure to answer in writing the following four questions:

a. What behavior did you start?
b. How did you start it?
c. How did it end?
d. What did this behavior get you?

Time 1 (write the time you started__________)

a. ____

b. ____

c. ____

d. ______________________________
____
____

Time 2 (write the time you started__________)

a. ______________________________
____
____

b. ______________________________
____
____

c. ______________________________
____
____

d. ______________________________
____
____

Time 3 (write the time you started__________)

a. ______________________________
____
____

b. ______________________________
____
____

c. ______________________________
____
____

d. ______________________________
____
____

Please check which of the following shows how you feel about this practice exercise:

a. Completely useless ________
b. Somewhat useless ________
c. So-so ________
d. Somewhat useful ________
e. Extremely useful ________

Explain in greater detail how you feel about this practice exercise and what you got out of it.

____
____
____
____
____

Concluding Feedback Form for School Conduct Problems

Name ______________________ Sex ________ Date ____________

The purpose of this concluding feedback form is to review whether this practice exercise was helpful to you or not.

____
____

1. Please check the answer that best fits how you feel about this practice exercise:

   a. I did not like working on this practice exercise at all. I wish I never saw it. ________
   b. I did not like this practice exercise at all, but I am glad I got to work on it. ________
   c. I am delighted I got a chance to work on this practice exercise. ________
   d. I am not only delighted about working on this practice exercise, but I wish all children who suffer from the same painful experience had a chance to work on it. ________

2. How helpful was it to work on this practice exercise? Please check the answer that applies to you:

a. Not helpful at all	______	c. Helpful	______
b. Somewhat helpful	______	d. Very helpful	______

3. Which practice exercise did you like best? Rank as No. 1 the one that you liked best, rank as No. 2 the one you liked next best, and so on; mark as N/A the ones you did not like at all or did not apply to you.

4. Why did you rank-order practice exercises the way you did?

Practice Exercises	*Rank-order*
a. Disruptive in class	________
b. Disrespectful and discourteous to others	________
c. Stealing or destroying others' property	________
d. Using excessive profanity (bad words) or verbal aggression	________
e. Uncooperative in school-related group activities	________
f. Not obeying commands from authority figures	________
g. Fighting others without provocation	________
h. Intimidating, bullying, or victimizing other students	________
i. Expressing extremely negative feelings about school	________
j. Testing classroom and school rules to extreme limits	________

____
____
____
____
____

5. Feel free to write any comments that might improve this practice exercise.

____
____
____
____
____

School Social Skills

The purpose of this practice exercise is to help you get along with grown-ups in better ways than you may have done in the past.

Practice Exercise 1. Relations with Adults

Name ______________________ Sex _______ Date ____________

The purpose of this practice exercise is to find out which relations skills you need to learn in order to deal positively and successfully with adults.

1. Below is a list of behaviors you need to learn to get along with grown-ups. Write what each behavior means to you. If you do not know it, look it up in a dictionary. If necessary, ask a grown-up to tell you what that behavior means, then write it down. Then give two examples of what each behavior means.

Behavior	*Definitions and Examples*
a. Follows verbal instructions	Example 1 ____________
____________	____________
____________	Example 2 ____________
____________	____________
b. Accepts criticism	Example 1 ____________
____________	____________
____________	Example 2 ____________
____________	____________
c. Accepts no for an answer	Example 1 ____________
____________	____________
____________	Example 2 ____________
____________	____________
d. Greets familiar adults	Example 1 ____________
____________	____________
____________	Example 2 ____________
____________	____________
e. Introduces self	Example 1 ____________
____________	____________
____________	Example 2 ____________
____________	____________

f. Makes requests ______________________ Example 1 ______________________
____
______________________ Example 2 ______________________
______________________ ______________________

g. Gives compliments ______________________ Example 1 ______________________
____
______________________ Example 2 ______________________
______________________ ______________________

h. Accepts compliments ______________________ Example 1 ______________________
____
______________________ Example 2 ______________________
______________________ ______________________

i. Makes conversation ______________________ Example 1 ______________________
____
______________________ Example 2 ______________________
______________________ ______________________

j. Apologizes ______________________ Example 1 ______________________
____
______________________ Example 2 ______________________
______________________ ______________________

k. Volunteers ______________________ Example 1 ______________________
____
______________________ Example 2 ______________________
______________________ ______________________

2. Now that you know what each behavior means, rank-order the behaviors you want to work on to learn to get along with grown-ups in better ways than you have done in the past. Rank as No. 1 the behavior you want to learn first, rank as No. 2 the behavior you want to learn next, and so on, until you have rank-ordered all the behaviors listed below according to how much you want to learn them.

Behaviors	*Rank-order*	*Behaviors*	*Rank-order*
a. Follows verbal instructions	________	g. Gives compliments	________
b. Accepts criticism	________	h. Accepts compliments	________
c. Accepts no for an answer	________	i. Makes conversation	________
d. Greets familiar adults	________	j. Apologizes	________
e. Introduces self	________	k. Volunteers	________
f. Makes requests	________		

3. Explain why you ranked ordered these behaviors the way you did.

____

____

____

____

Homework: During the coming week, think whether you do not want to change these behaviors and not get along with grown-ups, or whether you do want to learn to get along with grown-ups. What will happen to you if you do not get along with grown-ups? What will happen to you if you do learn how to get along with grown-ups? Write down your answers to these questions and give them to whoever is working with you on this practice exercise.

Final Follow-Up Form for School Social Skills Relations with Adults

Name ______________________ Sex ____ Date __________

The purpose of this form is to review whether this practice exercise was helpful to you or not.

1. Please check the answer that best fits how you feel about this practice exercise:

   a. I did not like working on this practice exercise at all. I wish I never saw it. ________
   b. I did not like this practice exercise at all, but I am glad I got to work on it. ________
   c. I am delighted I got a chance to work on this practice exercise. ________
   d. I am not only delighted about working on this practice exercise, but I wish all children who cannot get along with grown-ups had a chance to work on it. ________

2. How helpful was it to work on this practice exercise? Please check the answer that applies to you:

   a. Not helpful at all ______ c. Helpful ______
   b. Somewhat helpful ______ d. Very helpful ______

3. Which practice exercise did you like best? Rank as No. 1 the one that you liked best, rank as No. 2 the one you liked next best, and so on; mark as N/A the ones you did not like at all or did not apply to you.

Behaviors	*Rank-order*	*Behaviors*	*Rank-order*
a. Follows verbal instructions	________	g. Gives compliments	________
b. Accepts criticism	________	h. Accepts compliments	________
c. Accepts no for an answer	________	i. Makes conversation	________
d. Greets familiar adults	________	j. Apologizes	________
e. Introduces self	________	k. Volunteers	________
f. Makes requests	________		

4. Why did you rank-order the practice exercises the way you did?

____

____

____

____

____

5. Feel free to write any comments that might improve this practice exercise.

____

____

____

____

____

Practice Exercise 1. Peer Relations

Name ______________________________ Sex ___Date ______

The purpose of this practice exercise is to help you get along better with your classmates in school and on the playground.

The purpose of this practice exercise is to find out what behaviors make it very hard for you to get along with your classmates.

1. Below there is a list of behaviors that make it very hard for you to get along with your classmates. Explain what each behavior means; if necessary, ask a grown-up to tell you what that behavior means or look it up in a dictionary. Write down its meaning as you understand it and give two examples of the behavior.

Behavior	*Definitions and Examples*
a. Angry and hostile to classmates	Example 1 ______
______	______
______	Example 2 ______
______	______
b. Resists classmates' pressure	Example 1 ______
______	______
______	Example 2 ______
______	______
c. Reports classmates' behavior	Example 1 ______
______	______
______	Example 2 ______
______	______

2. How does each behavior make it hard for you to get along with your classmates? Explain and give two examples of how that behavior applies to you.

Behaviors	*Explanations and Examples*
a. Angry and hostile to classmates	Example 1 ______
______	______
______	Example 2 ______
______	______
b. Resists classmates' pressure	Example 1 ______
______	______
______	Example 2 ______
______	______
c. Reports classmates' behavior	Example 1 ______
______	______
______	Example 2 ______
______	______

3. What does each behavior get you? Explain what you gain from behaving in any of those three ways. Explain and give two examples of what you gain from that behavior.

Behavior Explanations and Examples

a. Angry and hostile to classmates Example 1 ____________

____________ ____________

____________ Example 2 ____________

____________ ____________

b. Resists classmates' pressure Example 1 ____________

____________ ____________

____________ Example 2 ____________

____________ ____________

c. Reports classmates' behavior Example 1 ____________

____________ ____________

____________ Example 2 ____________

____________ ____________

Homework: During the coming week, think about whether you want to get along with your classmates or whether you do not want to get along with them.

1. What will happen to you if you do not get along with them?

____

____

____

____

____

2. What will happen to you if you do get along with them?

____

____

____

____

____

Write down your answers and give them to whoever is working with you on this practice exercise.

Practice Exercise 1. School Rules

Name______________________________ Sex___Date__________

The purpose of this practice exercise is to help you follow school rules.

The purpose of this practice exercise is to find out whether you follow school rules or not.

1. What happens to you if you do not follow school rules? Check which answer applies to you best:

a. Reprimand from teacher	____	d. Transferred to a special school	____
b. Sent to principal's office	____	e. Not being promoted to next grade	____
c. Suspended from school	____	f. Other	____ (explain):

2. How often do you break school rules? Check which answer applies to you:

a. Almost every day	____	d. About once a month	____
b. Every other day	____	e. Once a year	____
c. At least once a week	____	f. Never	____

3. Below is a list of school rules that need to be followed if you want to do well in school. Of course, if you do not want to do well in school, you do not have to follow them. Regardless, you need to explain what each rule means to you. Explain and give two examples of what that rule means.

School Rule	*Explanations and Examples*
a. Responsibility with school supplies and property ____________	Example 1 ____________
____________	____________
____________	Example 2 ____________
____________	____________
b. Keeping good school attendance	Example 1 ____________
____________	____________
____________	Example 2 ____________
____________	____________
c. Following school dress code	Example 1 ____________
____________	____________
____________	Example 2 ____________
____________	____________

d. Keeping neat personal appearance ______________ Example 1 ______________
______________ Example 2 ______________
____

e. Walking quietly in school building ______________ Example 1 ______________
______________ Example 2 ______________
____

f. Not keeping dangerous weapons or drugs ______________ Example 1 ______________
______________ Example 2 ______________
____

g. Honesty ______________ Example 1 ______________
______________ Example 2 ______________
____

4. What happens to you if you break any of these rules? Please give a general result and then give two examples of what happens to you if you break any of these rules.

School Rules | *What Happens if You Break Them*

a. Responsibility with school supplies and property ______________ Example 1 ______________
______________ Example 2 ______________
____

b. Keeping good school attendance ______________ Example 1 ______________
______________ Example 2 ______________
____

c. Following school dress code ______________ Example 1 ______________
______________ Example 2 ______________
____

d. Keeping neat personal appearance ______________ Example 1 ______________
______________ Example 2 ______________
____

e. Walking quietly in school building Example 1 ______________

______________________________ ______________________________

______________________________ Example 2 ______________

______________________________ ______________________________

f. Not keeping dangerous weapons or drugs ______________ Example 1 ______________

______________________________ ______________________________

______________________________ Example 2 ______________

______________________________ ______________________________

g. Honesty Example 1 ______________

______________________________ ______________________________

______________________________ Example 2 ______________

______________________________ ______________________________

5. Do you enjoy breaking school rules? How does it make you feel when you break a school rule and you get punished for doing it? Please explain.

____

____

____

____

____

Homework: During the coming week, think whether you want to go on breaking school rules and being punished for it, or whether you want to quit breaking school rules.

1. What will happen to you if you keep breaking school rules?

____

____

____

2. What will happen to you if you do not break school rules?

____

____

____

It is up to you to make up your mind as to whether you want to go on breaking school rules or follow them. Nobody will do it for you and you will be the one who will be hurt by what you are doing. Write down your answers and give them to whoever is working with you on this practice exercise.

Practice Exercise 1. Classroom Behavior

Name ______________________________ Sex ___ Date _________

The purpose of this practice exercise on classroom behavior is to find out which behaviors get you into trouble in the classroom and in school.

The purpose of this practice exercise is to help you do better in the classroom and in school.

1. Below there is a list of behaviors you need to learn to get along with grown-ups. Write what each behavior means to you. If necessary, ask a grown-up to tell you what that behavior means, and then write it down. Give two examples of what each behavior means to you.

Behavior	*Meanings and Examples*
a. Listening to the eacher _________	Example 1 _____________________
______________________________	______________________________
______________________________	Example 2 _____________________
______________________________	______________________________
b. Participating in discussions	Example 1 _____________________
______________________________	______________________________
______________________________	Example 2 _____________________
______________________________	______________________________
c. Contributing to group projects	Example 1 _____________________
______________________________	______________________________
______________________________	Example 2 _____________________
______________________________	______________________________
d. Remaining on task ___________	Example 1 _____________________
______________________________	______________________________
______________________________	Example 2 _____________________
______________________________	______________________________
e. Completing homework assignments	Example 1 _____________________
______________________________	______________________________
______________________________	Example 2 _____________________
______________________________	______________________________

f. Asking permission

Example 1 ______________________

____

Example 2 ______________________

____

2. Now that you know what each behavior means, rank-order these behaviors according to the behavior you want to work on to learn to get along with grown-ups in better ways than you have done in the past. Rank as No. 1 the behavior you want to learn first, rank as No. 2 the behavior you want to learn next, and so on, until you have rank-ordered all the behaviors listed below according to how much you want to learn them.

Behaviors	*Rank-order*	*Behaviors*	*Rank-order*
a. Listening to the teacher	________	d. Remaining on tasks	________
b. Participating in discussions	________	e. Completing homework	________
c. Contributing to group projects	________	f. Asking permission	________

3. Explain why you rank-ordered these behaviors the way you did.

____
____
____
____
____

Homework: During the coming week, think about whether you want to change these behaviors and not behave well in class, or whether you do want to learn do well in class and in school.

1. What will happen to you if you do not do well in class and in school?

____
____
____
____

2. What will happen to you if you do well in class and in school?

____
____
____
____

Standard Practice Exercise No.____ for any School Social Skills Practice exercise

Title (name of behavior) ______________________________

Name ____________________________ Sex ______ Date _____

The purpose of this practice exercise is to understand more about how the behavior listed in the title above got you into trouble in school.

1. How does this behavior apply to you? Explain in detail.

____
____
____
____
____

2. How often do you behave this way?

   a. Practically every day _____
   b. Once a week _____
   c. A couple of times a month _____
   d. Once a month _____
   e. Once every 6 months _____
   f. Once a year _____
   g. Once every few years _____

   Explain further:

____
____
____
____
____

3. How did this behavior come about? Do you remember when it started? Check which answer fits best:

   a. When I was a child (younger than 5 years of age) _________
   b. When I was in elementary school _________
   c. When I was in middle school _________
   d. When I was in high school _________
   e. After high school _________
   f. Any other time _________

Explain further:

4. Are you pleased and proud of this behavior? If you are pleased and proud, write why.

5. Give three specific examples of how this behavior got you into trouble in school in the past.

   Example 1:

   Example 2:

   Example 3:

6. Give three specific examples of how this behavior gets you into trouble in school now

Example 1:

Example 2:

Example 3:

7. Give three specific examples of how this behavior will get you into trouble in school in the future.

Example 1:

Example 2:

Example 3:

____

____

____

____

____

Homework: Next week, plan to bring about or repeat this behavior at preset times (for instance, at 8 a.m., 12 noon, 4 or 7 p.m.) on at least 3 days (Monday, Wednesday, and Friday, or Tuesday, Thursday, and Saturday). It may sound strange to you to be asked to repeat this behavior. However, keep in mind that if you can start it, you can control it. If you can learn to control it, you may be able to let go of it. Otherwise, the behavior may come back when you least expect it; that is, the more you avoid this behavior now, the more it might haunt you in the future. For each time you start this behavior, write down what happened in detail. Make sure to answer in writing the following four questions:

a. What behavior did you start?
b. How did you start it?
c. How did it end?
d. What did this behavior get you?

Time 1 (write the time you started__________)

a. ____

b. ____

c. ____

d. ____

Time 2 (write the time you started__________)

a. ____

b. ____

____

____

c. ____

____

____

d. ____

____

____

Time 3 (write the time you started__________)

a. ____

____

____

b. ____

____

____

c. ____

____

____

d. ____

____

____

Check which of the following indicates how you feel about this practice exercise:

a. Completely useless _____
b. Somewhat useless _____
c. So-so _____
d. Somewhat useful _____
e. Extremely useful _____

Explain in greater detail how you feel about this practice exercise and what you got out of it.

____

____

____

____

____

Final Follow-Up Form for School Social Skills Classroom Behaviors

Name ______________________________ Sex _____ Date __________

The purpose of this practice exercise is to review whether this practice exercise was helpful to you or not.

1. Please select which statement best fits how you feel about this practice exercise:

   a. I did not like working on this practice exercise at all. I wish I never saw it. ________
   b. I did not like this practice exercise at all, but I am glad I got to work on it. ________
   c. I am delighted I got a chance to work on this practice exercise. ________
   d. I am not only delighted about working on this practice exercise, but I wish all children who cannot get along in the classroom had a chance to work on it. ________

2. How helpful was it to work on this practice exercise? Please check the answer that applies to you:

   a. Not helpful at all ____ c. Helpful ____
   b. Somewhat helpful ____ d. Very helpful ____

3. Which practice exercise did you like best? Rank as No. 1 the one that you liked best, rank as No. 2 the one you liked next best, and so on; mark as N/A the ones you did not like at all or did not apply to you.

Behaviors	*Rank order*	*Behaviors*	*Rank order*
a. Listening to the teacher	________	d. Remaining on tasks	________
b. Participating in discussions	________	e. Completing homework practice exercises	________
c. Contributing to group projects	________	f. Asking permission	________

4. Why did you rank-order the practice exercises the way you did?

____
____
____
____
____

5. Feel free to write any comments that might improve this practice exercise.

____
____
____
____
____

Unusual or Troublesome Behavior

The purpose of this practice exercise is to help you deal with unusual or troublesome behavior that might get you into trouble.

Practice Exercise 1. Unusual or Troublesome Behavior

Name ________________________ Sex _____ Date ________

The purpose of this practice exercise is to help you understand which behaviors seem unusual and seem to get you into trouble.

1. Below are unusual behaviors that can get you into trouble. Define them to the best of your ability. You may use a dictionary, or you may ask your teachers, friends, or whoever knows what each of these words means. Write down what you understand about what each word means to you and give two examples of that behavior

Unusual Behavior	*Definitions and Examples*
a. Irritability ______________	Example 1 ______________
______________	______________
______________	Example 2 ______________
______________	______________
b. Agitation ______________	Example 1 ______________
______________	______________
______________	Example 2 ______________
______________	______________
c. Lethargy______________	Example 1 ______________
______________	______________
______________	Example 2 ______________
______________	______________

d. Social withdrawal ______________ Example 1 ______________
______________ ______________
______________ Example 2 ______________
______________ ______________

e. Repetitions ______________ Example 1 ______________
______________ ______________
______________ Example 2 ______________
______________ ______________

f. Hyperactivity ______________ Example 1 ______________
______________ ______________
______________ Example 2 ______________
______________ ______________

g. Noncompliance ______________ Example 1 ______________
______________ ______________
______________ Example 2 ______________
______________ ______________

h. Inappropriate speech ______________ Example 1 ______________
______________ ______________
______________ Example 2 ______________
______________ ______________

2. Now that you have defined each word in the list above, rank-order these behaviors according to how troublesome they are for you. In the first column ("Yours"), rank as No. 1 the behavior that gets you into the most trouble, rank as No. 2 the behavior that gets you into trouble next, and so on, until you have ranked all the behaviors up to No. 8, the behavior that gets you into the least trouble.

Behavior	*Yours*	*Rank-orders Test Results*	*Difference*	*Final Rank-order*
a. Irritability	______	______	______	______
b. Agitation	______	______	______	______
c. Lethargy	______	______	______	______
d. Social withdrawal	______	______	______	______
e. Repetitions	______	______	______	______
f. Hyperactivity	______	______	______	______
g. Noncompliance	______	______	______	______
h. Inappropriate speech	______	______	______	______

3. Why did you rank-order your behaviors the way you did?

____

4. Now ask your teacher, counselor, or whoever is working with you on this practice exercise to write down the rank-order of these behaviors according to the test results about the same behaviors. How similar or different are your rank-orders from the rank-orders from the test results? Write why you think they are similar or different. Talk it over with your teachers and together come up with a final rank-order for these behaviors that will give you a way of working to improve them one behavior at a time. The behavior that has the final rank-order of No. 1 is what you will work on next week. The behavior that is rank-ordered as No. 2 is what you will work next, and so on, until all the unusual and troublesome behaviors are dealt with.

Homework: During the coming week, think whether you want to change your unusual or troublesome behavior or not.

1. What will happen to you if you do not change it?

2. What will happen to you if you do change it?

Standard Practice Exercise for Unusual or Troublesome Behavior

Practice exercise No. ____ Title of Behavior ____________________

Name ____________________________ Sex ______ Date __________

The purpose of this practice exercise is to understand more about the behavior listed above.

1. Explain in detail how the behavior listed above applies to you.

____
____
____
____
____

2. How often did this behavior get you into trouble? Check which answer applies to you:

a.	Practically every day	______	e.	Once every 6 months	______
b.	Once a week	______	f.	Once a year	______
c.	A couple of times a month	______	g.	Once every few years	______
d.	Once a month	______			

Explain further:

____
____
____
____
____

3. How did this behavior come about? Do you remember when you started it? Check which answer fits best:

a. When I was a child (younger than 5 years of age) ________
b. In elementary school ________
c. In middle school ________
d. In high school ________

Explain further when this behavior started.

____
____
____
____
____

4. How did this behavior get you in trouble? Explain.

____
____
____
____
____

5. Give three specific examples of how this behavior got you in trouble in the past.

Example 1:

Example 2:

Example 3:

6. Give three specific examples of how this behavior gets you in trouble now.

Example 1:

Example 2:

Example 3:

7. Give three specific examples of how this behavior will get you in trouble in the future.

Example 1:

Example 2:

Example 3:

Homework: During the coming week, pretend to repeat this behavior at preset times (for instance, at 8 a.m., 12 noon, 4 or 7 p.m.) on at least 3 days because if you can start it, you can stop it. Write down what you plan will happen in detail. For each time make sure to answer the following four questions:

(a) How did you start it?
(b) What followed?
(c) How did it end?
(d) What did this behavior get you?

Time 1 (write the time you started__________)

a. ____

____

____

b. ____

____

____

c. ____

____

____

d. ____

____

____

Time 2 (write the time you started__________)

a. ____

____

____

b. ____

____

____

c. ____

____

____

d. ____

____

____

Time 3 (write the time you started__________)

a. ____

____

____

b. ____

____

____

c. ____

____

____

d. ____

____

____

Check which of the following indicates what you got out of this practice exercise:

a. Completely useless _____
b. Somewhat useless _____
c. So-so _____
d. Somewhat useful _____
e. Extremely useful _____

Write down how you feel about this homework practice exercise and what you got out of it.

____
____
____
____
____

Concluding Follow-Up Form for Unusual or Troublesome Behavior

Name ______________________ Sex _______ Date ___________

The purpose of this final follow-up form is to review whether this practice exercise was helpful to you.

____

1. Which answer fits how you feel about this practice exercise?

   a. I did not like working on this practice exercise at all. I wish I never saw it. _______
   b. I did not like this practice exercise, but I am glad I got to work on it. _______
   c. I am happy I got a chance to work on this practice exercise. _______
   d. I am not only delighted about this practice exercise, but I wish all people in trouble with the law had a chance to work on it. _______

2. How helpful was it to work on this practice exercise? Please check the answer that applies to you:

   a. Not helpful at all _____
   b. Somewhat helpful _____
   c. Helpful _____
   d. Very helpful _____

3. Which practice exercise did you like best? Rank as No. 1 the one that you liked best, rank as No. 2 the one you liked next best, and so on, down to the one you did not like at all (No. 13).

Behavior	*Yours*	*Rank-orders Test Result*	*Difference*	*Final Rank-order*
a. Irritability	________	________	________	________
b. Agitation	________	________	________	________
c. Lethargy	________	________	________	________
d. Social withdrawal	________	________	________	________
e. Repetitions	________	________	________	________
f. Hyperactivity	________	________	________	________
g. Noncompliance	________	________	________	________
h. Inappropriate speech	________	________	________	________

4. Now have your teacher, counselor, or whoever is working with you on this practice exercise write down the rank-order of unusual or troublesome behaviors from the second test results. What are the differences between your rank-order and the rank-order from the test-results? Talk it over with the person who is helping you with this practice exercise and together come up with a final rank-order for these behaviors.

5. Now that you have completed this practice exercise, check which of these answers indicates how you feel about it. There is also space for you to explain further, if you want to:

   a. I did not like it at all, a waste of time. I wish I never saw this stupid practice exercise. ________
   b. I did not like it very much, but I want to go on with another practice exercise. ________
   c. I liked it and I want to go on with another practice exercise. ________
   d. I liked it a lot and I wish I had something like this practice exercise earlier. ________
   e. I liked it so much that I wish all young people could get something like this practice exercise to work on their problems. ________

6. Feel free to write any comments that might improve this practice exercise.

____
____
____
____
____
____
____
____
____
____
____

Adults

Butcher Treatment Planning Inventory (BTPI)

The purpose of this practice exercise is to help you become more aware of areas in your life that are perhaps relevant to the development of a specific treatment plan tailor-made for you.

Practice Exercise 1. Becoming Aware of Oneself

Name ______________________ Sex _______ Date ____________

The purpose of this practice exercise is to list some of the most common areas of your personality that are relevant to treatment planning. The remainder of this practice exercise consists of practice exercises that are drawn from this list.

1. Please define in writing what the areas of personality listed below mean to you. If necessary use a dictionary, ask a friend, or ask the professional you are working with at the present time. Give two examples that come to mind to complete each definition.

Areas of Personality to Define with Two Examples

____

____

a. Consistency of self-definition ____ Example 1 ______________

______________________ ______________________

______________________ Example 2 ______________

______________________ ______________________

b. Presentation of self ____________ Example 1 ______________

______________________ ______________________

______________________ Example 2 ______________

______________________ ______________________

c. Reason for seeking treatment ____ Example 1 ______________

______________________ ______________________

______________________ Example 2 ______________

______________________ ______________________

d. Closed-mindedness ____________ Example 1 ______________

______________________ ______________________

______________________ Example 2 ______________

______________________ ______________________

e. Problems in forming relationships ________________ Example 1 ________________ Example 2 ________________

f. Somatization of conflicts ________________ Example 1 ________________ Example 2 ________________

g. Low expectations of therapeutic benefit ________________ Example 1 ________________ Example 2 ________________

h. Self-oriented centeredness ________________ Example 1 ________________ Example 2 ________________

i. Lack of support ________________ Example 1 ________________ Example 2 ________________

j. Seriousness/depression/self-defeating behavior ________________ Example 1 ________________ Example 2 ________________

k. Disabling anxiety ________________ Example 1 ________________ Example 2 ________________

l. Intense anger expression ________________ Example 1 ________________ Example 2 ________________

m. Anger turned against the self ________________ Example 1 ________________ Example 2 ________________

n. Unusual thinking or bizarre beliefs Example 1 ____________________

________________________________ ____________________________

________________________________ Example 2 ____________________

________________________________ ____________________________

2. Now rank-order this list according to how much each area of personality applies to you and according to its strength and in comparison to other areas. Rank as No. 1 the area that applies to you the most, rank as No. 2 the area that applies to you second most, and so on, until the that applies to you the least (No. 14).

Areas	*Rank-order*
a. Consistency of self-description	______
b. Presentation of self	______
c. Reason for seeking treatment	______
d. Closed-mindedness	______
e. Problems in forming relationships	______
f. Somatization of conflicts	______
g. Low expectations of therapeutic benefit	______
h. Self-oriented centeredness	______
i. Lack of support	______
j. Seriousness/depression/self-defeating behavior	______
k. Disabling anxiety	______
l. Intense anger expression	______
m. Anger turned against the self	______
n. Unusual thinking or bizarre beliefs	______

3. Write why you ranked the list the way you just did.

____

____

____

____

____

4. Check which of the following indicates what you got out of this practice exercise:

a. Completely useless ______ d. Somewhat useful ______
b. Somewhat useless ______ e. Extremely useful ______
c. So-so ______

Homework: During the coming week, think about the areas listed above and write down how helpful or hurtful they are for you.

____
____
____
____
____

Standard Format for Most Practice Exercises in This Section

Practice Exercise No. ____: Title of Area, Behavior, or Troublesome thoughts: _____

Name ________________________ Sex _________ Date ___________

The purpose of this practice exercise is to understand more about the area listed in the title.

____

1. How is this area relevant to you? Explain in detail.

____
____
____
____
____
____

2. How often are you aware of this area? Check which answer applies to you:

a.	Practically every day	_____	e.	Once every 6 months	_____
b.	Once a week	_____	f.	Once a year	_____
c.	A couple of times a month	_____	g.	Once every few years	_____
d.	Once a month	_____	h.	Explain further:	_____

3. Can you remember how this area came about? Do you remember when you started becoming aware of it? Check which answer fits best:

a. When I was a child (younger than 5 years of age) _________
b. When I was in elementary school _________
c. When I was in middle school _________
d. When I was in high school _________
e. After high school _________
f. Any other time _________

4. Explain further:

5. Did this area ever get you in trouble? Explain.

9. Give three specific examples of how this area got you in trouble (if at all).

Example 1:

Example 2:

Example 3:

Homework: Next week, in order for you to become more aware of yourself ("Start it if you want to stop it!"), keep in mind the area you just worked on in this practice exercise, and plan, recall, or pretend to repeat the behavior in that area at preset times (for instance, at 8 a.m., 12 noon, 4 or 7 p.m.), at least three times. Write down what happened in detail. For each time make sure to answer in writing the following four questions:

(a) How did you start it?
(b) What followed?
(c) How did it end?
(d) What did this behavior get you?

Time 1 (write the time you started__________)

a. ____
____
____

b. ____
____
____

c. ____
____
____

d. ____
____
____

Time 2 (write the time you started__________)

a. ____
____
____

b. ____
____
____

c. ____
____
____

d. ____
____
____

Time 3 (write the time you started__________)

a. ____
____
____

b. ____
____
____

c. ____
____
____

d. ____
____
____

Check which of the following indicates what you got out of this practice exercise:

a. Completely useless ______
b. Somewhat useless ______
c. So-so ______
d. Somewhat useful ______
e. Extremely useful ______

Feel free to explain how you feel about the homework practice exercise and what you got out of it.

____
____
____
____
____
____
____
____
____
____
____
____

Concluding Feedback Form for Butcher Practice Exercise

Name ________________________ Sex ____ Date ______

The purpose of this concluding feedback form is to review whether this practice exercise was helpful to you or not.

1. Please check the answer that best fits how you feel about this practice exercise:

   a. I did not like working on this practice exercise at all. I wish I never saw it. ________
   b. I did not like this practice exercise at all, but I am glad I got to work on it. ________
   c. I am delighted I got a chance to work on this practice exercise. ________
   d. I am not only delighted about this practice exercise, but I wish all people who start psychological treatment would have a chance to work on it. ________

2. How helpful was it to work on this practice exercise? Please check the answer that applies to you:

a. Not helpful at all	_______	c. Helpful	_______
b. Somewhat helpful	_______	d. Very helpful	_______

3. Which practice exercise did you like best? Rank as No. 1 the one that you liked best, rank as No. 2 the one you liked next best, and so on, down to the one you did not like at all (No. 14).

Area	*Rank-order*
a. Consistency of self-description	________
b. Presentation of self	________
c. Reason for seeking treatment	________
d. Closed-mindedness	________
e. Problems in forming relationships	________
f. Somatization of conflicts	________
g. Low expectations of therapeutic benefit	________
h. Self-oriented centeredness	________
i. Lack of support	________
j. Seriousness/depression/self-defeating behavior	________
k. Disabling anxiety	________
l. Intense anger expression	________
m. Anger turned against the self	________
n. Unusual thinking or bizarre beliefs	________

4. Explain why you rank-ordered the practice exercises the way you did.

____

____

____

5. Which practice exercise was the most helpful to you? Sometimes what we like most is not necessarily the most helpful. Consequently, rank-order the practice exercises according to their helpfulness to you. Rank as No. 1 the most helpful, rank as No. 2 the next most helpful, and so on, down to the least helpful (No. 14).

Area	*Rank-order*
a. Consistency of self-description	________
b. Presentation of self	________
c. Reason for seeking treatment	________
d. Closed-mindedness	________
e. Problems in forming relationships	________
f. Somatization of conflicts	________
g. Low expectations of therapeutic benefit	________
h. Self-oriented centeredness	________

Area	*Rank-order*
i. Lack of support	________
j. Seriousness/depression/self-defeating behavior	________
k. Disabling anxiety	________
l. Intense anger expression	________
m. Anger turned against the self	________
n. Unusual thinking or bizarre beliefs	________

6. Explain why you rank-ordered the practice exercises the way you did.

____

____

7. Feel free to write any comments that might improve this practice exercise.

____

____

____

____

____

____

Single-Score Tests

Axis II Cluster C Internalizing Disorders

These disorders are included in Axis II Cluster C of the *Diagnostic and Statistical Manual of Mental Disorders* (DSM; American Psychiatric Association, 1994). They involve anxiety, depression, fear, and dependency that direct time and energies toward ruminating critically about or against the self, usually making others more important than oneself (L'Abate, 2005).

Beck Depression Inventory

The purpose of this practice exercise is to help you understand the nature of your depression. You will be asked to answer in writing many practice exercises containing a great many questions about the many behaviors that make up your troublesome thoughts. Of course, you do not have to answer any question or complete any practice exercise if you do not want to. Participation in working on this practice exercise is completely voluntary. It is completely up to you whether you want to learn more about yourself and whether you want professionals interested in your welfare to learn more about you. If you complete this practice exercise, it means that you do want to learn more about yourself and that you are interested in improving your troublesome thoughts.

Practice Exercise 1. Understanding Your Depression

Name ______________________________ Sex _____ Date ______

The purpose of this first practice exercise is to understand more about your troublesome thoughts. To learn more about yourself, you will need to explain what the behaviors listed below mean to you. Each behavior, together with other behaviors, very likely makes up your depression. To understand how these behaviors apply to you, you will need the help of a dictionary, of your attending professional, your relatives, your friends, or staff members, if you are at the present time in a clinical facility. Give two examples of each behavior as it applies to you.

Behaviors	*Definitions and Examples*
a. Seriousness ____________________	Example 1 ____________________
____________________	____________________
____________________	Example 2 ____________________
____________________	____________________
b. Pessimism ____________________	Example 1 ____________________
____________________	____________________
____________________	Example 2 ____________________
____________________	____________________
c. Past failures ____________________	Example 1 ____________________
____________________	____________________
____________________	Example 2 ____________________
____________________	____________________
d. Loss of pleasure ____________________	Example 1 ____________________
____________________	____________________
____________________	Example 2 ____________________
____________________	____________________
e. Guilt feelings ____________________	Example 1 ____________________
____________________	____________________
____________________	Example 2 ____________________
____________________	____________________
f. Feeling punished ____________________	Example 1 ____________________
____________________	____________________
____________________	Example 2 ____________________
____________________	____________________
g. Self-dislike ____________________	Example 1 ____________________
____________________	____________________
____________________	Example 2 ____________________
____________________	____________________

h. Self-criticalness ____________________
Example 1 ____________________
Example 2 ____________________

i. Suicidal thoughts ____________________
Example 1 ____________________
Example 2 ____________________

j. Crying ____________________
Example 1 ____________________
Example 2 ____________________

k. Agitation ____________________
Example 1 ____________________
Example 2 ____________________

l. Loss of interest ____________________
Example 1 ____________________
Example 2 ____________________

m. Indecisiveness ____________________
Example 1 ____________________
Example 2 ____________________

n. Worthlessness ____________________
Example 1 ____________________
Example 2 ____________________

o. Loss of energy ____________________
Example 1 ____________________
Example 2 ____________________

p. Changes in sleep ____________________
Example 1 ____________________
Example 2 ____________________

q. Irritability ____________________ Example 1 ____________________
____________________ ____________________
____________________ Example 2 ____________________
____________________ ____________________

r. Changes in appetite ____________________ Example 1 ____________________
____________________ ____________________
____________________ Example 2 ____________________
____________________ ____________________

s. Concentration difficulty ____________________ Example 1 ____________________
____________________ ____________________
____________________ Example 2 ____________________
____________________ ____________________

t. Tiredness and fatigue ____________________ Example 1 ____________________
____________________ ____________________
____________________ Example 2 ____________________
____________________ ____________________

u. Loss of interest in sex ____________________ Example 1 ____________________
____________________ ____________________
____________________ Example 2 ____________________
____________________ ____________________

2. Now that you have completed these definitions, it is important to find out how they apply to you. Rank order each behavior according to how much that particular behavior applies to you. Rank as No. 1 the behavior that applies to you the most, rank as No. 2 the behavior that applies to you next, and so on; mark as N/A the behaviors that do not apply to you at all.

Behaviors	*Rank-order*	*Behaviors*	*Rank-order*
a. Seriousness	________	l. Loss of interest	________
b. Pessimism	________	m. Indecisiveness	________
c. Past failures	________	n. Worthlessness	________
d. Loss of pleasure	________	o. Loss of energy	________
e. Guilt feelings	________	p. Changes in sleep	________
f. Punishment feelings	________	q. Irritability	________
g. Self-dislike	________	r. Changes in appetite	________
h. Self-criticalness	________	s. Concentration difficulty	________
i. Suicidal thoughts	________	t. Tiredness and fatigue	________
j. Crying	________	u. Loss of interest in sex	________
k. Agitation	________		

3. Why did you rank-order these behaviors the way you did?

____
____
____
____

4. Now that you have completed this practice exercise, write how you felt about it. Check which of these answers indicates how you felt about it. There is also space for you to explain further, if you want to:

   a. I did not like this practice exercise at all. I want to quit this stupid practice exercise. ______
   b. I did not like this practice exercise very much, but I want to go on with this practice exercise. ______
   c. I liked this practice exercise and I want to go on with this practice exercise. ______
   d. I liked this practice exercise a lot and I wish I had something like this practice exercise years ago. ______
   e. I liked it so much that I wish all people in psychiatric hospitals or in need of psychiatric help could get something like this practice exercise to work on. ______

Discuss your completed practice exercise with whoever has given it to you.

Homework: During the coming week, think more about these behaviors and whether you want to change the rank-order as listed above, or start working on the next practice exercise.

Standard Format for Most Internalizing Disorders

Practice Exercise No. ____: Name or Title of Behavior: ______________________
____

Name ________________________________ Sex ________ Date ______

The purpose of this practice exercise is to understand more about the behavior listed above.

1. How does this behavior apply to you? Explain in detail.

____
____
____
____
____

2. How often do you feel this behavior?

a. Practically every day	_____	e. Once every 6 months	_____
b. Once a week	_____	f. Once a year	_____
c. A couple of times a month	_____	g. Once every few years	_____
d. Once a month	_____		

3. Explain further:

____
____
____
____
____

4. How did this behavior come about? Do you remember when you started it? Check which answer fits best:

a. When I was a child (younger than 5 years of age)	_______
b. When I was in elementary school	_______
c. When I was in middle school	_______
d. When I was in high school	_______
e. After high school	_______
f. Any other time	_______

5. Explain further:

____
____
____
____
____
____

6. Was this behavior acceptable or unacceptable? Why? Explain.

____
____
____
____
____
____

7. Give three specific examples of how this behavior affects you in the present.

Example 1:

____
____
____
____

Example 2:

____
____
____
____

Example 3:

____
____
____
____

Homework: Next week plan to repeat this behavior at preset times (for instance, at 8 a.m., 12 noon, 4 or 7 p.m.) on at least 3 days (Monday, Wednesday, and Friday, or Tuesday, Thursday, and Saturday). If you can start it, you can stop it. Write down what happened in detail. For each time you start this behavior, make sure to answer in writing the following four questions:

a. How did you start it?
b. What followed?
c. How did it end?
d. What did this behavior get you?

Time 1 (write the time you started__________)

a. ____
____
____

b. ____
____
____

c. ____
____
____

d. ____

Time 2 (write the time you started__________)

a. ____

b. ____

c. ____

d. ____

Time 3 (write the time you started__________)

a. ____

b. ____

c. ____

d. ____

Check which of the following indicates how you feel about this practice exercise:

a. Completely useless _______
b. Somewhat useless _______
c. So-so _______
d. Somewhat useful _______
e. Extremely useful _______

Explain in greater detail how you feel about this practice exercise and what you got out of it.

____

Concluding Follow-Up Form for Beck Depression Inventory

Name ________________________________ Sex ____ Date _______

The purpose of this concluding follow-up form is to review whether this practice exercise was helpful to you or not.

1. Please check the answer that best fits how you feel about this practice exercise:

   a. I did not like working on this practice exercise at all. I wish I never saw it. ________
   b. I did not like this practice exercise at all, but I am glad I got to work on it. ________
   c. I am delighted I got a chance to work on this practice exercise. ________
   d. I am not only delighted about working on this practice exercise, but I wish all people with depression had a chance to work on it ________

2. How helpful was it to work on this practice exercise? Please check the answer that applies to you:

   a. Not helpful at all ____ c. Helpful ____
   b. Somewhat helpful ____ d. Very helpful ____

3. Which practice exercise did you like best? Rank as No. 1 the one that you liked best, rank as No. 2 the one you liked next best, and so on; mark as N/A the ones you did not like at all or did not apply to you.

Behaviors	*Rank-order*	*Behaviors*	*Rank-order*
a. Seriousness	________	l. Loss of interest	________
b. Pessimism	________	m. Indecisiveness	________
c. Past failures	________	n. Worthlessness	________
d. Loss of pleasure	________	o. Loss of energy	________
e. Guilt feelings	________	p. Changes in sleep	________
f. Punishment feelings	________	q. Irritability	________
g. Self-dislike	________	r. Changes in appetite	________
h. Self-criticalness	________	s. Concentration difficulty	________
i. Suicidal thoughts	________	t. Tiredness and fatigue	________
j. Crying	________	u. Loss of interest in sex	________
k. Agitation	________		

4. Sometimes what we like most is not necessarily the most helpful. Which practice exercise was the most helpful to you? Rank as No. 1 the most helpful, rank as No. 2 the next most helpful, and so on, down to the least helpful practice exercise; mark as N/A the practice exercises that did not apply to you.

Behaviors	*Rank-order*	*Behaviors*	*Rank-order*
a. Seriousness	________	l. Loss of interest	________
b. Pessimism	________	m. Indecisiveness	________
c. Past failures	________	n. Worthlessness	________
d. Loss of pleasure	________	o. Loss of energy	________
e. Guilty feelings	________	p. Changes in sleep	________
f. Punishment feelings	________	q. Irritability	________
g. Self-dislike	________	r. Changes in appetite	________
h. Self-criticalness	________	s. Concentration difficulty	________
i. Suicidal thoughts	________	t. Tiredness and fatigue	________
j. Crying	________	u. Loss of interest in sex	________
k. Agitation	________		

5. Explain why you rank-ordered these behaviors the way you did.

____
____
____
____
____

6. Feel free to write any comments or suggestions that might improve this practice exercise.

____
____
____
____
____

Beck Anxiety Inventory

The purpose of this practice exercise is to help you understand the nature of your anxiety. You will be asked to answer in writing many practice exercises containing a great many questions about the many behaviors that make up this troublesome thoughts. Of course, you do not have to answer any question or complete any practice exercise if you do not want to. Participation is completely voluntary. It is completely up to you whether you want to learn more about yourself and whether you want professionals interested in your welfare to learn more about you. If you complete this practice exercise, it means that you do want to learn more about yourself and that you are interested in improving your troublesome thoughts.

Practice Exercise 1. Understanding Your Anxiety

Name ________________________________ Sex ___ Date _____

The purpose of this first practice exercise is to understand more about your troublesome thoughts. To learn more about yourself, you will need to explain what the behaviors listed below mean to you. Each behavior, together with other behaviors, very likely makes up your anxiety. To understand how these behaviors apply to you, you will need the help of a dictionary, of your attending professional, your relatives, your friends, or staff members, if you are at the present time in a clinical facility. Give two examples to explain how each behavior applies to you.

Behaviors	*Definitions and Examples*
a. Feeling hot	Example 1 ______
______	______
______	Example 2 ______
______	______
b. Feeling wobbly	Example 1 ______
______	______
______	Example 2 ______
______	______
c. Feeling dizzy	Example 1 ______
______	______
______	Example 2 ______
______	______
d. Difficulty in breathing	Example 1 ______
______	______
______	Example 2 ______
______	______
e. Face flushed	Example 1 ______
______	______
______	Example 2 ______
______	______
f. Feeling scared	Example 1 ______
______	______
______	Example 2 ______
______	______
g. Unable to relax	Example 1 ______
______	______
______	Example 2 ______
______	______
h. Fearing the worst	Example 1 ______
______	______
______	Example 2 ______
______	______

i. Feeling terrified

____

____

____

Example 1 ____________________

____

Example 2 ____________________

____

j. Feeling nervous

____

____

____

Example 1 ____________________

____

Example 2 ____________________

____

k. Afraid to lose control

____

____

____

Example 1 ____________________

____

Example 2 ____________________

____

2. Now that you have completed these definitions, it is important to find out how they apply to you. Rank-order each behavior according to how much that particular behavior applies to you. Rank as No. 1 the behavior that applies to you the most, rank as No. 2 the behavior that applies to you next, and so on; mark as N/A the behaviors that do not apply to you at all.

Behaviors	*Rank-order*	*Behaviors*	*Rank-order*
a. Feeling hot	________	g. Unable to relax	________
b. Feeling wobbly	________	h. Fearing the worst	________
c. Feeling dizzy	________	i. Feeling terrified	________
d. Difficulty in breathing	________	j. Feeling nervous	________
e. Face flushed	________	k. Afraid to lose control	________
f. Feeling scared	________		

3. Write why you ranked your behaviors the way you did.

____

____

____

____

____

4. Now that you have completed this practice exercise, write how you felt about it. Check which of these answers indicates how you felt about it. There is also space for you to explain further, if you want to:

   a. I did not like this practice exercise at all. I want to quit this stupid practice exercise. ________
   b. I did not like this practice exercise very much, but I want to go on with this practice exercise. ________
   c. I liked this practice exercise and I want to go on with this practice exercise. ________

d. I liked this practice exercise a lot and I wish I had something like this practice exercise years ago. ________
e. I liked it so much that I wish all people in psychiatric hospitals or in need of psychiatric help could get something like this practice exercise to work on. ________

5. Discuss your completed practice exercise with whoever has given it to you.

Homework: During the coming week, think more about the behaviors covered by these words and whether you want to change the rank-order of these behaviors as listed above, or start working on the next practice exercise.

Concluding Feedback Form for Beck Anxiety Inventory

Name ______________________________ Sex _____ Date ______

The purpose of this concluding feedback form is to review whether this practice exercise was helpful to you or not.

1. Please check the answer that best fits how you feel about this practice exercise:

   a. I did not like working on this practice exercise at all. I wish I never saw it. ________
   b. I did not like this practice exercise at all, but I am glad I got to work on it. ________
   c. I am delighted I got a chance to work on this practice exercise. ________
   d. I am not only delighted about working on this practice exercise, but I wish all people with depression had a chance to work on it. ________

2. How helpful was it to work on this practice exercise? Please check the answer that applies to you:

   a. Not helpful at all ______
   b. Somewhat helpful ______
   c. Helpful ______
   d. Very helpful ______

3. Which practice exercise did you like best? Rank as No. 1 the one that you liked best, rank as No. 2 the one you liked next best, and so on; mark as N/A the ones you did not like at all or did not apply to you.

Behaviors	*Rank-order*	*Behaviors*	*Rank-order*
a. Feeling hot	________	g. Unable to relax	________
b. Feeling wobbly	________	h. Fearing the worst	________
c. Feeling dizzy	________	i. Feeling terrified	________
d. Difficulty in breathing	________	j. Feeling nervous	________
e. Face flushed	________	k. Afraid to lose control	________
f. Feeling scared	________		

4. Sometimes what we like most is not necessarily the most helpful. Which practice exercise was the most helpful to you? Rank as No. 1 the most helpful, rank as No. 2 the next most helpful, and so on, down to the least helpful practice exercise; mark as N/A the practice exercises that did not apply to you.

Behaviors	*Rank-order*	*Behaviors*	*Rank-order*
a. Feeling hot	________	g. Unable to relax	________
b. Feeling wobbly	________	h. Fearing the worst	________
c. Feeling dizzy	________	i. Feeling terrified	________
d. Difficulty in breathing	________	j. Feeling nervous	________
e. Face flushed	________	k. Afraid to lose control	________
f. Feeling scared	________		

5. Explain why you rank-ordered the practice exercises the way you did. How is this ranking different from how much you liked them? Please answer in detail.

____

____

____

____

____

6. Feel free to write any comments or suggestions that might improve this practice exercise.

____

____

____

____

____

Hamilton Anxiety Inventory

The purpose of this practice exercise is to help you understand the nature of your anxiety. You will be asked to answer in writing many practice exercises containing a great many questions about the many behaviors that make up your troublesome thoughts. Of course, you do not have to answer any question or complete any practice exercise if you do not want to. Participation is completely voluntary. It is completely up to you whether you want to learn more about yourself and whether you want professionals interested in your welfare to learn more about you. If you complete this practice exercise, it means that you do want to learn more about yourself and that you are interested in improving your troublesome thoughts.

Practice Exercise 1. Understanding Your Troublesome thoughts

Name ______________________ Sex ___ Date _____

The purpose of this practice exercise is to understand more about your troublesome thoughts. To learn more about yourself, you will need to explain what the behaviors and body parts listed below mean to you. Each behavior, together with other behaviors, very likely makes up your troublesome thoughts. To understand these behaviors and body parts, you will need the help of a dictionary, of your attending professional, your relatives, your friends, or staff members, if you are at the present time in a clinical facility. In addition to each definition, you need to give two examples of how that behavior or body part applies to you or how you understand it in your own words.

Behaviors and Body Parts	*Definitions and Examples*
a. Anxious mood	Example 1 ______
______	______
______	Example 2 ______
______	______
b. Tension	Example 1 ______
______	______
______	Example 2 ______
______	______
c. Muscles	Example 1 ______
______	______
______	Example 2 ______
______	______
d. Body sensations	Example 1 ______
______	______
______	Example 2 ______
______	______
e. Blood and veins	Example 1 ______
______	______
______	Example 2 ______
______	______
f. Respiration	Example 1 ______
______	______
______	Example 2 ______
______	______

g. Stomach ______ Example 1 ______ Example 2 ______

h. Sweating and perspiring ______ Example 1 ______ Example 2 ______

i. Nervous under pressure ______ Example 1 ______ Example 2 ______

j. Insomnia ______ Example 1 ______ Example 2 ______

k. Agitation ______ Example 1 ______ Example 2 ______

l. Mental anxiety ______ Example 1 ______ Example 2 ______

m. Body anxiety ______ Example 1 ______ Example 2 ______

n. Troublesome thoughts about health ______ Example 1 ______ Example 2 ______

o. Fear of losing self ______ Example 1 ______ Example 2 ______

2. Now that you have completed these definitions, it is important to find out how these behaviors and body parts apply to you. Rank-order each one according to how much that particular behavior or body part applies to you. Rank as No. 1 the one that applies to you the most, rank as No. 2 the one that applies to you next, and so on; mark as N/A the ones that do not apply to you at all.

Behaviors and Body Parts	*Rank-order*	*Behaviors and Body Parts*	*Rank-order*
a. Anxious mood		i. Nervous under pressure	________
b. Tension	________	j. Insomnia	________
c. Muscles	________	k. Agitation	________
d. Body sensations	________	l. Mental anxiety	________
e. Circulation	________	m. Body anxiety	________
f. Respiration	________	n. Troublesome thoughts about health	________
g. Stomach	________	o. Fear of losing self	________
h. Sweating and perspiring	________		

3. Write why you ranked the list the way you did.

____
____
____
____
____

4. Now that you have completed this practice exercise, check which of these answers indicates how you felt about it. There is also space for you to explain further, if you want to:

   a. I did not like this practice exercise at all. I want to quit this stupid practice exercise. ________
   b. I did not like this practice exercise very much, but I want to go on with it. ________
   c. I liked the practice exercises in this practice exercise and I willing to work on another practice exercise. ________
   d. I liked this practice exercise a lot and I wish I had something like this practice exercise years ago. ________
   e. I liked it so much that I wish all people in psychiatric hospitals or in need of psychiatric help could get something like this practice exercise to work on. ________

5. Discuss your completed practice exercise with whoever has given it to you.

Homework: During the coming week, think more about the exercise and whether you want to change the rank-orders listed above, or start working on the next practice exercise.

Concluding Feedback Form for Hamilton Anxiety Inventory

Name ________________________________ Sex _____ Date ______

The purpose of this form is to review whether this practice exercise was helpful to you or not.

1. Please check the answer that best fits how you feel about this practice exercise:

   a. I did not like working on this practice exercise at all. I wish I never saw it. _________
   b. I did not like this practice exercise at all, but I am glad I got to work on it. _________
   c. I am delighted I got a chance to work on this practice exercise. _________
   d. I am not only delighted about working on this practice exercise, but I wish all people with my troublesome thoughts had a chance to work on it _________

2. How helpful was it to work on this practice exercise? Please check the answer that applies to you:

a. Not helpful at all	____	c. Helpful	_____
b. Somewhat helpful	____	d. Very helpful	_____

3. Which practice exercise did you like best? Rank as No. 1 the one that you liked best, rank as No. 2 the one you liked next best, and so on; mark as N/A the ones you did not like at all or did not apply to you.

Behaviors and Body Parts	*Rank-order*	*Behaviors and Body Parts*	*Rank-order*
a. Anxious mood	_________	i. Nervous under pressure	_________
b. Tension	_________	j. Insomnia	_________
c. Muscles	_________	k. Agitation	_________
d. Body sensations	_________	l. Mental anxiety	_________
e. Circulation	_________	m. Body anxiety	_________
f. Respiration	_________	n. Troublesome thoughts about health	_________
g. Stomach	_________	o. Fear of losing self	_________
h. Sweating and perspiring	_________		

4. Explain why you rank-ordered the list the way you did.

____

____

____

____

5. Sometimes what we like most is not necessarily the most helpful. Which practice exercise was the most helpful to you? Rank as No. 1 the most helpful, rank as No. 2 the next most helpful, and so on, down to the least helpful practice exercise; mark as N/A the practice exercises that did not apply to you.

Behaviors and Body Parts	*Rank-order*	*Behaviors and Body Parts*	*Rank-order*
a. Anxious mood	________	i. Nervous under pressure	________
b. Tension	________	j. Insomnia	________
c. Muscles	________	k. Agitation	________
d. Body sensations	________	l. Mental anxiety	________
e. Circulation	________	m. Body anxiety	________
f. Respiration	________	n. Troublesome thoughts about health	________
g. Stomach	________	o. Fear of losing self	________
h. Sweating and perspiring	________		

6. Explain why you rank-ordered the list the way you did.

____

____

____

____

____

7. Feel free to write any comments or suggestions that might improve this practice exercise.

____

____

____

____

____

Hamilton Depression Inventory

The purpose of this practice exercise is to help you understand the nature of your depression. You will be asked to answer in writing many practice exercises containing a great many questions about the many behaviors that make up your troublesome thoughts. Of course, you do not have to answer any question or complete any practice exercise if you do not want to. Participation in working on this practice exercise is completely voluntary. It is completely up to you whether you want to learn more about yourself and whether you want professionals interested in your welfare to learn more about you. If you complete this practice exercise, it means that you do want to learn more about yourself and that you are interested in improving your troublesome thoughts.

Practice Exercise 1. Understanding Your Depression

Name ______________________________ Sex ___ Date ______

The purpose of this practice exercise is to understand more about your depression. To learn more about yourself, you will need to explain what the behaviors listed below mean to you. Each behavior, together with other behaviors, very likely makes up your depression. To understand these behaviors, you will need the help of a dictionary, or of your attending professional, your relatives, your friends, or staff members, if you are at the present time in a clinical facility. Give two examples of each definition.

Behaviors	*Definitions*
a. Depressed mood	Example 1 ______________
______________	______________
______________	Example 2 ______________
______________	______________
b. Feelings of guilt	Example 1 ______________
______________	______________
______________	Example 2 ______________
______________	______________
c. Thinking about suicide	Example 1 ______________
______________	______________
______________	Example 2 ______________
______________	______________
d. Insomnia	Example 1 ______________
______________	______________
______________	Example 2 ______________
______________	______________
e. Unable to work and act	Example 1 ______________
______________	______________
______________	Example 2 ______________
______________	______________
f. Motor retardation	Example 1 ______________
______________	______________
______________	Example 2 ______________
______________	______________

g. Feeling sexually inadequate

Example 1

Example 2

h. Loss of weight

Example 1

Example 2

i. Variations from day to night

Example 1

Example 2

j. Helplessness

Example 1

Example 2

k. Hopelessness

Example 1

Example 2

l. Worthlessness

Example 1

Example 2

m. Intellectual retardation

Example 1

Example 2

2. Now that you have completed these definitions, it is important to find out how they apply to you. Rank-order each behavior according to how much that particular behavior applies to you. Rank as No. 1 the behavior that applies to you the most, rank as No. 2 the behavior that applies to you next, and so on; mark as N/A the behaviors that do not apply to you at all.

Behaviors	*Rank-order*	*Behaviors*	*Rank-order*
a. Depressed mood	________	h. Loss of weight	________
b. Feelings of guilt	________	i. Variations during the day	________
c. Thinking about suicide	________	j. Helplessness	________
d. Insomnia	________	k. Hopelessness	________
e. Unable to work and act	________	l. Worthlessness	________
f. Motor retardation	________	m. Intellectual retardation	________
g. Feeling sexually inadequate	________		

3. Write why you ranked your behaviors the way you did.

____

____

____

____

____

4. Now that you have completed this practice exercise, write how you felt about it. Check which of these answers indicates how you felt about it. There is also space for you to explain further, if you want to:

   a. I did not like this practice exercise at all. I want to quit this stupid practice exercise. ________
   b. I did not like this practice exercise very much, but I want to go on with this practice exercise. ________
   c. I liked this practice exercise and I want to work on another practice exercise. ________
   d. I liked this practice exercise a lot and I wish I had something lke this years ago. ________
   e. I liked it so much that I wish all people with the same condition could get something like this practice exercise to work on. ________

4. Discuss your completed practice exercise with whoever has given it to you.

Homework: During the coming week, think more about the behaviors covered in this concluding feedback form and whether you want to change their rank-order as listed above, or start working on another practice exercise.

Concluding Feedback Form for Hamilton Depression Inventory

Name ________________________________ Sex _____ Date ______

The purpose of this concluding feedback form is to review whether this practice exercise was helpful to you or not.

1. Please check which answer best fits how you feel about this practice exercise:

   a. I did not like working on this practice exercise at all. I wish I never saw it. ________
   b. I did not like this practice exercise at all, but I am glad I got to work on it. ________
   c. I am delighted I got a chance to work on this practice exercise. ________
   d. I am not only delighted about working on this practice exercise, but I wish all people with the same condition had a chance to work on it. ________

2. How helpful was it to work on this practice exercise? Please check the answer that applies to you:

   a. Not helpful at ______ c. Helpful _____
   b. Somewhat helpful ______ d. Very helpful _____

3. Which practice exercise did you like best? Rank as No. 1 the one that you liked best, rank as No. 2 the one you liked next best, and so on; mark as N/A the ones you did not like at all or did not apply to you.

Behaviors	*Rank-order*	*Behaviors*	*Rank-order*
a. Depressed mood	________	h. Loss of weight	________
b. Feelings of guilt	________	i. Variations during the day	________
c. Thinking about suicide	________	j. Helplessness	________
d. Insomnia	________	k. Hopelessness	________
e. Unable to work and act	________	l. Worthlessness	________
f. Motor retardation	________	m. Intellectual retardation	________
g. Feeling sexually inadequate	________		

4. Explain why you rank-order the practice exercises the way you did.

____

____

____

____

____

5. Sometimes what we like most is not necessarily the most helpful. Which practice exercise was the most helpful to you? Rank as No. 1 the most helpful, rank as No. 2 the next most helpful, and so on, down to the least helpful practice exercise; mark as N/A the practice exercises that did not apply to you.

Behaviors	*Rank-order*	*Behaviors*	*Rank-order*
a. Depressed mood	________	h. Loss of weight	________
b. Feelings of guilt	________	i. Variations during the day	________
c. Thinking about suicide	________	j. Helplessness	________
d. Insomnia	________	k. Hopelessness	________
e. Unable to work and act	________	l. Worthlessness	________
f. Motor retardation	________	m. Intellectual retardation	________
g. Feeling sexually inadequate	________		

6. Explain why you rank-ordered the practice exercises the way you did.

____
____
____
____
____

7. Feel free to write any comments that might improve this practice exercise.

____
____
____
____
____

Other Troublesome Thoughts

The purpose of this practice exercise is to help you identify your major troublesome thoughts and help you deal with them. Usually there are two different types of troublesome thoughts: those related to self-criticism, and those related to overdependency on others. The evaluation form given below will help you identify which type is more pertinent to you or whether both troublesome thoughts are pertinent. Once a type of troublesome thought is identified, homework practice exercises are administered according to the results of the evaluation checklist given below.

Name __________________________ Age _____ Sex ____ Date _______

The purpose of this checklist is to find what kind of troublesome thoughts is affecting you at the present time. Please read the items below and rate them according to whether they apply to you most of the time, sometimes, or never.

Item	Most of the time	Some of the time	Never
1. Helplessness (feeling completely unable to cope or to deal with a situation)	_____	_____	_____
2. Feelings of worthlessness	_____	_____	_____
3. Loss (feeling completely lost and alone)	_____	_____	_____
4. Feelings of inferiority	_____	_____	_____
5. Abandonment (feeling abandoned and left out)	_____	_____	_____
6. Feeling guilty	_____	_____	_____
7. Comfort (not having anyone to comfort and support you)	_____	_____	_____
8. Feeling like a failure	_____	_____	_____
9. Closeness (not having anyone to be close to and to confide your hurts with)	_____	_____	_____
10. Fear of criticism	_____	_____	_____
11. Love and loss of love (unable to be loved by someone important to you)	_____	_____	_____
12. Perfectionism	_____	_____	_____
13. Protection (feeling no one looks after you)	_____	_____	_____
14. Afraid to make mistakes	_____	_____	_____
15. Nurturance (feeling without sufficient nurturance or care from anybody)	_____	_____	_____
16. Wanting acceptance and approval	_____	_____	_____
17. Rejection (being rejected by someone you love)	_____	_____	_____
18. Wanting to achieve well	_____	_____	_____
19. Overdependence (relying too much on someone else)	_____	_____	_____
20. Self-criticalness (being very hard on yourself)	_____	_____	_____

Instructions for Scoring*

Give two points for each checkmark under "Most of the time," one point for each checkmark under "Sometimes," and zero points for each checkmark under "Never." Then add up all the scores for the odd-numbered statements (1, 3, 5, etc.), and all the scores for the even-numbered statements (2, 4, 6, etc.). Write the totals below:

Totals for odd-numbered statements _____________

Totals for even-numbered statements _____________

* The professional should decide whether the scoring of this rating sheet is to be done by the respondent or by the professional.

If the total for odd-numbered statements is five or more points higher than the total for even-numbered statements, then your troublesome thoughts may stem primarily from depending too much on others. If your total for even-numbered statements is five or more points higher than the total for the odd-numbered statements, then your troublesome thoughts may stem primarily from being too self critical. If your two totals are within 1–4 points of each other, then your troublesome thoughts may stem from both depending too much on others and being too self-critical. Whatever the conclusion, regardless of your scores, rest assured that these troublesome thoughts are normal can be dealt successfully if they are discussed with those who care about you andif you keep on working on this practice exercise.

Practice Exercise 1. Too Many Troublesome Thoughts About Others

Name________________________________Sex __Date_______

1. This practice exercise is for people whose troublesome thoughts are related to breakups, rejections, and conflicts in their relationships with loved ones, past and present, are related to relying too much on others rather than on oneself. How does this practice exercise relate to your troublesome thoughts? Please comment.

____

____

____

____

____

2. These troublesome thoughts may be linked to a variety of past or present dependencies. Please read over the dependency troublesome thoughts that may have brought about your feeling overly serious, unhappy, and even miserable and bad about yourself. After you have read these troublesome thoughts, rank them in order of greatest importance to you. Rank as No. 1 the most important in its relationship to how you feel, rank as No. 2 the second most important as related to how you feel, and so on, down to the least important troublesome thought.

Troublesome Thoughts	*Rank-order*
a. Helplessness (feeling completely unable to cope or to deal with a situation)	________
b. Loss (feeling completely lost and alone)	________
c. Abandonment (feeling abandoned and left out)	________
d. Comfort (not having anyone to comfort and support you)	________
e. Closeness (not having anyone to be close to and to confide your hurts to)	________
f. Love and loss of love (unable to be loved by someone important to you)	________

Troublesome Thoughts	*Rank-order*
g. Protection (feeling you have no one to look after you)	________
h. Nurturance (feeling without sufficient nurturance or care from anybody)	________
I. Rejection (being rejected by someone you love)	________
l. Overdependence (relying too much on someone else)	________
m. Other (write your particular situation that is not listed above)	________

3. Pick the top five ranked dependency troublesome thoughts and write down how and why each of them is related to how you feel about yourself.

   Troublesome thoughts 1. ________________________________
   Troublesome thoughts 2. ________________________________
   Troublesome thoughts 3. ________________________________
   Troublesome thoughts 4. ________________________________
   Troublesome thoughts 5. ________________________________

4. Add whatever you want to make sure that the dependency troublesome thoughts listed above are the most important in relationship to how you feel. It is perfectly all right to change your rank-orders and include a troublesome thoughts that you had ranked differently earlier.

5. The rest of this practice exercise will help you deal with each of the dependency troublesome thoughts you have listed above. You will need to deal with each one once a week. Make sure that you make an appointment with yourself at a preset time at least 24 h ahead. If you have to change this appointment time for any reason, give yourself at least 24 h before working on each practice exercise.

Homework: Write any additional troublesome thoughts, feelings, or thoughts that come to mind during the coming week as you are thinking about dependency troublesome thoughts that lead to how you feel. Discuss these notes with your professional helper, if you have one, or with a friend.

Instructions: Under the title of this standard format for all the following practice exercises of this practice exercise, write the name of the self-critical attitude that is important to you. Start with the attitude rank-ordered as No. 1 for this practice exercise. In the practice exercise following this one, write the attitude ranked No. 2. Follow the same for all the next practice exercises of the attitudes ranked No. 3, No. 4, and No. 5. If you have ranked more than five self-critical attitudes and you want to work on them, write their name in the title of this standard format. This standard format is repeated from one week to another. The title of the practice exercise changes according to the rank-order you have written in the first practice exercise.

Standard Format for all Practice Exercises for Troublesome Thoughts

Practice Exercise No. ______Title of Troublesome thoughts ____________________

Name ___________________________________ Sex ______ Date __________

1. Write how the title of this practice exercise is related to how you feel.

____
____
____
____
____

2. Describe how this troublesome thoughts took place in your life from its very beginning.

____
____
____
____
____

3. What effects has this troublesome thoughts had on your life?

____
____
____
____
____

4. What did you learn from this troublesome thoughts?

____
____
____
____
____

5. How can you change this troublesome thoughts?

____
____
____
____
____

6. What part did you play in the influence of this troublesome thoughts on how you feel about yourself? Explain how you were, in part, responsible for allowing this troublesome thoughts to control your life.

____
____
____
____
____

7. During the next week, think about four possible ways of changing this troublesome thoughts for the better. What should you do to make sure that you will win rather than defeat yourself? You may want to talk these possible ways over with whoever is interested in your life and welfare.

Solution 1:

____
____
____
____
____

Solution 2:

____
____
____
____
____

Solution 3:

____
____
____
____
____

Solution 4:

____
____
____
____
____

Solution 5:

8. After you have made up your mind about which solution would work best for you and others, make sure you practice this solution until it becomes second nature to you. Write down which solution seems the best for you, why you selected it (pros and cons), and how you are going to practice it.

9. You need to practice this solution as soon as possible. Write down each instance when you practiced this solution. What happened?

Practice 1:

Practice 2:

Practice 3:

Practice 4:

10. Feel free to write whatever comments you want to make about this practice exercise and how it applies to you.

Once you have finished this practice exercise and are satisfied with the results, you may then use the same standard format to work on the next troublesome thoughts. Make sure you write the title of the troublesome thoughts at the top of this practice exercise. Note that we cannot go on to the next practice exercise unless this practice exercise is completed.

Practice Exercise 1. Ranking of Self-Critical Troublesome thoughts or Attitudes

Name ______________________ Sex ________ Date ________

1. This practice exercise is for people whose troublesome thoughts are related to poor or negative self-attitudes. How does this practice exercise apply to you?

2. Below you will find a list of self-critical troublesome thoughts or attitudes that are related to how you feel about yourself. Please read this list and rank these self-critical attitudes according to how they apply to you. Rank as No. 1 the attitude that applies to you the most, rank as No. 2 the attitude that applies to you second most, and so on, until the end. The last number would be assigned to the attitude that does not apply to you at all.

Self-Critical Attitudes	*Rank-order*
a. Feelings of worthlessness	________
b. Feelings of inferiority	________
c. Feeling guilty	________
d. Feeling like a failure	________
e. Fear of criticism	________
f. Perfectionism	________
g. Afraid to make mistakes	________
h. Wanting acceptance and approval	________
i. Wanting to achieve well	________
j. Self-criticalness (being very hard on yourself)	________
k. Other (write whatever critical self-attitude applies to you that is not listed above)	________

3. Pick the top five ranked self-critical attitudes that are most related to your depression and explain how and why this attitude is related to how you feel about yourself.

Attitude 1:

____
____
____
____

Attitude 2:

____
____
____
____

Attitude 3:

____
____
____
____

Attitude 4:

____
____
____
____
____

Attitude 5:

____

____

____

____

____

4. Add whatever you want to make sure that the self-critical attitudes listed above are the most important and are related to how you feel about yourself. It is perfectly all right to change your ranking and include another self-critical attitude that you had ranked earlier.

5. The rest of this practice exercise will help you deal with each of the self-critical attitudes listed above. You will deal with each one once a week. Make sure that you make an appointment with yourself at a preset time at least 24 h ahead. If you have to change this appointment time for any reason, give yourself at least 24 h to work on each practice exercise.

Homework: During the coming week, write down whatever feelings and thoughts come to you, as you keep thinking about this practice exercise and this practice exercise.

Instructions: Under the title of this standard format for all the following practice exercises of this practice exercise, write the self-critical attitude that is important to you. Start with the attitude rank-ordered as No. 1 for this practice exercise. In the practice exercise following this one, write the self-critical attitude ranked No. 2. Do the same for the next practice exercises ranked No. 3, No. 4, and No. 5. If you have ranked more than five self-critical attitudes and you want to work on them, feel free to write their name in the title of this standard format. This standard format is repeated from one week to another. The title of the practice exercise changes according to the rank-order you have written in the first practice exercise.

Standard Format for Self-Critical Practice Exercises

Practice Exercise No.______Title of Self-Critical Troublesome thoughts or Attitude

____

Name ________________________________ Sex ___ Date _______

The purpose of this practice exercise is to help you understand the nature of the self-critical troublesome thoughts or attitude written in the title of this practice exercise.

1. Write how the title of this practice exercise is related to how you feel about yourself.

____

____

____

____

2. Describe how this self-critical attitude developed in your life starting from its very beginning.

____

____

____

____

3. What effect has this self-critical attitude had on your life?

____

____

____

____

____

4. What did you learn from this self-critical attitude?

____

____

____

____

____

5. How can you change this self-critical attitude?

____

____

____

____

6. What part did you play in this self-critical attitude? Explain how you were, in part, responsible for allowing this self-critical attitude to control your life.

____

____

____

____

____

7. During the next week, think about four possible ways of changing this self-critical attitude for the better. What should you do to make sure that you will win rather than defeat yourself? You may want to talk these possible ways over with whoever is interested in your life and welfare.

Solution 1:

Solution 2:

Solution 3:

Solution 4:

8. After you have made up your mind about which solution would work best for you and others, make sure you practice this solution until it becomes second nature to you. Write down which solution seems the best for you and how you are going to practice it.

9. You need to practice this solution as soon as possible. Write down each instance when you practiced this solution. What happened?

Practice 1:

Practice 2:

Practice 3:

Practice 4:

10. Feel free to write whatever comments you want to make about this practice exercise and how it applies to you.

Once you have finished this practice exercise and are satisfied with the results, you may then use the same practice exercise format for the next troublesome thoughts. Note that we cannot go on to the next practice exercise unless this one is completed.

Axis II Cluster B Externalizing Personalities

These practice exercises are included among Axis II of Cluster B externalizing personalities according to the DSM. These personalities tend to discharge immediately verbally and nonverbally, expressing feelings directly through anger, acting out, aggression, hostility, and self-centered exhibitionism. They usually reject professional help because they are satisfied with themselves, making themselves more important than others, including professionals (L'Abate, 2005). Consequently, they reject any attempt to intervene in their conditions unless they are in a hospital or in jail.

Instructions for administration: After the first practice exercise, all subsequent ones follow the same format. Each personality part (one practice exercise per part) should be written in the title line of the practice exercises that follow the rank-order given by participants in the first practice exercise. This sequence may follow whatever criterion the professionals and the participants agree on. It can be either subjective or objective, taking into account the rank-order given by participants in the first practice exercise. This sequence could be changed by objective evaluation and negotiation between professionals and participants.

Anger Expression

The purpose of this practice exercise is to help you understand how you express your anger and how your anger expression may hurt you and others.

Practice Exercise 1. How I Express My Anger

Name________________________________Sex ___Date__________

The purpose of this first practice exercise is to determine whether and how you want to change your anger expression for the better. Answering this and other practice exercise may make you angry. You need to decide whether you want to stay angry or whether you want to improve on how you have expressed your anger up to now.

1. Below is a list of how anger is felt and expressed through a variety of ways. Check how much each expression applies to you: most of the time, sometimes, or never.

Anger Expressions	*Most of the Time*	*Sometimes*	*Never*
a. Fury	_______	_______	_______
b. Madness	_______	_______	_______
c. Rage	_______	_______	_______
d. Anger at self	_______	_______	_______
e. Anger at others	_______	_______	_______
f. Violence	_______	_______	_______
g. Aggravation	_______	_______	_______
h. Temper tantrums	_______	_______	_______
i. Hatred	_______	_______	_______
j. Hostility	_______	_______	_______
k. Fighting	_______	_______	_______
l. Frustration	_______	_______	_______
m. Annoyance	_______	_______	_______
n. Yelling	_______	_______	_______
o. Spite	_______	_______	_______
p. Bitterness	_______	_______	_______
q. Jealousy	_______	_______	_______
r. Impatience	_______	_______	_______
s. Upset	_______	_______	_______
t. Irritation	_______	_______	_______
u. Resentment	_______	_______	_______
v. Failure	_______	_______	_______
w. Humiliation	_______	_______	_______
x. Disturbed	_______	_______	_______
y. Indignant	_______	_______	_______
z. Disappointed	_______	_______	_______
aa. Tension	_______	_______	_______
bb. Discontent	_______	_______	_______
cc. Envy	_______	_______	_______
dd. Disgust	_______	_______	_______
ee. Depression	_______	_______	_______
ff. Sorrow	_______	_______	_______
gg. Fear	_______	_______	_______

Assign two points for each item rated "Most of the Time" and one point for each item rated "Sometimes" to obtain a total score that shows how intense or strong the anger expression is.

2. Which of these anger expressions would you like to change, if any? If you do not want to change any anger expression, and you are feeling angry now, then stop and do not go any further in this practice exercise. You do not need to change your anger expression if you do not want to.

On the other hand, if you do want to change your anger expression, rank-order the items according to which anger expression you want to change among all those listed below. Rank as No. 1 the expression you want to change the most, rank as No. 2 the reaction you want to change next, and so on; mark as N/A the anger expressions that you do not want or need to change or that do not apply to you.

Anger Expressions	*Rank-order*	*Anger Expressions*	*Rank-order*
a. Fury	________	r. Impatience	________
b. Madness	________	s. Upset	________
c. Rage	________	t. Irritation	________
d. Anger at self	________	u. Resentment	________
e. Anger at others	________	v. Failure	________
f. Violence	________	w. Humiliation	________
g. Aggravation	________	x. Disturbed	________
h. Temper tantrums	________	y. Indignant	________
i. Hatred	________	z. Disappointed	________
j. Hostility	________	aa. Tension	________
k. Fighting	________	bb. Discontent	________
l. Frustration	________	cc. Envy	________
m. Annoyance	________	dd. Disgust	________
n. Yelling	________	ee. Depression	________
o. Spite	________	ff. Sorrow	________
p. Bitterness	________	gg. Fear	________
q. Jealousy	________		

3. Explain why you rank-ordered the angry expressions the way you did.

____
____
____
____
____

Homework: During the coming week, keep thinking about how you express your anger. Make yourself pretend to express your anger by thinking about (a) what situation may arouse your anger, (b) how you would express your anger, and (c) how you would feel afterwards. Make an appointment with yourself for specific times (9 a.m., 12 noon, 7 p.m.) at least every other day and pretend to express your anger at least three times during the coming week. Write down what happened for the above issues a, b, and c.

Note: If you think that pretending to express your anger is silly, strange, or weird, think about the possibility that if you can start your anger expression, you may learn to stop it. Make sure that you write everything down and discuss your pretend situations with whoever is working with you on this practice exercise.

Time 1

a. ______________________________

____

____

b. ______________________________

____

____

c. ______________________________

____

____

Time 2

a. ______________________________

____

____

b. ______________________________

____

____

c. ______________________________

____

____

Time 3

a. ______________________________

____

____

b. ______________________________

____

____

c. ______________________________

____

____

Standard Practice Exercise Format for Anger Expression

Administer as many standard practice exercises as necessary before administering practice exercises on how to express anger positively.

Practice Exercise No.____ Type of Anger_________________________

Name________________________________Sex ____Date__________

The purpose of this practice exercise is to understand more about the type of anger expression listed above.

1. How does this anger expression apply to you? Explain in detail.

____

____

____

____

2. How often do you express your anger this way?

a.	Practically every day	______	e.	Once every 6 months	______
b.	Once a week	______	f.	Once a year	______
c.	A couple of times a month	______	g.	Once every few years	______
d.	Once a month	______			

3. Explain further:

____

____

____

____

4. How did you learn to express anger this way? Do you remember when you started it? Check which answer fits best:

   a. When I was a child (younger than 5 years of age) ____
   b. When I was in elementary school ____
   c. When I was in middle school ____
   d. When I was in high school ____
   e. After high school ____
   f. Any other time ____

5. Explain further:

6. Was this anger expression acceptable or unacceptable? Why? Explain.

7. Give three specific examples of how this anger expression affects you.

Example 1:

Example 2:

Example 3:

8. Give three specific examples of how this anger expression affects others.

   Example 1:

   ____
   ____
   ____
   ____
   ____

   Example 2:

   ____
   ____
   ____
   ____
   ____

   Example 3:

   ____
   ____
   ____
   ____
   ____

Homework: Next week, plan to repeat this anger expression at preset times (for instance, at 8 a.m., 12 noon, 4 or 7 p.m.) on at least 3 days (Monday, Wednesday, and Friday, or Tuesday, Thursday, and Saturday). If you can start it, you can stop it. Pretend to express your anger even if you do not feel like it.

Write down what happened in detail. For each time you start this reaction make sure to answer in writing the following four questions:

a. How did you start it?
b. What followed?
c. How did it end?
d. What did this reaction get you?

Time 1 (write the time you started__________)

a. ____
   ____

b. ____
   ____

c. ____
____

d. ____
____

Time 2 (write the time you started__________)

a. ____
____

b. ____
____

c. ____
____

d. ____
____

Time 3 (write the time you started__________)

a. ____
____

b. ____
____

c. ____
____

d. ____
____

Check which of the following indicates how you feel about this practice exercise:

a. Completely useless _____
b. Somewhat useless _____
c. So-so _____
d. Somewhat useful _____
e. Extremely useful _____

Explain in greater detail how you feel about this practice exercise and what you got out of it.

____
____
____
____
____
____
____
____

First Practice Exercise for How to Express Anger Positively

Practice Exercise No. ____Type of Anger____________________

Name ________________________________ Sex ____ Date ___________

The purpose of this practice exercise is to help you learn how to express anger in more positive ways than you may have done in the past.

1. To help you learn how to express your anger, it might be useful for you to explain what you understand about the many ways in which people can stop feeling angry. Below is a list of ways to stop feeling angry. Explain what you understand by each way, and give two examples of what you mean.

Ways to Stop Feeling Angry	*Explanation*
a. Do something soothing to calm down ______	Example 1 ______
______	Example 2 ______
b. Do something relaxing to calm down ______	Example 1 ______
______	Example 2 ______
c. Cool down as quickly as possible ______	Example 1 ______
______	Example 2 ______
d. Cool off as soon as possible ______	Example 1 ______
______	Example 2 ______
e. Try to relax ______	Example 1 ______
______	Example 2 ______

f. Try to calm myself as soon as possible ______	Example 1 ______
______	Example 2 ______
g. Try to simmer down ______	Example 1 ______
______	Example 2 ______
h. Reduce my anger as soon as possible ______	Example 1 ______
______	Example 2 ______
i. Control my urge to express angry feelings ______	Example 1 ______
______	Example 2 ______
j. Control my anger expression ______	Example 1 ______
______	Example 2 ______
k. Control my angry feelings ______	Example 1 ______
______	Example 2 ______
l. Stop myself from losing control ______	Example 1 ______
______	Example 2 ______
m. Keep my cool ______	Example 1 ______
______	Example 2 ______

n. Control myself ____________ Example 1 ____________
____________ ____________
____________ Example 2 ____________
____________ ____________

o. Do not lash out at what angers me Example 1 ____________
____________ ____________
____________ Example 2 ____________
____________ ____________

p. Try not to express my anger Example 1 ____________
____________ ____________
____________ Example 2 ____________
____________ ____________

q. Any other way to stop feeling angry (write what it is) ____________ Example 1 ____________
____________ ____________
____________ Example 2 ____________
____________ ____________

2. Rank-order the ways to stop feeling angry according to how much you would like to learn them. Rank as No. 1 the way that you would like to learn first, rank as No. 2 the way that you would like to learn next, and so on; mark as N/A the ways that do not apply to you or that are not preferable to you.

Ways to Stop Feeling Angry	*Rank-order*
a. Do something soothing to calm down	______
b Do something relaxing to calm down	______
c. Cool down as quickly as possible	______
d. Cool off as soon as possible	______
e. Try to relax	______
f. Try to calm myself as soon as possible	______
g. Try to simmer down	______
h. Reduce my anger as soon as possible	______
i. Control my urge to express angry feelings	______
j. Control my behavior	______
k. Control my angry feelings	______
l. Stop myself from losing my temper	______
m. Keep my cool	______
n. Control my temper	______
o. Do not lash out at what angers me	______
p. Try not to express my anger	______
q. Any other way (write what it is)	______

3. Explain why you ranked the ways to stop feeling angry the way you did.

____
____
____
____

Homework: During the coming week, think about all the ways that are available to you to control your anger expression.

Standard Practice Exercise for How to Stop Feeling Angry More Positively

Practice Exercise No.____Type of Expression______________________(fill in from the above list)

Name______________________________Sex ___Date__________

The purpose of this practice exercise is to help you become more specific, concrete, and practical in learning how to express your anger. Reducing your anger is easier said than done. The expression listed here may be general, vague, and not sufficient to learn how to control your anger. Consequently, in this practice exercise you will need to determine how each expression can apply to you.

1. Write at least three specific ways in which you could employ the expression listed in this practice exercise.

   a. ____
   ____
   ____

   b ____
   ____
   ____

   c. ____
   ____
   ____

2. List at least three examples of how you used the expression listed above to deal with your anger during the previous week
   Example 1:

____
____
____
____
____

Example 2:

Example 3:

3. What happened after you completed the expression you were supposed to use in this practice exercise? Explain in detail by

   a. Describing the situation,
   b. Describing how you expressed yourself, and
   c. Describing how you felt afterwards:

Explanation 1:

a.

b.

c.

Explanation 2:

a.

b.

c. ____
____
____

Explanation 3:

a. ____
____
____

b. ____
____
____

c. ____
____
____

Homework: During the coming week, note in writing whether the way you used in this practice exercise to control your anger, hostility, or aggression worked or did not work for you.

Concluding Follow-Up Form for Anger Expression

Name______________________________Sex _____Date_________

The purpose of this concluding follow-up form is to review whether this practice exercise was helpful to you or not.

1. Please check the answer that best fits how you feel about this practice exercise:

   a. I did not like working on this practice exercise at all. I wish I never saw it. _________
   b. I did not like this practice exercise at all, but I am glad I got to work on it. _________
   c. I am delighted I got a chance to work on this practice exercise. _________
   d. I am not only delighted about working on this practice exercise, but I wish all angry or aggressive people had a chance to work on it. _________

2. How helpful was it to work on this practice exercise? Please check the answer that applies to you:

a. Not helpful at all	_____	c. Helpful	_____
b. Somewhat helpful	_____	d. Very helpful	_____

3. Which practice exercise did you like best? Rank as No. 1 the one that you liked best, rank as No. 2 the one you liked next best, and so on; mark as N/A the ones you did not like at all or did not apply to you.

Anger Expressions	*Rank-order*	*Anger Expressions*	*Rank-order*
a. Fury	_________	r. Impatience	_________
b. Madness	_________	s. Upset	_________
c. Rage	_________	t. Irritation	_________
d. Anger at self	_________	u. Resentment	_________
e. Anger at others	_________	v. Failure	_________
f. Violence	_________	w. Humiliation	_________
g. Aggravation	_________	x. Disturbed	_________
h. Temper tantrums	_________	y. Indignant	_________
i. Hatred	_________	z. Disappointed	_________
j. Hostility	_________	aa. Tension	_________
k. Fighting	_________	bb. Discontent	_________
l. Frustration	_________	cc. Envy	_________
m. Annoyance	_________	dd. Disgust	_________
n. Yelling	_________	ee. Depression	_________
o. Spite	_________	ff. Sorrow	_________
p. Bitterness	_________	gg. Fear	_________
q. Jealousy	_________		

4. Why did you rank-order the practice exercises the way you did? Explain.

____

____

____

____

5. Sometimes what we like most is not necessarily the most helpful. Which practice exercise was the most helpful to you? Rank as No. 1 the most helpful, rank as No. 2 the next most helpful, and so on, down to the least helpful practice exercise; mark as N/A the practice exercises that did not apply to you.

Anger Expressions	*Rank-order*	*Anger Expressions*	*Rank-order*
a. Fury	_________	d. Anger at self	_________
b. Madness	_________	e. Anger at others	_________
c. Rage	_________	f. Violence	_________

Anger Expressions	*Rank-order*	*Anger Expressions*	*Rank-order*
g. Aggravation	________	u. Resentment	________
h. Temper tantrums	________	v. Failure	________
i. Hatred	________	w. Humiliation	________
j. Hostility	________	x. Disturbed	________
k. Fighting	________	y. Indignant	________
l. Frustration	________	z. Disappointed	________
m. Annoyance	________	aa. Tension	________
n. Yelling	________	bb. Discontent	________
o. Spite	________	cc. Envy	________
p. Bitterness	________	dd. Disgust	________
q. Jealousy	________	ee. Depression	________
r. Impatience	________	ff. Sorrow	________
s. Upset	________	gg. Fear	________
t. Irritation	________		

6. In going back to the practice exercises to help you stop feeling angry, which was most helpful among those administered to you? Rank as No. 1 the practice exercise that was most helpful to you, rank as No. 2 the practice exercise that was second most helpful, and so on, until all the practice exercises that were administered to you have been rank-ordered.

Ways to Control Anger	*Rank-order*
a. Do something soothing to calm down	________
b. Do something relaxing to calm down	________
c. Cool down as quickly as possible	________
d. Cool off as soon as possible	________
e. Try to relax	________
f. Try to calm myself as soon as possible	________
g. Try to simmer down	________
h. Reduce my anger as soon as possible	________
i. Control my urge to express angry feelings	________
j. Control my anger expression	________
k. Control my angry feelings	________
l. Stop myself from losing my temper	________
m. Keep my cool	________
n. Control myself	________
o. Do no lash out at what angers me	________
p. Try not to express my anger	________
q. Any other way (write what it is)	________

7. Explain why you rank-ordered these practice exercises the way you did.

____
____
____
____

8. Feel free to write any comments that might improve this practice exercise.

____
____
____
____
____

Self-Suffering (Masochism)

Practice Exercise 1. Understanding your Self-Suffering Personality

Name ______________________ Sex ___ Date _____

The purpose of this practice exercise is to understand more about this aspect of your personality. To learn more about yourself, you will need to explain what the parts listed below mean to you. Each part, together with other parts listed below, very likely makes up your personality.

1. To define these parts, you will need the help of a dictionary, your attending professional helper, your relatives, your friends, or staff members. For each part, add two examples that show your understanding of that part.

Parts	*Definitions and Examples*
a. Abstinent ______________	Example 1 ______________
______________	______________
______________	Example 2 ______________
______________	______________
b. Deferential ______________	Example 1 ______________
______________	______________
______________	Example 2 ______________
______________	______________

c. Diffident ____________________
____
____
____

Example 1 ____________________
____
Example 2 ____________________
____

d. Exaggerating ____________________
____
____
____

Example 1 ____________________
____
Example 2 ____________________
____

e. Undeserving ____________________
____
____
____

Example 1 ____________________
____
Example 2 ____________________
____

f. Discredited ____________________
____
____
____

Example 1 ____________________
____
Example 2 ____________________
____

g. Inverted ____________________
____
____
____

Example 1 ____________________
____
Example 2 ____________________
____

h. Dysphoric ____________________
____
____
____

Example 1 ____________________
____
Example 2 ____________________
____

2. Now that you have completed these definitions, it is important to find out how these parts apply to you. Rank-order each part according to how much it applies to you. Rank as No. 1 the part that applies to you the most, rank as No. 2 the part that applies to you next, and so on; mark as N/A the parts that may not apply to you.

Parts	*Rank-order*	*Parts*	*Rank-order*
a. Abstinent	________	e. Undeserving	________
b. Deferential	________	f. Discredited	________
c. Diffident	________	g. Inverted	________
d. Exaggerating	________	h. Dysphoric	________

3. Write why you rank-ordered these parts the way you did.

____
____
____
____
____

4. Now that you have completed this practice exercise, check which of these answers indicates how you feel about it. There is also space for you to explain further, if you want to:

   a. I did not like this practice exercise at all. I want to quit this stupid practice exercise. ________
   b. I did not like this practice exercise very much, but I want to go on with this practice exercise. ________
   c. I liked this practice exercise and I want to go on with this practice exercise. ________
   d. I liked this practice exercise a lot and I wish I had something like this practice exercise years ago. ________
   e. I liked it so much that I wish all people in trouble or in need of professional help could get something like this practice exercise to work on. ________

5. Discuss your completed practice exercise with whoever has given it to you.

Homework: During the coming week, think more about the parts you defined and rank-ordered and whether you want to change their rank-order as listed above, or start working on the next practice exercise.

Concluding Feedback Form for Self-Suffering Personality

Name ______________________ Sex ______ Date _______

The purpose of this concluding feedback form is to review whether this practice exercise was helpful to you or not.

1. Please check the answer that best fits how you feel about this practice exercise:

   a. I did not like working on this practice exercise at all. I wish I never saw it. ________
   b. I did not like this practice exercise at all, but I am glad I got to work on it. ________

c. I am delighted I got a chance to work on this practice exercise. ________
d. I am not only delighted about working on this practice exercise, but I wish all people with a personality like mine had a chance to work on it. ________

2. How helpful was it to work on this practice exercise? Please check the answer that applies to you:

a.	Not helpful at all	_____	c.	Helpful	_____
b.	Somewhat helpful	_____	d.	Very helpful	_____

3. Which practice exercise did you like best? Rank as No. 1 the one that you liked best, rank as No. 2 the one you liked next best, and so on; mark as N/A the ones you did not like at all or did not apply to you.

Parts		*Rank-order*	*Parts*		*Rank-order*
a.	Abstinent	________	e.	Undeserving	________
b.	Deferential	________	f.	Discredited	________
c.	Diffident	________	g.	Inverted	________
d.	Exaggerating	________	h.	Dysphoric	________

4. Explain why you rank-ordered these practice exercises the way you did.

____

____

____

____

____

5. Sometimes what we like most is not necessarily the most helpful. Which practice exercise was the most helpful to you? Rank as No. 1 the most helpful, rank as No. 2 the next most helpful, and so on, down to the least helpful practice exercise; mark as N/A the practice exercises that did not apply to you.

Parts		*Rank-order*	*Parts*		*Rank-order*
a.	Abstinent	________	e.	Undeserving	________
b.	Deferential	________	f.	Discredited	________
c.	Diffident	________	g.	Inverted	________
d.	Exaggerating	________	h.	Dysphoric	________

6. Explain why you rank-order these practice exercises the way you did.

____
____
____
____
____

7. Feel free to write any comments that might improve this practice exercise.

____
____
____
____
____

Help-Seeking (Dependent)

Practice Exercise 1. Understanding Your Help-Seeking Personality

Name ________________________________ Sex ___ Date _____

The purpose of this practice exercise is to understand more about your personality. To learn more about yourself, you will need to explain what the parts listed below mean to you. Each part, together with other parts listed below, very likely makes up your personality.

1. To understand these parts, you will need the help of a dictionary, your attending professional helper, your relatives, your friends, or staff members. For each part, add two examples that show your understanding of that part.

Parts	*Definitions and Examples*
a. Incompetent ________________	Example 1 ________________
________________	________________
________________	Example 2 ________________
________________	________________
b. Submissive ________________	Example 1 ________________
________________	________________
________________	Example 2 ________________
________________	________________

c. Naive ______________________ Example 1 ______________________

______________________ ______________________

______________________ Example 2 ______________________

______________________ ______________________

d. Introjected ______________________ Example 1 ______________________

______________________ ______________________

______________________ Example 2 ______________________

______________________ ______________________

e. Inept ______________________ Example 1 ______________________

______________________ ______________________

______________________ Example 2 ______________________

______________________ ______________________

f. Immature ______________________ Example 1 ______________________

______________________ ______________________

______________________ Example 2 ______________________

______________________ ______________________

g. Inchoate ______________________ Example 1 ______________________

______________________ ______________________

______________________ Example 2 ______________________

______________________ ______________________

h. Pacific ______________________ Example 1 ______________________

______________________ ______________________

______________________ Example 2 ______________________

______________________ ______________________

2. Now that you have completed these definitions, it is important to find out how these parts apply to you. Rank-order each part according to how much it applies to you. Rank as No. 1 the part that applies to you the most, rank as No. 2 the part that applies to you next, and so on; mark as N/A the parts that may not apply to you.

Parts	*Rank-order*	*Parts*	*Rank-order*
a. Incompetent	________	e. Inept	________
b. Submissive	________	f. Immature	________
c. Naive	________	g. Inchoate	________
d. Introjected	________	h. Pacific	________

3. Write why you rank-ordered these parts the way you did.

____

____

____

____

____

4. Now that you have completed this practice exercise, check which of these answers indicates how you feel about it. There is also space for you to explain further, if you want to:

   a. I did not like this practice exercise at all. I want to quit this stupid practice exercise. ________
   b. I did not like this practice exercise very much, but I want to go on with this practice exercise. ________
   c. I liked this practice exercise and I want to go on with this practice exercise. ________
   d. I liked this practice exercise a lot and I wish I had something like this practice exercise years ago. ________
   e. I liked it so much that I wish all people in trouble or in need of professional help could get something like this practice exercise to work on. ________

5. Discuss your completed practice exercise with whoever has given it to you.

Homework: During the coming week, think more about the parts you defined and rank-order and whether you want to change their rank-order as listed above, or start working on the next practice exercise.

Concluding Feedback Form for Help-Seeking Personality

Name ________________________________ Sex ______ Date _____

The purpose of this concluding feedback form is to review whether this practice exercise was helpful to you or not.

1. Please check the answer that best fits how you feel about this practice exercise:

   a. I did not like working on this practice exercise at all. I wish I never saw it. ________
   b. I did not like this practice exercise at all, but I am glad I got to work on it. ________

c. I am delighted I got a chance to work on this practice exercise. ________

d. I am not only delighted about working on this practice exercise, but I wish all people who need professional help had a chance to work on it. ________

2. How helpful was it to work on this practice exercise? Please check the answer that applies to you.

a. Not helpful at all	_____	c. Helpful	_____
b. Somewhat helpful	_____	d. Very helpful	_____

3. Which practice exercise did you like best? Rank as No. 1 the one that you liked best, rank as No. 2 the one you liked next best, and so on; mark as N/A the ones you did not like at all or did not apply to you.

Parts	*Rank-order*	*Parts*	*Rank-order*
a. Incompetent	________	e. Inept	________
b. Submissive	________	f. Immature	________
c. Naive	________	g. Inchoate	________
d. Introjected	________	h. Pacific	________

4. Explain why you rank-ordered these practice exercises the way you did.

____

____

____

____

____

5. Sometimes what we like most is not necessarily the most helpful. Which practice exercise was the most helpful to you? Rank as No. 1 the most helpful, rank as No. 2 the next most helpful, and so on, down to the least helpful practice exercise; mark as N/A the practice exercises that did not apply to you.

Parts	*Rank-order*	*Parts*	*Rank-order*
a. Incompetent	________	e. Inept	________
b. Submissive	________	f. Immature	________
c. Naive	________	g. Inchoate	________
d. Introjected	________	h. Pacific	________

6. Explain why you rank-ordered these practice exercises the way you did.

____
____
____
____
____

7. Feel free to write any comments that might improve this practice exercise.

____
____
____
____
____

Serious (Depressed)

Practice Exercise 1. Understanding Your Serious Personality

Name_______________Sex___Date_____

The purpose of this practice exercise is to understand more about your personality. To learn more about yourself, you will need to explain what the parts listed below mean to you. Each part, together with other parts listed below, very likely makes up your personality.

1. To understand these parts, you will need the help of a dictionary, your attending professional helper, your relatives, your friends, or staff members. For each part, add two examples that show your understanding of that part.

Parts	*Definitions and Examples*
a. Disconsolate _______________	Example 1 _______________
_______________	_______________
_______________	Example 2 _______________
_______________	_______________
b. Defenseless _______________	Example 1 _______________
_______________	_______________
_______________	Example 2 _______________
_______________	_______________

c. Pessimistic ____________________ Example 1 ____________________

d. Ascetic ____________________ Example 1 ____________________

Example 2 ____________________

e. Worthless ____________________ Example 1 ____________________

Example 2 ____________________

f. Forsaken ____________________ Example 1 ____________________

Example 2 ____________________

g. Depleted ____________________ Example 1 ____________________

Example 2 ____________________

h. Melancholic ____________________ Example 1 ____________________

Example 2 ____________________

2. Now that you have completed these definitions, it is important to find out how these parts apply to you. Rank-order each part according to how much it applies to you. Rank as No. 1 the part that applies to you the most, rank as No. 2 the part that applies to you next, and so on; mark as N/A the parts that may not apply to you.

Parts	*Rank-order*	*Parts*	*Rank-order*
a. Disconsolate	________	e. Worthless	________
b. Defenseless	________	f. Forsaken	________
c. Pessimistic	________	g. Depleted	________
d. Ascetic	________	h. Melancholic	________

3. Write why you rank-ordered these parts the way you did.

____

____

____

____

____

4. Now that you have completed this practice exercise, check which of these answers indicates how you feel about it. There is also space for you to explain further, if you want to:

   a. I did not like this practice exercise at all. I want to quit this stupid practice exercise. ______
   b. I did not like this practice exercise very much, but I want to go on with this practice exercise. ______
   c. I liked this practice exercise and I want to go on with this practice exercise. ______
   d. I liked this practice exercise a lot and I wish I had something like this practice exercise years ago. ______
   e. I liked it so much that I wish all people in trouble or in need of professional help could get something like this practice exercise to work on. ______

5. Discuss your completed practice exercise with whoever gave it to you.

Homework: During the coming week, think more about the parts you defined and rank-order and whether you want to change their rank-order as listed above, or start working on the next practice exercise.

Concluding Feedback Form for Serious Personality

Name________________________________Sex _____Date______

The purpose of this concluding feedback form is to review whether this practice exercise was helpful to you or not.

1. Please check the answer that best fits how you feel about this practice exercise:
   a. I did not like working on this practice exercise at all. I wish I never saw it. _______
   b. I did not like this practice exercise at all, but I am glad I got to work on it. _______
   c. I am delighted I got a chance to work on this practice exercise. _______

d. I am not only delighted about working on this practice exercise, but I wish all people who need professional help had a chance to work on it. ______

2. How helpful was it to work on this practice exercise? Please check the answer that applies to you.

a. Not helpful at all	____	c. Helpful	____
b. Somewhat helpful	____	d. Very helpful	____

3. Which practice exercise did you like best? Rank as No. 1 the one that you liked best, rank as No. 2 the one you liked next best, and so on; mark as N/A the ones you did not like at all or did not apply to you.

Parts	*Rank-order*	*Parts*	*Rank-order*
a. Disconsolate	________	e. Worthless	________
b. Defenseless	________	f. Forsaken	________
c. Pessimistic	________	g. Depleted	________
d. Ascetic	________	h. Melancholic	________

4. Explain why you rank-ordered these practice exercises the way you did.

____
____
____
____
____

5. Sometimes what we like most is not necessarily the most helpful. Which practice exercise was the most helpful to you? Rank as No. 1 the most helpful, rank as No. 2 the next most helpful, and so on, down to the least helpful practice exercise; mark as N/A the practice exercises that did not apply to you.

Parts	*Rank-order*	*Parts*	*Rank-order*
a. Disconsolate	________	e. Worthless	________
b. Defenseless	________	f. Forsaken	________
c. Pessimistic	________	g. Depleted	________
d. Ascetic	________	h. Melancholic	________

6. Explain why you rank-ordered these practice exercises the way you did.

____
____
____
____
____

7. Feel free to write any comments that might improve this practice exercise.

____

____

____

____

____

____

Selected Cluster B Personality Disorders

The purpose of the practice exercises in these practice exercises is to help participants understand the specific nature of their personalities. Participants are asked to answer in writing a great many questions about the parts that make up their special personalities. Participation in these practice exercises is completely voluntary. Working on these practice exercises is completely up to participants who want to learn more about themselves and who want professional helpers interested in their welfare to learn more about them. If participants complete the first practice exercise, it means that they do want to learn more about themselves and that they are interested in improving their personalities.

An attempt was made to give most personality disorders a positive connotation to avoid using psychiatric labels or jargon. Nevertheless, participants should be warned beforehand and understand in writing, by signing an informed consent form (Appendix A), that some of the parts that illustrate their personalities are quite negative, which participants might dislike. On the other hand, participants will need to confront and understand how these negative parts contribute to their dysfunctionalities. After this discussion and a practice exercise are completed, perhaps participants will be ready to start working on more positive aspects of their personalities (see Sect. 3 of this sourcebook). Note that schizotypal, borderline, and paranoid personalities do not have a practice exercise. However, the interested professional can replicate the format used here to reproduce additional practice exercises for these three personalities (Davis & Millon, 1999, p. 517).

Self-Interested (Narcissistic)

Practice Exercise 1. Understanding Your Self-interested Personality

Name_________________________________Sex_____Date______

The purpose of this practice exercise is to understand more about your personality. To learn more about yourself, you will need to explain what the parts listed below mean to you. Each part, together with other parts listed below, very likely makes up your overall personality.

1. To understand these parts, you will need the help of a dictionary, your attending professional helper, your relatives, your friends, or staff members. For each part, add two examples that show your understanding of that part.

Parts	*Definitions and Examples*
a. Haughty ____	Example 1 ____
	Example 2 ____
b. Exploitive ____	Example 1 ____
	Example 2 ____
c. Expansive ____	Example 1 ____
	Example 2 ____
d. Rationalizing ____	Example 1 ____
	Example 2 ____
e. Admirable ____	Example 1 ____
	Example 2 ____
f. Contrived ____	Example 1 ____
	Example 2 ____
g. Spurious ____	Example 1 ____
	Example 2 ____
h. Insouciant ____	Example 1 ____
	Example 2 ____

2. Now that you have completed these definitions, it is important to find out how these parts apply to you. Rank-order each part according to how much it applies to you. Rank as No. 1 the part that applies to you the most, rank as No. 2 the part that applies to you next, and so on; mark as N/A the parts that may not apply to you.

Parts	*Rank-order*	*Parts*	*Rank-order*
a. Haughty	________	e. Admirable	________
b. Exploitive	________	f. Contrived	________
c. Expansive	________	g. Spurious	________
d. Rationalizing	________	h. Insouciant	________

3. Write why you rank-ordered these parts the way you did.

____

____

____

____

____

4. Now that you have completed this practice exercise, check which of these answers indicates how you feel about it. There is also space for you to explain further, if you want to:

   a. I did not like this practice exercise at all. I want to quit this stupid practice exercise. ______
   b. I did not like this practice exercise very much, but I want to go on with this practice exercise. ______
   c. I liked this practice exercise and I want to go on with this practice exercise. ______
   d. I liked this practice exercise a lot and I wish I had something like this practice exercise years ago. ______
   e. I liked it so much that I wish all people in trouble or in need of professional help could get something like this practice exercise to work on. ______

5. Discuss your completed practice exercise with whoever has given it to you.

Homework: During the coming week, think more about the parts you defined and rank-ordered and whether you want to change their rank-order as listed above, or start working on the next practice exercise.

Concluding Feedback Form for Self-Interested Personality

Name________________________________Sex _____Date______

The purpose of this concluding feedback form is to review whether this practice exercise was helpful to you or not.

1. Please check the answer that best fits how you feel about this practice exercise:

   a. I did not like working on this practice exercise at all. I wish I never saw it. _______
   b. I did not like this practice exercise at all, but I am glad I got to work on it. _______
   c. I am delighted I got a chance to work on this practice exercise. _______
   d. I am not only delighted about working on this practice exercise, but I wish all people who need professional help had a chance to work on it. _______

2. How helpful was it to work on this practice exercise? Please check the answer that applies to you:

   a. Not helpful at all _______ c. Helpful _______
   b. Somewhat helpful _______ d. Very helpful _______

3. Which practice exercise did you like best? Rank as No. 1 the one that you liked best, rank as No. 2 the one you liked next best, and so on; mark as N/A the ones you did not like at all or did not apply to you.

Parts	*Rank-order*	*Parts*	*Rank-order*
a. Haughty	_________	e. Admirable	_________
b. Exploitive	_________	f. Contrived	_________
c. Expansive	_________	g. Spurious	_________
d. Rationalizing	_________	h. Insouciant	_________

4. Explain why you rank-ordered these practice exercises the way you did.

____
____
____
____
____

5. Sometimes what we like most is not necessarily the most helpful. Which practice exercise was the most helpful to you? Rank as No. 1 the most helpful, rank as No. 2 the next most helpful, and so on, down to the least helpful practice exercise; mark as N/A the practice exercises that did not apply to you.

Parts	*Rank-order*	*Parts*	*Rank-order*
a. Haughty	________	e. Admirable	________
b. Exploitive	________	f. Contrived	________
c. Expansive	________	g. Spurious	________
d. Rationalizing	________	h. Insouciant	________

6. Explain why you rank-ordered these practice exercises the way you did.

____
____
____
____
____

7. Feel free to write any comments that might improve this practice exercise.

____
____
____
____
____

Nonconformist (Negativistic)

Practice Exercise 1. Understanding Your Nonconformist Personality

Name________________________________Sex___Date_____

The purpose of this practice exercise is to understand more about your personality. To learn more about yourself, you will need to explain what the parts listed below mean to you. Each part, together with the other parts listed below, very likely makes up your unique personality.

1. To understand these parts, you will need the help of a dictionary, your attending professional helper, your relatives, your friends, or staff members. For each part, add two examples that show your understanding of that part.

Parts	*Definitions and Examples*
a. Resentful ________	Example 1 ________
________	________
________	Example 2 ________
________	________
b. Contrary ________	Example 1 ________
________	________
________	Example 2 ________
________	________
c. Skeptical ________	Example 1 ________
________	________
________	Example 2 ________
________	________
d. Displacing ________	Example 1 ________
________	________
________	Example 2 ________
________	________
e. Discontented ________	Example 1 ________
________	________
________	Example 2 ________
________	________
f. Vacillating ________	Example 1 ________
________	________
________	Example 2 ________
________	________
g. Divergent ________	Example 1 ________
________	________
________	Example 2 ________
________	________
h. Irritable ________	Example 1 ________
________	________
________	Example 2 ________
________	________

2. Now that you have completed these definitions, it is important to find out how these parts apply to you. Rank-order each part according to how much it applies to you. Rank as No. 1 the part that applies to you the most, rank as No. 2 the part that applies to you next, and so on; mark as N/A the parts that may not apply to you.

Parts	*Rank-order*	*Parts*	*Rank-order*
a. Resentful	_______	e. Discontented	_______
b. Contrary	_______	f. Vacillating	_______
c. Skeptical	_______	g. Divergent	_______
d. Displacing	_______	h. Irritable	_______

3. Write why you rank-ordered these parts the way you did.

____
____
____
____
____

4. Now that you have completed this practice exercise, check which of these answers indicates how you feel about it. There is also space for you to explain further, if you want to:

   a. I did not like this practice exercise at all. I want to quit this stupid practice exercise. _____
   b. I did not like this practice exercise very much, but I want to go on with this practice exercise. _____
   c. I liked this practice exercise and I want to go on with this practice exercise. _____
   d. I liked this practice exercise a lot and I wish I had something like this practice exercise years ago. _____
   e. I liked it so much that I wish all people in trouble or in need of professional help could get something like this practice exercise to work on. _____

5. Discuss your completed practice exercise with whoever has given it to you.

Homework: During the coming week, think more about the parts you defined and rank-order and whether you want to change their rank-order as listed above, or start working on the next practice exercise.

Concluding Feedback Form for Nonconformist Personality

Name________________________________Sex_____Date______

The purpose of this concluding feedback form is to review whether this practice exercise was helpful to you or not.

1. Please check the answer that best fits how you feel about this practice exercise:

   a. I did not like working on this practice exercise at all. I wish I never saw it. ________
   b. I did not like this practice exercise at all, but I am glad I got to work on it. ________
   c. I am delighted I got a chance to work on this practice exercise. ________
   d. I am not only delighted about working on this practice exercise, but I wish all people who need professional help had a chance to work on it. ________

2. How helpful was it to work on this practice exercise? Please check the answer that applies to you:

a. Not helpful at all	____	c. Helpful	____
b. Somewhat helpful	____	d. Very helpful	____

3. Which practice exercise did you like best? Rank as No. 1 the one that you liked best, rank as No. 2 the one you liked next best, and so on; mark as N/A the ones you did not like at all or did not apply to you.

Parts	*Rank-order*	*Parts*	*Rank-order*
a. Resentful	_________	e. Discontented	_________
b. Contrary	_________	f. Vacillating	_________
c. Skeptical	_________	g. Divergent	_________
d. Displacing	_________	h. Irritable	_________

4. Explain why you rank-ordered these practice exercises the way you did.

____
____
____
____
____
____

5. Sometimes what we like most is not necessarily the most helpful. Which practice exercise was the most helpful to you? Rank as No. 1 the most helpful, rank as No. 2 the next most helpful, and so on, down to the least helpful practice exercise; mark as N/A the practice exercises that did not apply to you.

Parts	*Rank-order*	*Parts*	*Rank-order*
a. Resentful	________	e. Discontented	________
b. Contrary	________	f. Vacillating	________
c. Skeptical	________	g. Divergent	________
d. Displacing	________	h. Irritable	________

6. Explain why you rank-ordered these practice exercises the way you did.

____
____
____
____
____

7. Feel free to write any comments that might improve this practice exercise.

____
____
____
____
____

Compelling (Compulsive)

Practice Exercise 1. Understanding Your Compelling Personality

Name________________________________Sex____Date_______

The purpose of this practice exercise is to understand more about your personality. To learn more about yourself, you will need to explain what the parts listed below mean to you. Each part, together with the other parts listed below, very likely makes up your personality.

1. To understand these parts, you will need the help of a dictionary, your attending professional helper, your relatives, your friends, or staff members. For each part, add two examples that show your understanding of that part.

Parts	*Definitions and Examples*
a. Disciplined ____________	Example 1 ____________
____________	____________
____________	Example 2 ____________
____________	____________
b. Respectful ____________	Example 1 ____________
____________	____________
____________	Example 2 ____________
____________	____________
c. Constricted ____________	Example 1 ____________
____________	____________
____________	Example 2 ____________
____________	____________
d. Reactive ____________	Example 1 ____________
____________	____________
____________	Example 2 ____________
____________	____________
e. Conscientious ____________	Example 1 ____________
____________	____________
____________	Example 2 ____________
____________	____________
f. Concealed ____________	Example 1 ____________
____________	____________
____________	Example 2 ____________
____________	____________
g. Compartmentalized ____________	Example 1 ____________
____________	____________
____________	Example 2 ____________
____________	____________
h. Solemn ____________	Example 1 ____________
____________	____________
____________	Example 2 ____________
____________	____________

2. Now that you have completed these definitions, it is important to find out how these parts apply to you. Rank-order each part according to how much it applies to you. Rank as No. 1 the part that applies to you the most, rank as No. 2 the part that applies to you next, and so on; mark as N/A the parts that may not apply to you.

Parts	*Rank-order*	*Parts*	*Rank-order*
a. Disciplined	__________	e. Conscientious	
b. Respectful	__________	f. Concealed	
c. Constricted	__________	g. Compartmentalized	
d. Reactive	__________	h. Solemn	

3. Write why you rank-ordered these parts the way you did.

____

____

____

____

____

4. Now that you have completed this practice exercise, check which of these answers indicates how you feel about it. There is also space for you to explain further, if you want to:

   a. I did not like this practice exercise at all. I want to quit this stupid practice exercise.______
   b. I did not like this practice exercise very much, but I want to go on with this practice exercise.______
   c. I liked this practice exercise and I want to go on with this practice exercise.______
   d. I liked this practice exercise a lot and I wish I had something like this practice exercise years ago.______
   e. I liked it so much that I wish all people in trouble or in need of professional help could get something like this practice exercise to work on.______

5. Discuss your completed practice exercise with whoever gave it to you.

Homework: During the coming week, think more about the parts you defined and rank-ordered and whether you want to change their rank-order as listed above, or start working on the next practice exercise.

Concluding Feedback Form for Compelling Personality

Name______________________________Sex______Date_______

The purpose of this concluding feedback form is to review whether this practice exercise was helpful to you or not.

1. Please check the answer that best fits how you feel about this practice exercise:

   a. I did not like working on this practice exercise at all. I wish I never saw it. _______
   b. I did not like this practice exercise at all, but I am glad I got to work on it. _______
   c. I am delighted I got a chance to work on this practice exercise. _______
   d. I am not only delighted about working on this practice exercise, but I wish all people who need professional help had a chance to work on it. _______

2. How helpful was it to work on this practice exercise? Please check the answer that applies to you.

   a. Not helpful at all ______ c. Helpful _______
   b. Somewhat helpful ______ d. Very helpful _______

3. Which practice exercise did you like best? Rank as No. 1 the one that you liked best, rank as No. 2 the one you liked next best, and so on; mark as N/A the ones you did not like at all or did not apply to you.

Parts	*Rank-order*	*Parts*	*Rank-order*
a. Disciplined	________	e. Conscientious	________
b. Respectful	________	f. Concealed	________
c. Constricted	________	g. Compartmentalized	________
d. Reactive	________	h. Solemn	________

4. Explain why you rank-ordered these practice exercises the way you did.

____
____
____
____
____
____

5. Sometimes what we like most is not necessarily the most helpful. Which practice exercise was the most helpful to you? Rank as No. 1 the most helpful, rank as No. 2 the next most helpful, and so on, down to the least helpful practice exercise; mark as N/A the practice exercises that did not apply to you.

Parts	*Rank-order*	*Parts*	*Rank-order*
a. Disciplined	_________	e. Conscientious	_________
b. Respectful	_________	f. Concealed	_________
c. Constricted	_________	g. Compartmentalized	_________
d. Reactive	_________	h. Solemn	_________

6. Explain why you rank-ordered these practice exercises the way you did.

____
____
____
____
____
____

7. Feel free to write any comments that might improve this practice exercise.

____
____
____
____
____
____

Unusual (Sadistic)

Practice Exercise 1. Understanding Your Unusual Personality

Name______________________________________Sex___Date_____

The purpose of this practice exercise is to understand more about your personality. To learn more about yourself, you will need to explain what the parts listed below mean to you. Each part, together with the other parts listed below, very likely makes up your personality.

1. To understand these parts, you will need the help of a dictionary, your attending professional helper, your relatives, your friends, or staff members. For each part, add two examples that show your understanding of that part.

Parts	*Definitions and Examples*
a. Precipitating ____________	Example 1 ____________
____________	____________
____________	Example 2 ____________
____________	____________
b. Abrasive ____________	Example 1 ____________
____________	____________
____________	Example 2 ____________
____________	____________
c. MDogmatic ____________	Example 1 ____________
____________	____________
____________	Example 2 ____________
____________	____________
d. Isolated ____________	Example 1 ____________
____________	____________
____________	Example 2 ____________
____________	____________
e. Combative ____________	Example 1 ____________
____________	____________
____________	Example 2 ____________
____________	____________
f. Pernicious ____________	Example 1 ____________
____________	____________
____________	Example 2 ____________
____________	____________
g. Eruptive ____________	Example 1 ____________
____________	____________
____________	Example 2 ____________
____________	____________
h. Hostile ____________	Example 1 ____________
____________	____________
____________	Example 2 ____________
____________	____________

2. Now that you have completed these definitions, it is important to find out how these parts apply to you. Rank-order each part according to how much it applies to you. Rank as No. 1 the part that applies to you the most, rank as No. 2 the part that applies to you next, and so on; mark as N/A the find parts that may not apply to you.

Parts	*Rank-order*	*Parts*	*Rank-order*
a. Precipitating	________	e. Combative	________
b. Abrasive	________	f. Pernicious	________
c. Dogmatic	________	g. Eruptive	________
d. Isolated	________	h. Hostile	________

3. Write why you rank-ordered these parts the way you did.

____

____

____

____

____

4. Now that you have completed this practice exercise, check which of these answers indicates how you feel about it. There is also space for you to explain further, if you want to:

   a. I did not like this practice exercise at all. I want to quit this stupid practice exercise. ______
   b. I did not like this practice exercise very much, but I want to go on with this practice exercise. ______
   c. I liked this practice exercise and I want to go on with this practice exercise. ______
   d. I liked this practice exercise a lot and I wish I had something like this practice exercise years ago. ______
   e. I liked it so much that I wish all people in trouble or in need of professional help could get something like this practice exercise to work on. ______

5. Discuss your completed practice exercise with whoever gave it to you.

Homework: During the coming week, think more about the parts you defined and rank-order and whether you want to change their rank-order as listed above, or start working on the next practice exercise.

Concluding Feedback Form for Unusual Personality

Name_______________________________Sex______Date______

The purpose of this concluding feedback form is to review whether this practice exercise was helpful to you or not.

1. Please check the answer that best fits how you feel about this practice exercise:

   a. I did not like working on this practice exercise at all. I wish I never saw it. _______
   b. I did not like this practice exercise at all, but I am glad I got to work on it. _______
   c. I am delighted I got a chance to work on this practice exercise. _______
   d. I am not only delighted about working on this practice exercise, but I wish all people who need professional help had a chance to work on it. _______

2. How helpful was it to work on this practice exercise? Please check the answer that applies to you:

   a. Not helpful at all ____ c. Helpful ____
   b. Somewhat helpful ____ d. Very helpful ____

3. Which practice exercise did you like best? Rank as No. 1 the one that you liked best, rank as No. 2 the one you liked next best, and so on; mark as N/A the ones you did not like at all or did not apply to you.

Parts	*Rank-order*	*Parts*	*Rank-order*
a. Precipitate	_________	e. Combative	_________
b. Abrasive	_________	f. Pernicious	_________
c. Dogmatic	_________	g. Eruptive	_________
d. Isolated	_________	h. Hostile	_________

4. Explain why you rank-ordered these practice exercises the way you did.

____
____
____
____
____

5. Sometimes what we like most is not necessarily the most helpful. Which practice exercise was the most helpful to you? Rank as No. 1 the most helpful, rank as No. 2 the next most helpful, and so on, down to the least helpful practice exercise; mark as N/A the practice exercises that did not apply to you.

Parts	*Rank-order*	*Parts*	*Rank order*
a. Precipitate	________	e. Combative	________
b. Abrasive	________	f. Pernicious	________
c. Dogmatic	________	g. Eruptive	________
d. Isolated	________	h. Hostile	________

6. Explain why you rank-ordered these practice exercises the way you did.

____
____
____
____
____
____

7. Feel free to write any comments that might improve this practice exercise.

____
____
____
____
____
____

Unpopular (Antisocial)

Practice Exercise 1. Understanding Your Unpopular Personality

Name________________________________Sex___Date_____

The purpose of this practice exercise is to understand more about your personality. To learn more about yourself, you will need to explain what the parts listed below mean to you. Each part, together with the other parts listed below, very likely makes up your personality.

1. To understand these parts, you will need the help of a dictionary, your attending professional helper, your relatives, your friends, or staff members. For each part, add two examples that show your understanding of that part.

Parts	*Definitions and Examples*
a. Impulsive ______	Example 1 ______
	Example 2 ______
b. Irresponsible ______	Example 1 ______
	Example 2 ______
c. Deviant ______	Example 1 ______
	Example 2 ______
d. Acting-out ______	Example 1 ______
	Example 2 ______
e. Autonomous ______	Example 1 ______
	Example 2 ______
f. Debased ______	Example 1 ______
	Example 2 ______
g. Unruly ______	Example 1 ______
	Example 2 ______
h. Callous ______	Example 1 ______
	Example 2 ______

2. Now that you have completed these definitions, it is important to find out how these parts apply to you. Rank-order each part according to how much it applies to you. Rank as No. 1 the part that applies to you the most, rank as No. 2 the part that applies to you next, and so on; mark as N/A the find parts that may not apply to you.

Parts	*Rank-order*	*Parts*	*Rank-order*
a. Impulsive	________	e. Autonomous	________
b. Irresponsible	________	f. Debased	________
c. Deviant	________	g. Unruly	________
d. Acting-out	________	h. Callous	________

3. Write why you rank-ordered these parts the way you did.

____
____
____
____
____

4. Now that you have completed this practice exercise, check which of these answers indicates how you feel about it. There is also space for you to explain further, if you want to:

   a. I did not like this practice exercise at all. I want to quit this stupid practice exercise. ______
   b. I did not like this practice exercise very much, but I want to go on with this practice exercise. ______
   c. I liked this practice exercise and I want to go on with this practice exercise. ______
   d. I liked this practice exercise a lot and I wish I had something like this practice exercise years ago. ______
   e. I liked it so much that I wish all people in trouble or in need of professional help could get something like this practice exercise to work on. ______

5. Discuss your completed practice exercise with whoever gave it to you.

Homework: During the coming week, think more about the parts you defined and rank-ordered and whether you want to change their rank-order as listed above, or start working on the next practice exercise.

Concluding Feedback Form for Unpopular Personality

Name_________________________________Sex _____Date_____

The purpose of this concluding feedback form is to review whether this practice exercise was helpful to you or not.

1. Please select which answer fits how you feel about this practice exercise:

   a. I did not like working on this practice exercise at all. I wish I never saw it. _______
   b. I did not like this practice exercise at all, but I am glad I got to work on it. _______
   c. I am delighted I got a chance to work on this practice exercise. _______
   d. I am not only delighted about working on this practice exercise, but I wish all people who need professional help had a chance to work on it. _______

2. How helpful was it to work on this practice exercise? Please check the answer that applies to you:

a. Not helpful at all	____	c. Helpful	____
b. Somewhat helpful	____	d. Very helpful	____

3. Which practice exercise did you like best? Rank as No. 1 the one that you liked best, rank as No. 2 the one you liked next best, and so on; mark as N/A the ones you did not like at all or did not apply to you.

Parts	*Rank-order*	*Parts*	*Rank-order*
a. Impulsive	_________	e. Autonomous	_________
b. Irresponsible	_________	f. Debased	_________
c. Deviant	_________	g. Unruly	_________
d. Acting-out	_________	h. Callous	_________

4. Explain why you rank-ordered these practice exercises the way you did.

____
____
____
____
____
____

5. Sometimes what we like most is not necessarily the most helpful. Which practice exercise was the most helpful to you? Rank as No. 1 the most helpful, rank

as No. 2 the next most helpful, and so on, down to the least helpful practice exercise; mark as N/A the practice exercises that did not apply to you.

Parts	*Rank-order*	*Parts*	*Rank-order*
a. Impulsive	________	e. Autonomous	________
b. Irresponsible	________	f. Debased	________
c. Deviant	________	g. Unruly	________
d. Acting-out	________	h. Callous	________

6. Explain why you rank-ordered these practice exercises the way you did.

____
____
____
____
____
____
____

7. Feel free to write any comments that might improve this practice exercise.

____
____
____
____
____
____
____

Exciting (Histrionic)

Practice Exercise 1. Understanding Your Exciting Personality

Name________________________________Sex___Date________

The purpose of this practice exercise is to understand more about your personality. To learn more about yourself, you will need to explain what the parts listed below mean to you. Each part, together with the other parts listed below, very likely makes up your personality.

1. To understand these parts, you will need the help of a dictionary, your attending professional helper, your relatives, your friends, or staff members. For each part, add two examples that show your understanding of that part.

Parts	*Definitions and Examples*
a. Dramatic ______	Example 1 ______
	Example 2 ______
b. Attention-seeking ______	Example 1 ______
	Example 2 ______
c. Flighty ______	Example 1 ______
	Example 2 ______
d. Dissociated ______	Example 1 ______
	Example 2 ______
e. Gregarious ______	Example 1 ______
	Example 2 ______
f. Shallow ______	Example 1 ______
	Example 2 ______
g. Disjointed ______	Example 1 ______
	Example 2 ______
h. Fickle ______	Example 1 ______
	Example 2 ______

2. Now that you have completed these definitions, it is important to find out how these parts apply to you. Rank-order each part according to how much it applies to you. Rank as No. 1 the part that applies to you the most, rank as No. 2 the part that applies to you next, and so on; mark as N/A the parts that may not apply to you.

Parts	*Rank-order*	*Parts*	*Rank-order*
a. Dramatic	__________	e. Gregarious	__________
b. Attention-seeking	__________	f. Shallow	__________
c. Flighty	__________	g. Disjointed	__________
d. Dissociated	__________	h. Fickle	__________

3. Write why you rank-ordered these parts the way you did.

____

____

____

____

____

4. Now that you have completed this practice exercise, check which of these statements indicates how you feel about it. There is also space for you to explain further, if you want to:

   a. I did not like this practice exercise at all. I want to quit this stupid practice exercise. ______
   b. I did not like this practice exercise very much, but I want to go on with this practice exercise. ______
   c. I liked this practice exercise and I want to go on with this practice exercise. ______
   d. I liked this practice exercise a lot and I wish I had something like this practice exercise years ago. ______
   e. I liked it so much that I wish all people in trouble or in need of professional help could get something like this practice exercise to work on. ______

5. Discuss your completed practice exercise with whoever gave it to you.

Homework: During the coming week, think more about the parts you defined and rank-ordered and whether you want to change their rank-order as listed above, or start working on the next practice exercise.

Concluding Feedback Form for Exciting Personality

Name________________________________Sex_____Date______

The purpose of this concluding feedback form is to review whether this practice exercise was helpful to you or not.

1. Please select the statement that best fits how you feel about this practice exercise:

   a. I did not like working on this practice exercise at all. I wish I never saw it. _______
   b. I did not like this practice exercise at all, but I am glad I got to work on it. _______
   c. I am delighted I got a chance to work on this practice exercise. _______
   d. I am not only delighted about working on this practice exercise, but I wish all people who need professional help had a chance to work on it. _______

2. How helpful was it to work on this practice exercise? Please check the answer that applies to you:

a. Not helpful at all	_____	c. Helpful	_____
b. Somewhat helpful	_____	d. Very helpful	_____

3. Which practice exercise did you like best? Rank as No. 1 the one that you liked best, rank as No. 2 the one you liked next best, and so on; mark as N/A the ones you did not like at all or did not apply to you.

Parts	*Rank-order*	*Parts*	*Rank-order*
a. Dramatic	_________	e. Gregarious	_________
b. Attention-seeking	_________	f. Shallow	_________
c. Flighty	_________	g. Disjointed	_________
d. Dissociated	_________	h. Fickle	_________

4. Explain why you rank-ordered these practice exercises the way you did.

____
____
____
____
____

5. Sometimes what we like most is not necessarily the most helpful. Which practice exercise was the most helpful to you? Rank as No. 1 the most helpful, rank as No. 2 the next most helpful, and so on, down to the least helpful practice exercise; mark as N/A the practice exercises that did not apply to you.

Parts	*Rank-order*	*Parts*	*Rank-order*
a. Dramatic	________	e. Gregarious	________
b. Attention-seeking	________	f. Shallow	________
c. Flighty	________	g. Disjointed	________
d. Dissociated	________	h. Fickle	________

6. Explain why you rank-ordered these practice exercises the way you did.

____
____
____
____
____

7. Feel free to write any comments that might improve this practice exercise.

____
____
____
____
____

Private (Avoidant)

Practice Exercise 1. Understanding Your Private Personality

Name________________________________Sex_______Date_______

The purpose of this practice exercise is to understand more about your personality. To learn more about yourself, you will need to explain what the parts listed below mean to you. Each part, together with the other parts listed below, very likely makes up your personality.

1. To understand these parts, you will need the help of a dictionary, your attending professional helper, your relatives, your friends, or staff members. For each part, add two examples that show your understanding of that part.

Parts	*Definitions and Examples*
a. Fretful ______	Example 1 ______
	Example 2 ______
b. Aversive ______	Example 1 ______
	Example 2 ______
c. Distracted ______	Example 1 ______
	Example 2 ______
d. Fantasy-oriented ______	Example 1 ______
	Example 2 ______
e. Alienated ______	Example 1 ______
	Example 2 ______
f. Vexatious ______	Example 1 ______
	Example 2 ______
g. Fragile ______	Example 1 ______
	Example 2 ______
h. Anguished ______	Example 1 ______
	Example 2 ______

2. Now that you have completed these definitions, it is important to find out how these parts apply to you. Rank-order each part according to how much it applies to you. Rank as No. 1 the part that applies to you the most, rank-order as No. 2 the part that applies to you next, and so on; mark as N/A the parts that may not apply to you.

Parts	*Rank-order*	*Parts*	*Rank-order*
a. Fretful	________	e. Alienated	________
b. Aversive	________	f. Vexatious	________
c. Distracted	________	g. Fragile	________
d. Fantasy-oriented	________	h. Anguished	________

3. Write why you rank-ordered these parts the way you did.

____

____

____

____

____

4. Now that you have completed this practice exercise, check which of these answers indicates how you feel about it. There is also space for you to explain further, if you want to:

   a. I did not like this practice exercise at all. I want to quit this stupid practice exercise. _____
   b. I did not like this practice exercise very much, but I want to go on with this practice exercise. _____
   c. I liked this practice exercise and I want to go on with this practice exercise. _____
   d. I liked this practice exercise a lot and I wish I had something like this practice exercise years ago. _____
   e. I liked it so much that I wish all people in trouble or in need of professional help could get something like this practice exercise to work on. _____

5. Discuss your completed practice exercise with whoever gave it to you.

Homework: During the coming week, think more about the parts you defined and rank-ordered and whether you want to change their rank-order as listed above, or start working on the next practice exercise.

Concluding Feedback Form for Private Personality

Name________________________________Sex ________Date__________

The purpose of this practice exercise is to review whether this practice exercise was helpful to you or not.

1. Please select the statement that best fits how you feel about this practice exercise:

   a. I did not like working on this practice exercise at all. I wish I never saw it. ________
   b. I did not like this practice exercise at all, but I am glad I got to work on it. ________
   c. I am delighted I got a chance to work on this practice exercise. ________
   d. I am not only delighted about working on this practice exercise, but I wish all people who need professional help had a chance to work on it. ________

2. How helpful was it to work on this practice exercise? Please check the answer that applies to you:

   a. Not helpful at all ______ c. Helpful ______
   b. Somewhat helpful ______ d. Very helpful ______

3. Which practice exercise did you like best? Rank as No. 1 the one that you liked best, rank as No. 2 the one you liked next best, and so on; mark as N/A the ones you did not like at all or did not apply to you.

Parts	*Rank-order*	*Parts*	*Rank-order*
a. Fretful	________	e. Alienated	________
b. Aversive	________	f. Vexatious	________
c. Distracted	________	g. Fragile	________
d. Fantasy-oriented	________	h. Anguished	________

4. Explain why you rank-ordered these practice exercises the way you did.

____
____
____
____
____

5. Sometimes what we like most is not necessarily the most helpful. Which practice exercise was the most helpful to you? Rank as No. 1 the most helpful, rank as No. 2 the next most helpful, and so on, down to the least helpful practice exercise; mark as N/A the practice exercises that did not apply to you.

Parts	*Rank-order*	*Parts*	*Rank-order*
a. Fretful	________	e. Alienated	________
b. Aversive	________	f. Vexatious	________
c. Distracted	________	g. Fragile	________
d. Fantasy-oriented	________	h. Anguished	________

6. Explain why you rank-ordered these practice exercises the way you did.

____
____
____
____
____

7. Feel free to write any comments that might improve this practice exercise.

____
____
____
____
____

Distinct (Schizoid)

Practice Exercise1. Understanding Your Distinct Personality

Name______________________________Sex______Date_______

The purpose of this practice exercise is to understand more about your personality. To learn more about yourself, you will need to explain what the parts listed below mean to you. Each part, together with the other parts listed below, very likely makes up your personality.

1. To understand these parts, define them with the help of a dictionary, your attending professional helper, your relatives, your friends, or staff members. For each part, add two examples that show your understanding of that part.

Parts	*Definitions and Examples*
a. Impassive ______	Example 1 ______
______	______
______	Example 2 ______
______	______
b. Unengaged ______	Example 1 ______
______	______
______	Example 2 ______
______	______
c. Impoverished ______	Example 1 ______
______	______
______	Example 2 ______
______	______
d. Intellectualizing ______	Example 1 ______
______	______
______	Example 2 ______
______	______
e. Complacent ______	Example 1 ______
______	______
______	Example 2 ______
______	______
f. Meager ______	Example 1 ______
______	______
______	Example 2 ______
______	______
g. Undifferentiated ______	Example 1 ______
______	______
______	Example 2 ______
______	______
h. Apathetic ______	Example 1 ______
______	______
______	Example 2 ______
______	______

2. Now that you have completed these definitions, it is important to find out how these parts apply to you. Rank-order each part according to how much it applies to you. Rank as No. 1 the part that applies to you the most, rank-order as No. 2 the part that applies to you next, and so on; mark as N/A the parts that may not apply to you.

Parts	*Rank-order*	*Parts*	*Rank-order*
a. Impassive	________	e. Complacent	________
b. Unengaged	________	f. Meager	________
c. Impoverished	________	g. Undifferentiated	________
d. Intellectualizing	________	h. Apathetic	________

3. Write why you rank-ordered these parts the way you did.

____

____

____

____

____

4. Now that you have completed this practice exercise, check which of these statements indicates how you feel about it. There is also space for you to explain further, if you want to:

   a. I did not like this practice exercise at all. I want to quit this stupid practice exercise. ______
   b. I did not like this practice exercise very much, but I want to go on with this practice exercise. ______
   c. I liked this practice exercise and I want to go on with this practice exercise. ______
   d. I liked this practice exercise a lot and I wish I had something like this practice exercise years ago. ______
   e. I liked it so much that I wish all people in trouble or in need of professional help could get something like this practice exercise to work on. ______

5. Discuss your completed practice exercise with whoever gave it to you.

Homework: During the coming week, think more about the parts you just defined and rank-ordered and whether you want to change that rank-order-order or start working on the next practice exercise.

Concluding Feedback Form for Distinctive Personality

Name______________________________Sex _______Date________

The purpose of this concluding feedback form is to review whether this practice exercise was helpful to you or not.

1. Please select the statement that best fits how you feel about this practice exercise:

   a. I did not like working on this practice exercise at all. I wish I never saw it. _______
   b. I did not like this practice exercise at all, but I am glad I got to work on it. _______
   c. I am delighted I got a chance to work on this practice exercise. _______
   d. I am not only delighted about working on this practice exercise, but I wish that people who need professional help had a chance to work on it. _______

2. How helpful was it to work on this practice exercise? Please check the answer that applies to you.

   a. Not helpful at all _______ c. Helpful _______
   b. Somewhat helpful _______ d. Very helpful _______

3. Which practice exercise did you like best? Rank as No. 1 the one that you liked best, rank as No. 2 the one you liked next best, and so on; mark as N/A the ones you did not like at all or did not apply to you.

Parts	*Rank-order*	*Parts*	*Rank-order*
a. Impassive	_______	e. Complacent	_______
b. Unengaged	_______	f. Meager	_______
c. Impoverished	_______	g. Undifferentiated	_______
d. Intellectualizing	_______	h. Apathetic	_______

4. Explain why you rank-ordered these practice exercises the way you did.

____
____
____
____
____

5. Sometimes what we like most is not necessarily the most helpful. Which practice exercise was the most helpful to you? Rank as No. 1 the most helpful, rank as No. 2 the next most helpful, and so on, down to the least helpful practice exercise; mark as N/A the practice exercises that did not apply to you.

Parts	*Rank-order*	*Parts*	*Rank-order*
a. Impassive	________	e. Complacent	________
b. Unengaged	________	f. Meager	________
c. Impoverished	________	g. Undifferentiated	________
d. Intellectualizing	________	h. Apathetic	________

6. Explain why you rank ordered these practice exercises the way you did.

____
____
____
____
____

7. Feel free to write any comments that might improve this practice exercise.

____
____
____
____
____

Mixed Internalizing and Externalizing Personalities

Practice exercises included here are based on factor analyses that did not distinguish between internalizing and externalizing personalities.

Personality Disorders: Form 1992

Practice Exercise 1. Understanding Your Personality

Name______________________________Sex__________Date__________

The purpose of this practice exercise is to understand more about your personality. To learn more about yourself, you will need to explain what the parts listed below mean to you. Each part, together with the other parts, very likely makes up your overall personality.

1. To understand these parts, you will need the help of a dictionary, your attending professional helper, your relatives, your friends, or staff members, if you are presently in a clinical facility. Give two examples for each definition to make sure each part is understood correctly.

Parts	*Definitions and Examples*
a. Affective lability ______	Example 1 ______
______	______
______	Example 2 ______
______	______
b. Anxiousness ______	Example 1 ______
______	______
______	Example 2 ______
______	______
c. Compulsivity ______	Example 1 ______
______	______
______	Example 2 ______
______	______
d. Conduct problems ______	Example 1 ______
______	______
______	Example 2 ______
______	______
e. Diffidence ______	Example 1 ______
______	______
______	Example 2 ______
______	______
f. Identity problems ______	Example 1 ______
______	______
______	Example 2 ______
______	______
g. Insecure attachments ______	Example 1 ______
______	______
______	Example 2 ______
______	______
h. Interpersonal disesteem ______	Example 1 ______
______	______
______	Example 2 ______
______	______
i. Intimacy problems ______	Example 1 ______
______	______
______	Example 2 ______
______	______

j. Narcissism ____________________ Example 1 ____________________

____________________ ____________________

____________________ Example 2 ____________________

____________________ ____________________

k. Passive oppositionality ____________________ Example 1 ____________________

____________________ ____________________

____________________ Example 2 ____________________

____________________ ____________________

l. Rejection ____________________ Example 1 ____________________

____________________ ____________________

____________________ Example 2 ____________________

____________________ ____________________

m. Restricted expression ____________________ Example 1 ____________________

____________________ ____________________

____________________ Example 2 ____________________

____________________ ____________________

n. Social avoidance ____________________ Example 1 ____________________

____________________ ____________________

____________________ Example 2 ____________________

____________________ ____________________

o. Sensation (stimulation) seeking Example 1 ____________________

____________________ ____________________

____________________ Example 2 ____________________

____________________ ____________________

p. Suspiciousness ____________________ Example 1 ____________________

____________________ ____________________

____________________ Example 2 ____________________

____________________ ____________________

2. Now that you have completed these definitions, it is important to find out how they apply to you. Rank-order each part according to how much that part applies to you. Rank as No. 1 the part that applies to you the most, rank as No. 2 the part that applies to you next, and so on; mark as N/A the parts that do not apply to you at all.

Parts		*Rank-order*	*Parts*		*Rank-order*
a.	Affective lability	________	i.	Intimacy problems	________
b.	Anxiousness	________	j.	Narcissism	________
c.	Compulsivity	________	k.	Passive oppositionality	________
d.	Conduct problems	________	l.	Rejection	________
e.	Diffidence	________	m.	Restricted expression	________
f.	Identity problems	________	n.	Social avoidance	________
g.	Insecure attachments	________	o.	Sensation seeking	________
h.	Interpersonal disesteem	________	p.	Suspiciousness	________

3. Write why you rank-ordered these parts the way you did.

____
____
____
____
____

4. Now that you have completed this practice exercise, check which of these answers indicates how you feel about it. There is also space for you to explain further, if you want to:

   a. I did not like this practice exercise at all. I want to quit this stupid practice exercise. _____
   b. I did not like this practice exercise very much, but I want to go on with this practice exercise. _____
   c. I liked this practice exercise and I want to go on with this practice exercise. _____
   d. I liked this practice exercise a lot and I wish I had something like this practice exercise years ago. _____
   e. I liked it so much that I wish all people in trouble and in need of professional help could get something like this practice exercise to work on. _____

5. Discuss your completed practice exercise with whoever gave it to you.

Homework: During the coming week, think more about the parts covered by these words and whether you want to change the rank-order of these words as listed above, or start working on the next practice exercise.

Concluding Feedback Form for Personality Form 1992

Name______________________________Sex _______Date________

The purpose of this concluding feedback form is to review whether this practice exercise was helpful to you or not.

1. Please select the statement that best fits how you feel about this practice exercise:

    a. I did not like working on this practice exercise at all. I wish I never saw it. _____
    b. I did not like this practice exercise at all, but I am glad I got to work on it. _____
    c. I am delighted I got a chance to work on this practice exercise. _____
    d. I am not only delighted about working on this practice exercise, but I wish people who need professional help had a chance to work on it. _____

2. How helpful was it to work on this practice exercise? Please check the answer that applies to you:

a. Not helpful at all	____	c. Helpful	_____
b. Somewhat helpful	____	d. Very helpful	_____

3. Which practice exercise did you like best? Rank as No. 1 the one that you liked best, rank as No. 2 the one you liked next best, and so on; mark as N/A the ones you did not like at all or did not apply to you.

Parts	*Rank-order*	*Parts*	*Rank-order*
a. Affective lability	_________	i. Intimacy problems	_________
b. Anxiousness	_________	j. Narcissism	_________
c. Compulsivity	_________	k. Passive oppositionality	_________
d. Conduct problems	_________	l. Rejection	_________
e. Diffidence	_________	m. Restricted expression	_________
f. Identity problems	_________	n. Social avoidance	_________
g. Insecure attachments	_________	o. Sensation seeking	_________
h. Interpersonal disesteem	_________	p. Suspiciousness	_________

4. Explain why you rank-order these practice exercises the way you did.

____
____
____
____
____

5. Sometimes what we like most is not necessarily the most helpful. Which practice exercise was the most helpful to you? Rank as No. 1 the most helpful, rank as No. 2 the next most helpful, and so on, down to the least helpful practice exercise; mark as N/A the practice exercises that did not apply to you.

Parts	*Rank-order*	*Parts*	*Rank-order*
a. Affective lability	________	i. Intimacy problems	________
b. Anxiousness	________	j. Narcissism	________
c. Compulsivity	________	k. Passive oppositionality	________
d. Conduct problems	________	l. Rejection	________
e. Diffidence	________	m. Restricted expression	________
f. Identity problems	________	n. Social avoidance	________
g. Insecure attachments	________	o. Sensation seeking	________
h. Interpersonal disesteem	________	p. Suspiciousness	________

6. Explain why you rank-ordered these practice exercises the way you did.

____
____
____
____
____

7. Feel free to write any comments that might improve this practice exercise.

____
____
____
____
____

Personality Disorders: Form 1989

Practice Exercise 1. Understanding Your Personality

Name________________________________Sex______Date________

The purpose of this practice exercise is to understand more about your personality. To learn more about yourself, you will need to explain what the parts listed below mean to you. Each part, together with the other parts, very likely makes up your overall personality.

1. To understand these parts, you will need the help of a dictionary, of your attending professional, your relatives, your friends, or staff members, if you are at the present time in a clinical facility. To make sure you understand each part, give two examples to show how each part is understood.

Parts	*Definitions and Examples*
a. Compulsivity ________________	Example 1 ________________
	Example 2 ________________
b. Conduct problems ________________	Example 1 ________________
	Example 2 ________________
c. Diffidence ________________	Example 1 ________________
	Example 2 ________________
d. Identity problems ________________	Example 1 ________________
	Example 2 ________________
e. Insecure attachment ________________	Example 1 ________________
	Example 2 ________________

f. Intimacy problems ____________ Example 1 ____________

Example 2 ____________

g. Narcissism ____________ Example 1 ____________

Example 2 ____________

h. Suspiciousness ____________ Example 1 ____________

Example 2 ____________

i. Affective lability ____________ Example 1 ____________

Example 2 ____________

j. Passive oppositionality ____________ Example 1 ____________

Example 2 ____________

k. Perceptual cognitive distortion __ Example 1 ____________

Example 2 ____________

l. Rejection ____________ Example 1 ____________

Example 2 ____________

m. Self-harming parts ____________ Example 1 ____________

Example 2 ____________

n. Restricted expression ______________ Example 1 ______________
______________ ______________
______________ Example 2 ______________
______________ ______________

o. Social avoidance ______________ Example 1 ______________
______________ ______________
______________ Example 2 ______________
______________ ______________

p. Sensation seeking ______________ Example 1 ______________
______________ ______________
______________ Example 2 ______________
______________ ______________

q. Interpersonal disesteem ______________ Example 1 ______________
______________ ______________
______________ Example 2 ______________
______________ ______________

r. Anxiousness ______________ Example 1 ______________
______________ ______________
______________ Example 2 ______________
______________ ______________

2. Now that you have completed these definitions, it is important to find out how they apply to you. Rank-order each part according to how much that particular part applies to you. Rank as No. 1 the part that applies to you the most, rank as No. 2 the part that applies to you next, and so on; mark as N/A the parts that do not apply to you.

Parts	*Rank-order*	*Parts*	*Rank-order*
a. Compulsivity	_______	k. Perceptual cognitive distortion	_______
b. Conduct problems	_______	l. Rejection	_______
c. Diffidence	_______	m. Self-harming parts	_______
d. Identity problems	_______	n. Restricted expression	_______
e. Insecure attachment	_______	o. Social avoidance	_______
f. Intimacy problems	_______	p. Sensation seeking	_______
g. Narcissism	_______	q. Interpersonal disesteem	_______
h. Suspiciousness	_______	r. Anxiousness	_______
i. Affective lability	_______		
j. Passive oppositionality	_______		

3. Write why you rank-ordered these parts the way you did.

____
____
____
____
____

4. Now that you have completed this practice exercise, check which answer indicates how you feel about it. There is also space for you to explain further, if you want to:

   a. I did not like this practice exercise at all. I want to quit this stupid practice exercise. _____
   b. I did not like this practice exercise very much, but I want to go on with this practice exercise. _____
   c. I liked this practice exercise and I want to go on with this practice exercise. _____
   d. I liked this practice exercise a lot and I wish I had something like this practice exercise years ago. _____
   e. I liked it so much that I wish all people in trouble or in need of professional help could get something like this practice exercise to work on. _____

5. Discuss your completed practice exercise with whoever gave it to you.

Homework: During the coming week, think more about the parts covered by these words and whether you want to change their rank-order as listed above, or you want to start working on the next practice exercise.

Concluding Feedback Form for Personality Form 1989

Name________________________________Sex _______Date________

The purpose of this concluding feedback form is to review whether this practice exercise was helpful to you or not.

1. Please check the answer that best fits how you feel about this practice exercise:

   a. I did not like working on this practice exercise at all. I wish I never saw it. _____
   b. I did not like this practice exercise at all, but I am glad I got to work on it. _____
   c. I am delighted I got a chance to work on this practice exercise. _____
   d. I am not only delighted about working on this practice exercise, but I wish all people with troubles who need professional help had a chance to work on it. _____

2. How helpful was it to work on this practice exercise? Please check the answer that applies to you:

a.	Not helpful at all	_______	c.	Helpful	_______
b.	Somewhat helpful	_______	d.	Very helpful	_______

3. Which practice exercise did you like best? Rank as No. 1 the one that you liked best, rank as No. 2 the one you liked next best, and so on; mark as N/A the ones you did not like at all or did not apply to you.

Parts		*Rank-order*	*Parts*		*Rank-order*
a.	Compulsivity	_______	k.	Perceptual cognitive distortion	_______
b.	Conduct problems	_______	l.	Rejection	_______
c.	Diffidence	_______	m.	Self-harming parts	_______
d.	Identity problems	_______	n.	Restricted expression	_______
e.	Insecure attachment	_______	o.	Social avoidance	_______
f.	Intimacy problems	_______	p.	Sensation seeking	_______
g.	Narcissism	_______	q.	Interpersonal disesteem	_______
h.	Suspiciousness	_______	r.	Anxiousness	_______
i.	Affective lability	_______			
j.	Passive oppositionality	_______			

4. Explain why you rank-ordered these practice exercises the way you did.

____

____

____

____

____

5. Sometimes what we like most is not necessarily the most helpful. Which practice exercise was the most helpful to you? Rank as No. 1 the most helpful, rank as No. 2 the next most helpful, and so on, down to the least helpful practice exercise; mark as N/A the practice exercises that did not apply to you.

Parts		*Rank-order*	*Parts*		*Rank-order*
a.	Compulsivity	_______	e.	Insecure attachment	_______
b.	Conduct problems	_______	f.	Intimacy problems	_______
c.	Diffidence	_______	g.	Narcissism	_______
d.	Identity problems	_______	h.	Suspiciousness	_______

Parts	*Rank-order*	*Parts*	*Rank-order*
i. Affective lability	_______	n. Restricted expression	_______
j. Passive oppositionality	_______	o. Social avoidance	_______
k. Perceptual cognitive distortion	_______	p. Sensation seeking	_______
		q. Interpersonal disesteem	_______
l. Rejection	_______	r. Anxiousness	_______
m. Self-harming parts	_______		

6. Explain why you rank-ordered the practice exercises the way you did.

____

____

____

____

____

7. Feel free to write any comments that might improve this practice exercise.

____

____

____

____

____

Personality Disorders: Form 1990

Practice Exercise 1. Understanding Your Personality

Name_______________________________Sex______Date________

The purpose of this practice exercise is to understand more about your personality. To learn more about yourself, you will need to explain what the parts listed below mean to you. Each part, together with he other parts, very likely makes up your personality.

1. To define and understand these parts, you will need the help of a dictionary, your attending professional, relatives, friends, or staff members, if you are at the present time in a clinical facility. To make sure you understand each part, give two examples to show how each part is understood.

Parts	*Definitions and Examples*
a. Suicide proneness ________	Example 1 ________
	Example 2 ________
b. Self-derogation ________	Example 1 ________
	Example 2 ________
c. Anhedonia ________	Example 1 ________
	Example 2 ________
d. Instability ________	Example 1 ________
	Example 2 ________
e. Hypersensitivity ________	Example 1 ________
	Example 2 ________
f. Anger/aggression ________	Example 1 ________
	Example 2 ________
g. Pessimism ________	Example 1 ________
	Example 2 ________
h. Negative affect ________	Example 1 ________
	Example 2 ________
i. Suspiciousness ________	Example 1 ________
	Example 2 ________

j. Self-centered exploitation ______ Example 1 ______
______ ______
______ Example 2 ______
______ ______

k. Passive-aggressiveness ______ Example 1 ______
______ ______
______ Example 2 ______
______ ______

l. Dramatic exhibitionism ______ Example 1 ______
______ ______
______ Example 2 ______
______ ______

m. Grandiose egocentrism ______ Example 1 ______
______ ______
______ Example 2 ______
______ ______

n. Social isolation ______ Example 1 ______
______ ______
______ Example 2 ______
______ ______

o. Emotional coldness ______ Example 1 ______
______ ______
______ Example 2 ______
______ ______

p. Dependency ______ Example 1 ______
______ ______
______ Example 2 ______
______ ______

q. Conventionality-rigidity ______ Example 1 ______
______ ______
______ Example 2 ______
______ ______

r. Impulsivity ______ Example 1 ______
______ ______
______ Example 2 ______
______ ______

s. High energy ______________ Example 1 ______________
______________ ______________
______________ Example 2 ______________
______________ ______________

t. Antisocial part ______________ Example 1 ______________
______________ ______________
______________ Example 2 ______________
______________ ______________

u. Strange thoughts ______________ Example 1 ______________
______________ ______________
______________ Example 2 ______________
______________ ______________

2. Now that you have completed these definitions, it is important to find out how these parts apply to you. Rank-order each part according to how much that particular part applies to you. Rank as No. 1 the part that applies to you the most, rank-order as No. 2 the part that applies to you next, and so on; mark as N/A the parts that do not apply to you.

Parts	*Rank-order*	*Parts*	*Rank-order*
a. Suicide proneness	________	m. Grandiose egocentrism	________
b. Self-derogation	________	n. Social isolation	________
c. Anhedonia	________	o. Emotional coldness	________
d. Instability	________	p. Dependency	________
e. Hypersensitivity	________	q. Conventionality-rigidity	________
g. Pessimism	________	r. Impulsivity	________
h. Negative affect	________	s. High energy	________
i. Suspiciousness	________	t. Antisocial part	________
j. Self-centered exploitation	________	u. Strange thoughts	________
k. Passive-aggressiveness	________		
l. Dramatic exhibitionism	________		

3. Write why you rank-ordered the parts the way you did.

____
____
____
____
____

4. Now that you have completed this practice exercise, check which of these answers indicates how you feel about it. There is also space for you to explain further, if you want to:

a. I did not like this practice exercise at all. I want to quit this stupid practice exercise. ________
b. I did not like this practice exercise very much, but I want to go on with this practice exercise. ________
c. I liked this practice exercise and I want to go on with this practice exercise. ________
d. I liked this practice exercise a lot and I wish I had something like this practice exercise years ago. ________
e. I liked it so much that I wish all people in trouble or in need of professional help could get something like this practice exercise to work on. ________

5. Discuss your completed practice exercise with whoever gave it to you.

Homework: During the coming week, think more about these parts and whether you want to change their rank-order as listed above, or you want to start working on the next practice exercise.

Concluding Feedback Form for Personality Form 1990

Name________________________________Sex ________Date__________

The purpose of this concluding feedback form is to review whether this practice exercise was helpful to you or not.

1. Please check the answer that best fits how you feel about this practice exercise:

   a. I did not like working on this practice exercise at all. I wish I never saw it. ________
   b. I did not like this practice exercise at all, but I am glad I got to work on it. ________
   c. I am delighted I got a chance to work on this practice exercise. ________
   d. I am not only delighted about working on this practice exercise, but I wish all people who need professional help had a chance to work on it. ________

2. How helpful was it to work on this practice exercise? Please check the answer that applies to you:

   a. Not helpful at all ________ c. Helpful ________
   b. Somewhat helpful ________ d. Very helpful ________

3. Which practice exercise did you like best? Rank as No. 1 the one that you liked best, rank as No. 2 the one you liked next best, and so on; mark as N/A the ones you did not like at all or did not apply to you.

Behaviors	*Rank-order*	*Behaviors*	*Rank-order*
a. Suicide proneness	_____	l. Dramatic exhibitionism	_____
b. Self-derogation	_____	m. Grandiose egocentrism	_____
c. Anhedonia	_____	n. Social isolation	_____
d. Instability	_____	o. Emotional coldness	_____
e. Hypersensitivity	_____	p. Dependency	_____
g. Pessimism	_____	q. Conventionality-rigidity	_____
h. Negative affect	_____	r. Impulsivity	_____
i. Suspiciousness	_____	s. High energy	_____
j. Self-centered exploitation	_____	t. Antisocial part	_____
k. Passive-aggressiveness	_____	u. Strange thoughts	_____

4. Explain why you rank-ordered the practice exercises the way you did.

5. Sometimes what we like most is not necessarily the most helpful. Which practice exercise was the most helpful to you? Rank as No. 1 the most helpful, rank as No. 2 the next most helpful, and so on, down to the least helpful practice exercise; mark as N/A the practice exercises that did not apply to you.

Parts	*Rank-order*	*Parts*	*Rank-order*
a. Suicide proneness	_____	l. Dramatic exhibitionism	_____
b. Self-derogation	_____	m. Grandiose egocentrism	_____
c. Anhedonia	_____	n. Social isolation	_____
d. Instability	_____	o. Emotional coldness	_____
e. Hypersensitivity	_____	p. Dependency	_____
g. Pessimism	_____	q. Conventionality-rigidity	_____
h. Negative affect	_____	r. Impulsivity	_____
i. Suspiciousness	_____	s. High energy	_____
j. Self-centered exploitation	_____	t. Antisocial part	_____
k. Passive-aggressiveness	_____	u. Strange thoughts	_____

6. Explain why you rank-ordered the practice exercises the way you did.

7. Feel free to write any comments that might improve this practice exercise.

Multiple Score Tests

Personality Dimensions from the Minnesota Multiphasic Personality Inventory-2

The purpose of the practice exercises in this practice exercise is to help you deal with, understand, and even control some personality characteristics that may work against you rather than for you. These personality characteristics should have been pinpointed and identified by previous testing.

Practice Exercise 1. Anxiety

Name________________________________ Sex______Date________

1. What does anxiety mean for you? Define it as it applies especially to you.

2. In the list of problems with anxiety given below, explain in detail which of them applies especially to you and give two examples to show you understand what anxiety means.

Problems	*Explanations and Examples*
a. Tension ______	Example 1 ______
______	______
______	Example 2 ______
______	______
b. Physical problems in general ______	Example 1 ______
______	______
______	Example 2 ______
______	______
c. Physical problems in particular: i. Heart pounding ______	Example 1 ______
	______
______	Example 2 ______
______	______
ii. Shortness of breath ______	Example 1 ______
______	______
______	Example 2 ______
______	______
iii. Loose bowels ______	Example 1 ______
______	______
______	Example 2 ______
______	______
iv. Sweating ______	Example 1 ______
______	______
______	Example 2 ______
______	______
v. Any other physical problem not listed above ______	Example 1 ______
	______
______	Example 2 ______
______	______
d. Trouble with sleep ______	Example 1 ______
______	______
______	Example 2 ______
______	______

e. Worries about ________________ Example 1 ________________

________________ Example 2 ________________

f. Trouble concentrating ________________ Example 1 ________________

________________ Example 2 ________________

g. Fears of: ________________ Example 1 ________________

i. Losing my mind ________________ Example 2 ________________

ii. Not making it in life ________________ Example 1 ________________

________________ Example 2 ________________

iii. Losing my family ________________ Example 1 ________________

________________ Example 2 ________________

iv. Losing my job ________________ Example 1 ________________

________________ Example 2 ________________

v. Losing my friends ________________ Example 1 ________________

________________ Example 2 ________________

vi. Any other fear (describe in detail) ________________ Example 1 ________________

________________ Example 2 ________________

3. Rank-order these problems with anxiety according to how strong they are for you. Rank as No. 1 the problem that is the strongest and affects you the most, rank as No. 2 the problem that is next strongest, and so on; mark as N/A the problems that do not affect you at all.

Problems	*Rank-order*	*Problems*	*Rank-order*
a. Tension	________	d. Trouble with sleep	________
b. Physical problems in general	________	e. Worries about	________
		f. Trouble concentrating	________
c. Physical problems in particular:	________	g. Fears of:	
		i. Losing my mind	________
i. Heart pounding	________	ii. Not making it in life	________
ii. Shortness of breath	________	iii. Losing my family	________
iii. Loose bowels	________	iv. Losing my job	________
iv. Sweating	________	vi. Any other fear (described above)	________
v. Any other physical problem not listed above	________		

3. Now explain why you rank-ordered these problems the way you did.

____

____

____

____

____

Homework: During the coming week, think about your problems with anxiety and whether you want to change their rank-order or keep it the same. Feel free to change the rank-order if you feel it is more specific about problems with your anxiety.

Standard Format for Anxiety

Practice Exercise No. ____________Name of Problem____________

Name__________________________ Sex________ Date__________

The purpose of this and other practice exercises is to help you learn to control your problems with anxiety, one problem at a time. To achieve this goal, go back to the rank-ordering of problems with anxiety completed in the previous practice exercise. Write in the space above the problem you ranked as No. 1. Your next practice exercise will consist of the problem ranked No. 2, and so on, until you have completed a practice exercise for each feeling that you rank-ordered. Use this same format for all the other practice exercises, following the rank-order given in the first practice exercise. Before you start answering, be sure to make as many copies of this practice exercise as the number of rank-ordered problems given in the preceding practice exercise.

1. How does this problem apply to you? Please explain in detail.

____
____
____
____
____

2. How often do you feel this problem?

a.	Practically every day	_____	d.	Once a month	_____
b.	Once a week	_____	e.	Once every 6 months	_____
c.	A couple of times a month	_____	f.	Once a year	_____
			g.	Once every few years	_____

3. Please explain further:

____
____
____
____
____

4. How did this problem come about? Do you remember how it started? Check which answer fits best:

   a. When I was a child (younger than 5 years of age) _____
   b. When I was in elementary school _____
   c. When I was in middle school _____
   d. When I was in high school _____
   e. After high school _____
   f. Any other time _____

5. Please explain further:

____
____
____
____
____

6. Was this problem acceptable or unacceptable? Why? Explain.

7. Give three specific examples of how this particular problem affected you in the past.

Example 1:

Example 2:

Example 3:

8. Give three specific examples of how this problem affects you in the present.

Example 1:

Example 2:

Example 3:

9. Give three specific examples of how this problem will affect you in the future.

Example 1:

Example 2:

Example 3:

Homework: During the next week, make sure you make regular appointments with yourself to work on your rank-ordered problems (for instance, on Monday, Wednesday, and Friday night at 8 o'clock). Make sure that no one will bother you so that you can concentrate on this problem. During this time (either 30 or 60minute, depending on how long you want to work on this problem), try to concentrate on the problem that you are working on. Make it as real as you can in your mind. As soon as you feel the problem coming on, start answering the questions asked below. The idea here is for you to start the problem rather than for you to try to stop it. Remember: If you want to stop your problem, in your mind, start it in your mind! If you can start it, you can stop it. For each time you start this problem, make sure to answer in writing the following four questions:

a. How did you start it?
b. What followed?
c. How did it end?
d. What did this problem get you?

Time 1 (write the time you started__________)

a. ______________________________

____

____

b. ______________________________

____

____

c. ______________________________

____

____

d. ______________________________

____

____

Time 2 (write the time you started__________)

a. ______________________________

____

____

b. ______________________________

____

____

c. ______________________________

____

____

d. ______________________________

____

____

Time 3 (write the time you started__________)

a. ____
____
____

b. ____
____
____

c. ____
____
____

d. ____
____
____

Check which of the following indicates how you feel about this practice exercise:

a.	Completely useless	______	d.	Somewhat useful	______
b.	Somewhat useless	______	e.	Extremely useful	______
c.	So-so	______			

Explain in greater detail how you feel about this practice exercise and what you got out of it.

____
____
____
____
____

Bring this completed practice exercise and your written notes to your professional helper.

Practice Exercise 1. Fears

Name ______________________________Sex_____ Date_______

1. What do fears mean for you? Define them the best you can.

____
____
____
____
____

2. After you have defined them in general, define those things or situations listed below. Give two examples to show that you understand that fear. Feel free to use a dictionary to understand fully the meaning of each characteristic quality.

Fearful Things or Situations	*Definitions and Examples*
a. Blood ______________	Example 1 ______________
______________	______________
______________	Example 2 ______________
______________	______________
b. High places ______________	Example 1 ______________
______________	______________
______________	Example 2 ______________
______________	______________
c. Money ______________	Example 1
______________	______________
______________	Example 2 ______________
______________	______________
d. Snakes ______________	Example 1 ______________
______________	______________
______________	Example 2 ______________
______________	______________
e. Mice ______________	Example 1 ______________
______________	______________
______________	Example 2 ______________
______________	______________
f. Spiders ______________	Example 1 ______________
______________	______________
______________	Example 2 ______________
______________	______________
g. Dogs ______________	Example 1 ______________
______________	______________
______________	Example 2 ______________
______________	______________

h. Other animals (________________) ____

Example 1 ____

Example 2 ____

i. Leaving home ____

Example 1 ____

Example 2 ____

j. Fire ____

Example 1 ____

Example 2 ____

k. Storms (thunder, lightning, etc.) ____

Example 1 ____

Example 2 ____

l. Water ____

Example 1 ____

Example 2 ____

m. Dark places ____

Example 1 ____

Example 2 ____

n. Being indoors ____

Example 1 ____

Example 2 ____

o. Being outdoors ____

Example 1 ____

Example 2 ____

p. Dirt ______________________ Example 1 ______________________

______________________ ______________________

______________________ Example 2 ______________________

______________________ ______________________

q. Any other fear not listed above. What is it? (______________) Example 1 ______________________

______________________ Example 2 ______________________

______________________ ______________________

2. Which of the following things or situations upsets you the most? Rank-order them in the order that they upset you. Rank as No. 1 the object or troublesome thoughts that upsets you the most, rank as No. 2 the one that upsets you next, and so on; mark as N/A the ones that do not upset you at all and that do not apply to you.

Fearful Objects or Troublesome thoughts	*Rank-order*
a. Blood	________
b. High places	________
c. Money	________
d. Snakes	________
e. Mice	________
f. Spiders	________
g. Dogs	________
h. Other animals (__________)	________
i. Leaving home	________
j. Fire	________
k. Storms (thunder, etc.)	________
l. Water	________
m. Dark places	________
n. Being indoors	________
o. Being outdoors	________
p. Dirt	________
q. Any other fear not listed above What is it? (______________)	________

3. Explain why you rank-ordered your fears the way you did.

____

____

____

____

____

Homework: During the next week, keep thinking about your fears and whether you should rank-order differently from the way you did. Feel free to change the rank-order if appropriate.

Standard Format for Fears

Practice Exercise No. ____Title of Feared Thing or Situation_______

Name________________________________ Sex_____Date__________

The purpose of this and other practice exercises is to help you learn to control your fears, one at a time. To achieve this goal, go back to the rank-ordering of your fears completed in the previous practice exercise. Write in the space above the fear you ranked as No. 1. Your next practice exercise will consist of the fear ranked No. 2, and so on, until you have completed a practice exercise for each fear that you rank-ordered. Use this very same format for all the other practice exercises following the rank-order given in the first practice exercise. Before you start answering, be sure to make as many copies of this practice exercise as the number of rank-ordered fears given in the preceding practice exercise.

1. How does this fear apply to you? Please explain in detail.

____

____

____

____

____

2. How often do you feel this fear?

   a. Practically every day _______
   b. Once a week _______
   c. A couple of times a month _______
   d. Once a month _______
   e. Once every 6 months _______
   f. Once a year _______
   g. Once every few years _______

3. Please explain further:

____

____

____

____

____

4. How did this fear come about? Do you remember how it started? Check which answer fits best:

   a. When I was a child (younger than 5 years of age) ________
   b. When I was in elementary school ________
   c. When I was in middle school ________
   d. When I was in high school ________
   e. After high school ________
   f. Any other time ________

5. Please explain further:

____
____
____
____
____

6. Was this fear acceptable or unacceptable? Why? Explain.

____
____
____
____
____

7. Give three specific examples of how this fear affected you in the past.

   Example 1:

____
____
____
____
____

   Example 2:

____
____
____
____
____

Example 3:

8. Give three specific examples of how this fear affects you in the present.

Example 1:

Example 2:

Example 3:

9. Give three specific examples of how this particular fear will affect you in the future.

Example 1:

Example 2:

____

____

____

____

____

____

Example 3:

____

____

____

____

____

Homework: During the next week, make regular appointments with yourself to work on your fearful thing or situation (for instance, on Monday, Wednesday, and Friday nights at 8 o'clock). Make sure that no one will bother you in order for you to concentrate on this problem. During this time (either 30 or 60 minutes, depending on how long you want to work on this fear), try to concentrate on the fear that you are working on. Make it as real as you can in your mind. As soon as you feel this specific fear coming on, start answering the questions asked below. The idea here is for you to start the fear rather than for you to try to stop it. Remember: If you want to stop your fear in your mind, start it in your mind! If you can start it, you can stop it. For each time you start this particular fear, make sure to answer the following four questions:

a. How did you start it?
b. What followed?
c. How did it end?
d. What did this fear get you?

Time 1 (write the time you started__________)

a. ____

____

____

b. ____

____

____

c. ____

____

____

d. ______________________________
____
____

Time 2 (write the time you started__________)

a. ______________________________
____
____

b. ______________________________
____
____

c. ______________________________
____
____

d. ______________________________
____
____

Time 3 (write the time you started__________)

a. ______________________________
____
____

b. ______________________________
____
____

c. ______________________________
____
____

d. ______________________________
____
____

Check which of the following indicates how you feel about this practice exercise:

a.	Completely useless	______	d.	Somewhat useful	______
b.	Somewhat useless	______	e.	Extremely useful	______
c.	So-so	______			

Explain in greater detail how you feel about this practice exercise and what you got out of it.

____

____

____

____

____

Bring this completed practice exercise and your written notes to your professional helper.

Practice Exercise 1. Obsessiveness

Name______________________________Sex________Date__________

This troublesome thoughts shows itself in different ways. The purpose of this practice exercise is to find those ways and learn to control them, if possible.

1. Define the ways listed below in which obsessiveness shows itself in everyday behavior. Give two specific examples of how each way shows itself in your behavior.

Obsessions	*Examples*
a. Trouble in making decisions_____	Example 1 ____________
____________________	____________________
____________________	Example 2 ____________
____________________	____________________
b. Thinking too much about issues and problems__________	Example 1 ____________
	____________________
____________________	Example 2 ____________
____________________	____________________
c. Causing others to be impatient with me and my ways________	Example 1 ____________
	____________________
____________________	Example 2 ____________
____________________	____________________
d. Trouble with changes________	Example 1 ____________
____________________	____________________
____________________	Example 2 ____________
____________________	____________________

e. Any other obsession (write what it is)______________________
____
____

Example 1 ______________________
____
Example 2 ______________________
____

2. Pick the obsession that is the strongest in your mind (specify:______) and answer the following questions about it.

a. How often does it take place? Check which answer applies:

i. Daily _____
ii. Weekly _____
iii. Monthly _____
iv. Rarely _____
v. Explain how it takes place.

____
____
____

b. How strongly does this obsession affect:

i. Your life in general?

____
____
____

ii. Your marriage or your relationships with the opposite sex?

____
____
____

iii. Your parents?

____
____
____

iv. Your children?

____
____
____

v. Your friends?

____

____

____

vi. Your work?

____

____

____

vii. Your leisure time?

____

____

____

3. If you have more than one obsession, write the second one here (____________) and answer the same questions about it.

a. Check how often it takes place:

i. Daily _____
ii. Weekly _____
iii. Monthly _____
iv. Rarely _____
v. Please explain how it takes place: _____

____

____

____

b. How strongly does this obsession affect:

i. Your life in general?

____

____

____

ii. Your marriage or your relationships with the opposite sex?

____

____

____

iii. Your parents?

____
____
____

iv. Your children?

____
____
____

v. Your friends?

____
____
____

vi. Your work?

____
____
____

vii. Your leisure time?

____
____
____

8. If you have another obsession, write it here (____________) and answer the same questions asked of the two previous obsessions.

9. There is the possibility that your obsessive behavior comes about from an inability to connect and to link feelings, thinking, and actions together. What do you think of this possibility? If you think that this possibility may apply to you, comment on the various relationships within yourself between:

   a. Thinking and acting

____
____
____

b. Acting and feelings

___

___

___

c. Thinking and feelings

___

___

___

Homework: Part of this homework practice exercise may not make sense for you. However, try to follow these instructions. First, decide whether you want your obsession(s) to control you or whether you want to learn to control your obsession(s). If you want your obsession(s) to control you, go no further. You do not need to complete this practice exercise. If you want to learn how to control your obsession(s), you will need to follow these instructions consistently.

Step 1: Set specific times when you can start to think about your obsession(s). At the beginning, these times may have to be closely spaced, according to how often you think about your obsession(s). For instance, if you obsess twice a day, start obsessing at least once every hour for 12 h a day for a week, if at all possible. However, this time you must write what you are obsessing about as long as you can stand it. It does not matter if you repeat yourself. In fact, the more you repeat yourself, the better off you will be.

Step 2: See if, in the second week, you can start decreasing how often you can obsess every day. Instead of 12 times a day, could you go down to ten times a day for a week, always at prearranged times? In this case, you may want to obsess every hour and a half rather than every hour. It is important that you follow the schedule you set beforehand, that is, if you have planned the day before to obsess on the hour every hour, except for mealtimes. Use a clock or timer to remind you of obsessing right at the time you planned and not at any other time. Keep writing what you are obsessing about as long as possible, even if you repeat yourself, as many times as possible.

Step 3: If you are successful in performing this practice exercise for the second week, see if you can set the goal of decreasing your obsessing to eight times for the third week, always at preset times.

Step 4: If you have completed the previous step, see if you can now decrease your obsessing to six times for the fourth week, decreasing it every week after you have been able to perform this task for at least a week.

Note: Do not try to rush and go faster than necessary. It may be dangerous for you to go faster than the instructions given above! Keep track of how well you follow your schedule and discuss it with your professional helper.

Practice Exercise 1. Depression

Name________________________________Sex____Date______

Depression means a lot of different things to different people. The purpose of this practice exercise is to decrease your depression.

1. What does depression mean to you? Define it and describe it as you see it.

____

____

____

____

____

2. Below is a list of feelings that are related to depression. Please expand on all of them by using two examples to show you have understood what that feeling is.

____

____

____

____

____

Feelings	*Expansions and Examples*
a. Feeling blue _______________	Example 1 _______________
_______________________	_______________________
_______________________	Example 2 _______________
_______________________	_______________________
b. Uncertainty about the future ____	Example 1 _______________
_______________________	_______________________
_______________________	Example 2
_______________________	_______________________

c. Uninterested in living ______________________________
____
____
Example 1 ______________________________
Example 2 ______________________________

d. Brooding ______________________________
____
____
Example 1 ______________________________
Example 2 ______________________________

e. Unhappiness ______________________________
____
____
Example 1 ______________________________
Example 2 ______________________________

f. Crying often ______________________________
____
____
Example 1 ______________________________
Example 2 ______________________________

g. Feeling hopeless and empty ______________________________
____
____
Example 1 ______________________________
Example 2 ______________________________

h. Thinking of killing myself ______________________________
____
____
Example 1 ______________________________
Example 2 ______________________________

i. Wishing to be dead ______________________________
____
____
Example 1 ______________________________
Example 2 ______________________________

j. Sinfulness and lack of forgiveness
____
____
Example 1 ______________________________
Example 2 ______________________________

k. Lacking supports ______________________________
____
____
Example 1 ______________________________
Example 2 ______________________________

l. Another feelings not listed above. What is it? ____________________ ____________________ ____________________

Example 1 ____________________ ____________________

Example 2 ____________________ ____________________

3. Now rank-order these feelings based on how strong they are for you. Rank as No. 1 the strongest feeling for you, rank as No. 2 the second strongest feeling, and so on; mark as N/A the feelings that do not apply to you.

Feelings	*Rank-order*
a. Feeling blue	________
b. Uncertainty about the future	________
c. Uninterested in living	________
d. Brooding	________
e. Unhappiness	________
f. Crying often	________
g. Feeling hopeless and empty	________
h. Thinking of killing myself	________
i. Wishing to be dead	________
j. Sinfulness and lack of forgiveness	________
k. Lacking supports	________
l. Another feeling (____________)	________

3. Explain why you rank-ordered these feelings the way you did.

____
____
____
____
____

Homework: During the next week, think about your rank-order of feelings and change that order if you feel it did not accurately represent how you feel.

Standard Format for Feelings of Depression

Practice Exercise No. _____Title of Feeling____________________

Name____________________________ Sex_____Date__________

The purpose of this and other practice exercises is to help you learn to control your feelings of depression, one at a time. To achieve this goal, go back to the rank-ordering of your feelings completed in the previous practice exercise. Write in the space above the feeling you ranked as No. 1. Your next practice exercise will consist of the feeling ranked No. 2, and so on, until you have completed a practice exercise for each feeling that you rank-ordered. Use this same format for all the other practice exercises following the rank-order given in the first practice exercise. Before you start answering, be sure to make as many copies of this practice exercise as the number of rank-ordered feelings given in the previous practice exercise.

1. How does this feeling apply to you? Please explain in detail.

____
____
____
____
____

2. How often do you feel this feeling?

   a. Practically every day ________
   b. Once a week ________
   c. A couple of times a month ________
   d. Once a month ________
   e. Once every 6 months ________
   f. Once a year ________
   g. Once every few years ________

3. Please explain further:

____
____
____
____
____

4. How did this feeling come about? Do you remember when it started? Check which answer fits best:

   a. When I was a child (younger than 5 years of age) ________
   b. When I was in elementary school ________
   c. When I was in middle school ________
   d. When I was in high school ________
   e. After high school ________
   f. Any other time ________

5. Please explain further:

6. Was this feeling acceptable or unacceptable? Why? Explain.

7. Give three specific examples of how this feeling affected you in the past.

   Example 1:

   Example 2:

   Example 3:

8. Give three specific examples of how this feeling affects you in the present.

   Example 1:

Example 2:

Example 3:

9. Give three specific examples of how you want this feeling to affect you in the future.

Example 1:

Example 2:

Example 3:

Homework: During the next week, make regular appointments with yourself to work on your rank-ordered feelings (for instance, on Monday, Wednesday, and Friday night at 8 o'clock). Make sure that no one will bother you in order for you to concentrate on this feeling. During this time (either 30 or 60 minute, depending on how long you want to work on this feeling), try to concentrate on the feeling that you are working on. Make it as real as you can in your mind. As soon as you feel the feeling coming on, start answering the questions asked below. The idea here is for you to start the feeling rather than for you to try to stop it. Remember: If you want to stop your feeling in your mind, start it in your mind! If you can start it, you can stop it. Write down what happened in detail. For each time you start this feeling, make sure to answer the following four questions:

a. How did you start it?
b. What followed?
c. How did it end?
d. What did this problem get you?

Time 1 (write the time you started__________)

a. ______________________________

____

____

b. ______________________________

____

____

c. ______________________________

____

____

d. ______________________________

____

____

Time 2 (write the time you started__________)

a. ______________________________

____

____

b. ______________________________

____

____

c. ______________________________

____

____

d. ____
____
____

Time 3 (write the time you started__________)

a. ____
____
____

b. ____
____
____

c. ____
____
____

d. ____
____
____

Check which of the following indicates how you feel about this practice exercise:

a. Completely useless _______ d. Somewhat useful _______
b. Somewhat useless _______ e. Extremely useful _______
c. So-so _______

Explain in greater detail how you feel about this practice exercise and what you got out of it.

____
____
____
____
____

Bring this completed practice exercise and your written notes to your professional helper.

Practice Exercise 1. Compulsions

Name________________________________ Sex_____ Date _______

Compulsions are behaviors that repeat themselves often and unnecessarily without your control. In fact, these behaviors control you. Which compulsion controls your life?

1. Define each compulsion and give two examples of each.

Compulsions	*Definitions and Examples*
a. Hand washing ______	Example 1 ______
______	______
______	Example 2 ______
______	______
b. Hoarding (collecting things)	Example 1 ______
______	______
______	Example 2 ______
______	______
c. Counting ______	Example 1 ______
______	______
______	Example 2 ______
______	______
d. Buying/shopping ______	Example 1 ______
______	______
______	Example 2 ______
______	______
e. Other compulsions: what is it?	Example 1 ______
______	______
______	Example 2 ______
______	______

2. Pick the compulsion that applies to you the most and describe it in detail.

______

______

______

______

______

3. Describe in detail what you feel and think and what happens to you before, during, and after you have given in to this compulsion.

   a. Before

______

______

______

b. During

c. After

4. How often does this compulsion take place?

a. Daily	________	c. Monthly	________
b. Weekly	________	d. Rarely	________

5. Please explain in greater detail how often it takes place.

6. How strongly does this compulsion affect:

   a. Your life in general?

   b. Your partner or your relationships with the opposite sex?

   c. Your parents?

d. Your children?

e. Your friends?

f. Your work?

g. Your leisure time?

7. If you have more than one compulsion, describe the others by answering questions 2 through 6 above.

8. There is the possibility that compulsive behavior comes about from our inability to connect and to link feelings, thinking, and actions together. What do you think of this possibility? If you think that it may apply to you, please comment on the various relationships within yourself between:

   a. Thinking and acting

   b. Acting and feelings

   c. Thinking and feelings

Homework: Part of this homework practice exercise may not make sense for you. However, try to follow these instructions. First, you have to decide whether you want your compulsion to control you or whether you want to learn to control your compulsion. If you want your compulsion to control your life, go no further. You do not need to complete this practice exercise. If you want to learn how to control your compulsion, you will need to follow these instructions consistently.

Step 1. You need to set specific times when you can start to work on your compulsion. At the beginning, these times may have to be closely spaced, according to how often you perform your compulsion. For instance, if you hand wash ten times a day, set 12 times when you are going to wash your hands, at least once every hour on the hour for 12 h a day for a week. However, it is crucial that you record and log how often and how many times you washed your hands each day.

Step 2. In the second week, you can start decreasing how often you wash your hands every day. Instead of 12 times a day, could you go down to ten times a day for a week, always at prearranged times? In this case, you may want to wash your hands every hour and a half rather than every hour. It is important that you follow the schedule you set beforehand; that is, if you have planned from the day before to wash your hands on the hour every hour, except for mealtimes, use a clock or timer to remind you of washing your hands right at the time you planned and not at any other time. Again log and record how often and how many times you have washed your hands each day.

Step 3. In the third week, see if you can set the goal of decreasing your hand washing to eight times a day for a week always at preset times. Keep track of how well you follow your schedule.

Step 4. In the fourth week, see if you can now decrease your hand washing to six times a day for a week. Thereafter, decrease your schedule by two hand washings every week after you have been able to perform this task for at least a week. But do not try to rush and go faster than necessary. It may be dangerous for you to go faster than the instructions given above.

Discuss your records with your professional helper.

Practice Exercise 1. Health Troublesome thoughts

Name ________________________________ Sex_____Date______

The purpose of this practice exercise is to find whether some of your health troublesome thoughts are due to actual physical causes or whether they are produced from emotional tensions without proved medical causes.

1. Circle how often and how strongly these physical troublesome thoughts worried or affected you. Circle only those troublesome thoughts that apply to you:

Frequency: How often?
Everyday = 4; Once a week = 3; Once a month = 2; Once a year = 1; Never = 0.
Intensity: How strong?
Very strong = 3; Somewhat strong = 2; a bit strong = 1; Not strong at all = 0.

	Frequency					Intensity			
1. Gastrointestinal									
a. Constipation	4	3	2	1	0	3	2	1	0
b. Nausea and vomiting	4	3	2	1	0	3	2	1	0
c. Stomach trouble	4	3	2	1	0	3	2	1	0
d. Other (_______)	4	3	2	1	0	3	2	1	0
2. Neurological									
a. Convulsions	4	3	2	1	0	3	2	1	0
b. Dizziness	4	3	2	1	0	3	2	1	0
c. Fainting spells	4	3	2	1	0	3	2	1	0
d. Paralysis	4	3	2	1	0	3	2	1	0
e. Other (_______)	4	3	2	1	0	3	2	1	0
3. Sensory problems									
a. Hearing	4	3	2	1	0	3	2	1	0
b. Vision	4	3	2	1	0	3	2	1	0
c. Smell	4	3	2	1	0	3	2	1	0
d. Balance	4	3	2	1	0	3	2	1	0
4. Cardiovascular system									
a. Heart	4	3	2	1	0	3	2	1	0
b. Chest pains	4	3	2	1	0	3	2	1	0
c. Other (_______)	4	3	2	1	0	3	2	1	0
5. Skin	4	3	2	1	0	3	2	1	0
6. Pains	4	3	2	1	0	3	2	1	0
a. Headaches	4	3	2	1	0	3	2	1	0
b. Neck	4	3	2	1	0	3	2	1	0
c. Lower back	4	3	2	1	0	3	2	1	0
d. Other (_______)	4	3	2	1	0	3	2	1	0
7. Respiration									
a. Coughing	4	3	2	1	0	3	2	1	0
b. Hay fever	4	3	2	1	0	3	2	1	0
c. Asthma	4	3	2	1	0	3	2	1	0
d. Emphysema	4	3	2	1	0	3	2	1	0
e. Other (_______)	4	3	2	1	0	3	2	1	0

8. What have you done about these troublesome thoughts? Please describe in detail.

9. What have you done about feeling healthy and keeping healthy?

10. What have you done about your diet?

11. What have you done about exercising regularly?

12. What have you done about your mental and emotional attitude towards your body?

13. What is the relationship between your physical troublesome thoughts and painful past events in your life?

14. What is the relationship between your physical troublesome thoughts and stressful events in your present life?

15. Of all the things you have been asked above, what can you change and how are you going to change it?

____
____
____
____
____

16. When is the last time you received a thorough physical examination?

____
____
____
____
____

17. If you have not had a complete physical examination in the last 2 years, get one before going any further with this or other practice exercises.

Homework: During the next week, think more about physical troublesome thoughts that have a demonstrated medical basis and troublesome thoughts that have no medical basis. Make an appointment with yourself at least 24 h in advance at a specific time and place. If there are some troublesome thoughts that do not have a demonstrated medical basis, pick the one that stresses you the most and answer in writing questions 8–15. After completing the answers to this first troublesome thoughts, repeat this process for any other troublesome thoughts that does not have a demonstrated medical basis. Be sure to follow medical prescriptions for all those troublesome thoughts that are medically demonstrated. Discuss your answers with your professional helper.

Practice Exercise 1. Unusual Thinking

Name ______________________ Sex__________ Date______

Unusual thinking may entail different things for different people The purpose of this practice exercise is to learn more about the nature of your unusual thinking.

1. In what way is your thinking unusual?

____
____
____
____
____

2. Have you experienced hallucinations or visions of any kind recently? For instance, have you:

    a. Heard something very unusual or strange? What?

____

____

____

        i. When?
        ii. How often have you heard it?

Every day	______
Every other day	______
Once or twice a week	______
Once every 2 weeks	______
Once a month	______
Once a year	______
Less than once a year	______

        iii. Can you control what you heard? Yes____ No____

    b. Seen something very unusual or strange? What?

____

____

____

        i. When?

____

____

____

        ii. How often have you seen it?

Every day	______
Every other day	______
Once or twice a week	______
Once every 2 weeks	______
Once a month	______
Once a year	______
Less than once a year	______

        iii. Can you control what you have seen? Yes____ No_____

c. Smelled something that you have never smelled before? What?

____
____
____

i. When?

____
____
____

ii. How often have you smelled it?

Every day	______	Once a month	______
Every other day	______	Once a year	______
Once or twice a week	______	Less than once a year	______
Once every 2 weeks	______		

iii. Can you control what you have smelled? Yes____ No_____

3. Describe any strange or peculiar thoughts that have come into your head lately. What are they?

____
____
____
____
____

a. When do you have these thoughts?

____
____
____

b. How often do these thoughts come into your head?

Every day	______	Once a month	______
Every other day	______	Once a year	______
Once or twice a week	______	Less than once a year	______
Once every 2 weeks	______		

c. Can you control these thoughts? Yes____ No____

4. Do you find that you cannot trust anybody these days and that you are suspicious or fearful that:

a.	Others may speak ill of you	Yes____	No____
b.	Others are plotting against you	Yes____	No____
c.	Someone is trying to poison you	Yes____	No____
d.	Someone is trying to hurt you or your reputation	Yes____	No____
e.	Somebody is trying to cheat you	Yes____	No____
f.	Somebody is after you	Yes____	No____
g.	Someone has it in for me	Yes____	No____

5. Do you think that you are on a special mission? Yes____ No____

   a. If yes, what is this special mission about?

____
____
____

   b. What will you get if and when you finish this special mission?

____
____
____

5. Do you think you have received special powers? Yes____ No_____

   a. If yes, who granted you these powers?

____
____
____

   b. What do these special powers consist of?

____
____
____

Homework: If you want to keep hearing, seeing, or smelling strange things or if you want to keep having peculiar thoughts and stay suspicious of others, going on your special mission, or keeping your special powers, do nothing more. You do not need to do this homework practice exercise. However, if you want to get rid of strange and peculiar things or thoughts, follow these instructions.

Step 1. Make three appointments with yourself next week at preset times, such as Tuesday, Thursday, and Saturday at 9 p.m., for at most 1 h. Set a clock or timer to make sure that you spend just 1 h with yourself and write down whatever comes into your mind. If the things listed above come into your head at other times, write a brief note on a piece of paper and use it during your next appointment.

Step 2. During this hour, try to hear, see, smell, or think whatever you have experienced lately. As you make yourself start these things, write down everything you see, hear, smell, feel, and think in as much detail as you can. If you cannot write, talk into a tape-recorder. Bring your notes or tapes to your professional helper and ask whether there is medication that could help avoid all your unusual thinking.

Practice Exercise 1. Anger

Name ___________ Sex____Date______

The purpose of this and other practice exercises is to help you control and express your anger in more constructive and positive ways than you may have done in the past.

1. Anger and hostility show themselves in various ways. Define and write in detail what, how, when, and how often you get angry. Feel free to use a dictionary if you need help with these definitions.

   a. Irritability

      What is it? Define it:

____

____

____

      How? (Give an example):

____

____

____

      When?

____

____

____

      How often?

____

____

____

How strong?

b. Grouchiness

What is it? Define it:

How? (Give an example):

When?

How often?

How strong?

c. Impatience

What is it? Define it:

How? (Give an example):

When?

How often?

How strong?

d. Hotheadedness

What is it? Define it:

How? (Give an example):

When?

How often?

How strong?

e. Annoyance

What is it? Define it:

How? (Give an example):

When?

How often?

How strong?

f. Stubbornness

What is it? Define it:

How? (Give an example):

When?

How often?

How strong?

g. Swearing

What is it? Define it:

How? (Give an example):

When?

How often?

How strong?

h. Smashing or breaking things

What is it? Define it:

How? (Give an example):

When?

How often?

How strong?

i. Loss of control, temper tantrums

What is it? Define it:

How? (Give an example):

When?

How often?

How strong?

j. Verbal abuse of others

What is it? Define it:

How? (Give an example):

When?

How often?

How strong?

k. Physical abuse of others

What is it? Define it:

How? (Give an example):

When?

How often?

How strong?

____
____
____

l. Any other way to express anger peculiar to you

What is it? Define it:

____
____
____

How? (Give an example):

____
____
____

When?

____
____
____

How often?

____
____
____

How strong?

____
____
____

3. Rank-order these terms by how often and how strong you show that particular form of anger. Pick the worst way you show anger and give it a rank-order of No. 1. Then pick the next worst and give it a rank-order of No. 2, and so on; mark as N/A the forms of anger that do not present a problem for you.

Anger	*Rank-order*	*Anger*	*Rank-order*
a. Irritability	________	d. Hotheadedness	________
b. Grouchiness	________	e. Annoyances	________
c. Impatience	________	f. Stubbornness	________

Anger	*Rank-order*	*Anger*	*Rank-order*
g. Swearing	________	j. Verbal abuse of others	________
h. Smashing or breaking things	________	k. Physical abuse of others	________
i. Loss of control, temper tantrums	________	l. Your peculiar way to show anger	________

4. Explain why you rank-ordered these forms of anger the way you did.

____
____
____
____
____

Homework: During the coming week, think about how you have rank-ordered the ways anger is expressed. Feel free to change that order if you feel it is closer to the ways you show and express anger. Be sure to discuss your completed practice exercise with your professional helper.

Standard Practice Exercise for Anger

Practice Exercise No. _____ Title of Angry Behavior ______________

Name____________________________Sex__________Date________

The purpose of this and other practice exercises is to help you learn to control your angry feelings, one angry feeling at a time. To achieve this goal, go back to the rank-ordering of your angry feelings completed in the previous practice exercise. Write in the space above the angry feeling you ranked as No. 1.Your next practice exercise will consist of the angry feeling you ranked as No. 2, and so on, until you have completed a practice exercise for each feeling that you rank-ordered. Use this same format for all the other practice exercises following the rank-order given in the first practice exercise. Before you start answering, be sure to make as many copies of this practice exercise as the number of rank-ordered angry feelings given in the previous practice exercise.

1. How does this angry feeling apply to you? Please explain in detail.

____
____
____
____
____

2. How often do you express this angry feeling?
   a. Practically every day ______
   b. Once a week ______
   c. A couple of times a month ______
   d. Once a month ______
   e. Once every 6 months ______
   f. Once a year ______
   g. Once every few years ______

3. Please explain further:

____
____
____
____
____

4. How did this angry feeling come about? Do you remember when it started? Check which answer fits best:

   a. When I was a child (younger than 5 years of age) ______
   b. When I was in elementary school ______
   c. When I was in middle school ______
   d. When I was in high school ______
   e. After high school ______
   f. Any other time ______

5. Please explain further:

____
____
____
____
____

6. Was this angry feeling acceptable or unacceptable? Why? Explain.

____
____
____
____
____

7. Give three specific examples of how this angry feeling affected you in the past.

Example 1:

Example 2:

Example 3:

8. Give three specific examples of how this angry feeling affects you in the present.

Example 1:

Example 2:

Example 3:

____
____
____
____
____

9. Give three specific examples of how this angry feeling will affect you in the future.

Example 1:

____
____
____
____
____

Example 2:

____
____
____
____
____

Example 3:

____
____
____
____
____

Homework: During the next week, make regular appointments with yourself to work on this practice exercise (for instance, on Monday, Wednesday, and Friday nights at 8 o'clock). Make sure that no one will bother you in order for you to concentrate on this practice exercise. During this time (either 30 or 60 minute, depending on how long you want to work on this feeling angry), try to concentrate on the specific feeling of anger that you are working on. Make it as real as you can in your mind. As soon as you feel that angry feeling coming on, start answering the questions asked below. The idea here is for you to start the angry feeling rather than for you to try to stop it. Remember: If you want to stop your angry feelings in your mind, start them in your mind! If you can start it, you can stop it. Write down what happened in detail. For each time you start this angry feeling, make sure to answer in writing the following four questions:

a. How did you start it?
b. What followed?
c. How did it end?
d. What did this feeling angry get you?

Time 1 (write the time you started__________)

a ____
____
____

b ____
____
____

c ____
____
____

d ____
____
____

Time 2 (write the time you started__________)

a ____
____
____

b ____
____
____

c ____
____
____

d ____
____
____

Time 3 (write the time you started__________)

a ____
____
____

b ____
____
____

c ____
____
____

d ____
____
____

Check which of the following indicates how you feel about this practice exercise:

a. Completely useless _____ d. Somewhat useful _____
b. Somewhat useless _____ e. Extremely useful _____
c. So-so _____

Explain in greater detail how you feel about this practice exercise and what you got out of it.

____
____
____
____
____
____

Bring this completed practice exercise and your written notes to your professional helper.

Practice Exercise 1. Cynicism

Name ____________ Sex____Date_____

Cynicism means a lot of things. Some of these things may apply to you and some may not. Determine which of these things apply to you and which do not by answering the questions below.

1. Distrust of others

   a. Are you distrustful of others? Yes_____ No_____
   b. If yes, how distrustful are you? A lot_____ Some_____ A little _____
   c. What is it that you distrust? ______________________
   d. Whom do you distrust the most? ______________________
   e. Whom do you distrust next? ______________________
   f. Whom do you distrust the least? ______________________
   g. How does this distrust affect you?

   ____
   ____
   ____

2. Negativity and negative motivation

   a. How negative are you? A lot_____ Some_____ A little______
   b. What are you negative about?

   ____
   ____
   ____

   c. What does your negativity get you?

   ____
   ____
   ____

   d. How did you learn to think negatively?

   ____
   ____
   ____

   e. Give an example of your negativity and what it got you in the end.

   ____
   ____
   ____

   f. How can you learn to replace your negative feelings with positive feelings? If you do not know, ask your professional helper for suggestions.

   ____
   ____
   ____

3. Most people are honest because they fear being caught.

   a. This statement, if you believe it to be true, would mean that you believe that most people are dishonest. Is that what you believe? Yes_____ No____
   b. What does honesty mean to you?

   ____
   ____
   ____

   c. While we cannot control other people's honesty and there is little we can do about it, except to make sure they behave honestly with us, there is a great deal we can do to make sure we strive to be as honest as possible. Why?

4. People cannot be relied upon.

   a. Why not?

   b. What past painful experiences have led you to believe that statement to be true?

   c. If you cannot rely on other people, can other people rely on you? If so, why should they?

   d. Instead of making a general statement, would it be better to say that some people can be relied upon and some cannot? Please comment.

5. Friendliness cannot be trusted.

   a. If you believe this statement to be true, you must have felt let down a lot. What experiences led you to believe the truth of that statement? List at least three painful experiences that led you to believe not to trust friendliness.

   Experience 1:

Experience 2:

____
____
____

Experience 3:

____
____
____

b. Between friendliness on one extreme and coldness on the other, can you find a middle point where you can be yourself without turning people off?

____
____
____

6. Distance from others is the best policy.

a. Do you believe this statement to be true or false?
b. If you believe this statement to be true, why do you?

____
____
____

c. What would be the outcome for you by always keeping distance from others?

____
____
____

d. Rather than making one flat statement for everybody, could you agree that there are some people that we want to keep distant from us. On the other hand, there are people who we need to be close to and we want them to be close to us? What kind of people do you want to keep distant from?

____
____
____

e. Why?

f. What kind of people would you like to be close to? Why?

7. People are out to take advantage of others.

   a. Do you believe this statement to be true or false?
   b. If you believe this statement to be true, what experiences in your past led you to believe it to be true?

   c. What kind of people are more likely to take advantage of you?

   d. What kind of people are more likely not to take advantage of you?

   e. What do you think about this statement: Certain people are more likely to take advantage of us if we let them.

8. Rank-order the above statements from items 3–7 according to the how much they apply to you and how much you believe the statement to be true. Rank as No. 1 the statement that applies to you the most and that you believe to be most true, rank as No. 2 the next statement that you believe to apply to you, and so on; mark as N/A the statements that do not apply to you.

Statement	*Rank-order*
a. Most people are honest because they fear being caught.	________
b. People cannot be relied upon.	________
c. Friendliness cannot be trusted.	________
c. Distance from others is the best policy.	________
d. People are out to take advantage of others.	________

9. Explain why you rank-ordered these statements the way you did.

____

____

____

____

____

Homework: During the coming week, think about how you have rank-ordered these statements and feel free to change that order if you feel that that change is closer to the way you think.

Standard Practice Exercise for Cynicism

Practice Exercise No.___ Title of Cynical Statement ______________

Name______________________________Sex_____Date___________

The purpose of this and other practice exercises is to help you learn to control your cynical thinking, one statement at a time. To achieve this goal, go back to the rank-ordering of the statements completed in the previous practice exercise. Write in the space above the statement you ranked as No. 1. Your next practice exercise will consist of the statement ranked as No. 2, and so on, until you have completed a practice exercise for each statement. Use this same format for all the other practice exercises following the rank-order given in the first practice exercise. Before you start answering, be sure to make as many copies of this practice exercise as the number of rank-ordered statements given in the previous practice exercise.

1. How does this statement apply to you? Please explain in detail.

____

____

____

____

____

2. How often do you express this statement?

a.	Practically every day	_____	e.	Once every 6 months	_____
b.	Once a week	_____	f.	Once a year	_____
c.	A couple of times a month	_____	g.	Once every few years	_____
d.	Once a month	_____			

3. Please explain further:

____
____
____
____
____

4. How did this statement come about? Do you remember how it started? Check which answer fits best:

   a. When I was a child (younger than 5 years of age) ______
   b. When I was in elementary school ______
   c. When I was in middle school ______
   d. When I was in high school ______
   e. After high school ______
   f. Any other time ______

5. Please explain further:

____
____
____
____
____

6. Was this statement acceptable or unacceptable? Why? Explain.

____
____
____
____
____

7. Give three specific examples of how this statement affected you in the past.

Example 1:

Example 2:

Example 3:

8. Give three specific examples of how this statement affects you in the present.

Example 1:

Example 2:

Example 3:

9. Give three specific examples of how this statement will affect you in the future.

Example 1:

Example 2:

Example 3:

Homework: During the next week, make regular appointments with yourself to work on this practice exercise (For instance, Monday, Wednesday, and Friday nights at 8 o'clock). Make sure that no one will bother you in order for you to concentrate on this practice exercise. During this time (either 30 or 60 minute, depending on how long you want to work on this practice exercise), try to concentrate on the statement that you are working on. Make it as real as you can in your mind. As soon as you feel you have this statement in your mind, start answering the questions asked below. The idea here is for you to start thinking rather than for you to try to stop thinking. Remember: If you want to stop your cynical thinking in your mind, start it in your mind! If you can start it, you can stop it. Write down what happened in detail. For each time you start thinking cynically, make sure to answer the following four questions:

a. How did you start it?
b. What followed?
c. How did it end?
d. What did this statement get you?

Time 1 (write the time you started__________)

a. ______________________________
____
____

b. ______________________________
____
____

c. ______________________________
____
____

d. ______________________________
____
____

Time 2 (write the time you started__________)

a. ______________________________
____
____

b. ______________________________
____
____

c. ______________________________
____
____

d. ______________________________
____
____

Time 3 (write the time you started__________)

a. ______________________________
____
____

b. ______________________________

____

____

c. ____

d. ____

Check which of the following indicates how you feel about this practice exercise:

a.	Completely useless	_____	d.	Somewhat useful	_____
b.	Somewhat useless	_____	e.	Extremely useful	_____
c.	So-so	_____			

Explain in greater detail how you feel about this practice exercise and what you got out of it.

____

Bring this completed practice exercise and your written notes to your professional helper.

Practice Exercise 1. Antisocial Practices

Name____________________Sex_____Date__________

The purpose of this and other practice exercises is to help you control your antisocial behaviors. As you know, that is not an easy goal. You will need to work on this practice exercise as well and as completely as you can.

1. List the discipline or conduct problems you had during your school years.

____

2. Have you ever been in trouble with the law? How and how much?

a. When?

b. Where?

3. How much stealing have you done in the past?

a. When?

b. Where?

4. How much shoplifting have you done in the past?

a. When?

b. Where?

5. How much lying have you done in the past?

a. When?

b. Where?

6. Have you ever set a fire? To what?

a. When?

b. Where?

7. Any other antisocial practice not listed above:

a. What?

b. When?

c. Where?

8. One of the major attitudes that produces antisocial behavior is: "I know better."

a. How does this attitude apply to you?

b. How did you develop it?

c. What did this attitude get you?

d. How can you change this attitude if it gets you into trouble?

____
____
____

9. A second attitude that leads to antisocial behavior is: "I won't be caught."

   a. How does this attitude apply to you?

   ____
   ____
   ____

   b. How did you develop it?

   ____
   ____
   ____

   c. What did this attitude get you?

   ____
   ____
   ____

   d. How can you change this attitude if it gets you into trouble?

   ____
   ____
   ____

10. Rank-order the antisocial behaviors listed below according to how much and how often you practiced that behavior. Rank as No. 1 the behavior that was the most common in your practice, rank as No. 2 the behavior that was next common, and so on; mark as N/A the behaviors that do not apply to you.

Antisocial Behaviors	*Rank-order*
a. Discipline or conduct problems in school	________
b. In trouble with the law	________
c. Stealing	________
d. Shoplifting	________
e. Lying	________
f. Setting fires	________
g. Any other behavior (________________)	________

Homework: During the coming week, think more about how you behaved in the past and what that behavior got you.

1. Was it rewarding?

____
____
____
____
____

2. Was it helpful?

____
____
____
____
____

3. Did you enjoy it?

____
____
____
____
____

4. What did that behavior get you?

____
____
____
____
____

Standard Practice Exercise for Antisocial Practices

Practice Exercise No.____ Title of Behavior______________________

Name______________________________Sex_____Date___________

The purpose of this and other practice exercises is to help you learn to control your antisocial practices, one behavior at a time. To achieve this goal, go back to thinking of the behaviors completed in the previous practice exercise. Write in the space above the behavior you ranked as No. 1. Your next practice exercise will consist of the behavior rank-ordered No. 2, and so on, until you have completed a practice exercise for each behavior that you rank-ordered. Use this same format for all the other practice exercises following the rank-order given in the first practice exercise. Before you start answering, however, be sure to make as many copies of this practice exercise as the number of rank-ordered statements given in the preceding practice exercise.

1. How does this behavior apply to you? Please explain in detail.

____

____

____

____

____

2. How often did you behave this way?

   a. Practically every day ________
   b. Once a week ________
   c. A couple of times a month ________
   d. Once a month ________
   e. Once every 6 months ________
   f. Once a year ________
   g. Once every few years ________

3. Please explain further:

____

____

____

____

____

4. How did this behavior come about? Do you remember how it started? Check which answer fits best:

   a. When I was a child (younger than 5 years of age) ________
   b. When I was in elementary school ________
   c. When I was in middle school ________
   d. When I was in high school ________
   e. After high school ________
   f. Any other time ________

5. Please explain further:

6. Was this behavior acceptable or unacceptable? Why? Explain.

7. Give three specific examples of how this behavior affected you in the past.

Example 1:

Example 2:

Example 3:

8. Give three specific examples of how this behavior affects you in the present.

Example 1:

Example 2:

Example 3:

9. Give three specific examples of how this behavior will affect you in the future.

Example 1:

Example 2:

Example 3:

____
____
____
____
____

Homework: During the next week, make regular appointments with yourself to work on this practice exercise (for instance, on Monday, Wednesday, and Friday nights at 8 o'clock). Make sure that no one will bother you in order for you to concentrate on this practice exercise. During this time (either 30 or 60 minute), depending on how long you want to work on this practice exercise) try to recall behaviors that got you into trouble. As soon as you feel you have this behavior in your mind, start answering the questions asked below. The idea here is for you to start thinking rather than to try to stop thinking. Remember: If you want to stop your behavior in your mind, start it in your mind! If you can start it in your mind, perhaps you can stop it outside of your mind. Write down what happened in detail. For each time you start thinking about this past behavior, make sure to answer in writing the following four questions:

a. How did you start it?
b. What followed?
c. How did it end?
d. What did this behavior get you?

Time 1 (write the time you started__________)

a. ____
____
____

b. ____
____
____

c. ____
____
____

d. ____
____
____

Time 2 (write the time you started__________)

a. ____
____
____

b. ____
____
____

c. ____
____
____

d. ____
____
____

Time 3 (write the time you started__________)

a. ____
____
____

b. ____
____
____

c. ____
____
____

d. ____
____
____

Check which of the following choices indicates how you feel about this practice exercise:

a. Completely useless __________ d. Somewhat useful __________
b. Somewhat useless __________ e. Extremely useful __________
c. So-so __________

Explain in greater detail how you feel about this practice exercise and what you got out of it.

____
____
____
____

Bring this completed practice exercise and your written notes to your professional helper.

Practice Exercise 1. Type A Personality

Name______________________________Sex_____Date___________

Type A personality is a label used for individuals who are otherwise described as workaholics. This troublesome thoughts means an intense and burning involvement and investment in work. Work is the major source of satisfaction in their lives at the expense of other aspects of their personality and of other people in their lives.

Answer the following questions. Be sure to match numbers and letters on your answer sheets with the same numbers and letters on this practice exercise. It might take more than one sitting to answer all the questions found in this practice exercise. Make sure to make appointments to work on installments of this practice exercise at least 24 h in advance and no longer than 1 h at a time. You will need more than one appointment to complete this practice exercise.

1. Are you a type A personality? In what way?

2. How is work the most important priority in your life?

   a. How did you develop this priority?
   b. How does this priority affect:
      i. The rest of your life?
      ii. Your marriage (if you are married)?
      iii. Your children (if you have any)?
      iv. The rest of your family (parents, siblings, in laws)?
      v. Your friends (if you have any)?
      vi. Your leisure time (if you have any)?

2. One characteristic of type A personalities is "drivenness."

   a. How does this label apply to you?
   b. How did you develop this drivenness?
   c. Can you enjoy doing nothing?
   d. How would you feel if you did nothing?
   e. Do you feel that you have to justify your existence? Why?
   f. Can you enjoy your vacations?
   g. Do you take work with you when you go on vacations?
   h. Do you have headaches on Sundays?

2. Another characteristic of type A personalities is "immediacy," that is, never leave to tomorrow what can be done today!

   a. How does this characteristic apply to you?
   b. Ho.w did you develop this characteristic?
   c. What does this characteristic get:

i. You?
ii. Your wife/husband/partner (if you have one)?
iii. Your children (if you have any)?
iv. The rest of your family (parents, siblings, in laws)?
v. Your friends (if you have any)?
vi. Your leisure time?

4. One of the major effects of drivenness and immediacy may be a deficit in awareness of other people's needs, wants, and desired. Sometimes this attitude is expressed in the phrase, "Don't interrupt when I am interrupting!"

   a. How does this phrase apply to you?
   b. Are you able to listen to others (rather than to yourself)?
   c. Are your feelings, thoughts, and action more important than the feelings, thoughts, and actions of others? Why?
   d. How would reply to this proverb: "No person is an island unto oneself"?

5. Another characteristic of type A personalities is a restriction in time perspective, as if life is too short and time is also short.

   a. How does this perspective apply to you?
   b. How did you develop this restricted time perspective?
   c. How does this perspective affect you?
   d. How does it affect your family?
   e. How does it affect your friends?
   f. How does it affect your leisure time?

6. Another characteristic of type A personalities is the belief that "bluntness is the best policy."

   a. How does this characteristic apply to you?
   b. How does it affect your family?
   c. How does it affect your friends?
   d. How does it affect your relationships with the people you work with?
      i. Your subordinates?
      ii. Your peers?
      iii. Your superiors?

7. Many of the previous characteristics bring about a pattern of using and manipulating others for your own gains and profits.

   a. How does this pattern apply to you?
   b. How did you develop it?
   c. Who do you use?
   d. How do you manipulate others?
   e. What does this pattern get you?

8. One of the major characteristic goals of type A personalities is to achieve success through hard work. Success, however, is defined in terms of externals, such as:

   a. Money: What does it mean to you?
   b. Material rewards (objects, things): What do they mean to you?
   c. Intangibles, like fame and glory: What do they mean to you?

9. If your sense of self-importance and self-esteem comes from all these externals, how are you going to feel if or when they are no longer available to you, as in retirement or old age?

Homework: During the next week, keep a daily diary of all your thoughts troublesome thoughting the following topics:

a. How is work your most important priority in your life?
b Who gets short-changed by this priority?
c. What other priorities in your life get short-changed?
d. How does your drivenness effect others?
e. What makes you think you are invulnerable to heart attack, burnout, or breakdown?
f. Why do you need everything now? Why can't you wait until tomorrow?
g. What will happen to you and to your family if you keep up the pace you have been following thus far?
h. Why should people be nice to you if you are not to them?
i. If your self-esteem is linked to externals, what would happen to you if and when these externals disappear?
j. Are money, things, fame, and glory more important than what your spouse, children, and family think of you?

If you cannot write about all of these topics in one sitting, take one topic at a time each week and think about it for the whole week, writing everything that comes to mind at preset and regular appointments with yourself, for no longer than 1 h. It is doubtful whether you will be able to change if you do not follow these instructions: writing at regularly preset times for no longer than 1 h.

Practice Exercise 1. Low Self-Esteem

Name______________________________Sex_____Date___________

There are many ways of not feeling good about oneself. Here are 11 harmful and hurtful beliefs about oneself. How do they apply to you?

1. I do not like myself.

a. How does this belief apply to you?

b. How did you develop it?

c. Why do you believe it?

2. I am not important.

a. How does this belief apply to you?

b. How did you develop it?

c. Why do you believe it?

3. I am not good-looking enough.

a. How does this belief apply to you?

b. How did you develop it?

c. Why do you believe it?

4. I am not bright enough.

 a. How does this belief apply to you?

 b. How did you develop it?

 c. Why do you believe it?

5. I am not rich enough.

 a. How does this belief apply to you?

 b. How did you develop it?

c. Why do you believe it?

6. I am clumsy.

   a. How does this belief apply to you?

   b. How did you develop it?

   c. Why do you believe it?

7. I am awkward.

   a. How does this belief apply to you?

   b. How did you develop it?

   c. Why do you believe it?

8. I am useless.

   a. How does this belief apply to you?

   ____
   ____
   ____

   b. How did you develop it?

   ____
   ____
   ____

   c. Why do you believe it?

   ____
   ____
   ____

9. I am a burden to others.

   a. How does this belief apply to you?

   ____
   ____
   ____

   b. How did you develop it?

   ____
   ____
   ____

   c. Why do you believe it?

   ____
   ____
   ____

10. I am afraid of what others think of me.

   a. How does this belief apply to you?

   ____
   ____
   ____

b. How did you develop it?

c. Why do you believe it?

11. Negativity controls me.

 a. How does this belief apply to you?

 b. How did you develop it?

 c. Why do you believe it?

12. There are two major characteristics about all of the previous 11 statements, one you will agree with, the second you will not:

 a. At one time in your life you decided to think negatively about yourself or to believe what others may have said negatively about you. The decision to believe negatively about yourself, however, was entirely yours.
 b. What do you think about this statement?

 c. None of the negative statements listed above have anything to do with the external, objective reality. However, you have made them your reality, deciding to believe about yourself negatively rather than positively.

d. What do you think about this statement?

____

____

____

13. The power to think negatively or positively about yourself is entirely yours. You have the power to choose. What will you choose? You have to decide whether you want negativity or positivity about yourself to control your life. If you want to go on thinking negatively about yourself, the rest of this practice exercise will not help you. However, if you want to learn to think positively about yourself, you may want to complete this practice exercise.

14. Rank-order each of the 11 beliefs in order of how they apply to you. Rank as No. 1 the belief that applies to you the most, rank as No. 2 the belief that applies to you next, and so on; mark as N/A the beliefs that do not apply to you.

Belief	*Rank-order*
1. I do not like myself	________
2. I am not important	________
3. I am not good-looking enough	________
4. I am not bright enough	________
5. I am not rich enough	________
6. I am clumsy	________
7. I am awkward	________
8. I am useless	________
9. I am a burden to others	________
10. I am afraid of what others think of me	________
11. Negativity controls me	________

Homework: During the coming week, think about how you have rank-ordered those beliefs about yourself. Feel free to change the order if you feel that that change would reflect more accurately how you feel about yourself.

Standard Practice Exercise for Low Self-Esteem

Practice Exercise No.____ Name of Belief________________________

Name______________________________Sex_____Date____________

The purpose of this and other practice exercises is to help you learn to decrease your beliefs in low self-esteem, one belief at a time. To achieve this goal, go back to the rank-ordering of the beliefs completed in the previous practice exercise. Write in the space above the belief you ranked as No. 1. Your next practice exercise will consist of the belief rank-ordered No. 2, and so on, until you have completed a practice exercise for each belief that you rank-ordered.Use this same format for all the other practice exercises following the rank-order given in the first practice exercise. Before you start answering, however, be sure to make as many copies of this practice exercise as the number of rank-ordered statements given in the previous practice exercise.

1. How does this belief apply to you? Please explain in detail.

____
____
____
____
____

2. How often do you feel this belief?

   a. Practically every day ________
   b. Once a week ________
   c. A couple of times a month ________
   d. Once a month ________
   e. Once every 6 months ________
   f. Once a year ________
   g. Once every few years ________

3. Please explain further:

____
____
____
____
____

4. How did this belief come about? Do you remember when it started? Check which answer fits best:

   a. When I was a child (younger than 5 years of age) ________
   b. When I was in elementary school ________
   c. When I was in middle school ________
   d. When I was in high school ________
   e. After high school ________
   f. Any other time ________

5. Please explain further:

6. Was this belief acceptable or unacceptable? Why? Explain.

7. Give three specific examples of how this belief affected you in the past.

Example 1:

Example 2:

Example 3:

8. Give three specific examples of how this belief affects you in the present.

Example 1:

Example 2:

Example 3:

9. Give three specific examples of how this belief will affect you in the future.

Example 1:

Example 2:

Example 3:

Homework: During the next week, make regular appointments with yourself to work on this practice exercise (for instance, on Monday, Wednesday, and Friday nights at 8 o'clock). Make sure that no one will bother you in order for you to concentrate on this practice exercise. During this time (either 30 or 60 minute, depending on how long you want to work on this practice exercise, try to concentrate on this belief. As soon as you feel you have this belief in your mind, start answering the questions asked below. The idea here is for you to start thinking rather than to try to stop thinking about it. Remember: If you want to stop thinking of yourself as being low in self-esteem, start thinking positively in your mind! If you can start it in your mind, perhaps you can stop it outside of your mind. Write down what happened in detail. For each time you start thinking about this belief, make sure to answer in writing the following four questions:

a. How did you start thinking about it?
b. What followed?
c. How did it end?
d. What did this belief get you?

Time 1 (write the time you started__________)

a ______________________________
____
____

b ______________________________
____
____

c ______________________________
____
____

d ______________________________
____
____

Time 2 (write the time you started__________)

a ______________________________
____
____

b ______________________________
____
____

c ______________________________
____
____

d ______________________________
____
____

Time 3 (write the time you started__________)

a ____

____

____

b ____

____

____

c ____

____

____

d ____

____

____

Check which of the following choices indicates how you feel about this practice exercise:

a.	Completely useless	______	d.	Somewhat useful	______
b.	Somewhat useless	______	e.	Extremely useful	______
c.	So-so	______			

Explain in greater detail how you feel about this practice exercise and what you got out of it.

____

____

____

____

____

Bring this completed practice exercise and your written notes to your professional helper.

Practice Exercise 1. Social Discomfort

Name______________________________Sex_____Date____________

Being socially uncomfortable means a variety of things to different people. The purpose of this and other practice exercises is to help you become more comfortable socially.

1. What does it mean to you to be uncomfortable socially?

____

____

____

____

____

2. We use a variety of reasons to explain why we are socially uncomfortable. Answer all of the reasons below whether they apply to you or not:

   a. Shyness
      i. This is one of the main reasons used to explain social discomfort. How does it apply to you?
      ii. How shy are you? A great deal________ Some________ Not at all ______
      iii. If your answer is "A great deal" or "Some," explain how this shyness developed in you:

      ____
      ____
      ____

      iv. What does shyness get you?

      ____
      ____
      ____

   b. Fear of being discovered
      i. How strong is this fear? Very strong __________ Strong __________ Not at all strong _____
      ii. What are you afraid that people will discover in you?

      ____
      ____
      ____

      iii. What are you afraid will happen if or when they discover what you do not want them to find out?

      ____
      ____
      ____

      iv. What is the worst that could happen to you after they discover it?

      ____
      ____
      ____

v. Has it ever happened to you and, if so, how?

____

____

____

vi. What happens if what they discovered is not true?

____

____

____

c. I like my company better than the company of others.
   i. Why is the company of others so uncomfortable to you?

____

____

____

   ii. How did this fear develop in you?

____

____

____

   iii. What is the worst that could happen to you if you developed some acquaintances or, worse, some friendships?

____

____

____

d. I am afraid of getting close to people.
   i. How afraid are you? A lot____ Some_____ Not at all____
   ii. If your answer is "A lot" or "Some," how did this fear develop in you?

____

____

____

   iii. What is the worst that could happen if you learned to get close to people?

____

____

____

e. If people discover what a stupid (awkward, clumsy, ugly, etc.) person I am, they won't have anything to do with me.
   i. How did you develop this idea?

____
____
____

   ii. What does this idea get you?

____
____
____

   iii. Why is what people think of you so important?

____
____
____

   iv. Why can't you think on your own two feet?

____
____
____

f. Parties are awful.
   i. Why?

____
____
____

   ii. Aren't you entitled to fun and pleasure?

____
____
____

   iii. Why not?

____
____
____

iv. How are you going to meet people and make friends?

g. I do not like crowds.
   i. Why not?

   ii. What does this dislike get you?

   iii. What is the worst that could happen to you if you were in a crowd?

h. Give your own reason for social discomfort. If none of the reasons given above apply to you, please explain what your social discomfort consists of and what causes it in you?

   i. How did this idea develop in you?

   ii. What does this reason get you?

Rank-order each of these eight reasons in order of how much they apply to you. Rank as No. 1 the reason that applies to you the most, rank as No. 2 the reason that applies to you next, and so on, down to the reasons that applies to you the least; mark as N/A the reasons that do not apply to you at all.

Reasons		*Rank-order*
a.	Shyness	________
b.	Fear of being discovered	________
c.	I like my company better than the company of others.	________
d.	I am afraid of getting close to people.	________
e.	If people discover what a stupid person I am, they won't have anything to do with me.	________
f.	Parties are awful.	________
g.	I do not like crowds.	________
h.	Your own peculiar (and very likely negative) reason	________

Homework: During the coming week, think about your rank-order of all the negative reasons you believe about yourself. Feel free to change that rank-order if you think it is not an accurate representation of you.

Standard Practice Exercise for Social Discomfort

Practice Exercise No.____ Title of Reason______________________

Name______________________________Sex_____Date___________

The purpose of this and other practice exercises is to help you learn to improve your social discomfort, one reason at a time. To achieve this goal, go back to the rank-ordering of reasons completed in the previous practice exercise. Write in the space above the reason you ranked as No. 1. Your next practice exercise will consist of the reason ranked as No. 2, and so on, until you have completed a practice exercise for each reason that you rank-ordered. Use this same format for all the other practice exercises following the rank-order given in the first practice exercise. Before you start answering, however, be sure to make as many copies of this practice exercise as the number of rank-ordered statements given in the previous practice exercise.

1. How does the reason for feeling socially uncomfortable apply to you? Please explain in detail.

____

____

____

____

____

2. How often do you use this reason for feeling socially uncomfortable?

   a. Practically every day ________
   b. Once a week ________
   c. A couple of times a month ________
   d. Once a month ________
   e. Once every 6 months ________
   f. Once a year ________
   g. Once every few years ________

3. Please explain further:

____
____
____
____
____

4. How did this reason for feeling socially uncomfortable come about? Do you remember when it started? Check which answer fits best:

   a. When I was a child (younger than 5 years of age) ________
   b. When I was in elementary school ________
   c. When I was in middle school ________
   d. When I was in high school ________
   e. After high school ________
   f. Any other time ________

5. Please explain further:

____
____
____
____
____

6. Was this reason for feeling socially uncomfortable acceptable or unacceptable? Why? Explain.

____
____
____
____
____

7. Give three specific examples of how this reason affected you in the past.

Example 1:

Example 2:

Example 3:

8. Give three specific examples of how this reason affects you in the present.

Example 1:

Example 2:

Example 3:

____
____
____
____
____

9. Give three specific examples of how this reason will affect you in the future.

Example 1:

____
____
____
____
____

Example 2:

____
____
____
____
____

Example 3:

____
____
____
____
____

Homework: During the next week, make regular appointments with yourself to work on this practice exercise (for instance, on Monday, Wednesday, and Friday nights at 8 o'clock). Make sure that no one will bother you in order for you to concentrate on this practice exercise. During this time (either 30 or 60 minute, depending on how long you want to work on this practice exercise), try to concentrate on the reason for your social discomfort. As soon as you feel you have this reason in your mind, start answering the questions asked below. The idea here is for you to start thinking rather than to try to stop thinking. Remember: If you want to stop thinking of yourself as being a social misfit, start thinking positively in your mind! If you can start it in your mind, perhaps you can stop it outside of your mind. Write down what happened in detail about a social situation where you felt the reason for feeling uncomfortable. Make sure to answer in writing the following four questions:

a. How did you start this reason for feeling socially uncomfortable?
b. What followed?
c. How did it end?
d. What did this reason get you?

Time 1 (write the time you started__________)

a. ______________________________
____
____

b. ______________________________
____
____

c. ______________________________
____
____

d. ______________________________
____
____

Time 2 (write the time you started__________)

a. ______________________________
____
____

b. ______________________________
____
____

c. ______________________________
____
____

d. ______________________________
____
____

Time 3 (write the time you started__________)

a. ______________________________
____
____

b. ______________________________
____
____

c. ______________________________
____
____

d. ____
____
____

Check which of the following choices indicates how you feel about this practice exercise:

a. Completely useless ________ d. Somewhat useful ________
b. Somewhat useless ________ e. Extremely useful ________
c. So-so ________

Explain in greater detail how you feel about this practice exercise and what you got out of it.

____
____
____
____
____

Bring this completed practice exercise and your written notes to your professional helper.

Practice Exercise 1. Family Problems

Name______________________________Sex_____Date___________

Please write in detail which of the problems listed below describe your family best. Be sure that the numbers and letters on your answer sheets match those on this practice exercise. You will need more than one sitting to answer all these questions. Make an appointment with yourself at least 24 h in advance for no longer than 1 h at a time.

1. Arguments and fights

   a. How do these arguments and/or fights happen?
   b. How often do these fights and/or arguments take place?

      i. At least once a day ________
      ii. At least once a week ________
      iii. At least once a month ________
      iv. Rarely ________
      v. Never ________

   c. How strong are these arguments/fights?

      i. Very strong ________

ii. Strong ________
iii. Not strong ________
iv. Not strong at all ________

d. How long do these arguments/fights last?

i. One hour at most ________
ii. More than 1 h ________
iii. Hours ________
iv. A whole day ________
v. A week ________
vi. A month ________
vii. Months ________
viii. Years ________

e. What are these arguments/fights about?
f. What are the results of these arguments/fights?

i. Very positive ________
ii. Positive ________
iii. Neither positive or negative ________
iv. Negative ________
v. Very negative ________

g. Please explain and expand on the nature of your choice in Question f.

2. Inability to show love

a. How is this inability to love shown in your family?
b. How did this inability to love develop in your family?
c. In some families the inability to love is shown through giving but not getting or receiving it.
d. How does this statement apply to your family?
e. In some families the inability to love is shown through getting and receiving love rather than giving it.

How does this statement apply to your family?

f. What are some of the ways that your family fails to show love? Which of the following apply to you?

Please explain and expand:

i. Abuse. Underline which: physical, verbal, chemical, alcohol, other
ii. Neglect. Underline which: lack of attention, busyness, incompetence, other

   iii. Stress on doing and performing at the expense of being together and available emotionally to each other
   iv. Stress on things and money at the expense of being together and available emotionally to each other
   v. Stress on togetherness and being available emotionally for each other at the expense of doing or having
   vi. Any other way that is not listed above

3. Unpleasantness

   a. How is this unpleasantness shown in your family?
   b. What does this unpleasantness do to your family?
   c. Does anybody gain anything from this unpleasantness?

4. Anger and hate

   a. How are anger and hate shown in your family?
   b. What are the results of anger and hate in your family?
   c. How did anger and hate develop in your family?

5. Abuse and neglect in childhood

   a. How much of your present family problems are due or related to childhood experiences?

      i. A great deal ________
      ii. Some ________
      iii. Not at all ________

   b. If your answer is i or ii, please expand on these past painful experiences
   c. Has the pain of these experiences ever been shared in the family?

      i. No, never ________
      ii. Sometimes ________
      iii. Only when we are upset ________
      iv. Other (please explain and expand)

6. Family of origin

   a. Where do these problems come from?

      i. Parents ________
      ii. Grandparents ________
      iii. In-laws ________
      iv. Other (please explain)

b. What kind of problems have been present in your family of origin?
c. What have these problems done to your family?

7. Present relationships

   a. What kind of problems exist in your present family relationships?
   b. What do these problems do to you?
   c. What do these problems do to your partner (companion, mate, spouse, etc.)?

8. Problems peculiar to your family

   a. What kind of problems exist in your family that were not listed or considered above?
   b. How did these problems develop?
   c. What do these problems do to you?

9. Rank-order the problems presented above in terms of how strong they are for you and your family. Rank as No. 1 the problem that affects your family the most, rank as No. 2 the problem that affects your family next, and so on, down to the problem that affects your family the least.

Problem	*Rank-order*
1. Arguments and fights	________
2. Inability to show love	________
3. Unpleasantness	________
4. Anger and hate	________
5. Abuse and neglect in childhood	________
6. Family of origin	________
7. Present relationships	________
8. Problems peculiar to your family	________

Homework: Next week, think about your rank-orders of the previous practice exercise. Feel free to change that order if you think it would be more accurate of your family problems.
Standard Practice Exercise for Family Problems

Practice exercise No.____ Name of Problem____________________

Name______________________________Sex_____Date___________

The purpose of this and other practice exercises is to help you learn to improve how you think about your family problems, one problem at a time. To achieve this goal, go back to the rank-ordering of problems completed in the previous practice exercise. Write in the space above the problem you ranked as No. 1. Your next practice exercise will consist of the problem rank-ordered No. 2, and so on, until you have completed a practice exercise for each problem that you rank-ordered. Use this same format for all the other practice exercises following the rank-order given in the first practice exercise. Before you start answering, however, be sure to make as many copies of this practice exercise as the number of rank-ordered statements given in the previous practice exercise.

1. How does this problem apply to you? Please explain in detail.

____
____
____
____
____

2. How often does this problem take place?

a.	Practically every day	_____	d.	Once a month	_____
b.	Once a week	_____	e.	Once every 6 months	_____
c.	A couple of times a month	_____	f.	Once a year	_____
			g.	Once every few years	_____

3. Please explain further:

____
____
____
____
____

4. How did this problem come about? Do you remember when it started? Check which answer fits best:

   a. When I was a child (younger than 5 years of age) ______
   b. When I was in elementary school ______
   c. When I was in middle school ______
   d. When I was in high school ______
   e. After high school ______
   f. Any other time ______

5. Please explain further:

____
____
____
____
____

6. Was this problem acceptable or unacceptable? Why? Explain.

7. Give three specific examples of how this problem affected you in the past.

Example 1:

Example 2:

Example 3:

8. Give three specific examples of how this problem affects you in the present.

Example 1:

Example 2:

Example 3:

9. Give three specific examples of how this problem will affect you in the future.

Example 1:

Example 2:

Example 3:

Homework: During the next week, make regular appointments with yourself to work on this practice exercise (for instance, on Monday, Wednesday, and Friday nights at 8 o'clock). Make sure that no one will bother you in order for you to concentrate on this practice exercise. During this time (either 30 or 60 minute, depending on how long you want to work on this practice exercise), try to concentrate on this family problem. As soon as you feel you have this reason in your mind, start answering the questions asked below. The idea here is for you to start thinking rather than to try to stop thinking. Remember: If you want to stop thinking of your family problems, start thinking positively in your mind! If you can start it in your mind, perhaps you can stop it outside of your mind. Write down what happened in detail about a past family problem related to this practice exercise. Make sure to answer in writing the following four questions:

a. How did you start this specific problem?
b. What followed?
c. How did it end?
d. What did this family problem get you?

Time 1 (write the time you started__________)

a. ____
____
____

b. ____
____
____

c. ____
____
____

d. ____
____
____

Time 2 (write the time you started__________)

a. ____
____
____

b. ____
____
____

c. ____
____
____

d. ____
____
____

Time 3 (write the time you started__________)

a. ____
____
____

b. ____
____
____

c. ____
____
____

d. ____
____
____

Check which of the following choices shows how you feel about this practice exercise:

a.	Completely useless	_____	d.	Somewhat useful	_____
b.	Somewhat useless	_____	e.	Extremely useful	_____
c.	So-so	_____			

Explain in greater detail how you feel about this practice exercise and what you got out of it.

____
____
____
____
____

Bring this completed practice exercise and your written notes to your professional helper.

Practice Exercise 1. Work Interference

Name_______________________________Sex_____Date___________

There are many ways of interfering with work performance. Answer the following questions. Be sure that the numbers and letters on your answer sheets match those on this practice exercise. You may need more than one sitting to answer all these questions. For each sitting, make an appointment with yourself at least 24 h in advance and no longer than 1 h.

Please write about each of the following ways:

1. Low self-confidence

   a. What does your low self-confidence consist of?
   b. How did you develop it?
   c. What does this low self-confidence say about you as a person?
   d. How does your low self-confidence relate to your work performance?

2. Trying too hard to please others

   a. Why are making others more important than you?
   b. What does pleasing others get you?
   c. How did learn to please others at your expense?
   d. How would you react to the statement, "To please others means killing oneself"?

3. Trouble concentrating

   a. How troublesome is your inability to concentrate?
   b. How is your trouble in concentrating related to your work performance?
   c. How did this trouble in concentrating develop?

4. Conflicts with authority

   a. What kind of conflicts with authority do you have?
   b. How did these conflicts with authority develop?
   c. How do these conflicts affect your work performance?

5. Conflicts with coworkers

   a. What kind of conflicts with coworkers do you have?
   b. How did these conflicts with coworkers develop?
   c. How do these conflicts affect your work performance?

6. Unable to make decisions

   a. How are you unable to make decisions?
   b. What kind of decisions do you have trouble making?
   c. How does this inability to make decisions affect your work performance?

7. Uptight and unable to relax

   a. How uptight and unable to relax are you?
   b. How did this uptightness and inability to relax develop?
   c. How much are this uptightness and inability to relax affecting your work performance?

i. A great deal ________
ii. Some ________
iii. Not at all ________

8. Lack of family support for career choice

   a. How did this lack of support for you career choice develop?
   b. Does your lack of family support in career choice apply also to other parts of your life? How?
   c. Why do you lack family support in your career choice?
   d. How does this lack of family support affect your work performance?

9. Questions about career

   a. What questions about your career do you have?
   b. How did these questions develop?
   c. Why do you have these questions?
   d. How do these questions affect your work performance?

10. Another way not listed above

    a. What way not listed above interferes with your work performance?
    b. How does it affect your work performance?
    c. How did it develop?

11. Now rank-order all of the above ways according to the degree of interference with work. Rank as No. 1 the way that most interferes with your work performance, rank as No. 2 the way that interferes next, and so on down to the way that interferes least.

Ways	*Rank-order*
1. Low self-confidence	________
2. Trying too hard to please others	________
3. Trouble concentrating	________
4. Conflicts with authority	________
5. Conflicts with coworkers	________
6. Unable to make decisions	________
7. Uptight and unable to relax	________
8. Lack of family support for career choice	________
9. Questions about career	________
10. Another way not listed above-	________

Homework: During the coming week, think about the rank-orders of ways that interfere with your work. Feel free to change that rank-order if you think that it is more accurate of how you think about your work.

Standard Practice Exercise for Work Interference

Practice Exercise No.____ Title of Way ________________________

Name______________________________Sex_____Date___________

The purpose of this and other practice exercises is to help you learn to improve how you think about your ways of work interference, one way at a time. To achieve this goal, go back to the rank-ordering of problems completed in the previous practice exercise. Write in the space above the problem you ranked as No. 1. Your next practice exercise will consist of the way you rank-ordered No. 2, and so on, until you have completed a practice exercise for each way that you rank-ordered. Use this same format for all the other practice exercises following the rank-order given in the first practice exercise. Before you start answering, however, be sure to make as many copies of this practice exercise as the number of rank-ordered statements given in the previous practice exercise.

1. How does this way of work interference apply to you? Please explain in detail.

____

____

____

____

____

2. How often does this way take place?

a.	Practically every day	____	e.	Once every 6 months	____
b.	Once a week	____	f.	Once a year	____
c.	A couple of times a month	____	g.	Once every few years	____
d.	Once a month	____			

3. Please explain further:

____

____

____

____

____

4. How did this way come about? Do you remember when it started? Check which answer fits best:

a. When I was a child (younger than 5 years of age) ______
b. When I was in elementary school ______
c. When I was in middle school ______

d. When I was in high school ______
e. After high school ______
f. Any other time ______

5. Please explain further:

6. Was this way acceptable or unacceptable? Why? Explain.

7. Give three specific examples of how this way affected you in the past.

Example 1:

Example 2:

Example 3:

8. Give three specific examples of how this way affects you in the present.

Example 1:

Example 2:

Example 3:

9. Give three specific examples of how this way will affect you in the future.

Example 1:

Example 2:

Example 3:

Homework: During the next week, make regular appointments with yourself to work on this practice exercise (for instance, on Monday, Wednesday, and Friday nights at 8 o'clock). Make sure that no one will bother you in order for you to concentrate on this practice exercise. During this time (either 30 or 60 minute, depending on how long you want to work on this practice exercise), try to concentrate on this way. As soon as you feel you have this way in your mind, start answering the questions asked below. The idea here is for you to start thinking rather than to try to stop thinking. Remember: If you want to stop thinking about what interferes with your work, start thinking positively in your mind! If you can start it in your mind, perhaps you can stop it outside of it. Write down what happened in detail about the way related to this practice exercise. Make sure to answer in writing the following four questions:

a. How did you start this specific way?
b. What followed?
c. How did it end?
d. What did this way get you?

Time 1 (write the time you started__________)

a. ____
____
____

b. ____
____
____

c. ____
____
____

d. ____
____
____

Time 2 (write the time you started__________)

a. ____
____
____

b. ____
____
____

c. ____
____
____

d. ____
____
____

Time 3 (write the time you started__________)

a. ____
____
____

b. ____
____
____

c. ____
____
____

d. ____
____
____

Check which of the following choices indicates how you feel about this practice exercise:

a. Completely useless _____ d. Somewhat useful _____
b. Somewhat useless _____ e. Extremely useful _____
c. So-so _____

Explain in greater detail how you feel about this practice exercise and what you got out of it.

____
____
____
____
____

Bring this completed practice exercise and your written notes to your professional helper.

Practice Exercise 1. Negative Treatment Indicators

Name______________________________Sex_____Date___________

The purpose of this and other practice exercises is to see whether you can change attitudes that interfere with your welfare and the welfare of those you love and who love you

Below there is a list of various negative, self-defeating, and destructive attitudes that make professional help very difficult. See which of these attitudes apply to you, but try to answer as many as you can, even though that attitude may not apply to you.

1. Negative attitudes toward receiving help from others in general

a. What are these attitudes in you?
b. How did these negative attitudes develop in you?
c. With what troublesome thoughts would you accept help?
d. With what troublesome thoughts would you not accept help?

2. No one can understand me or my problems. I am the only one who can.

   a. Why do you think so?
   b. How did this attitude develop in you?
   c. You can use your hopelessness to destroy you or to improve you. Which is your choice and why do you chose it?

3. I do not need anybody to help me solve my problems.

   a. Have you ever heard the expression: "No person is an island unto oneself"? What does it mean to you?
   b. How did you develop this destructive attitude?
   c. What have you done to solve your problems by yourself?
   d. How successful were you?

4. I know better.

   a. What does this attitude get you?
   b. How did you develop it?
   c. If you know better than anyone else, no one can ever tell you anything. Is that right? Please comment
   d. Why is being right more important to you than being close to people you love and who love you, and being happy, successful, effective, competent, etc.?

5. Doctors are incompetent and they are just in for the money.

   a. Every profession has its share of incompetents. Are there any incompetent people where you work? How do you spot them?
   b. What does this attitude get you?
   c. Do you get your sense of importance by putting other people down?
   d. This attitude says that you elected yourself judge and jury of others; what happens when others do it to you?

6. My problems belong to me and to no one else

   a. How did this attitude develop in you?
   b. What do you get by holding on to your problems?
   c. Are you the only one who has these problems?
   d. Should other people hold onto them as you do?
   e. What would happen to them then?

7. I like my life the way it is. I do not care what others think.

   a. No matter what the price is?
   b. No matter how it affects those who love you?
   c. How did you develop such a negative attitude?
   d. Apparently you are thinking only or mainly of yourself. What would happen if everybody thought the way you do?

8. I cannot change, nor want to change, my life.

   a. Why do you feel so hopeless?
   b. How did you develop such hopelessness?
   c. What does this hopelessness do to you? What do you get?

9. No one can help me.

   a. Why do you feel that way?
   b. How did you develop such a negative attitude?
   c. What does this attitude do to you? What does it get you?

10. I like trouble in my life, because as long as there is trouble, I do not have to take responsibility for my behavior; it's much more convenient to blame others!

    a. How did you develop such a negative attitude?
    b. What does this attitude get you?
    c. What does this attitude do to those who care for you?

11. My car can be fixed but I cannot be fixed.

    a. What makes you think you cannot be fixed?
    b. Do you know of anything in nature or in your experience that fixes itself?
    c. If you cannot ask for help and want to stay the same, what would those who love you do?
    d. Please comment on the following: "If I cannot change, why should anybody else?"

12. Cars are machines. I am human and I cannot be fixed.

    a. What does this attitude consist of?
    b. How did it develop?
    c. What did it get you?
    d. What does it get those who love you?

13. Any other attitude of your choice

a. What does this attitude consist of?
b. How did it develop?
c. What did it get you?
d. What does it get those who love you?

14. Any other attitude of your choice

a. What does this attitude consist of?
b. How did it develop?
c. What did it get you?
d. What does it get those who love you?

15. Now you have at least two choices. One choice is to do absolutely nothing. Keep on doing exactly what you have been doing all along. Do not change in any way possible! Think, however, if you can, about these two statements:

a. We make our choices, we pay our price. What will be the natural outcome of these negative attitudes to you and to those whom you love and who love you?
b. Only strong people ask for help, because weak people cannot. What does this statement mean and how does it apply to you?

16. Rank-order the list of negative attitudes given below according to how much you use it in your life. Rank each attitude according to its strength and in comparison to other negative attitudes. Rank as No. 1 the strongest negative attitude, rank as No. 2 the second, and so on; mark as N/A the attitudes that do not apply to you.

Negative Attitude	*Rank-order*
1. Negative attitudes toward receiving help from others in general	________
2. No one can understand me or my problems	________
3. I do not need anybody to help me solve my problems	________
4. I know better than anybody else	________
5. Doctors are incompetent and they are in it for the money	________
6. My problems belong to me and to no one else	________
7. I like my life the way it is. I do not care what others think	________
8. I cannot change, nor want to change, my life	________
9. No one can help me	________
10. I like trouble in my life	________
11. My car can be fixed but I cannot be fixed	________
12. Cars are machines. I am human and I cannot be fixed	________
13. Any other attitude of your choice (____________________)	________
14. Any other attitude of your choice (____________________)	________

Homework: During the coming week, think about how you have rank-ordered these attitudes and feel free to change the rank-order in ways you feel may fit you better.

Standard Practice Exercise for Negative Attitudes

Practice exercise No.____ Name of Attitude ____________________

Name______________________________Sex_____Date___________

The purpose of this and other practice exercises is to help you learn to improve your attitudes, one attitude at a time. To achieve this goal, go back to the rank-ordering of attitudes completed in the preceding practice exercise. Write in the space above the attitude you ranked as No. 1. Your next practice exercise will consist of the attitude rank-ordered No. 2, and so on, until you have completed a practice exercise for each attitude that you rank-ordered. Use this same format for all the other practice exercises following the rank-order given in the first practice exercise. Before you start answering, however, be sure to make as many copies of this practice exercise as the number of rank-ordered statements given in the previous practice exercise.

1. How does this attitude apply to you? Please explain in detail.

____

____

____

____

____

2. How often does this attitude take place?

   a. Practically every day ______
   b. Once a week ______
   c. A couple of times a month ______
   d. Once a month ______
   e. Once every 6 months ______
   f. Once a year ______
   g. Once every few years ______

3. Please explain further:

____

____

____

____

____

4. How did this attitude come about? Do you remember when it started? Check which answer fits best:

   a. When I was a child (younger than 5 years of age) ______
   b. When I was in elementary school ______
   c. When I was in middle school ______

d. When I was in high school ______
e. After high school ______
f. Any other time ______

5. Please explain further:

____
____
____
____
____

6. Was this attitude acceptable or unacceptable? Why? Explain.

____
____
____
____
____

7. Give three specific examples of how this attitude affected you in the past.

Example 1:

____
____
____
____
____

Example 2:

____
____
____
____
____

Example 3:

____
____
____
____
____

8. Give three specific examples of how this attitude affects you in the present.

Example 1:

Example 2:

Example 3:

9. Give three specific examples of how this attitude will affect you in the future.

Example 1:

Example 2:

Example 3:

____
____
____
____
____

Homework: During the next week, make regular appointments with yourself to work on this practice exercise (for instance, on Monday, Wednesday, and Friday nights at 8 o'clock). Make sure that no one will bother you in order for you to concentrate on this practice exercise. During this time (either 30 or 60 minute, depending on how long you want to work on this practice exercise), try to concentrate on this attitude. As soon as you feel you have this attitude in your mind, start answering the questions asked below. The idea here is for you to start thinking rather than to try to stop thinking. Remember: If you want to stop thinking of your negative attitudes, you start thinking positively in your mind! If you can start it in your mind, perhaps you can stop it outside of it. Write down what happened in detail about the attitude related to this practice exercise. Make sure to answer the following four questions:

a. How did you start this specific attitude?
b. What followed?
c. How did it end?
d. What did this attitude get you?

Time 1 (write the time you started__________)

a. ____
____
____

b. ____
____
____

c. ____
____
____

d. ____
____
____

Time 2 (write the time you started__________)

a. ____
____
____

b. ____
____
____

c. ____
____
____

d. ____
____
____

Time 3 (write the time you started__________)

a. ____
____
____

b. ____
____
____

c. ____
____
____

d. ____
____
____

Check which of the following choices indicates how you feel about this practice exercise:

a. Completely useless ______
b. Somewhat useless ______
c. So-so ______
d. Somewhat useful ______
e. Extremely useful ______

Explain in greater detail how you feel about this practice exercise and what you got out of it.

____
____
____
____
____

Bring this completed practice exercise and your written notes to your professional helper.

Personality Dimensions from the Five-Factor Model of Personality (Neuroticism Extraversion Openness [NEO] Inventory)

The purpose of this practice exercise is to help you deal with personality characteristics or qualities that may work against you rather than for you. These characteristic should have been pin-pointed and identified by previous testing.

Practice Exercise 1. Low Agreeableness

Name________________________________ Sex_____ Date____

The purpose of this practice exercise it to help you better understand personal characteristics or qualities that may work against you rather than for you.

1. Low agreeableness is made up of the characteristics or personal qualities listed below. Define each term, using a dictionary or asking for help from others. Write down what each characteristic means to you, and give two examples to show you understand the meaning of each characteristic.

Characteristics	*Definitions and Examples*
a. Cynicism ____________________	Example 1 ____________________
______________________________	______________________________
______________________________	Example 2 ____________________
______________________________	______________________________
b. Doubt ______________________	Example 1 ____________________
______________________________	______________________________
______________________________	Example 2 ____________________
______________________________	______________________________
c. Inability to trust friends or family	Example 1 ____________________
______________________________	______________________________
______________________________	Example 2 ____________________
______________________________	______________________________
d. Quarrelsomeness ____________	Example 1 ____________________
______________________________	______________________________
______________________________	Example 2 ____________________
______________________________	______________________________
e. Readiness to pick fights _______	Example 1 ____________________
______________________________	______________________________
______________________________	Example 2 ____________________
______________________________	______________________________

f. Exploitive (conning) of others ___	Example 1 ___
___	___
___	Example 2 ___
___	___
g. Manipulative of others ___	Example 1 ___
___	___
___	Example 2 ___
___	___
h. Lying ___	Example 1 ___
___	___
___	Example 2 ___
___	___
i. Rude and inconsiderate manner toward others ___	Example 1 ___
	___
___	Example 2 ___
___	___
j. Limiting social support ___	Example 1 ___
___	___
___	Example 2 ___
___	___
k. Lacking of respect for conventions	Example 1 ___
___	___
___	Example 2 ___
___	___
l. Trouble with the law ___	Example 1 ___
___	___
___	Example 2 ___
___	___
m. Inflated and grandiose sense of self	Example 1 ___
___	___
___	Example 2 ___
___	___
n. Arrogance ___	Example 1 ___
___	___
___	Example 2 ___
___	___

2. Rank-order these characteristics according to how you think they apply to you. Rank as No. 1 the characteristic that applies to you the most, rank as No. 2 the characteristic that applies to you next, and so on, down to the characteristic that applies to you the least (No. 14).

Characteristic	*Rank-order*
a. Cynicism	_________
b. Doubt	_________
c. Inability to trust friends or family	_________
d. Quarrelsomeness	_________
e. Readiness to pick fights	_________
f. Exploitive (conning) of others	_________
g. Manipulative of others	_________
h. Lying	_________
i. Rude and inconsiderate manner toward others	_________
j. Limiting social support	_________
k. Lacking of respect for social conventions	_________
l. Trouble with the law	_________
m. Inflated and grandiose sense of self	_________
n. Arrogance	_________

Homework: During the next week, think on whether you want to go on being very disagreeable or whether you want to be more effective in your relationships with others. It is very difficult sometimes to be agreeable and effective at the same time. What do you think? Write down your answer and discuss it with whoever is working with you on this practice exercise.

Standard Practice Exercise for All Personality Characteristics

Practice Exercise No. _____Title of Characteristic ________________

Name____________________________ Sex________ Date________

The purpose of this practice exercise it to help you better understand personal characteristics or qualities that may work against you rather than for you. Fill in the characteristic from the above list, starting with the one you ranked as No. 1.

1. What does the title of this practice exercise mean to you?

   a. Write down what you understand by this characteristic.
   b. If you are not familiar with it, you may be familiar with similar words.

c. Write down what words come to your mind to understand what is meant by this characteristic.
d. Which of these words applies to you, as you see yourself? Choose words you recognize and write down what they mean to you:

2. Write down when and how this characteristic applies to you. Write down as many instances as you can remember, where this characteristic applies to your behavior, the more instances the better.

3. What happened when you behaved in a manner described by this characteristic? Write in detail what the result was for you and for others who were involved with you.

4. How did you learn to behave in this way?

   a. Did you learn by yourself or did someone you knew behave the same way?
   b. Write down how and who thought you how to behave in this way.

5. Do you want to behave this way for the rest of your life or do you want to change?

   a. If you want to go on behaving the same way, you may as well stop writing.
   b. If you want to change this behavior for the better, go on with this practice exercise.
   c. What is your choice?

6. Give one or more reasons for whatever choice you make:

   a. I want to quit this practice exercise because __________.
   b. I want to go on with this practice exercise because __________.

Homework: If you choose to go on with this practice exercise, you should pat yourself on the back. You made a decision that might help you behave in more acceptable and comfortable ways with those you love and who love you as well as your neighbors, friends, and strangers. To go on with this program you will need to follow these instructions for next week: Keep track in writing of at least three situations when you behaved in a manner described by the title of this practice exercise. Write down (a) how the situation came about; (b) what your behavior consisted of, that is, how you behaved; and (c) what result did you get from behaving the way you did.

First situation: ____

Second situation: ____

Third situation: ____

Also during this coming week, try to behave in a manner opposite from the title of this practice exercise for at least three times, writing down what happened in the same way you did above:

First situation: ____

Second situation: ____

Third situation: ____

1. Now read back your answers to the three situations.

   a. Which of these situations was best for you?
   b. What results did you get from behaving one way or another?
   c. Choose what behavior was best for you: behaving according to the title of this practice exercise or the opposite?
   d. Are there choices in between these two extremes? Write down at least three possible choices available to you that you could follow in the future:

First choice: ____

Second choice: ____

Third choice: ____

2. During the coming week, think which of these choice is best for you, and write down the behavior you want to follow. Choose a behavior

   a. that is not hurtful to you and others and that is helpful to you and others;
   b. that is pleasing to you and others; and
   c. that you can be proud of.

Practice Exercise 1. High Agreeableness

Name______________________________ Sex________ Date_______

The purpose of this practice exercise it to help you better understand personal characteristics or qualities that may work against you rather than for you.

1. High agreeableness is made up by the following characteristics or personal qualities. Using a dictionary or asking others, define each characteristic as you understand it and give two examples to show you understand the meaning of each characteristic.

Characteristics	*Definitions and Examples*
a. Gullibility ____________________	Example 1 ____________
______________________________	______________________
______________________________	Example 2 ____________
______________________________	______________________
b. Indiscriminate trust of others ____	Example 1 ____________
______________________________	______________________
______________________________	Example 2 ____________
______________________________	______________________
c. Excessive candor and generosity ___	Example 1 ____________
______________________________	______________________
______________________________	Example 2 ____________
______________________________	______________________
d. Putting yourself down __________	Example 1 ____________
______________________________	______________________
______________________________	Example 2 ____________
______________________________	______________________
e. Inability to stand up to others and fight back ______________	Example 1 ____________
	______________________
______________________________	Example 2 ____________
______________________________	______________________
f. Easily taken advantage of ________	Example 1 ____________
______________________________	______________________
______________________________	Example 2 ____________
______________________________	______________________

2. Rank-order these characteristics according to how much they apply to you. Rank as No. 1 the characteristic that applies to you the most, rank as No. 2 the characteristic that applies to you next, and so on, down to the characteristic that applies to you the least.

Characteristics	*Rank-order*
a. Gullibility	________
b. Indiscriminate trust of others	________
c. Excessive candor and generosity	________
d. Putting yourself down	________
e. Inability to stand up to others and fight back	________
f. Easily taken advantage of	________

Homework: During the next week, think about whether you want to go on being very agreeable or whether you want to be more effective in your relationships with others. It is very difficult sometimes to be agreeable and effective at the same time. What do you think? Write down your answer and discuss it with whoever is working with you on this practice exercise.

Practice Exercise 1. Low Conscientiousness

Name____________________________ Sex________ Date________

The purpose of this practice exercise it to help you better understand personal characteristics or qualities that may work against you rather than for you.

1. Low conscientiousness is made up of at least the seven characteristics listed below. Next to each characteristic, write down what it means. Use a dictionary or ask others for assistance. Give two examples to show that you understand the characteristic.

Characteristics	*Definitions and Examples*
a. Underachievement ______________	Example 1 ______________
________________________________	________________________________
________________________________	Example 2 ______________
________________________________	________________________________
b. Not fulfilling intellectual or artistic potential ______________	Example 1 ______________
	________________________________
________________________________	Example 2 ______________
________________________________	________________________________
c. Poor academic performance relative to ability ______________	Example 1 ______________
	________________________________
________________________________	Example 2 ______________
________________________________	________________________________
d. Disregard of rules and responsibilities ______________	Example 1 ______________
	________________________________
________________________________	Example 2 ______________
________________________________	________________________________
e. Trouble with the law ______________	Example 1 ______________
________________________________	________________________________
________________________________	Example 2 ______________
________________________________	________________________________

f. Unable to discipline (or control) self____________ Example 1 ____________ Example 2 ____________

g. Personal and occupational aimlessness____________ Example 1 ____________ Example 2 ____________

2. Rank-order these characteristic according to how much they apply to you. Rank as No. 1 the characteristic that applies to you the most, rank as No. 2 the characteristic that applies to you next, and so on, down to the characteristic that applies to you the least.

Characteristics	*Rank-order*
a. Underachievement	______
b. Not fulfilling intellectual or artistic potential	______
c. Poor academic performance relative to ability	______
d. Disregard of rules and responsibilities	______
e. Trouble with the law	______
f. Unable to discipline (or control) self	______
g. Personal and occupational aimlessness	______

Homework: During the next week, think about whether you want to be very low in conscientiousness or whether you want to be effective in your relationships with others. It is very difficult sometimes to be low in conscientiousness and effective at the same time. What do you think? Write down your answer and discuss it with whoever is working with you on this practice exercise.

Practice Exercise 1. High Conscientiousness

Name____________ Sex______ Date______

The purpose of this practice exercise it to help you better understand personal characteristics or qualities that may work against you rather than for you.

1. High conscientiousness is made up of the characteristics or personal qualities listed below. Define each one, using a dictionary or asking others for assistance. Write down what you understand each characteristic means, and give two examples to show you understand it.

Characteristics	*Definitions and Examples*
a. Overachievement ______	Example 1 ______ Example 2 ______
b. Workaholic absorption in job or cause to the exclusion of family, social, and personal interests ______	Example 1 ______ Example 2 ______
c. Compulsiveness ______	Example 1 ______ Example 2 ______
d. Excessive cleanliness, tidiness, and attention to detail ______	Example 1 ______ Example 2 ______
e. Rigid self-discipline ______	Example 1 ______ Example 2 ______
f. Inability to set tasks and responsibilities aside and relax ______	Example 1 ______ Example 2 ______
g. Lack of spontaneity ______	Example 1 ______ Example 2 ______
h. Overly scrupulous in moral behavior ______	Example 1 ______ Example 2 ______

2. Rank-order these characteristics of high conscientiousness according to how much they apply to you. Rank as No. 1 the characteristic that applies to you the most, rank as No. 2 the characteristic that applies to you next, and so on, down to the characteristic that applies to you the least.

Characteristics	*Rank-order*
a. Overachievement	________
b. Workaholic absorption	________
c. Compulsiveness	________
d. Excessive cleanliness	________
e. Rigid self-discipline	________
f. Inability to set tasks aside and relax	________
g. Lack of spontaneity	________
h. Overly scrupulous in moral behavior	________

Homework: During the next week, think about whether you want to go on being very conscientious or whether you want to be effective in your relationships with others. It is very difficult sometimes to be very conscientious and effective at the same time. What do you think? Write down your answer and discuss it with whoever is working with you on this practice exercise.

Practice Exercise 1. Introversion

Name________________________Sex________Date________

The purpose of this practice exercise it to help you better understand personal characteristics or qualities that may work against you rather than for you.

1. Introversion is made up of the characteristics or personal qualities listed below. Define each one, using a dictionary or asking others for assistance. Give two examples to show you understand each characteristic.

Characteristics	*Definitions and Examples*
a. Social isolation ________________	Example 1 ________________
________________________	________________________
________________________	Example 2 ________________
________________________	________________________
b. Interpersonal detachment ________	Example 1 ________________
________________________	________________________
________________________	Example 2 ________________
________________________	________________________

c. Lack of support networks ________ Example 1 ________
________________ ________________
________________ Example 2 ________
________________ ________________

d. Flatness of feelings and emotions Example 1 ________
________________ ________________
________________ Example 2 ________
________________ ________________

e. Lack of joy and zest in life ________ Example 1 ________
________________ ________________
________________ Example 2 ________
________________ ________________

f. Reluctance to assert self ________ Example 1 ________
________________ ________________
________________ Example 2 ________
________________ ________________

g. Unwilling to assume leadership roles ________ Example 1 ________
________________ ________________
________________ Example 2 ________
________________ ________________

h. Social inhibition ________ Example 1 ________
________________ ________________
________________ Example 2 ________
________________ ________________

i. Shyness ________ Example 1 ________
________________ ________________
________________ Example 2 ________
________________ ________________

2. Rank-order these characteristics according to how they apply to you. Rank as No. 1 the characteristic that applies to you the most, rank as No. 2 the characteristic that applies to you next, and so on, down to the characteristic that applies to you the least.

Characteristics	*Rank-order*
a. Social isolation	________
b. Interpersonal detachment	________
c. Lack of support networks	________

Characteristics	*Rank-order*
d. Flattened feelings and emotions	________
e. Lack of joy and zest for life	________
f. Reluctance to assert self	________
g. Unwilling to assume leadership roles	________
h. Social inhibition	________
i. Shyness	________

Homework: During the next week, think about whether you want to go on being introverted or whether you want to be effective in your relationships with others. It is very difficult sometimes to be introverted and effective at the same time. What do you think? Write down your answer and discuss it with whoever is working with you on this practice exercise.

Practice Exercise 1. Extroversion

Name________________________Sex________Date______

The purpose of this practice exercise it to help you better understand personal characteristics or qualities that may work against you rather than for you.

1. Extroversion is made up of the characteristics or personal qualities listed below. Define each one, using a dictionary or asking others for assistance. Give two examples to show you understand each characteristic.

Characteristics	*Definitions and Examples*
a. Excessive talking ____________	Example 1 ____________
____________	____________
____________	Example 2 ____________
____________	____________
b. Inappropriate self-disclosure ____	Example 1 ____________
____________	____________
____________	Example 2 ____________
____________	____________
c. Social friction ____________	Example 1 ____________
____________	____________
____________	Example 2 ____________
____________	____________
d. Inability to spend time alone ____	Example 1 ____________
____________	____________
____________	Example 2 ____________
____________	____________

e. Attention seeking ______________ Example 1 ______________

______________ ______________

______________ Example 2 ______________

______________ ______________

f. Overly dramatic expression of emotions ______________ Example 1 ______________

______________ ______________

______________ Example 2 ______________

______________ ______________

g. Reckless excitement seeking ______ Example 1 ______________

______________ ______________

______________ Example 2 ______________

______________ ______________

h. Inappropriate attempts to dominate and control others ______________ Example 1 ______________

______________ ______________

______________ Example 2 ______________

______________ ______________

2. Rank-order these characteristics according to how much they apply to you. Rank as No. 1 the characteristic that applies to you the most, rank as No. 2 the characteristic that applies to you next, and so on, down to the characteristic that applies to you the least.

Characteristics	*Rank-order*
a. Excessive talking	________
b. Inappropriate self-disclosure	________
c. Social friction	________
d. Inability to spend time alone	________
e. Attention seeking	________
f. Overly dramatic expression of emotions	________
g. Reckless excitement seeking	________
h. Inappropriate attempts to dominate others	________

Homework: During the next week, think about whether you want to go on being highly extroverted or whether you want to be effective in your relationships with others. It is very difficult sometimes to be highly extroverted and effective at the same time. What do you think? Write down your answer and discuss it with whoever is working with you on this practice exercise.

Practice Exercise 1. Low Neuroticism

Name______________________________Sex_______Date________

The purpose of this practice exercise it to help you understand personal characteristics or qualities that may work against you rather than for you.

1. Low neuroticism is made up of the characteristics or personal qualities listed below. Define each one, using a dictionary or asking others for assistance. Give two examples to show you understand each characteristic.

Characteristics	*Definitions and Examples*
a. Inadequate troublesome thought about health matters __________	Example 1 __________
__________	Example 2 __________
b. Inadequate troublesome thoughts about social adjustment __________	Example 1 __________
__________	Example 2 __________
c. Emotional blandness (avoidance of either high or low feelings) __________	Example 1 __________
__________	Example 2 __________

2. Rank-order these characteristics according to how much they apply to you. Rank as No. 1 the characteristic that applies to you the most, rank as No. 2 the characteristic that applies to you next, and rank as No. 3 the characteristic quality that applies to you the least.

Characteristics	*Rank-order*
a. Inadequate troublesome thought about health matters	________
b. Inadequate troublesome thought about social adjustment	________
c. Emotional blandness	________

Homework: During the next week, think about whether you want to go on denying certain aspects of yourself or whether you want to be more effective in your relationships with yourself and others. It is hard sometimes to deny one characteristic and to be effective at the same time. What do you think? Write down your answer and discuss it with whoever is working with you on this practice exercise.

Practice Exercise 1. High Neuroticism

Name________________________________Sex________Date_______

The purpose of this practice exercise it to help you better understand personal characteristics or qualities that may work against you rather than for you.

1. High neuroticism is made up of the characteristics or personal qualities listed below. Define each one, using a dictionary or asking others for assistance. Give two examples to show you understand each characteristic.

Characteristics	*Definitions and Examples*
a. Chronic negative feelings:	Example 1 ______________________
i. Anxiety	________________________________
________________________________	Example 2 ______________________
________________________________	________________________________
ii. Fearfulness	Example 1 ______________________
________________________________	________________________________
________________________________	Example 2 ______________________
________________________________	________________________________
iii. Tension	Example 1 ______________________
________________________________	________________________________
________________________________	Example 2 ______________________
________________________________	________________________________
iv. Irritability	Example 1 ______________________
________________________________	________________________________
________________________________	Example 2 ______________________
________________________________	________________________________
v. Anger	Example 1 ______________________
________________________________	________________________________
________________________________	Example 2 ______________________
________________________________	________________________________
vi. Dejection	Example 1 ______________________
________________________________	________________________________
________________________________	Example 2 ______________________
________________________________	________________________________

vii. Hopelessness ____________ Example 1 ____________
______________________________ ______________________________
______________________________ Example 2 ____________
______________________________ ______________________________

viii. Guilt ____________ Example 1 ____________
______________________________ ______________________________
______________________________ Example 2 ____________
______________________________ ______________________________

ix. Shame ____________ Example 1 ____________
______________________________ ______________________________
______________________________ Example 2 ____________
______________________________ ______________________________

b. Inability to tolerate frustration or unpleasantness ____________ Example 1 ____________
______________________________ Example 2 ____________
______________________________ ______________________________

c. Irrational beliefs ____________ Example 1 ____________
______________________________ ______________________________
______________________________ Example 2 ____________
______________________________ ______________________________

d. Unrealistic expectations ____________ Example 1 ____________
______________________________ ______________________________
______________________________ Example 2 ____________
______________________________ ______________________________

e. Perfectionistic demands on self ___ Example 1 ____________
______________________________ ______________________________
______________________________ Example 2 ____________
______________________________ ______________________________

f. Unwarranted pessimism ____________ Example 1 ____________
______________________________ ______________________________
______________________________ Example 2 ____________
______________________________ ______________________________

g. Unfounded body troublesome thoughts ____________ Example 1 ____________
______________________________ Example 2 ____________
______________________________ ______________________________

h. Helplessness ______________________ Example 1 ______________________
______________________ ______________________
______________________ Example 2 ______________________
______________________ ______________________

i. Dependence on others for emotional support ______________________ Example 1 ______________________
______________________ ______________________
______________________ Example 2 ______________________
______________________ ______________________

j. Dependence on others for decision making ______________________ Example 1 ______________________
______________________ ______________________
______________________ Example 2 ______________________
______________________ ______________________

2. Rank-order these characteristics according to how much they apply to you. Rank as No. 1 the characteristic that applies to you the most, rank as No. 2 the characteristic that applies to you next, and so on, down to the characteristic that applies to you the least.

Characteristics	*Rank-order*
a. Chronic negative feelings:	
i. Anxiety	________
ii. Fearfulness	________
iii. Tension	________
iv. Irritability	________
v. Anger	________
vi. Dejection	________
vii. Hopelessness	________
viii. Guilt	________
ix. Shame	________
b. Inability to tolerate frustration or unpleasantness	________
c. Irrational beliefs	________
d. Unrealistic expectations	________
e. Perfectionistic demands on self	________
f. Unwarranted pessimism	________
g. Unfounded body troublesome thoughts	________
h. Helplessness	________
i. Dependence on others for emotional support	________
j. Dependence on others for decision making	________

Homework: During the next week, think about whether you want to go on being highly neurotic or whether you want to be effective in your relationships with yourself and with others. It is very difficult sometimes to be highly neurotic and effective at the same time. What do you think? Write down your answer and discuss it with whoever is working with you on this practice exercise.

Practice Exercise 1. Low Openness

Name______________________________Sex_________Date_________

The purpose of this practice exercise it to help you better understand personal characteristics or qualities that may work against you rather than for you.

1. Low openness is made up of the characteristics or personal qualities listed below. Define each one, using a dictionary or asking others for assistance. Give two examples to show you understand each characteristic.

Characteristics	*Definitions and Examples*
a. Difficulty adapting to social or personal change __________	Example 1 __________ Example 2 __________
b. Low tolerance in understanding different viewpoints __________	Example 1 __________ Example 2 __________
c. Low tolerance in understanding different lifestyles __________	Example 1 __________ Example 2 __________
d. Emotional blandness __________	Example 1 __________ Example 2 __________
e. Inability to understand and express own feelings __________	Example 1 __________ Example 2 __________
f. Constricted range of interests __________	Example 1 __________ Example 2 __________

g. Insensitivity to art and beauty ____ Example 1 ____________________

________________________________ ________________________________

________________________________ Example 2 ____________________

________________________________ ________________________________

h. Excessive conformity to authority Example 1 ____________________

________________________________ ________________________________

________________________________ Example 2 ____________________

________________________________ ________________________________

2. Rank-order these characteristics according to how much they apply to you. Rank as No. 1 the characteristic that applies to you the most, rank as No. 2 the characteristic that applies to you next, and so on, down to the characteristic that applies to you the least.

Characteristics	*Rank-order*
a. Difficulty adapting to social or personal change	________
b. Low tolerance in understanding different viewpoints	________
c. Low tolerance in understanding different lifestyles	________
d. Emotional blandness	________
e. Inability to understand and express own feelings	________
f. Constricted range of interests	________
g. Insensitivity to art and beauty	________
h. Excessive conformity to authority	________

Homework: During the next week, think about whether you want to go on not being very open or whether you want to be effective in your relationships with others. It is very difficult sometimes not to be open and be effective at the same time. What do you think? Write down your answer and discuss it with whoever is working with you on this practice exercise.

Practice Exercise 1. High Openness

Name__________________________Sex________Date__________

The purpose of this practice exercise it to help you better understand personal characteristics or qualities that may work against you rather than for you.

1. High openness to experience is made up of the characteristics or personal qualities listed below. Define each one, using a dictionary or asking others for assistance. Give two examples to show you understand each characteristic.

Characteristics	*Definitions and Examples*
a. Preoccupation with fantasy and day dreaming ______	Example 1 ______ Example 2 ______
b. Lack of practicality ______	Example 1 ______ Example 2 ______
c. Eccentric thinking (e.g., belief in ghosts, reincarnation, UFOs) ______	Example 1 ______ Example 2 ______
d. Diffuse identity ______	Example 1 ______ Example 2 ______
e. Changing goals ______	Example 1 ______ Example 2 ______
f. Joining a religious cult ______	Example 1 ______ Example 2 ______
g. Susceptibility to nightmares and to states of altered consciousness ______	Example 1 ______ Example 2 ______
h. Social rebelliousness and nonconformity ______	Example 1 ______ Example 2 ______
i. Interference with social or vocational advancement ______	Example 1 ______ Example 2 ______

2. Rank-order these characteristics according to how much they apply to you. Rank as No. 1 the characteristic that applies to you the most, rank as No. 2 the characteristic that applies to you next, and so on, down to the characteristic that applies to you the least.

Characteristics	*Rank-order*
a. Preoccupation with fantasy and daydreaming	________
b. Lack of practicality	________
c. Eccentric thinking	________
d. Diffuse identity	________
e. Changing goals	________
f. Joining religious cult	________
g. Susceptibility to nightmares and altered states	________
h. Social rebelliousness and nonconformity	________
i. Interference with social or vocational advancement	________

Homework: During the next week, think about whether you want to go on being very open or whether you want to be effective in your relationships with others. It is very difficult sometimes to be very open and effective at the same time. What do you think? Write down your answer and discuss it with whoever is working with you on this practice exercise.

Next to Last Practice Exercise for Each Characteristic: Developing and Checking on a Plan

Name____________________________Sex______Date__________

The purpose of this practice exercise is to help you better understand personal characteristics or qualities that may work against you rather than for you.

1. Following what you have written at the end of the last practice exercise, write down a plan for how you will behave in the future. If you cannot do it by yourself, ask the help of someone you know who cares about you, whether a relative, a friend, or a professional counselor. Before starting on your plan, complete the following sentences by writing a characteristic you do not like about yourself or others:

   a. When someone is __________________________ with me, I will ________.

   b. When someone is __________________________with me, I will ________.

   c. When someone is ________________________________ with me, I will ________.

2. Complete the following sentences:

   a. I plan to behave (write down the behavior you will follow) ______________________________ when ______________________________.

   b. I plan to behave (write down the behavior you will follow) ______________________________ when ______________________________.

   c. I plan to behave (write down the behavior you will follow) ______________________________ when ______________________________.

3. Now that you have written down a plan on how to behave, apply it next week and write down what happened in at least three situations.

   First situation: ______________________________
   Second situation: ______________________________
   Third situation: ______________________________

2. Did your plan work? If it worked well, go on and apply it again and again. If the plan did not work well, what happened? Why did the plan not work well? What part of the plan do you need to change to behave the way you planned? Write down what you need to change to get an improved plan to behave the way you planned.

Homework: Next week, apply your changed plan in at least three situations and write down

a. what happened;
b. how you behaved; and
c. what the result was in each situation:
   First situation: ______________________________
   Second situation: ______________________________
   Third situation: ______________________________

6. What did you learn from the changes you made in your plan?

Last Practice Exercise: Checking and Rechecking on the Plan

Name______________________________Sex________Date____________

The purpose of this practice exercise it to check on whether this practice exercise was helpful to you in any way.

1. It is important that you check on whether your plan worked or not. If it worked, do not change it. If it did not work, perhaps you may need to talk with someone you trust who may help you develop a better plan. If you do not check with someone, it will be impossible to find out what went wrong in your plan.

2. Write down what you learned by talking with someone you trust about your plan to behave in a helpful, pleasing, and prideful manner.
3. How can you change your plan to put what you just learned into it? Write down what you want to do to change your plan.
4. If necessary, you may repeat some of the practice exercises done in the past weeks but with a changed plan. See if it helped.
5. Did working on this practice exercise help you or not? Write down how this practice exercise helped you and how it did not help.

Personality Dimensions from the Personality Assessment Inventory (PAI)

The purpose of this practice exercise is to help you deal with, understand, and even enjoy some personality dimensions that may work against you rather than for you. These personality dimensions should have been pinpointed and identified by previous testing. When working on the questionnaires, make sure that the numbers on your answer sheet match the numbers and letters on the practice exercise.

Practice Exercise 1. Somatic Complaints

Name____________________________Sex______Date______________

The purpose of this practice exercise is to learn more about any complaints that you may have about your body.

1. List as many physical complaints as you have experienced in order of severity from the one that has lasted longest and more intensely down to the one that did not last very long and was less intense.
2. Troublesome Thoughts list.
3. Take the troublesome thought that has been the most bothersome and troublesome to you and answer the following questions about it:
4. When did this troublesome thought start?
5. Can you remember any other significant event in your life that was close to the beginning of this troublesome thought?
6. How often does it bother you?
7. How intense is this troublesome thought?
8. How much does this troublesome thought interfere with your:

   a. Home life
   b. Work
   c. Leisure time activities
   d. Sex life
   e. Social life
   f. Anything else?

9. What have you done to get rid of this troublesome thought? Write down all the various cures you have followed or doctors that you have consulted to get rid of this troublesome thought.

10. How much does this troublesome thought cause you to lose control of yourself?

    a. Most of the time ________
    b. Sometimes ________
    c. Never ________

11. What kind of feelings and emotions does this troublesome thought elicit in you, and what kind of feelings and emotions have you experienced about the lack of results from seeking treatment?

Homework: During the next week, keep track of all the troublesome thoughts you are feeling, and write down the troublesome thought, the exact time of occurrence, and whatever proceeded or followed your becoming aware of that troublesome thought.

Practice Exercise 2. Tracking Troublesome thoughts

Name________________________________Sex________Date___________

The purpose of this practice exercise is to learn more about your physical troublesome thoughts:

1. List as many physical complaints as you have experienced in order of severity from the one that has lasted longest and more intensely down to the one that did not last very long and was less intense.
2. Troublesome thoughts list.
3. Take the troublesome thought that has been the most bothersome and troublesome to you and answer the following questions about it:
4. When did this troublesome thought start?
5. Can you remember any other significant event in your life that was close to the beginning of this troublesome thought?
6. How often does it bother you?
7. How intense is this troublesome thought?
8. How much does this troublesome thought interfere with your:

    a. Home life
    b. Work
    c. Leisure time activities
    d. Sex life
    e. Social life
    f. Anything else?

9. What have you done to get rid of this troublesome thought? Write down all the various cures you have followed or doctors that you have consulted to get rid of this troublesome thought.
10. How much does this troublesome thought cause you to lose control of yourself?

    a. Most of the time _______
    b. Sometimes _______
    c. Never _______

11. What kind of feelings and emotions does this troublesome thought elicit in you, and what kind of feelings and emotions have you experienced about the lack of result from seeking treatment?

Homework: During the coming week, continue to keep track of your troublesome thoughts. This time, however, write down what kind of feelings you experience as you become aware of each troublesome thought.

Practice Exercise 1. Conversion Troublesome Thoughts

Name____________________________Sex______Date____________

The purpose of this practice exercise is to find out more about physical complaints for which no physical basis can be found.

1. List as many complaints of body sensations as you have experienced for which there does not seem to be a physical basis. List them in order of severity from the one that has lasted longest and more intensely than any other troublesome thought down to the one that did not last very long and was less intense.
2. Troublesome thoughts list.
3. Now take the troublesome thought that has been the most bothersome and troublesome to you and answer the following questions about it:
4. When did this troublesome thought start?
5. Can you remember any other significant event in your life that was close to the beginning of this troublesome thought?
6. How often does it bother you?
7. How intense is this troublesome thought?
8. How much does this troublesome thought interfere with your:

    a. Home life
    b. Work
    c. Leisure time activities
    d. Sex life
    e. Social life
    f. Anything else?

9. What have you done to get rid of this troublesome thought? Write down all the various cures you have followed or doctors that you have consulted to get rid of this troublesome thought:
10. How much does this troublesome thought cause you to lose control of yourself?

    a. Most of the time ________
    b. Sometimes ________
    c. Never ________

11. What kind of feelings and emotions does this troublesome thought elicit in you, and what kind of feelings and emotions have you experienced about the lack of result from seeking treatment?

Homework: During the coming week, keep track of every time you are becoming aware of each troublesome thought. Write down the exact time of occurrence, its duration, and whatever feelings were present before, during, and after you became aware of that troublesome thought.

Standard Practice Exercise for Troublesome Thoughts

This practice exercise can be repeated with all other troublesome thoughts that follow after the first and second troublesome thoughts.

Practice Exercise No.____Title of Troublesome thoughts:____________________

Name________________________________Sex_______Date___________

The purpose of this practice exercise is to learn more about the troublesome thought that is bothering you the most after the one you have considered in the previous practice exercise.

Answer the following questions about the complaint listed above:

1. When did this troublesome thought start?
2. Can you remember any other significant event in your life that was close to the beginning of this troublesome thought?
3. How often does it bother you?
4. How intense is this troublesome thought?
5. How much does this troublesome thought interfere with your:

    a. Home life
    b. Work
    c. Leisure time activities
    d. Sex life
    e. Social life

f. Anything else?

6. What have you done to get rid of this troublesome thought? Write down all the various cures you have followed or doctors that you have consulted to get rid of this troublesome thought:
7. How much does this troublesome thought cause you to lose control of yourself?

   a. Most of the time ___________
   b. Sometimes ___________
   c. Never ___________

8. What kind of feelings and emotions does this troublesome thought elicit in you, and what kind of feelings and emotions have you experienced about the lack of result from seeking treatment?

Homework: During the coming week, write down each time you become aware of each troublesome thought, registering when you became aware of it, its nature, duration, intensity, and what feelings you experienced at the time.

Practice Exercise 1. Somatization

Name________________________________Sex_____Date__________

The purpose of this practice exercise is to learn more about your troublesome thoughts with your body sensations.

1. List as many physical complaints troublesome thoughting your general health or fatigue as you have experienced. List them in order of severity from the one that has lasted longest and more intensely than any other troublesome thought down to the one that did not last very long and was less intense.
2. Troublesome thoughts list.
3. Now take the troublesome thought that has been the most bothersome and troublesome to you and answer the following questions about it:
4. When did this troublesome thought start?
5. Can you remember any other significant event in your life that was close to the beginning of this troublesome thought?
6. How often does it bother you?
7. How intense is this troublesome thought?
8. How much does this troublesome thought interfere with your:

   a. Home life
   b. Work
   c. Leisure time activities
   d. Sex life
   e. Social life
   f. Anything else?

9. What have you done to get rid of this troublesome thought? Write down all the various cures you have followed or doctors that you have consulted to get rid of this troublesome thought.
10. How much does this troublesome thought cause you to lose control of yourself?

    a. Most of the time ______
    b. Sometimes ______
    c. Never ______

11. What kind of feelings and emotions does this troublesome thought elicit in you, and what kind of feelings and emotions have you experienced about the lack of result from seeking treatment?
12. How does this complaint about your health affect your state of depression or anxiety? Please write as long as it is necessary to explain in detail.

Homework: During the coming week, write down each time you become aware of each troublesome thought, registering when you became aware of it, its nature, duration, intensity, and what feelings you experienced at the time.

Standard Practice Exercise for Troublesome Thoughts about Physical Sensations and your Body

This practice exercise can be used repeatedly to deal with multiple bodily troublesome thoughts.

Practice Exercise No.___Title of Physical Sensation_______________

Name______________________________Sex______Date_________

The purpose of this practice exercise is to learn more about your bodily sensations.

Answer the following questions about the sensation listed in the title of this practice exercise:

1. When did this troublesome thought start?
2. Can you remember any other significant event in your life that was close to the beginning of this troublesome thought?
3. How often does it bother you?
4. How intense is this troublesome thought?
5. How much does this troublesome thought interfere with your:

a. Home life
b. Work
c. Leisure time activities
d. Sex life
e. Social life
f. Anything else?

6. What have you done to get rid of this troublesome thought? Write down all the various cures you have followed or doctors that you have consulted to get rid of this troublesome thought:
7. How much does this troublesome thought cause you to lose control of yourself?

a.	Most of the time	________
b.	Sometimes	________
c.	Never	________

8. What kind of feelings and emotions does this troublesome thought elicit in you, and what kind of feelings and emotions have you experienced about the lack of result from seeking treatment?

Homework: During the coming week, write down each time you become aware of each troublesome thought, registering when you became aware of it, its nature, duration, intensity, and what feelings you experienced at the time.

Practice Exercise 1. Health Troublesome Thoughts

Name____________________________________Sex____Date_______

The purpose of this and other practice exercises is to learn more about your worries about your health.

1. List as many worries about your health and physical problems as you have experienced that (1) take a great deal of your time, thinking and talking about them; (2) affect how your feel about yourself; and (3) make you feel like a disabled person. List these worries in order of severity, from the one that has lasted longest and more intensely, down to the one that did not last as long and was less intense.
2. Troublesome thoughts list.
3. Now take the troublesome thought that has been the most bothersome and troublesome to you and answer the following questions about it:
4. When did this troublesome thought start?
5. Can you remember any other significant event in your life that was close to the beginning of this troublesome thought?
6. How often does this troublesome thought bother you?
7. How strong is this troublesome thought?
8. How much does this troublesome thought interfere with your:

a. Home life
b. Work
c. Leisure time activities
d. Sex life
e. Social life
f. Anything else?

9. What have you done to get rid of this troublesome thought? Write down all the various cures you have followed or doctors that you have consulted to get rid of this troublesome thought:
10. How much does this troublesome thought cause you to lose control of yourself?

a.	Most of the time	________
b.	Sometimes	________
c.	Never	________

11. What kind of feelings and emotions does this troublesome thought elicit in you, and what kind of feelings and emotions have you experienced about the lack of result from seeking treatment?

Homework: During the coming week, write down each time you become aware of each troublesome thought, writing down the exact time you became aware of it, its nature, duration, intensity, and what feelings you experienced at the time.

Standard Practice Exercise for Health Troublesome Thoughts

This practice exercise can be used repeatedly to deal with multiple bodily troublesome thoughts.

Practice Exercise No. ___ Title of Troublesome thoughts ________________

Name_____________________________Sex______Date___________

The purpose of this practice exercise is to learn more about your troublesome thoughts about your health.

Answer the following questions about the troublesome thought in the title of this practice exercise.

1. When did this troublesome thought start?
2. Can you remember any other significant event in your life that was close to the beginning of this troublesome thought?

3. How often does this troublesome thought bother you?
4. How strong is this troublesome thought?
5. How much does this troublesome thought interfere with your:

   a. Home life
   b. Work
   c. Leisure time activities
   d. Sex life
   e. Social life
   f. Anything else?

6. What have you done to get rid of this troublesome thought? Write down all the various cures you have followed or doctors that you have consulted to get rid of this troublesome thought.
7. How much does this troublesome thought cause you to lose control of yourself?

   a. Most of the time _______
   b. Sometimes _______
   c. Never _______

8. What kind of feelings and emotions does this troublesome thought elicit in you, and what kind of feelings and emotions have you experienced about the lack of result from seeking treatment?

Homework: During the coming week, write down each time you become aware of each troublesome thought, registering when you became aware of it, its nature, duration, intensity, and what feelings you experienced at the time.

Practice Exercise 1. Defining Anxiety

Name________________________________Sex______Date________

The purpose of this and other practice exercises is to help you learn more about your anxiety and possibly learn to control it.

1. What does anxiety mean to you? Define it as it applies especially to you.

____
____
____

2. How often do you experience these feelings?

   a. All the time _______
   b. Often _______
   c. Occasionally _______
   d. Seldom _______
   e. Other (please explain): _______

3. How long do they last?

a.	Years	______	d.	Days	______
b.	Months	______	e.	Hours	______
c.	Weeks	______	f.	Other (please explain):	______

4. How intense are these feelings?

a.	Extreme	______	c.	Mild	______
b.	Moderate	______	e.	Other (please explain):	______

5. Rank-order the following feelings or problems in the order of most troublesome to least troublesome according to how you feel. Rank as No. 1 the feeling or problem that is generally the worst, rank as No. 2 the feeling or problem that is generally second worst, and so on, down to the least troublesome feeling or problem.

Feelings		*Rank-order*
a.	Tension (shaky, restless, tight muscles or tired)	______
b.	Heart pounding or palpitations	______
c.	Shortness of breath	______
d.	Nausea, diarrhea, or abdominal distress	______
e.	Sweating or clammy hands	______
f.	Other physical problems	______
g.	Sleep problems	______
h.	In regard to concerning	______
i.	Trouble concentrating	______
j.	Fear of losing my mind	______
k.	Fear of not making it in life	______
l.	Fear of losing my job	______
m.	Fear of failing in school	______
n.	Fear of losing my friends	______
o.	Irritability	______
p.	Other fears______	______

6. Why did you select the feeling or problem that you rated as the most uncomfortable? What makes this feeling or problem seem so bad?
7. How did this feeling or problem develop? What events and thoughts have contributed to the development of this feeling or problem?
8. How has your family contributed to this feeling or problem? What does this feeling or problem do to your family?
9. How does this feeling or problem upset other areas of your life (e.g., friends, work, leisure, school)?
10. What memories do you have of experiencing this problem or feeling? What was happening?

Homework: Now you must make up your mind. Do you want to learn to control your anxiety, or do you want your anxiety to control you? If you want your anxiety to control you, do nothing and go on as you have always done in the past. If you want to learn to control your anxiety, maybe this homework may be of help to you.

During the next week, make an appointment with yourself (at least 24 h ahead) every other day at regular times for regular periods of time, for instance, Tuesday, Thursday and Saturday at 9 p.m. for 30–60 minute. During these times make sure that you can work on your anxiety without anyone or anything disturbing you. Remember, that if you want to learn to stop your anxiety, you need to start and stop it at preset, regular times.

During each of these appointments, pay attention to the feeling you selected to write about during this week's practice exercise. Go back to a time when you strongly felt this emotion (you may feel it in the present).

As soon as you feel this feeling, begin to write down whatever you feel or whatever comes to mind that relates to it or that is brought forth by your experiencing and staying with the feeling. Try to make yourself stay with the feeling during the length of the practice exercise.

Discuss your notes with your professional helper each week after you complete your practice exercise.

After you finish with this anxiety feeling, use the same procedure for the next anxiety feeling. Try to stay with the same feeling for the entire week. Switch to another feeling the next week if you can.

Standard Practice Exercise for Anxiety

Practice Exercise No.____Title of Feeling: ______________________

Name____________________________Sex_______Date__________

The purpose of this practice exercise is to learn more about your anxiety. Answer the following questions about the feeling listed above.

1. How did this feeling or problem develop? What events and thoughts have contributed to the development of this feeling or problem?
2. How has your family contributed to this feeling or problem? What does this feeling or problem do to your family?
3. How does this feeling or problem upset other areas of your life (e.g., friends, work, leisure, school)?
4. What memories do you have of experiencing this problem or feeling? What was happening?

Homework: During the next week, make an appointment with yourself (at least 24 h ahead) every other day at regular times for regular periods of time, for instance,

Tuesday, Thursday and Saturday at 9 p.m. for 30–60 minute. During these times make sure that you can work on this specific feeling without anyone or anything disturbing you. During each of these appointments pay attention to the feeling selected for this practice exercise to write about during this week's practice exercise. Go back to a time when you strongly felt this emotion (you may feel it in the present). As soon as you feel this feeling, begin to write down whatever you feel or whatever comes to mind that relates to it or that is brought forth by your experiencing and staying with the feeling. Try to make yourself stay with the feeling during the length of the practice exercise.

Practice Exercise 1. Obsessions-Compulsions

Name_______________________________Sex______Date_________

The purpose of this and other practice exercises is to help you learn to cope with your obsessions or compulsions.

1. Define what you understand as an obsession. If necessary, look it up in a dictionary or consult a friend.
2. Define what you understand as a compulsion. If necessary, look it up in a dictionary or consult a friend.
3. For purposes of understanding whether you suffer from either obsessions or compulsions, three lists of characteristics that break down each troublesome thought are given below. Define each term as you understand it. If necessary, consult a dictionary or a friend. After writing down these definitions, check whether that characteristic applies to you not at all, sometimes, or most of the time. If necessary, consult someone who knows you very well to see whether a characteristic applies to you or not.

	Not at all	*Applies to me: Sometimes*	*Most of the Time*	*Rank-order*
A. External characteristics:				
i. Overorganized	________	________	________	________
ii. Dutiful	________	________	________	________
iii. Work-oriented	________	________	________	________
iv. Conscientious	________	________	________	________
v. Disciplined	________	________	________	________
vi. Perfectionistic	________	________	________	________
vii. Rule-bound	________	________	________	________
viii. Detail-oriented	________	________	________	________
ix. Achievement-oriented	________	________	________	________

	Not at all	*Applies to me: Sometimes*	*Most of the Time*	*Rank-order*
x. Controlling	________	________	________	________
xi. Very proper	________	________	________	________
xii. Any other characteristic not listed above (__________)	________	________	________	________
B. Internal characteristics:				
i. Fault-finding	________	________	________	________
ii. Self-doubting	________	________	________	________
iii. Self-critical	________	________	________	________
iv. Worrisome	________	________	________	________
v. Needing approval	________	________	________	________
vi. Fearful of disapproval	________	________	________	________
vii. Guilt-ridden	________	________	________	________
viii. Fearful of expressing hostility	________	________	________	________
ix. Any other characteristic not listed above (__________)	________	________	________	________
C. Interpersonal characteristics:				
i. Inflexible	________	________	________	________
ii. Formal	________	________	________	________
iii. Pedantic	________	________	________	________
iv. Dogmatic	________	________	________	________
v. Serious	________	________	________	________
vi. Lacking in spontaneity	________	________	________	________
vii. Any other characteristic not listed above (__________)	________	________	________	________

2. Now go back to those characteristics that you have checked as applying to you most of the time and rank-order them in order of importance to you. Rank as No. 1 the characteristic that applies to you the most, rank as No. 2 the characteristic that applies to you second, and so on down the list of characteristics that apply to you most of the time. If you have not listed anything under "Most of the time," go over those that apply to you "Sometimes" and rank-order them as indicated above.

Homework: During the coming week, go back to your rank-orderings and change them if you feel it is appropriate to do so.

Standard Practice Exercise for Obsessions and Compulsions

Practice Exercise No.___ O/C Characteristic____________________

Name____________________________Sex_______Date_________

The purpose of this and all other practice exercises is to teach how to cope with your obsessions or compulsions.

1. Write how the characteristic cited above in the title of this practice exercise applies to you.
2. What advantages do you get from this characteristic?
3. What disadvantages do you get from this characteristic?
4. How did this characteristic develop within yourself?
5. How is this characteristic similar or different from that of family members, parents, caregivers, siblings, or other important relatives who influenced you a great deal?
6. Do you want to keep this characteristic, or do you want to leave it behind you? Why?
7. What would happen to you if you kept it?
8. What would happen to you if you left it behind?
9. How would you change it if you kept it?
10. How would you replace it if you left it behind?
11. The major decision you have to make now is whether this characteristic controls you or whether you control it.
12. What are the advantages of it controlling you versus your controlling it?
13. What will it take for you to learn to control it? Write down a plan that you believe will give you greater control over it, if that is what you want. Discuss this plan with your counselor or friend, changing it according to his or her advice, and try it out for at least a week to see whether it works or not. If this plan does not work, try to develop another plan with the help of a counselor or friend.

Practice Exercise 1. Phobias

Name_________________________Sex_______Date____________

The purpose of this and other practce exercises is to help you cope with your fears or phobias in better ways than you have done before.

1. Do fears or phobias interfere with significant parts of your life? If so, how?
2. Fears and phobias mean that you have to keep constant watch over what you are afraid of to avoid contact with it. Write down how this constant watching limits your life activities.

3. What kind of phobias control you? Please specify whether your phobias involve:

   a. Social situations
   b. Public transportation
   c. Heights
   d. Enclosed spaces
   e. Specific objects
   f. Specific animals
   g. Any other situation not included in the list above

4. It is important to know whether you suffer from one intense phobia rather than a variety of phobias.

   a. Which is it?
   b. The major issue here is whether you want this phobia to control you, or whether you want to learn to control it.
   c. What is your choice? Why?

5. If you want to learn to control this phobia or many phobias, you need to write in detail about the phobia that affects you the most.

   a. How did this phobia develop over time?
   b. How did it snowball to take control of you?
   c. What have you done to achieve control over it?

Homework: If you want to learn to control this phobia, you will need to make specific appointments with yourself (e.g., 7 p.m. for 1 h) to start this phobia when you want it. If you want to learn to stop it, you need to learn to start it. If you can learn to start it, you can learn to stop it. However, you will need to write down what is happening to you when you allow yourself to start it. Discuss your writing with your professional helper.

Standard Practice Exercise for Phobias

Practice Exercise No.___Name of Phobia________________________

Name______________________________Sex________Date___________

Please write in detail about the phobia that is listed above in the title of this practice exercise.

1. How does this phobia interfere with significant parts of your life?
2. This phobia means that you have to keep constant watch over what you are afraid of to avoid contact with it. Write down how this constant watching limits your life activities.

3. How much does this phobia control you?
4. The major issue here is whether you want this phobia to control you, or whether you want to learn to control it. What is your choice? Why?
5. If you want to learn to control this phobia or other phobias, you need to write about the phobia that affects you the most in detail.

   a. How did this phobia develop over time?
   b. How did it snowball to take control of you?
   c. What have you done to achieve control over it?

Homework: If you want to learn to control this phobia you will need to make specific appointments with yourself (e.g., 7 p.m. for 1 h) to start this phobia when you want it. If you want to learn to stop it, you need to learn to start it. If you can learn to start it you can learn to stop it. However, you will need to write down what is happening to you when you allow yourself to start it. Discuss your writing with your professional helper.

Practice Exercise 1. Traumatic Stress

Name______________________________Sex________Date__________

The purpose of this practice exercise is to learn more about stresses that have hurt you severely.

1. Write down what experience of a disturbing traumatic event in the past is still distressing you.
2. Does this event produce recurrent episodes of anxiety? If yes, how? If not how does it affect you?
3. Has this event left you changed or damaged in some fundamental way? Write down how this event affected you.
4. Possible traumatic events involve:

   a. Victimization
   b. Rape
   c. Abuse
      i. Physical
      ii. Verbal
      iii. Sexual (incest, fondling, genital touching, anal intercourse)
   d. Combat experiences
   e. Life-threatening accidents
   f. Natural disasters, e.g., earthquakes
   g. Any other event not included above, name it:

5. Tell in detail what happened as you remember it, not leaving anything out.
6. What feelings are related to this event? Can you write about them in detail?
7. Have you discussed this event with anybody?

8. What were the reactions of the person you discussed this event with?
9. Have you been able to grieve about the painfulness of this event? If yes, how? If not, why not?
10. Allow yourself to express whatever feelings you have with someone you trust who can understand and discuss with you the pain of this event, whether it is your helper, friend, or family member.

Homework: During the coming week, write down how you feel whenever someone you trust understands you. Write down also how you feel whenever you do not feel understood.

Practice Exercise 1. Hyperactivity or Drivenness

Name_______________________________Sex________Date__________

The purpose of this and other practice exercises is to learn more about your hyperactivity or drivenness.

1. We need to determine how often this troublesome thought is present in you. Does it apply to you never, sometimes, or most of the time? If necessary, check with someone who knows you very well to see whether and how these characteristics apply to you.

	Not at all	*Sometimes*	*Most of the Time*	*Rank-order*
A. Activity level, evidenced by:				
i. Keeping busy all the time	______	______	______	______
ii. Involving a wide range of activities	______	______	______	______
iii. In a driven but somewhat disorganized manner	______	______	______	______
iv. With accelerated thought processes	______	______	______	______
B. Grandiosity, made up of:				
i. Inflated self-esteem or sense of importance	______	______	______	______
ii. Expansiveness	______	______	______	______
iii. Beliefs of having exceptionally high levels of common skills	______	______	______	______
iv. Beliefs bordering on the delusional in terms of having special and unique talents that will lead to fame and fortune	______	______	______	______

	Not at all	Sometimes	Most of the Time	Rank-order
C. Irritability, where relationships with others are strained due to:	______	______	______	______
i. Your frustrations with the inability or unwillingness of those around you to keep up with your plans, demands, and possibly unrealistic ideas	______	______	______	______
ii. At the extreme, this irritability may result in accusations that significant others are attempting to thwart your plans for success and achievement.	______	______	______	______

2. After you have checked those characteristics that apply to you most of the time, rank-order them according to how much they describe you. Rank as No. 1 the one that describes you best, rank as No. 2 the one that describes you second best, and so on, until you have rank-ordered all the characteristics that apply to you most of the time. Then do the same for the characteristics that apply to you sometimes.

Homework: During the coming week, make an appointment with yourself for a definite, preset time (no longer than 1 h) to think about how these characteristics control you, and to decide whether you want to learn to control them.

Standard Practice Exercise for Hyperactivity and Drivenness

Practice Exercise No.___Title of Behavior_______________________

Name_________________________________Sex______Date_________

What is your decision about whether the characteristic named in the title of this practice exercise should control you or whether you want to learn to control it? If you want to stay the same and not change, you do not need to complete these practice exercises. If you have decided you want to change and you want to learn to control this characteristic, go on with this practice exercise.

1. How did this characteristic develop over time? Can you write about how it began and how it took over your life?

____

____

____

2. How did this characteristic develop from your family relationships? Did anyone in your family have this characteristic? How?

____

____

____

3. What are the advantages of this characteristic?

____

____

____

4. What are the disadvantages of this characteristic?

____

____

____

Homework: Develop a plan for learning to control this characteristic over time. If necessary, talk with your professional helper to develop this plan. If you do not have any help, talk with a friend to see whether he or she can help you develop a plan.

Practice Exercise 1. Extreme Doubts and No Confidence in Others

Name______________________________Sex______Date________

The purpose of this and other practice exercise is to help you understand how extreme doubt and no confidence in others may be destructive to you.

1. To understand this troublesome thought, we need to determine to what extent it is made up of characteristics that control you. Do these characteristics apply to you never, sometimes, or most of the time?

	Not at all	Sometimes	Most of the Time	Rank-order
A. Hypervigilance, consists of:				
i. Close monitoring of the environment for evidence that others are trying to harm or discredit you in some devious way	______	______	______	______
ii. Questioning and not trusting the motives of those around you, despite the nature or history of the relationship in question	______	______	______	______
B. Ideas of persecution:				
i. Quick to feel that you have been treated inequitably	______	______	______	______
ii. Belief that there is a concerted effort by others to undermine your interests or your welfare	______	______	______	______
C. Resentment:				
i. You are likely to be easily insulted or slighted	______	______	______	______
ii. Typically responding by holding grudges toward others	______	______	______	______
iii. Inclined to attribute your misfortunes to the neglect of others	______	______	______	______
iv. Discrediting successes of others as being the result of luck or favoritism	______	______	______	______
v. Being envious of others	______	______	______	______
vi. Disinclined to assist others in achieving goals and successes	______	______	______	______

2. After you have checked those characteristics that apply to you most of the time, rank-order them according to which characteristic describes you best. Rank as No. 1 the one that describes you best, rank as No. 2 the one that describes you second best, and so on, until you have rank-ordered all the characteristics that apply to you most of the time. Then do the same for the characteristics that apply to you sometimes.

Homework: During the next week, make an appointment with yourself for a definite, preset time (no longer than 1 h) to think about how these characteristics control you, and to decide whether you want to learn to control them.

Standard Practice Exercises for Extreme Doubts and No Confidence in Others

Use the same standard practice exercise as you used for hyperactivity, but change the title of the behavior.

Practice Exercise 1. Unusual Thinking

Name________________________________Sex______Date________

The purpose of this and other practice exercise is to understand in greater detail the nature of your thinking.

1. To understand and help you with your unusual thinking, you need to check which characteristics apply to you never, sometimes, or most of the time. You may need the help of a professional to answer some of these items.

	Not at all	*Sometimes*	*Most of the Time*	*Rank-order*
A. Psychotic experiences, made up of:				
i. Unusual perceptions and sensations	______	______	_____	_____
ii. Magical thinking	______	______	_____	_____
iii. Unusual ideas that may involve delusional beliefs	______	______	_____	_____
iv. Hallucinations	______	______	_____	_____
Auditory (ears)	______	______	_____	_____
Visual (eyes)	______	______	_____	_____
B. Social detachment				
i. Socially isolated	______	______	_____	_____
ii. Few close or warm interpersonal relationships	______	______	_____	_____
iii. Having difficulty in interpreting normal nuances of interpersonal behavior that provide meaning to personal relationships	______	______	_____	_____

	Not at all	Sometimes	Most of the Time	Rank-order
iv. Social isolation and emotional detachment may serve to decrease the sense of discomfort that is fostered by interpersonal contact	____	____	____	____
C. Thought disorder				
i. Thought processes marked by confusion and difficulties in concentration	____	____	____	____
ii. Severe depression due to:	____	____	____	____
Brain injury or disease	____	____	____	____
Effects of medication	____	____	____	____
v. Consequences of drug or alcohol abuse	____	____	____	____

2. After you have checked those characteristics that apply to you most of the time, rank-order them according to which characteristic describes you best. Rank as No. 1 the one that describes you best, rank as No. 2 the one that describes you second best, and so on, until you have rank-ordered all the characteristics that apply to you most of the time. Then do the same for the characteristics that apply to you sometimes.

Homework: During the next week, make an appointment with yourself for a definite, preset time (no longer than 1 h) to think about how these characteristics control you, and to decide whether you want to learn to control them. Write down what you have concluded, and discuss it with your professional helper.

Standard Practice Exercises for Unusual Thinking

Use the same standard practice exercise as you used for hyperactivity, but change the title of the behavior.

Practice Exercise 1. Borderline Characteristics

Name______________________________Sex________Date____________

1. To understand and help you with your borderline characteristics of behavior, you need to check which characteristics apply to you never, sometimes, or most of the time.

	Not at all	*Some-times*	*Most of the Time*	*Rank-order*
A. Affective instability made up of:				
i. Highly responsive emotionally	_____	_____	_____	____
ii. Rapid and extreme mood swings (rather than more cyclic mood changes as seen in mood disorders)	_____	_____	_____	____
iii. Episodes of poorly controlled anger	_____	_____	_____	____
B. Identity problems				
i. Uncertain about major life issues	_____	_____	_____	____
ii. Little sense of purpose	_____	_____	_____	____
iii. Feeling empty, bored, or unfulfilled	_____	_____	_____	____
C. Negative relationships				
i. History of involvement in ambivalent intense and unstable relationships	_____	_____	_____	____
ii. Often feel resentful and betrayed by people who were once close to you	_____	_____	_____	____
D. Self-harm				
i. Impulsive in areas that have high potential for negative consequences	_____	_____	_____	____
ii. Excessive spending	_____	_____	_____	____
iii. Unsafe or promiscuous sex	_____	_____	_____	____
iv. Substance abuse	_____	_____	_____	____
v. Ineffective social and occupational performance	_____	_____	_____	____
vi. At risk for self-mutilation and suicidal behavior	_____	_____	_____	____

2. After you have checked those characteristics that apply to you most of the time, rank-order them according to which characteristic describes you best. Rank as No. 1 the one that describes you best, rank as No. 2 the one that describes you second best, and so on, until you have rank-ordered all the characteristics that apply to you most of the time. Then do the same for the characteristics that apply to you sometimes.

Homework: During the next week, make an appointment with yourself for a definite, preset time (no longer than 1 h) to think about how these characteristics control you, and to decide whether you want to learn to control them. Write down what you conclude and discuss it with your professional helper.

Standard Practice exercises for Borderline Personality

Use the same format as you used for the standard practice exercise for hyperactivity, but change the title.

Practice Exercise 1. Antisocial Characteristics

Name______________________________Sex_____Date______

The purpose of this practice exercise is to understand the nature of your antisocial characteristics.

1. To understand and help you with your antisocial characteristics of behavior, you need to check which characteristics apply to you never, sometimes, or most of the time.

	Not at all	*Some-times*	*Most of the Time*	*Rank-order*
a. A conduct disorder during adolescence	____	____	____	____
b. Involvement in illegal occupations	____	____	____	____
c. Engagement in criminal acts involving	____	____	____	____
d. Theft	____	____	____	____
e. Destruction of property	____	____	____	____
f. Physical aggression toward others	____	____	____	____
g. Little regard for others or of the opinion of the society around you	____	____	____	____
i. Desire to satisfy your own goals and impulses	____	____	____	____
j. Taking advantage of others, even those who are closest to you	____	____	____	____
k. Little responsibility for the property of others	____	____	____	____
l. Little loyalty to your acquaintances	____	____	____	____
m. No remorse of a long-lasting nature	____	____	____	____
n. Little importance for your roles as spouse, parent, or employee	____	____	____	____
o. Reckless and potentially dangerous to yourself and to those around you	____	____	____	____
p. Craving excitement and stimulation				
q. Easily bored by routine or convention	____	____	____	____

2. After you have checked those characteristics that apply to you most of the time, rank-order them according to which characteristic describes you best. Rank as No. 1 the one that describes you best, rank as No. 2 the one that describes you

second best, and so on, until you have rank-ordered all the characteristics that apply to you most of the time. Then do the same for the characteristics that apply to you sometimes.

Homework: During the next week, make an appointment with yourself for a definite, preset time (no longer than 1 h) to think about how these characteristics control you, and to decide whether you want to learn to control them.

Standard Practice Exercises for Antisocial Characteristics

Use the same format of practice exercise as you used for hyperactivity, but change the title.

Practice Exercise 1. Aggression

Name________________________________Sex______Date________

1. To understand and help you with your aggressive characteristics, you need to check which characteristics apply to you never, sometimes, or most of the time.

	Not at all	*Some-times*	*Most of the Time*	*Rank-order*
A. Aggressive attitudes:				
i. Easily angered	____	____	____	____
ii. Having difficulty controlling expression of your anger	____	____	____	____
iii. Likely to be perceived by others as being hostile and readily provoked	____	____	____	____
B. Verbal aggression				
i. Not easily intimidated by confrontation	____	____	____	____
ii. Verbally aggressive (critical, insulting, or threatening) with little provocation	____	____	____	____
iii. Displaying anger as soon as it is experienced	____	____	____	____
C. Physical aggression				
i. Prone to physical display of anger	____	____	____	____
ii. Including damage to property	____	____	____	____
iii. Physical fights	____	____	____	____
iv. Threats of violence	____	____	____	____

	Not at all	Some-times	Most of the Time	Rank-order
v. Intimidating others by your temper	____	____	____	____
vi. Potential for violence	____	____	____	____

2. Now you need to rank-order these characteristics according to how much they apply to you. Rank as No. 1 the characteristic that applies to you the most, rank as No. 2 the characteristic that applies to you second, and so on; mark as N/A the characteristics that do not apply to you.

Homework: During the coming week, write down all instances of aggression that you have been involved with. Write down what led to that situation, what happened, and what the outcome was.

Standard Practice Exercise for Aggression

Use the same format of practice exercise as you used for hyperactivity, but change the title.

Practice Exercise 1. Suicidal Ideation

Suicidal ideation consists of thoughts and ideas relating to death and suicide, ranging from hopelessness to general and vague thoughts of dying and suicide, with concrete plans for the suicidal act. Use any of the depression practice exercises contained in this sourcebook.

Stress

Identify the nature of life stressors and find the most suitable practice exercise to deal with them, such as anxiety, depression, or any other troublesome thought that is specific to the respondent. When in doubt, to learn more about the individual, use either anxiety-related practice exercises or the self-awareness practice exercise contained in this sourcebook.

Nonsupport

The perception of lack of social support from available or unavailable social relationships, family members, friends, and neighbors entails identifying the presence of other factors, including loneliness, anxiety, depression, moodiness, or even paranoia. Practice exercises relevant to any of these factors are available in this sourcebook.

Treatment Resistance or Rejection

Two practice exercises are available in this sourcebook. One deals with the negative treatment indicators content scale of the MMPI-2. Another deals with treatment rejection, the Butcher Treatment Planning Inventory (BTPI)

Dominance

This scale measures the extent to which one is controlling, submissive, or autonomous in interpersonal relationships. Other characteristics may need to be identified before settling on a practice exercise that would help decrease it. For instance, dominance often is present in either impulsive or driven individuals, who would profit from social training or practice exercises for externalization disorders available in this sourcebook.

Fear of Closeness (Warmth)

Fear of closeness means lacking in empathic, affectionate, sociable, or sympathetic characteristics. There is fear of engaging in intimate relationships, or rejecting them and having no confidence in them. These characteristics develop within the context of an unfeeling personality that has little patience with faults of others, and who is uninterested in making commitments to personal relationships. It may represent also denial of dependency. It is suggested that perhaps this kind of characteristic be dealt with through focused distance writing, asking respondents to write for 20 minute a day for four consecutive days about hurts and traumas that have not been disclosed or discussed with anyone heretofore. An alternative suggestion would be the administration of the intimacy for couples practice exercise available in this sourcebook.

Couples

Improving Relationships

Instructions for professionals:

1. Administer the Relationship Assessment Test (RAT) to each partner.
2. Add up the points for each area to see which areas have the highest degree of discrepancy between partners.
3. Choose which areas are the most troublesome, and discuss the findings with the couple. If necessary have the partners rank-order the six areas from most troublesome to least troublesome, independently of the test results.

4. Assign pertinent practice exercises, beginning with the most troublesome areas and ending with the least troublesome ones.
5. Upon completion of Practice Exercise No. 6, ask the couple to develop their own practice exercise for maintaining the relationship.
6. Readminister the RAT to see whether any changes have taken place of a result of this program.

Relationship Assessment Test (RAT)

On a scale from 1 to 5, agree or disagree with the following statements as they apply to you. Circle the appropriate number: 1 = disagree completely; 2 = disagree; 3 = neutral; 4 = agree; 5 = agree completely.

A. Personal values

1.	I believe in keeping traditions alive	1	2	3	4	5
2.	My independence is important to me	1	2	3	4	5
3.	Family is important to me	1	2	3	4	5
4.	I want my partner's respect	1	2	3	4	5
5.	If you work for something, you appreciate it more	1	2	3	4	5
6.	Parents and elders are to be respected	1	2	3	4	5
7.	A college education is needed to get a good job	1	2	3	4	5
8.	Religion or faith helps one through hard times	1	2	3	4	5
9.	Nice houses reflect the value of the owners	1	2	3	4	5
10.	Expensive cars are symbols of good taste	1	2	3	4	5

B. Expectations

1.	The man should be head of the household	1	2	3	4	5
2.	A woman should work at home	1	2	3	4	5
3.	The man should share household chores	1	2	3	4	5
4.	I thought we would live in the country	1	2	3	4	5
5.	Love can overcome all problems	1	2	3	4	5
6.	Males have more freedom and choices in life	1	2	3	4	5
7.	Females have more freedom and choices in life	1	2	3	4	5
8.	Men make better leaders	1	2	3	4	5
9.	A woman is expected to bear children for her man	1	2	3	4	5
10.	I expect(ed) financial security by age 30	1	2	3	4	5

C. Beliefs

1.	Lovers automatically know how each other feels	1	2	3	4	5
2.	Nagging is the best way to get something done.	1	2	3	4	5
4.	An argument ends when the other admits fault	1	2	3	4	5
5.	I must be an achiever to be worthwhile	1	2	3	4	5
6.	It is terrible if the house is not cleaned daily	1	2	3	4	5
7.	It would be awful if my partner stops loving me	1	2	3	4	5
8.	I must be perfect so that others think I am smart	1	2	3	4	5
9.	If my children misbehave, I must be a bad parent	1	2	3	4	5
10.	My ideas are usually correct	1	2	3	4	5

D. Anger

1.	I am in charge of my anger	1	2	3	4	5
2.	I am able to show anger without violence	1	2	3	4	5
3.	I take responsibility for my anger	1	2	3	4	5
4.	My partner does things to make me angry	1	2	3	4	5
5.	I can control others by showing my anger	1	2	3	4	5
6.	My family says I embarrass them when I am angry	1	2	3	4	5
7.	I feel guilty after one of my tantrums	1	2	3	4	5
8.	I can't help myself when I get angry	1	2	3	4	5
9.	I get angry when others don't do what I say	1	2	3	4	5
10.	I often hurt the feelings of those I care about	1	2	3	4	5

E. Power

To indicate how comfortable you are with each item, circle 1 for very comfortable, 2 for somewhat comfortable, or 3 for not at all comfortable.

1.	Responsibilities are assigned	1	2	3
2.	Authority is used	1	2	3
3.	Finances and money are handled	1	2	3
4.	Vacations or recreational events are planned	1	2	3
5.	Acceptable behavior is defined	1	2	3
6.	We deal with parents and siblings	1	2	3
7.	Major decisions are made	1	2	3
8.	Household chores are divided	1	2	3
9.	Decisions are carried out	1	2	3
10.	We decide to have social contacts	1	2	3

F. Sex and intimacy

1.	I am comfortable with sexuality and lovemaking	1	2	3
2.	Sex is important to me	1	2	3
3.	I can talk about sex with my partner	1	2	3
4.	My partner understands if I ever say no to sex	1	2	3

5.	Sex is becoming routine and boring for me	1	2	3
6.	I like to touch my partner	1	2	3
7.	I enjoy being touched by my partner	1	2	3
8.	I like to be held even if sex doesn't follow	1	2	3
9.	I share my sexual fantasies with my partner	1	2	3
10.	I make time for sex and lovemaking	1	2	3

This practice exercise is designed to work on your relationship. As you complete the practice exercises given to you, be honest about your feelings. Even though you may feel uncomfortable doing the practice exercises in the beginning, the process will become more natural as you progress.

It is important to set aside at least 1 h a week to make positive changes in your relationship. You must make a commitment to work toward that goal.

This is an opportunity to be truthful to yourself about your relationship, so do not try to hide your true feelings. There are no trick questions and there are no right or wrong answers.

Practice Exercise 1. Values

Name________________________Sex_______Date_____________

The purpose of this homework practice exercise is to clarify your values in relationship to the values of your partner. Think about objects, events, or activities that you consider most important to you. Be sure to match the numbers and letters of your answer sheets with those in these practice exercises.

1. Prepare two lists of values; one list represents your own (Mine), and the other one represents what you think your partner values (Partner's). List them in order of negotiability, according to four levels of negotiability:

    a. Nonnegotiable (e g., killing, stealing, etc.)
    b. Nonnegotiable but with some exceptions (e.g., having a glass of wine even though you may not drink alcoholic beverages)
    c. Negotiable issues and problems that need to be negotiated anew with your partner, such as the areas included in this practice exercise or not included in it.
    d. Not needing negotiation (e. g., brushing your teeth, buying your clothes, etc.).

2. During the coming week, compare your lists with those of your partner.

    a. Write down your impressions of the lists. Do not discuss your impressions with your partner yet.
    b. Wait until both of you have gone over your respective lists.
    c. Set a specific appointment time (at least 24 h ahead) when you will discuss your reactions to each other's lists.

3. Note (always in writing) agreements between your lists and those of your partner.
4. Note which disagreements exist among the lists.

5. Note the accuracy of your perception of your partner's values
6. Note what opposite ideas exist between you and your partner.
7. Note what similar ideas exist between you and your partner
8. At the preset (at least 24 h in advance) appointment time, exchange your lists and notes and discuss areas of disagreement and agreement. Write down which areas of disagreement exist between you two.

Homework: During the coming week, write down a plan on how disagreements between you two could be dealt with and possibly resolved. Make another appointment (at least 24 h in advance) and compare and contrast (pros and cons) each other's plan, coming up with a master plan that includes ideas from each other's plan.

Practice Exercise 2. Expectations

Name______________________________Sex_____Date___________

The purpose of this practice exercise is to clarify your expectations of yourself and of your partner.

1. Complete the following sentences:

   a. As a woman (man) I must ____
   ____

   b. If I had the courage, I would ______________________________________
   ____

   c. If you knew me, you would think ___________________________________
   ____

   d. I would like to ____
   ____

   e. I want to ____
   ____

   f. I need ____
   ____

   g. My daydreams focus on ____
   ____

   h. I dream of ____
   ____

   i. I expect ____

   j. I hope____
   ____

   k. In the future ____
   ____

2. Write about problems in your role as a man (woman).
3. Write about problems in your role as a partner.
4. Write about your problems in your role as a parent.
5 Write about the last time you felt your partner treated you fairly and respectfully.
6. Write what your reaction was to his/her behavior.
7. Write about the last time your partner treated you unfairly or disrespectfully.
8. Write what your reaction was to her/his behavior.
9. Make an appointment (24 h in advance) to discuss and compare your answers with your partner.

Homework: During the following week, write down each time you feel that you do something that is not your responsibility. Then set a time when you and your partner will switch roles in your roles as homemaker and as parent. This practice exercise may mean that the one who is working full-time may have a week off for "vacation." Record what happens, and write down your feelings about the switch in roles.

Practice Exercise 3. Beliefs

Name______________________________Sex______Date____________

The purpose of this practice exercise is to clarify your beliefs and to discuss them with your partner.

1. For the next 3 days, state your belief (how you feel, what your think, and how you behave) in regard to each belief listed below. State what might be a better or more helpful belief.

____

____

____

____

2. Rank-order your beliefs according to their importance to you. Rank as No. 1 the belief that in most important in your life, rank as No. 2 the belief that is second in your life, and so on; mark as N/A the beliefs that might not be important to you.

Belief	*Rank-order*	*Belief*	*Rank-order*
a. Sex	________	g. Friends	________
b. Personal appearance	________	h. Relatives	________
c. Home	________	i. Religion	________
d. Love	________	j. Politics	________
e. Children	________	k. Partner	________
f. Career (work, job)	________	l. Money	________

3. Explain why you rank-ordered your beliefs the way you did.

____
____
____
____
____

4. Complete this sentence: "If I were to change my beliefs, the danger would be________."

____
____
____
____

Homework: Next week, think and write down how and why you should change beliefs that do not work well for you.

Practice Exercise 4. Anger

Name _______________________ Sex____ Date__________

The purpose of this practice exercise is to understand how anger affects your relationship.

1. What do you do when you become angry?

____
____
____
____

2. How do those around you react to your anger?

____
____
____
____

3. How do you react to their reactions?

____
____
____
____

4. Complete the following sentences:

   a. I feel angry when my partner ____
   ____

   b. I get angry about ____
   ____

   c. Anger is ____
   ____

   d. Anger ____
   ____

5. List the number of times in the last few weeks that you have become angry with each of the following people:

   a. Partner ______ How did you express your anger?
   b. Child ________ How did you express your anger?
   c. Mother ______ How did you express your anger?
   d. Father _______ How did you express your anger?
   e. Other________ How did you express your anger?

6. What usually happens when you lose control?
7. What will happen if you do not learn to control your anger?
8. Give three reasons why you should control your anger.
9. Why do you want to control your anger now?
10. List other ways to express your anger.
11. What does this anger do to you and your partner?
12. How do you use anger to control your relationship?
13. How do you react when others become angry with you?
14. List the number of times in the last few weeks that the following people were angry with you:

    a. Mate ______ How was the anger expressed?
    b. Child ______ How was the anger expressed?
    c. Mother ______ How was the anger expressed?
    d. Father ______ How was the anger expressed?
    e. Other __________ How was the anger expressed?

Homework: During the following week, write down every time you become angry: (1) what situation led to your anger; (2) what the anger was about; (3) how you expressed your anger; (4) what was the outcome of your anger; and (5) how your could have dealt with the situation in a more constructive, helpful fashion.

Practice Exercise 5. Power

Name____________________________Sex______Date____________

The purpose of this practice exercise is to learn more about how power is discussed in your relationship.

Power consists of two separate behaviors: (1) who makes decisions, and (2) who carries out the decisions about (a) finances; (b) information (books, TV, videotapes, movies, restaurants, entertainment, etc.); (c) chores, errands, responsibilities; and (d) goods and possessions.

1. Who makes the decisions and who carries them out?

2. Who decides what in your relationship?

3. How do you separate authority from responsibility?

4. What are some decisions that you and your partner have made in the last 4 weeks that both of you were happy with?

5. What are some decisions that you and your partner have made in the last 4 weeks that you were unhappy with?

____

____

____

____

6. How does your partner show that your ideas mean something to him/her?

____

____

____

____

7. Do you give in to your partner to prevent an argument? How does that make you feel?

____

____

____

____

8. What do you do to get your way?

____

____

____

____

9. What are some decisions you are responsible for?

____

____

____

____

Homework: During the next week, at a specified time, hold a 30 minute meeting with your partner. Write down your ideas about how an issue could be solved, and compare lists. After talking about all options, pick one that you can agree on.

Practice Exercise 6. Sex and Sexuality

Name________________________________Sex_____Date____________

The purpose of this practice exercise is to increase the chances that sex and sexuality improve in your relationship, if they do need improvement.

1. What initially attracted you to your partner?

____
____
____
____

2. Give a brief description of your dating.

____
____
____
____

3. What is the difference between sex and sexuality?

____
____
____
____

4. What do you think makes a good lover?

____
____
____
____

5. List the strengths in your sexual relationship.

____
____
____
____

6. List the weaknesses in your sexual relationship.

____
____
____
____

7. What pleases your partner sexually?

____
____
____
____

8. What pleases you sexually?

____
____
____
____

9. Are you willing to experiment? If so, what would you like to do sexually that you have not done before?

____
____
____
____

Homework: During the next week, talk with your partner about ways you both could make the sexual side of your relationship more satisfying. Write them down and discuss them with each other.

Relationship Conflict

The purpose of this practice exercise is to decrease conflicts between partners.

Practice Exercise 1. Arguments

Name________________________________Sex______Date_________

The purpose of this practice exercise is to learn more about how you argue. Be sure that the numbers and letters in your answer sheets match those in this practice exercise.

1. Check how often arguments take place in your relationship:
   a. Almost every day ______
   b. About every other day ______
   c. Once or twice a week ______
   d. A couples of times a month ______
   e. Once every 2–3 months ______

2. How intense (strong) are these arguments?
   a. Very, very strong ______
   b. Strong enough to upset us ______
   c. Somewhat strong ______
   d. Not very strong ______

3. How long do these arguments last?
   a. Minutes______(explain)
   b. Hours______(explain)
   c. Days_____(explain)
   d. Weeks_______(explain)

4. How are these arguments started? Write down how your arguments begin and develop.
5. How do your arguments get out of hand? That is, how do they become stronger or more intense?
6. What are the results of these arguments? That is, how do they end?
7. What have you done up to the present to decrease these arguments?
8. Was whatever you have done to decrease these arguments successful? If yes, why? If no, why not?
9. How do you feel after each argument? Write down in detail your feelings after each argument.

Homework: During the next week, try to start as many arguments as possible. If you want to learn to control your arguments, to end or to improve them, you should be able to start them. If you know how to start them and you practice enough times, eventually you may be able to learn to stop them.

As soon as you see that an argument is coming or inevitable, make sure you start a tape-recorder to record as much of the argument as possible. In the absence of a tape-recorder, make sure to write down (1) how the argument started; (2) how heated (strong) it was; (3) what it was about; (4) how it ends; and (5) what the results were. Write down also the feelings that you experienced before, during, and after each argument. Bring your tape or written notes to your counselor or therapist.

Note to professionals: The couple should be congratulated or thanked for finishing this homework practice exercise. Tape or notes should be returned to the couple with the prescription to listen to the tape or to find out from the notes the destructive patterns of responding that are peculiar to each individual, such as (1) using the pronoun "You" coupled with "never" or "always," rather than the pronouns "I" or "We"; (2) reading the partner's mind ("I know what you are thinking, feeling, etc."); (3) bringing up painful events from the past, as if the past could be changed; (4) ultimatums ("If you do not stop ____ by the end of the week, I will leave you") coupled with blackmail or bribery; (5) making excuses to justify one's behavior but not allowing similar excuses for the partner; (6) other patterns, such as, for instance, (a) distracting by changing topic or focusing on an issue that is irrelevant to the argument at hand, (b) walking out on the confrontation, (c) getting out of hand and using coercion and manipulation to win the argument, and (d) any other pattern not listed above.

The couple should be encouraged to continue arguing to find out more about themselves in ways that would not come out if they were not arguing. Other positive refraining of the arguing pertains to the professional helper's personal style and experience. After the couple brings back whatever individual patterns are peculiar to each, the helper could prescribe that each partner continue with that pattern. However, the partner should monitor, that is, write down, every time the pattern is used.

Practice Exercise 2. Avoidance

Name________________________________Sex_____Date__________

The purpose of this practice exercise is to learn how stop avoiding each other.

Answer the following questions in writing:

1. How does avoidance take place in your relationship?

____
____
____
____

2. Who avoids whom?

____
____
____
____

3. Who avoids what? What are specific areas of avoidance in your relationship?

____
____
____
____

4. Why is avoidance used?

____
____
____
____

5. What does avoidance contribute to the relationship?

____
____
____
____

6. Does it mean that avoidance is one way to avoid painful confrontations?

____

____

____

____

7. Does it mean that avoidance is one way of sweeping the problem under the rug so that nothing is ever solved or resolved between you two?

____

____

____

____

____

Homework: During the next week, spend some time thinking about and writing down all of the advantages and disadvantages that are related to avoidance of issues and problems in the relationship. What would happen to the relationship if all issues in it were avoided? Make an appointment with your partner (at least 24 h in advance) to compare, contrast, and discuss your answers to the questions asked in this practice exercise.

Practice Exercise 3. Communication Difficulties

Name________________________________ Sex______Date_________

The purpose of this practice exercise is to understand how you fail to communicate in your relationship.

1. Check which difficulties in communication exist in your relationship. Check all that apply to the relationship in your opinion:

Difficulty	*Rank-order*
a. Blaming rather than supporting	_________
b. Discounting the partner's feelings and thinking rather than affirming them	_________
c. Avoidance rather than approach of issues	_________
d. Anger, contempt, and resentment rather than understanding, support, and help	_________
e. Immediacy, responding to the partner immediately without thinking rather than thinking before responding	_________
f. Withdrawing and leaving any confrontation rather than staying with it until a mutually agreeable solution is found	_________
g. Losing one's temper and jumping to conclusions rather than keeping control of oneself and allowing the partner to express himself or herself	_________

Difficulty	*Rank-order*
h. Not listening rather than listening	________
i. Inability to communicate either feelings or thoughts rather than being able to communicate both feelings and thoughts	________
j. Unwillingness to communicate at all rather that wanting to communicate no matter how painful the topic may be	________
k. Any other difficulty not listed above	________

1. Now that you have checked which communication difficulties are present in your relationships, rank-order them according to their level of difficulty. Rank as No. 1 the one that entails the greatest difficulty, rank as No. 2 the second most difficult area, and so on, until you have rank-ordered all of the difficulties listed above; mark as N/A the difficulties that do not apply. Bring these rank-orderings to your professional or discuss them with your partner by appointment made at least 24 h in advance, never on the spur of the moment.

   Note to professionals: If relevant, pick the difficulty ranked as No. 1 and ask the couple to elaborate on it on the basis of their developmental background, that is, similar patterns of communicating from their parents, the payoff of each difficulty, etc. If necessary, assign each difficulty as homework in order for the couple to be able to achieve better control of it. The principle behind this suggestion is the same as other principles of control: (1) If you want to stop it, learn to start it! (2) Approach what you have avoided. (3) Write down in detail what happened, as often as necessary.

Practice Exercise 4. Disconfirmation

Name________________________________Sex_____ Date_________

The purpose of this practice exercise is to understand how disconfirmation takes place in your relationship.

1. What does disconfirmation mean to you? (Hint: Look it up in a dictionary.)

____

____

____

____

2. What would you like to happen in this relationship? What is the opposite of disconfirmation?

____

____

____

____

3. How does disconfirmation take place in your relationship? Check all that apply:

Disconfirmation	*Rank-order*
a. Sarcasm	________
b. Put downs	________
c. Not listening	________
d. Verbal abuse, like name-calling	________
e. Withdrawing and avoiding	________
f. Criticisms	________
g. Ignoring	________
h. Physical abuse, like hitting or shoving	________
i. Nagging	________
j. Any other disconfirmation not listed above. What is it? (________________________)	________

4. Rank-order the disconfirmations listed above according to how extreme and painful they are to you. Rank as No. 1 the most painful, rank as No. 2 the next most painful, and so on; mark as N/A the disconfirmations that do not apply to the relationship.
5. By appointment 24 h in advance, compare, contrast, and discuss your answers with your partner and see whether you can find any agreement in how each of you disconfirms and discounts the other. Discuss how disconfirmation and discounting are destructive to your relationship. Write down your conclusions and bring them to your helper.

   Note to professionals: In addition to discussing the pattern with this couple, one could go into the historical-developmental events that were related to this pattern, including how the family of origin used the same pattern and how each partner feels discounted by the other in a way that replicates patterns in the family of origin.

Practice Exercise 5. Painful Deterioration in the Relationship

Name______________________________Sex______Date_________

The purpose of this practice exercise is to learn more about how your relationship is deteriorating.

1. How is this relationship deteriorating? Explain in detail.
2. How do you feel about this deterioration?

____

____

____

3. What contributed to this deterioration?

____

____

____

4. Sometimes deterioration in a relationship develops because the partners care so much for each other that each has given up the self for the other one. Consequently, once the self has been given up, each partner starts to think negatively about the partner's behavior, allowing the partner's behavior to occupy all of his or her time and energy. This deterioration can be observed very readily by counting how often each of you is using the "You" pronoun instead of the "I" and "We" pronouns. To check on this possibility, write down all the statements that you have made to you partner containing the "You" pronoun. If you like, in addition, you may record how often your partner is using the "You" pronoun in talking with you. If both of you can complete this exercise, you may want to make an appointment (at least 24 h in advance) to see and compare what kind of results each of you has obtained.
5. Another possibility, which is not exclusive of the previous one, consists of trying to discuss your individual hurts about this deterioration. Sometimes one partner hurts much more than the other, and the one who does not hurt is unable or unwilling to listen to the partner's hurt feelings. If when the one who hurts discusses this feeling with the partner and the partner indicates that he or she is not interested in hearing about these feelings, perhaps the relationship is irretrievably broken, since there does not seem to be any potential for intimacy. If we cannot discuss our hurts with our partner, why stay married?
6. Another variation on the same theme consists of both of you spending 15–20 minute a day for 4 or 5 days writing down all the hurts that you have accumulated in your lifetime. After finishing these lists, you should make an appointment (at least 24 h in advance) with each other and discuss your lists, allowing for whatever reactions these lists elicit from each other. After discussing these reactions, you need to decide whether you want to continue discussing each other's hurts or whether you want to separate. One of you may deny or minimize any hurts. He or she may prefer to keep distant and not discuss any hurts with anybody, remaining a loner away from intimate relationships. If this is what one of you wants, perhaps marriage is not for that person.
7. There are other possibilities available if you want them. Bring your lists and notes to your professional helper and discuss them with him or her.

Practice Exercise 6. Emotional Coercion/Intimidation

Name________________________________Sex______Date__________

The purpose of this practice exercise is to learn how coercion and intimidation affect this relationship.

1. What does coercion/intimidation mean to you? Define both words to the best of your ability. If necessary, consult a dictionary or ask a friend for help in defining both terms.

____
____
____

2. How is coercion/intimidation taking place in your relationship?

____
____
____

3. How did this pattern come about?

____
____
____

4. What are the results of this pattern on each of you and on your relationship?

____
____
____

5. Whoever uses coercion/intimidation wants to control or manipulate the one who does not use this pattern. What do you think about this possibility? How does it apply to your relationship?

____
____
____

Homework: During the next week, record how many times this pattern takes place. Write down in detail (1) what brought it about, (2) how it progressed, and (3) what the outcome was in each instance. Bring your notes to your professional helper.

Practice Exercise 7. Verbal Attack

Name__________________________Sex____ Date_________

The purpose of this practice exercise is to understand how verbal abuse and attack takes place in your relationship.

1. How is verbal attack taking place in your relationship?

____
____
____
____

2. What does verbal attack consist of? Write in detail whatever makes up this pattern.

____
____
____
____

3. How often does verbal attack take place?

   a. More than once a day ________
   b. At least once a day ________
   c. Once or twice a week ________
   d. Once or twice a month ________
   e. Once in a while ________

4. What is the purpose of verbal attack? Check as many as apply:

   a. To control the partner ________
   b. To put down the partner and put oneself up ________
   c. To discount the partner to elevate oneself ________
   d. This is the only way of relating known to the abuser ________
   e. To make the abused partner feel inadequate and unimportant ________
   f. "It was good for my father, it was good for my mother and is good enough for me" ________
   g. This is the only way for the abuser to relieve frustrations ________
   h. This is the only way for the abuser to feel important ________
   i. The responsibility for the abuse resides inside the abused partner ("It's all your fault!") and not in the abuser ________
   j. Any other excuse used to justify the abuse (write what it is) ________

5. The one who is the victim of abuse and attack has to deal with the abuser, who will deny the importance and intensity of the attack. What excuses are used to justify the attack? Write as many as can be remembered.

____
____
____
____

Homework: During the coming week, write down and list any verbal attack received: (1) what seems to bring it about, (2) what it consists of, and (3) what was the outcome. Bring these notes to your professional helper.

Practice Exercise 8. Physical Abuse

Name______________________________ **Sex**_____**Date**_________

Note to professionals: Usually verbal abuse takes place together with physical abuse. Nonetheless, conceivably, there may be physical abuse without verbal abuse, but very rarely. Hence, the previous practice exercise should be given before handing this one to the couple.

The purpose of this practice exercise is to understand how physical abuse is taking place in your relationship.

1. What does physical abuse consist of? Write down in detail what makes up this abuse.

____
____
____
____
____

2. How often does it take place?

   a. More than once a day ____
   b. Once every couple of days ____
   c. A couple of times a week ____
   d. At least once a week ____
   e. A couple of times a month ____
   f. Once in 2–3 months _____
   g. Once or twice a year _____

3. What is the result of the abuse?

____
____
____
____
____

4. What happens after the abuse?

a. What does the abused one do?

b. What does the abuser do?

5. Were the police ever called?

6. If the police were called, what happened?

7. If the police were not called, what happened?

8. Why were the police not called?

____
____
____
____
____

9. Did the abused partner ever leave the house?

____
____
____
____
____

Note: In cases of physical abuse, it is important for each partner to receive help separately, by joining groups specifically set up for these purposes. If such groups are not available, the major decision is whether the abuser is willing to take responsibility and own up to his or her abuse. If the abuser refuses to ask for help (for whatever reasons), the abused one should do whatever is necessary to protect himself or herself as well as the children (if there are any). Protection may mean leaving the house, calling the police, going to a shelter for battered partners, asking the local department of children and families for help, or calling the health department, one's clergy, or a lawyer.

Practice Exercise 9. Threats

Name________________________________Sex____ Date_________

The purpose of this practice exercise is to learn more about what kind of threats take place in your relationship.

1. What do threats consist of in this relationship? Write down all the threats made as far back as you can remember.

____
____
____
____
____

2. How often are these threats made?

a. Every day	_______	e. Once every other week	_______
b. very other day	_______	f. Once a month	_______
c. A couple of times a week	_______	g. Once every few months	_______
d. Once a week	_______		

3. What brings these threats up?

____

____

____

____

____

4. Are these threats ever carried out? If yes, how? If no, why not?

____

____

____

____

____

5. Were threats a common way of relating in your family background? Who used them the most in your family?

____

____

____

____

____

6. Do threats produce the desired result? If yes, how?

____

____

____

____

____

7. Why are threats used? What are the reasons for using them?

____

____

____

____

____

Homework: During the next week, record all the threats made in your relationship. Make sure to write down (1) what brought them about, (2) how they were voiced, and (3) their outcome or result. Bring these notes to your professional helper.

Practice Exercise 10. Threatened Use of Weapons

Name________________________________ Sex____Date_________

Note: If weapons are used in the house and threats have been made about their use, and if an improvement in the relationship is desired, the one who uses them should bring them to a police station for safekeeping. Unless this procedure is followed, there is little hope that professional help will be available except for the one who has been threatened. Threat of actual or potential use should be taken very seriously. The one who has been threatened must do whatever it takes to protect himself or herself and the children.

Whatever is written about threatened use of weapons applies to their use. Unless they are deposited at the police department for safekeeping, the partner who does not use weapons should take whatever steps are necessary to safeguard his or her safety as well as the safety of the children.

Practice Exercise 11. Communication

Name________________________________Sex_____ Date_________

The same practice exercise as for difficulties in communication could be used here.

Practice Exercise 12. Undesirable Habits

Name________________________________Sex_____ Date_________

The purpose of this practice exercise is to learn more about how undesirable habits affect your relationship.

1. What habits do you not like in yourself?

____

____

____

____

____

2. What habits do you not like in your partner?

____

____

____

____

____

3. Why are these habits undesirable?

____

____

____

____

____

4. Are you willing to change your undesirable habit(s) if your partner is willing to give up his or her undesirable ones? Why?

____

____

____

____

____

Homework: Make an appointment with your partner at least 24 h in advance and discuss your lists of undesirable habits. Rank-order these habits from the most undesirable to the more acceptable. Rank as No. 1 the most undesirable habit, and write down what could be done to either stop it or to change it in a way that makes it more acceptable to the partner. If you have time, do the same with undesirable habit No. 2. Otherwise, make another appointment to see whether what you have decided about undesirable habit No. 1 is working or not. If it is, go on to a plan for No. 2. If it is not working, ask for help from your professional helper.

Practice Exercise 13. Choices (Preferences)

Name______________________________ Sex____Date_________

The purpose of this practice exercise is to understand your personal choices and how they affect your relationship.

1. Choice means whatever you like and want in contrast to what you do not like or want. List what your likes and dislikes are on two separate pages.
2. Once you have made this list, rank-order your likes and dislikes according to what you like and want first, second, etc. Do the same with your dislikes, rank-ordering first the dislikes you do not want at all down to the dislikes that may be acceptable under certain conditions.
3. Once you have completed these lists of likes and dislikes, think whether each like has been fulfilled or not.

    a. If it has not been fulfilled, what will it take for you to fulfill it?

    ____
    ____
    ____

    b. What will you need to do to get what you want and like?

    ____
    ____
    ____

    c. What plan can you prepare to see that you get what you want?

    ____
    ____
    ____

4. Choices are made in terms of what is most important to you. Rank-order the following choices according to their importance to you. Rank as No. 1 the choice that is most important to you, rank as No. 2 the next most important choice, and so on, down to the least important choice:

Choices	*Rank-order*
a. Self	________
b. Partner	________
c. Child(ren)	________
d. Parents	________
e. Siblings	________
f. Relatives (uncle, aunts)	________

Choices	*Rank-order*
g. In-laws	_________
h. Friends	_________
i. Boss	_________
j. Coworkers	_________
k. Neighbors	_________
l. Others (_____________)	_________

5. Why did you rank-order the way you did? Explain in detail why you chose the way you did.

____
____
____
____
____

6. There are other rank-orderings that are relevant to our choices, and that is, whether we prefer work to leisure time activities or home over work, etc. Rank-order which of these choices is most preferable to you. Rank as No. 1 your first choice, rank as No. 2 your second choice, and so on; mark as N/A the choices that do not apply to you.

Choice	*Rank-order*
a. Family over work	_________
b. Family over leisure time	_________
c. Work over leisure time	_________
d. Leisure time over family	_________
e. Leisure time over work	_________
f. Family over work	_________
g. Children over partner	_________
h. Leisure over work	_________
i. Parent(s) over partner	_________
j. Friends over family	_________
k. Money over family	_________
l. Things over family	_________
m. TV over family	_________
n. Drinking over family	_________
o. Work over family	_________
p. Other (_______________)	_________

7. Why did you rank-order these choices the way you did?

____
____
____
____
____

Homework:

1. Make an appointment with your partner at least 24 h in advance.
2. Contrast and compare your answers with those of your partner.
3. Discuss any similarities and differences in your choices.
4. Discuss what the outcome is bound to be for each choice you have made.
5. Bring your answers and notes to your professional helper and discuss with him or her what helpful or hurtful choices may be for you and for your relationship.

Practice Exercise 14. The Nature of Relationships

Name________________________________ Sex____Date_________

The purpose of this practice exercise is to understand more about your relationships.

1. Circle from 10 to 1 the relationships listed below, where 10 represents most satisfactory relationships and 1 represents the least satisfactory relationships. Omit any relationship that does not apply to you.

	Satisfactory <------------------- *Unsatisfactory*									
a. Your partner	10	9	8	7	6	5	4	3	2	1
b. Your child	10	9	8	7	6	5	4	3	2	1
c. Your parents	10	9	8	7	6	5	4	3	2	1
d. Your siblings	10	9	8	7	6	5	4	3	2	1
e. Your in-laws	10	9	8	7	6	5	4	3	2	1
f. Your friends	10	9	8	7	6	5	4	3	2	1
g. Your neighbors	10	9	8	7	6	5	4	3	2	1
h. Your boss	10	9	8	7	6	5	4	3	2	1
i. Your coworkers	10	9	8	7	6	5	4	3	2	1
j. Anyone else (____________)	10	9	8	7	6	5	4	3	2	1

2. Write down the nature of your relationship with those you have rated as unsatisfactory. What can you do to make these relationships more satisfactory?

____
____
____
____
____

Homework: Check with your partner or helper to develop a plan to make your unsatisfactory relationships more satisfactory for you. (1) Write this plan down. (2) What are its advantages and disadvantages? (3) See if you can apply your plan or parts of your plan. Ask for help if necessary.

Practice Exercise 15. Responsibilities

Name________________________________ Sex____Date__________

The purpose of this practice exercise is to learn more about responsibilities in your relationship.

1. What responsibilities do you have? List them below
   a. House
      i ______________________________
      ii ______________________________
      iii ______________________________
      iv ______________________________
      v ______________________________
   b. Work
      i ______________________________
      ii ______________________________
      iii ______________________________
      iv ______________________________
      v ______________________________
   c. Leisure time
      i ______________________________
      ii ______________________________
      iii ______________________________
      iv ______________________________
      v ______________________________

2. Which responsibilities do you enjoy and why?

3. Which responsibilities you do not enjoy and why?

4. Who makes decisions in your home and who carries out these decisions? Who has the authority to make decisions, and who has the responsibility to carry out those decisions?

5. Who decides what is done in your home? ______________________

   a. Why is it done this way?

   b. Is this arrangement satisfactory for you? If yes, why? If no, why not?

6. Who decides what is done at work?

____

____

____

____

7. Who decides what is done in your leisure time?

____

____

____

____

8. Is the authority to make decisions matched by who is responsible to carry them out? Is there a difference between who makes decisions and who carries them out?

____

____

____

____

9. What is the outcome of an imbalance between authority and responsibility?

____

____

____

____

10. If there is an imbalance between authority and responsibility, what is its outcome on the relationship?

____

____

____

____

Homework: During next week write down (1) who makes decisions, (2) what the decisions are about, (3) who carries these decisions out, and (4) what is the outcome of this arrangement on the relationship.

Practice Exercise 16. Values

Name______________________________ Sex____ Date________

The purpose of this practice exercise is to learn more about your values and how they affect your relationship.

1. Values relate to what is important to you. During the next week, take 15–20 minute a day for as many days as it is necessary to write down what is important to you. After you have finished this list, prioritize it. Rank as No. 1 whoever or whatever is most important to you; rank as No. 2 whoever or whatever is second in importance, and so on, until you have rank-ordered each item in your list.
2. Discuss your list with your partner and respond to his or her list of values if he or she has one.

    a. Why is someone or something so important to you?

    ____
    ____
    ____

    b. Why is someone or something so important to your partner?

    ____
    ____
    ____

3. What are the outcomes that develop from each value?

    ____
    ____
    ____
    ____
    ____

    a. Lists the advantages and disadvantages that are related or relevant to each value.

    ____
    ____
    ____

    b. List the advantages and disadvantages of each value for your relationship with each other:

    ____
    ____
    ____

4. Values vary from nonnegotiable to negotiable.

   a. Which value is nonnegotiable for you and why?

   ____
   ____
   ____

   b. Which is negotiable under certain conditions (which conditions and why?)

   ____
   ____
   ____

   c. Which value is completely negotiable and why?

   ____
   ____
   ____

   d. Which values do not need negotiation?

   ____
   ____
   ____

5. Which values need changing and why?

____
____
____
____
____

6. What will happen if you do not change some of your values?

____
____
____
____
____

7. What will happen if you do change some values?

____
____
____
____
____

Homework: It is important that you think seriously about some of the issues brought up by this practice exercise. During the next week, think about how you have answered some questions and how you would like to change your answers. After you are sure that you can live with your answers, make an appointment (at least 24 h ahead of time) with your partner and discuss your reactions to each other's answers. Keep notes about your discussion and bring them to your professional helper.

Couple Satisfaction

The purpose of this practice exercise is to improve your satisfaction, either in the marriage or in a committed couple relationship.

Practice Exercise 1. Defining Marital Satisfaction

Name_______________________Sex_____ Date________

The purpose of this practice exercise is to help you define the nature of couple satisfaction by making sure that you understand and discuss with each other the meaning of each dimension that makes up such satisfaction.

1. Below are listed the various dimensions that cover a range of couple satisfaction-dissatisfaction. Define each dimension, using a dictionary if necessary, and give two examples of how that dimension is shown concretely in your relationship.

Dimensions	*Meanings and Examples*
a. Affective or emotional communication ________________	Example 1 ________________
______________________	______________________
______________________	Example 2 ________________
______________________	______________________
b. Aggression ________________	Example 1 ________________
______________________	______________________
______________________	Example 2 ________________
______________________	______________________

c. Conflict over child rearing _______ Example 1 ______________________
______________________________________ ______________________________
______________________________________ Example 2 ______________________
______________________________________ ______________________________

d. Conventionalization ____________ Example 1 ______________________
______________________________________ ______________________________
______________________________________ Example 2 ______________________
______________________________________ ______________________________

e. Disagreements about finances (money) __________________ Example 1 ______________________
______________________________________ ______________________________
______________________________________ Example 2 ______________________
______________________________________ ______________________________

f. Dissatisfaction with children _____ Example 1 ______________________
______________________________________ ______________________________
______________________________________ Example 2 ______________________
______________________________________ ______________________________

g. Family history of distress _______ Example 1 ______________________
______________________________________ ______________________________
______________________________________ Example 2 ______________________
______________________________________ ______________________________

h. Global distress _________________ Example 1 ______________________
______________________________________ ______________________________
______________________________________ Example 2 ______________________
______________________________________ ______________________________

i. Inconsistency _________________ Example 1 ______________________
______________________________________ ______________________________
______________________________________ Example 2 ______________________
______________________________________ ______________________________

j. Problem-solving communication Example 1 ______________________
______________________________________ ______________________________
______________________________________ Example 2 ______________________
______________________________________ ______________________________

k. Role orientation _______________ Example 1 ______________________
______________________________________ ______________________________
______________________________________ Example 2 ______________________
______________________________________ ______________________________

l. Time together ________________ Example 1 ____________________

________________________________ ________________________________

________________________________ Example 2 ____________________

________________________________ ________________________________

m. Sexual dissatisfaction __________ Example 1 ____________________

________________________________ ________________________________

________________________________ Example 2 ____________________

________________________________ ________________________________

2. Rank-order dimensions according to how troublesome they are to you in this relationship. Rank as No 1 the dimension that is the most troublesome to you; rank as No. 2 the dimension that is next troublesome to you, and so on; mark as N/A the dimensions that may not be troublesome to you at all or that do not apply to this relationship.

Dimensions	*Rank-orders* Mine	Partner	Joint
a. Affective or emotional communication	_____	_____	_____
b. Aggression	_____	_____	_____
c. Conflict over child rearing	_____	_____	_____
d. Conventionalization	_____	_____	_____
e. Disagreements over finances (money)	_____	_____	_____
f. Dissatisfaction with children	_____	_____	_____
g. Family history of distress	_____	_____	_____
h. Global distress	_____	_____	_____
i. Inconsistency	_____	_____	_____
j. Problem-solving communication	_____	_____	_____
k. Role orientation	_____	_____	_____
l. Time together	_____	_____	_____
m. Sexual dissatisfaction	_____	_____	_____

3. Why did you rank-order these dimensions the way you did?

____

____

____

____

____

Homework: During the coming week, make an appointment with your partner and go over your definitions and your rank-orders. Record your partner's rank-orders in the appropriate column above, and add both to achieve a joint rank-order. Take notes while you are discussing (comparing and contrasting) your answers. Give your completed practice exercises and your notes to the professional who is assisting you with this practice exercise. You will need to reconcile your rank-orders with the rank-orders received from answering the test given at the outset of this program. Whatever order you agree with will determine the order of future practice exercises.

Practice Exercise 1. Aggregression

Name_____________________________Sex__________ Date__________

The purpose of this practice exercise is to understand how aggression is affecting your relationship negatively.

1. How does aggression take place in your relationship? Explain in detail.

____
____
____
____
____

2. How did you learn to be aggressive or nonaggressive?

____
____
____
____
____

3. What do you get out of being or not being aggressive?

____
____
____
____
____

4. What does aggression or nonaggression mean to your partner?

____
____
____
____
____

7. How does aggression or nonaggression affect your relationship with:

   a. Children ______________________
   b. Parents ______________________
   c. Siblings ______________________
   d. In-laws ______________________
   e. Friends ______________________
   f. Neighbors ______________________
   g. Boss ______________________
   h. Coworkers ______________________
   i. Anyone else you know who may have been affected by this patern

   ____

8. If aggression or nonaggression (indicate which) is a problem for you, do you want to continue with it or do you want to give it up? If you want to keep it, you do not need to complete this practice exercise. However, if you are troublesome thoughted about it and want to change, follow the homework assigned below.

Homework: During the next week, record in writing or with a tape recorder all the instances in which you either behaved aggressively or were unable to deal with the aggression of your partner. Make sure to record what was said or done in detail, and bring your notes or tapes to your next counseling or therapy session.

Practice Exercise 19. Global Distress

Name______________________Sex________ Date__________

The purpose of this practice exercise is to understand how much distress is present in your relationship.

1. Describe the overall nature of your distress.

   a. What does it consist of?

____
____
____
____
____

b. Break it down into its parts and in detail.

____

____

____

____

____

c. How does this distress affect:

   i. Yourself ______________________
   ii. Partner ______________________
   iii. Children ______________________
   iv. Parents ______________________
   v. In-laws ______________________
   vi. Siblings ______________________
   vii. Friends ______________________
   viii. Coworkers ______________________
   ix. Anybody else (name them) ______________________

2. Is this distress something that you have always experienced in the past or is it more related to present circumstances in your relationship?

   a. If your distress was also present in the past, describe the circumstances that were responsible for your becoming distressed.

____

____

____

____

____

   b. Describe the present circumstances that are responsible for your distress.

____

____

____

____

____

3. What have you done thus far to deal with this distress?

____

____

____

____

____

4. Has anything you have tried in the past to deal with your distress worked?

____
____
____
____
____

5. If you are working on this pattern presently, it looks like previous efforts to deal with distress have not worked. Is that correct?

____
____
____
____
____

6. If so, what have you done to discuss this distress with your partner?

____
____
____
____
____

7. If you have tried to discuss your distress with your partner, what has happened?

____
____
____
____
____

8. Many couples do not know how to discuss their distresses with their partners. As a result they keep a lot of feelings bottled up inside.

   a. Is this the case with you? Yes______ No______
   b. Is this the case with your partner? Yes______ No_____
   c. If "a" is yes, with whom do you discuss your distress?

____
____
____

d. If "b" is yes, with whom does your partner discuss his or her distress?

____
____
____

9. How do you feel when someone who cares for you listens to your distress?

____
____
____
____
____

10. How do you feel when someone who claims to care for you does not listen to your distress?

____
____
____
____
____

11. Do you listen to the distress of your partner?

a. If yes, what happens?

____
____
____

b. If no, what happens?

____
____
____

Homework: During the next week, take 15–20 minute a day for 4 days to write down all of the distresses that you have experienced in the present and in the past. Bring your notes to your next counseling or therapy session.

Practice Exercise 20. Affective Communication

Name______________________________ Sex_______Date_________

The purpose of this practice exercise is to understand how you and your partner communicate emotionally.

1. By affective communication is meant all the verbal and nonverbal signals that partners give each other to express their care for each other. This pattern is also called affection (nonverbal) and understanding (verbal). How does this pattern apply to you and to your relationship?

2. How do you communicate affection and understanding to your partner?

   a. Write how affection is communicated nonverbally.

   b. Write how understanding is communicated verbally.

3. How does your partner communicate affection and understanding to you?

4. How do you fail to communicate affection and understanding to your partner?

5. How does your partner fail to communicate affection and understanding to you?

____
____
____
____
____

6. Do you want more affection and better communication with your partner? If yes, why? If no, why not?

____
____
____
____
____

7. Affective communication or miscommunication may develop from patterns of disaffection listed below. Rank-order these patterns in order of troublesome thought to you. Rank as No. 1 the pattern you are most troublesome thoughted about, rank as No. 2 the next pattern of troublesome thought, and so on, down to the last pattern of least troublesome thought to you.

Patterns of Disaffection	*Rank-orders*		
	Mine	Partner	Joint
a. Minimal affection for one's partner	______	______	______
b. Minimal understanding for one's partner	______	______	______
c. Absence of common interests	______	______	______
d. Absence of shared leisure activities	______	______	______
e. General dissatisfaction with the relationship	______	______	______
f. Inclination toward separation or divorce	______	______	______
g. Other (name)________________	______	______	______

8. After you have finished your rank-orders and completed this practice exercise, check with your partner and record his or her rank-orders of the same patterns of dissatisfaction. Add both rank-orders together and write about each pattern according to the joint rank-order listed above. Describe in full and in detail.

   a. Minimal affection for one's partner. Joint rank-order ______
      i. How did this pattern arise?

____
____
____

ii. How did this pattern develop?

___

___

___

iii. What effect has this pattern had on your overall relationship?

___

___

___

b. Minimal understanding of one's partner. Joint rank-order ___

i. How did this pattern arise?

___

___

___

ii. How did this pattern develop?

___

___

___

iii. What effect has this pattern had on your overall relationship?

___

___

___

c. Absence of common interests. Joint rank-order ___

i. How did this pattern arise?

___

___

___

ii. How did this pattern develop?

___

___

___

iii. What effect has this pattern had on your overall relationship?

____
____
____

d. Absence of shared leisure activities. Joint rank-order______
   i. How did this pattern arise?

____
____
____

   ii. How did this pattern develop?

____
____
____

   iii. What effect has this pattern had on your overall relationship?

____
____
____

e. General dissatisfaction with the relationship. Joint rank-order ______
   i. How did this pattern arise?

____
____
____

   ii. How did this pattern develop?

____
____
____

   iii. What effect has this pattern had on your overall relationship?

____
____
____

f. Inclination toward separation and divorce. Joint rank-order ______
   i. How did this pattern arise?

____
____
____

   ii. How did this pattern develop?

____
____
____

   iii. What effect has this pattern had on your overall relationship?

____
____
____

g. Other (name)____
   Joint rank-order______
   i. How did this pattern arise?

____
____
____

   ii. How did this pattern develop?

____
____
____

   iii. What effect has this pattern had on your overall relationship?

____
____
____

9. What are the major issues on which you disagree?

____
____
____
____
____

10. Did you and your partner ever sit down (by appointment only) and discuss these issues, rather than discussing them when you are mad, sad, or frustrated? If yes, what happened? If no, why not?

____
____
____
____
____

Homework: What can you do to improve this kind of communication in your relationship? Write down a plan that you would like to follow to improve affection and understanding in your relationship, if that is what you want. No plan can work unless your partner is willing and able to develop a plan of his or her own. If such a plan has been written individually by both of you, make an appointment with each other and compare and contrast your respective plans. See if you can put together both plans into a single one. Keep notes of whatever happened at this meeting and bring them to your next counseling or therapy session.

Practice Exercise 21. Problem-Solving Communication

Name______________________ Sex_______ Date_________

The purpose of this practice exercise is to understand how you and your partner solve problems together or separately.

1. Problem-solving communication deals with how a couple is able or unable to solve and resolve differences in feelings, opinions, and behavior. How does this pattern apply to your relationship? Are you and your partner able to solve and resolve differences? If you are able to do so, then this practice exercise is inappropriate for you. However, if you not able to solve and resolve differences, complete this practice exercise.

2. Write how you and your partner are unable to reconcile differences.

____
____
____
____
____

   a. In what areas are these differences more pronounced?

____
____
____

b. Why are you unable to reach an agreement?

3. What is the process whereby the two of you fail to reach an agreement?

4. Usually, couples are not able to reconcile differences because they keep on "reacting" to each other rather than "proacting." Write down what you understand by these words.

   a. Reacting

   b. Proacting

   c. How much are your difficulties in reconciling differences dues to reactivity rather than responsiveness to each other?

5. If reactivity is not present in your communication, sometimes evasiveness, withdrawal, and avoidance may be present. One of you may want to approach an issue, while the other may want to avoid it. How does this pattern apply to your relationship?

6. If your problems in communicating affection and understanding are not covered by the previous points, describe the process of failing to communicate.

   a. What happens when one of you fails to communicate affection and understanding? What does your partner do or say?

____
____
____

   b. How does this failure get out of hand into a full-blown argument or fight?

____
____
____

   c. How does your argument end? What is the result of your failure to be affectionate and understanding?

____
____
____

Homework: How were affection and understanding communicated in your family of origin? Write in full and in detail about how this process took place. If necessary, check with a family member to make sure that you are describing this process correctly. Make an appointment with your partner and exchange your notes about what you learned about affection and understanding from your family of origin. Keep notes about your reactions to this exchange, and bring them to your next counseling or therapy session.

Practice Exercise 1. Time Together

Name________________________________ Sex______Date__________

The purpose of this practice exercise is to check on how much time you and your partner spend together.

1. This pattern entails a lack of common interests and dissatisfaction with the characteristic quality and quantity of either leisure time together or work time. How much does it apply to your relationship?

   a. A great deal ______
   b. Some ___________
   c. Not at all ________

2. What interests do you have or not have in common in your relationship?

   a. Interests in common

____
____
____

   b. Interests that only one partner has

____
____
____

3. How did this pattern develop in your relationship?

____
____
____
____
____

4. What is the outcome of little time spent together?

____
____
____
____
____

5. You would like:

   a. Much more time together ____
   b. More time together _________
   c. Less time together __________
   d. Much less time together _____

6. Why? What are the reasons for your choice?

____
____
____
____
____

7. What have you done to improve the quantity and characteristic quality of time spent together?

____
____
____
____
____

8. Did you succeed? If yes, how? If no, why not?

____
____
____
____
____

Homework: During the next week, add up how much time you actually spend together day by day for the whole week. After a week, make an appointment with your partner at least 24 h in advance and compare each other's time measurements. Write down a summary of your ensuing discussion or conclusions, and bring your notes to the next counseling or therapy session.

Practice Exercise 22. Disagreements Over Finances

Name______________________ Sex________Date_________

The purpose of this practice exercise is to understand how you and your partner agree or disagree about how money is spent in your household.

1. This pattern deals with discord over money and management of financial matters. How much does this pattern apply to you?

   a. A great deal ______
   b. Some ___________
   c. Not at all ________

2. If you have checked "a" or "b," go on with this practice exercise. If you have checked "c," you may need to become aware of why this may be deemed a problem.

____
____
____
____
____

3. Write in detail about how money and management of financial matters is a problem in your relationship.

4. Is it possible that one of you exaggerates the importance of the problem and that the other minimizes it or and even denies it?

5. If you and your partner are at opposite extremes of how to deal with money, in that one of you exaggerates and the other minimizes or denies it, are you also on opposite extremes in other areas of your relationship? List as many areas in which you feel you and your partner are at opposite extremes in your relationship.

6. What do money and possessions mean to you? Explain fully the meaning, both symbolic and real, of both.

   a. Money

   b. Possessions

7. Is it possible that conflict over financial matters may hide feelings that have not been fully expressed in the relationship?

8. If that is the case (and it might not be), what is the nature of these feelings? Could you express them in writing and in detail?

9. Are you ready to discuss these feelings with your partner?

   a. What are you afraid might happen if you did?

   b. What might happen if you did not?

   c. Which of these two alternatives is more constructive for the relationship and why?

Homework: During the next week, give some thought to the possibility that money matters may be used as a way of distracting yourself from getting in touch with and expressing hidden feelings that you might be afraid to express otherwise. In addition, write down any argument you might have had during the week about money and possessions. Why are you letting these matters control the relationship?

Practice Exercise 1. Sexual Dissatisfaction

Name______________________________ Sex______Date_________

The purpose of this practice exercise is to understand why there is sexual satisfaction or dissatisfaction in your relationship.

1. Dissatisfaction relates to the frequency and characteristic quality of intercourse and other sexual activitkies. How much does it apply to you?

   a. A great deal ____
   b. Some _________
   c. Not at all ______

2. What is unsatisfactory about sex and sexuality in your relationship? Write in full and in detail.

____
____
____
____
____

3. What is the meaning of sex and sexuality for you? Write in full and in detail.

____
____
____
____
____

4. Is sex performance-oriented (doing it) or is presence-oriented, that is, being together without demands for perfection, performance, production, or problem solving? Do you use sex as physical release or as a way of coming together emotionally?

____
____
____
____
____

5. Have you and your partner ever discussed all the anxieties, fears, and emotions relating to past sexual activities before you two met? If yes, how? If no, why not?

6. Is there unspoken or unfinished business about sex and sexuality in your relationship that was present before you met? If so, can you write about it, or do you feel too ashamed and guilty to write about it?

7. Have you ever told each other what you especially enjoy about sex and sexuality?

8. Are there certain taboos that each of you are setting to limit sex and sexuality in your relationship?

9. How free are you to talk about this topic with your partner?

Homework: During the next week, make two or three appointments with each other before you go to bed. Plan to pleasure each other without using your genital organs. Flip a coin to decide who should go first in being pleasured. The one who is designated as the "pleasurer" should spread a cream or lotion on the partner's body. Spend time caressing and touching your partner's body (except for the genital areas). Ask for feedback from your partner about what is pleasurable and what is nonpleasurable during this activity. Alternate the role of "pleasuree" and "pleasurer" the next time you get together to repeat this activity. The purpose of this activity is to decrease any performance anxiety and improve the closeness and meaning of sex and sexuality. If one partner becomes sexually aroused by this activity, try to avoid having intercourse then and there. Instead, make an appointment specifically devoted to that purpose. Keep pleasuring separate from sexuality as long as you can to increase the chance of eventually both sides coming together in more ways than one.

Practice Exercise 1. Role Orientation

Name______________________________ Sex_____Date_________

The purpose of this practice exercise is to understand your orientation toward the various roles that are needed to fulfill a relationship.

1. This pattern means the adoption of a traditional versus a nontraditional view of marriage and the parental gender roles. On a scale from 1 to 10, rate your relationship on how traditional or nontraditional it is.

Extremely traditional 1 2 3 4 5 6 7 8 9 10 Extremely nontraditional

2. Explain why you rated your relationship the way you did.

____
____
____
____
____

3. Do you like your relationship the way you rated it? If yes, why? If not, how would you like it to be? Rate how you would like it to be ideally.

Extremely traditional 1 2 3 4 5 6 7 8 9 10 Extremely nontraditional

4. What do you need to do to make your relationship closer to what you would like it to be? Write down a plan or ideas on how you could make your relationship more satisfactory to you.

____
____
____
____
____

5. How cooperative do you think your partner will be in implementing a plan to improve your relationship? Rate this degree of expectation below:

Very cooperative 1 2 3 4 5 6 7 8 9 10 Very uncooperative

Homework: During the next week, spend time and energy writing down the steps of a plan to improve your role orientation by defining what it means for you to be an effective partner.

Practice Exercise 2. Defining Role Orientation

Name______________________________ Sex________Date__________

1. Define each role listed below, and give two examples of that role. If necessary, use a dictionary to help you understand fully the meaning of each role.

Role	*Definition*
a. Person	______________________________
b. Partner	______________________________
c. Parent	______________________________
d. Provider	______________________________
e. Caregiver	______________________________
f. Homemaker	______________________________

Role	*Definition*
g. Worker	______________________________
	______________________________
	______________________________
h. Hobbyist	______________________________
	______________________________
	______________________________
i. Other	______________________________
(__________)	______________________________
	______________________________

2. Now rank-order these roles according to their importance to you. Rank as No. 1 the role that is the most important to you, rank as No. 2 the role that is second in importance to you, and so on, down to the least important role.

Role	*Rank-order*	*Role*	*Rank-order*
a. Person	_________	f. Homemaker	_________
b. Partner	_________	g. Worker	_________
c. Parent	_________	h. Hobbyist	_________
d. Provider	_________	i. Other __________	_________
e. Caregiver	_________		

3. From these rank-orders, develop a plan of how to reconcile these roles with your partner and with other responsibilities. After you have completed the rank-orderings and developed a tentative plan, make an appointment with your partner and discuss each other's notes, rank-orders, and discrepancies between your respective rank-orders. See if you can begin to develop a plan that is agreeable to both of you. Keep notes of your conclusions, and bring them to your next counseling or therapy session.

Practice Exercise 1. Family History of Distress and Trouble

Name______________________________ Sex_______Date_________

The purpose of this practice exercise is to understand the influence that your family of origin has had on your present relationship.

1. Present relationship dissatisfaction may reflect an unhappy childhood and disharmony in your parents' marriages and extended family. How much does this statement it apply to you?

   a. A great deal ____
   b. Some _________
   c. Not at all ______

If your answer is "c," you might not need to go any further with this practice exercise.

2. Spend 15–20 minute a day for 4 days writing down how painful these experiences were for you, listing all hurtful experiences and how they affected you in the long run.

Day 1

____
____
____
____
____

Day 2

____
____
____
____
____

Day 3

____
____
____
____
____

Day 4

____
____
____
____
____

3. How much are you now repeating in your relationship the same kind of patterns you learned from your family of origin?

a. A great deal ______
b. Some __________
c. Not at all ________

4. If you checked “a” or “b,” how do you feel about this possibility?

____
____
____
____
____

5. If intimacy were defined as discussing past and present hurts as well as discussing fears of being hurt in the future, how much does this definition apply to your relationship?

   a. A lot __________
   b. Somewhat ______
   c. Not at all _______

6. If intimate relationships were to be classified according to the following styles, how does each style apply to your past or present relationship?

   a. Abusive-apathetic (neglectful), verbally and nonverbally. No intimacy is possible here.

____
____
____

   b. Reactive-repetitive, where each partner responds immediately and negatively to the other partner’s words or deeds in a way that escalates to abuse or neglect or anger, frustration, and eventual withdrawal. Intimacy here is occasional and sporadic.

____
____
____

   c. Creative-proactive, where each partner is committed to the enhancement of self and of the other. Intimacy is possible and present here.

____
____
____

7. Which of these styles describes relationships in your family of origin? Elaborate on your choice.

____
____
____
____

8. Which of these styles describes your present relationship? Elaborate.

____
____
____
____

9. How can you break away from the influence of your family of origin without rejecting members of your family? What choices are possible to you?

____
____
____
____

Homework: During the next week, for 15–20 minute a day for 4–5 days write down possible ways of not letting your family of origin control and influence your life and destiny. After you have finished this homework, make an appointment with your partner to discuss, compare, and contrast your answers to the same practice exercise. Keep notes of this meeting, and bring them to your next counseling or therapy session.

Practice Exercise 1. Dissatisfaction with Children

Name______________________________ Sex________Date__________

The purpose of this practice exercise is to understand possible satisfaction and dissatisfaction with your children.

1. This pattern indicates that there are many disappointments in your parent–child relationships. How much does this statement apply to you?

   a. A great deal ____
   b. Some _________
   c. Not at all ______

2. If you answer "c," you do not need to go any further. However, if your answer is either "a" or "b," write about the nature of disappointments and problems in your relationship with your children.

____
____
____
____

3. What kind of role does your behavior play in the development of these disappointments and problems?

____
____
____
____

4. Parent–child problems arise from various possibilities. Check which possibility applies to you:

   a. Parenting is an individual issue, where both parents are not able to work as partners in dealing with the children. Partners did not develop an effective parenting plan and, instead, parented the children as separate individuals, without any plan.

____
____
____

   b. Parents are at opposite extremes in the soft-hard dimension, with one partner playing the "nice" role through "yea-saying" without setting clear limits, while the other partner plays the "nasty" role through "nay-saying" and limit setting.

____
____
____

   c. Parents are too busy arguing and fighting with each other to spend any time to devote themselves to parenting.

____
____
____

d. What other possibilities are specific to you and your partner as parents that are not included in the three possibilities given above? Write about them in detail.

____

____

____

5. Have you ever spent any time thinking about parenting as one of the most, if not the most, responsible task of life? What are your feelings and thoughts on this matter?

____

____

____

____

____

6. You, like most of us, have taken classes in practically any area of knowledge. However, no classes were ever taken in parenting.
   a. Is that conclusion correct?

____

____

____

   b. The only parenting we are aware of and experienced is the parenting we received from our parents. If that parenting was inadequate, how can we assume we know better than our parents? What are your feelings and thoughts on this matter?

____

____

____

Homework: During the next week, make an appointment with your partner and together try to find out what parenting courses or programs are available in your community. Use your counselor or therapist to get help in this area. If no course on parenting is available in your community, find a popular book on the subject and try to learn from it to develop a parenting plan together with your partner. If necessary, see if you can develop a parenting study group to discuss and seek help from other parents on how to parent in better ways than you may have done in the past. A Planned Parenting practice exercise in available in Sect. 4 of this sourcebook.

Practice Exercise 1. Conflicts Over Child Rearing

Name_______________________ Sex__________ Date__________

The purpose of this practice exercise is to understand the nature of conflicts over raising children in your relationship. This practice exercise deals with conflicts that may exist between partners in regard to parenting practices and parental responsibilities.

1. How much does this practice exercise apply to you?

   a. A great deal ________
   b. Some ________
   c. Not at all ________

2. If you checked "a" or "b," go on with this practice exercise. If you checked "c," you will need to discuss this issue further with your partner and your professional helper, especially if your partner disagrees with your views on this matter.

____
____
____
____
____

3. What is the nature of conflicts that exist between you and your partner in regard to children? Write about these conflicts in detail.

____
____
____
____
____

4. Is this a major bone of contention between you two, or are there other areas of conflict underlying this issue?

____
____
____
____
____

5. How much of these conflicts repeat patterns existing in your family of origin? Check which answer applies to you.

   A great deal _____
   Somewhat ______
   Not at all _______

a. How did child rearing take place in your family of origin?

b. How similar are your parenting styles to those in your family of origin?

6. These conflicts may represent the fact that neither one of you has been able to clarify priorities in regard to:

   a. Selfhood: How important do you feel you are?

   b. Partnership: How important does it feels to you?

   c. Parenthood: How important does it feels to you?

7. Answer how you feel about each of the following statements:

   a. Selfhood is the backbone of a partnership.

   b. A partnership is the backbone of parenting.

c. Parenting is to be performed by both partners.

8. How do these statements apply to differences in parenting styles between you and your partner?

9. These conflicts indicate that perhaps your priorities may be unclear or unqualified. For instance, where would you put yourself in regard to the partnership and parenthood? First, second, or third?

10. If you put selfhood second or third to either partnership or parenthood, perhaps many of your child-rearing conflicts may stem from the possibility that you may have given up part of your self to put most of your energy into the parenting before the partnership.

a. If you are not clear about your importance, how will your partner as well as your children learn to see themselves as important?

b. If you put yourself down or allow your partner to put you down, what are your children going to learn from this pattern?

____

____

____

c. How do you guess your partner is reacting to these issues?

____

____

____

Homework: During the next week, write down how many times you have put the partnership and parenthood ahead of yourself. After recording in detail how you let yourself down, make an appointment with your partner to discuss each other's notes. Keep progress notes and conclusions of your appointment, and bring them to your next counseling or therapy session.

Practice Exercise 1. Inconsistency

Name______________________________ Sex______ Date_________

The purpose of this practice exercise is to receive more information about how consistent or inconsistent you are in your relationship.

1. The title of this practice exercise covers a variety of behaviors listed below. Rank-order these factors according to how troublesome thoughted you are about them. Rank as No. 1 the factor that is of greatest troublesome thought to you, rank as No. 2 the next factor of troublesome thought, and so on, with the last factor being of least troublesome thought. After you have finished with your rank-orders, check with your partner and write down his or her rank-orders. Add both rank-orders to derive a joint rank-order.

Behaviors	*Rank-orders*		
	Mine	Partner's	Joint
a. General inability to solve differences	_____	_____	_____
b. Misinterpretations of each other's views	_____	_____	_____
c. Propensity to perceive disagreements as personal criticisms	_____	_____	_____
d. Escalation of minor differences into major conflicts	_____	_____	_____
e. Saying one thing and doing another	_____	_____	_____
f. Being in good humor one day and in bad humor another day without any explanation	_____	_____	_____
g. Being capricious and thoughtless about your partner's needs	_____	_____	_____
h. Black is white and white is black	_____	_____	_____

Behaviors	*Rank-orders*		
	Mine	Partner's	Joint
i. Lying and deception, not knowing which is the truth	_____	_____	_____
j. Being affectionate one day and hostile the next day without apparent reason	_____	_____	_____
k. Name a pattern of inconsistency not listed above ________________________________	_____	_____	_____

2. Give specific examples of your inconsistency related to any or all of the factors listed above.

a. ____

____

____

b. ____

____

____

c. ____

____

____

d. ____

____

____

e. ____

____

____

f. ____

____

____

g. ____

____

____

h. ____

____

____

i. ____

____

____

j. ____

____

____

k. ____

____

____

3. Give specific examples of inconsistency in your partner related to any or all of the factors listed above.

a. ______________________________
____
____

b. ______________________________
____
____

c. ______________________________
____
____

d. ______________________________
____
____

e. ______________________________
____
____

f. ______________________________
____
____

g. ______________________________
____
____

h. ______________________________
____
____

i. ______________________________
____
____

j. ______________________________
____
____

k. ______________________________
____
____

4. What do you have to do to decrease your inconsistency in your relationship? How do you contribute to this inconsistency?

____
____
____
____
____

5. What, do you guess, does your partner do in regard to his or her inconsistency? How does he or she contribute to it?

6. What do you want to do to improve your inconsistency?

   a. What have you done in the past?

   b. What would you like to do in the future?

   c. Describe in detail.

6. How did you agree to disagree and why?

7. Are issues of inconsistency hiding some more serious underlying issues within yourself or between you two?

____
____
____
____
____

Homework: During the next week, check on the two columns marked Mine and Partner's instances in which either you or your partner have been inconsistent. Also write down what made up this inconsistency, with whatever may have led to it and what happened at and after the end of that episode. Complete as many instances as there are present in your relationship.

a. Instance of inconsistency ______________________
b. Pattern ______________________
c. What led into it? ______________________
d. What happened? ______________________
e. How did it end? ______________________
f. How did you feel during and after this instance? __________

Concluding Follow-Up Form for Couple Satisfaction

Name ______________________ Sex_____Date_______

The purpose of this concluding feedback form is to review whether the practice exercises in this practice exercise were helpful to you.

1. Which answer best fits how you feel about this practice exercise?

   a. I did not like working on this practice exercise at all. I wish I never saw it. _________
   b. I did not like this practice exercise, but I am glad I got to work on it. ___________
   c. I am happy I got a chance to work on this. _________
   d. I am not only delighted about this practice exercise, but I wish all couples could get it. ___________

2. How helpful was it to work on this practice exercise? Please check the answer that applies to you.

   a. Not helpful at all ________
   b. Somewhat helpful _______
   c. Helpful _______________
   d. Very helpful ___________

3. Which practice exercise did you like best that was the most helpful to you? Rank as No. 1 the one that you liked best, rank as No. 2 the one you liked next best, and so on; mark as N/A the ones you did not like at all or did not apply to you.

Dimensions	*Rank-orders*		
	Mine	Partner	Joint
a. Affective or emotional communication	_____	_____	_____
b. Aggression	_____	_____	_____
c. Conflict over child rearing	_____	_____	_____
d. Conventionalization	_____	_____	_____
e. Disagreements over money	_____	_____	_____
f. Dissatisfaction with children	_____	_____	_____
g. Family history of distress	_____	_____	_____
h. Global distress	_____	_____	_____
i. Inconsistency	_____	_____	_____
j. Problem-solving communication	_____	_____	_____
k. Role orientation	_____	_____	_____
l. Time together	_____	_____	_____
m. Sexual dissatisfaction	_____	_____	_____

4. Explain why you have rank-ordered the practice exercises the way you did.

____
____
____
____
____
____
____
____

5. Make an appointment with your partner and write down in the appropriate column your partner's rank-orders. Discuss (compare and contrast) whatever differences you may find in your individual rank-orders.

6. After completion of this practice exercise, check which of these answers indicates how you felt about it. There is also space for you to explain further, if you want to:

   a. I did not like it at all, a waste of time. I wish I never saw this stupid practice exercise._______
   b. I did not like it very much, but I want to go on with another practice exercise._______
   c. I liked it and I want to go on with another practice exercise. _______
   d. I liked it a lot and I wish I had something like this practice exercise earlier.

   ____

e. I liked it so much that I wish all couples could get something like this practice exercise to work on. _______

7. How could this practice exercise be improved? Do you have any suggestions? Feel free to write whatever could improve this practice exercise.

____
____
____
____
____

Families

Family Profile Form (FPF)

The purpose of this practice exercise is to help your family members learn from one another rather than to change anybody's feelings, opinions, or behaviors.

Practice Exercise 1. Definitions and Examples

Name ______________________________ Sex _____ Date ________

The purpose of this practice exercise is to learn how your family sees itself along a variety of dimensions.

1. Define each dimension of family life by using a dictionary or asking other family members, friends, or relatives. For each definition give at least two examples of how that definition applies to your family.

Dimensions	*Definitions and Examples*
a. Description	Example 1: ____________
____________	____________
____________	Example 2: ____________
____________	____________
b. Evaluation	Example 1: ____________
____________	____________
____________	Example 2: ____________
____________	____________

c. Self-expression
____
____
____

Example 1: ______________________
____
Example 2: ______________________
____

d. Reflection
____
____
____

Example 1: ______________________
____
Example 2: ______________________
____

e. Touching
____
____
____

Example 1: ______________________
____
Example 2 ______________________
____

f. Brainstorming
____
____
____

Example 1: ______________________
____
Example 2: ______________________
____

g. Play
____
____
____

Example 1: ______________________
____
Example 2: ______________________
____

h. Negotiation
____
____
____

Example 1: ______________________
____
Example 2: ______________________
____

i. Role taking
____
____
____

Example 1: ______________________
____
Example 2: ______________________
____

3. Now that you have completed the definitions of these dimensions and given examples of how they apply to your family, rank-order these dimensions according to how they apply to your family. Rank as No. 1 the dimension that applies to your family the most, rank as No. 2 the dimension that applies second, and so on, down to the dimension that applies to your family very little or not at all.

Dimensions	*Rank-order*	*Dimensions*	*Rank-order*
a. Description	________	f. Brainstorming	________
b. Evaluation	________	g. Play	________

Dimensions	*Rank-order*	*Dimensions*	*Rank-order*
c. Self-expression	________	h. Negotiation	________
d. Reflection	________	i. Role taking	________
e. Touching	________		

4. Why did you rank-order these dimensions the way you did?

____
____
____
____
____

Homework: During the coming week, before you meet with your family for a family meeting, think about why you rank-ordered the dimensions listed above the way you did. If you need to change this rank-order, do so and write down why you changed it.

Standard Practice Exercise for Family Dimensions

Exercise No. ____Title of Dimension: ____________________

Name ______________________________ Sex _____Date _______

The purpose of this practice exercise is to understand more about the dimension listed in the title.

1. How does this dimension apply to your family? Explain in detail.

____
____
____
____
____

2. How often does this dimension take place in your family?

a. Practically every day	_____	e. Once every 6 months	_____
b. Once a week	_____	f. Once a year	_____
c. A couple of times a month	_____	g. Once every few years	_____
d. Once a month	_____		

3. Please explain further:

____

4. How did this dimension come about? Do you remember when it started? Check which answer fits best:

   a. When I was a child (younger than 5 years of age) _____
   b. When I was in elementary school _____
   c. When I was in middle school _____
   d. When I was in high school _____
   e. After high school _____
   f. Any other time _____

5. Please explain further:

6. Give three specific examples of how this dimension gets your family in trouble.

   Example 1:

   Example 2:

   Example 3:

Homework: Next week, in order for you to learn more about yourself and your family, plan to repeat this dimension as a family at preset, prearranged times (for instance, at 8 a.m., 12 noon, 4 or 7 p.m.) on at least 3 days (on Monday, Wednesday, and Friday, or Tuesday, Thursday, and Saturday). Write down what happened in detail. For each time make sure to answer in writing the following four questions:

a. How did you start it?
b. What followed?
c. How did it end?
d. What did this dimension get you?

Time 1 (write time you started __________)

a. ______________________________
____
____

b. ______________________________
____
____

c. ______________________________
____
____

d. ______________________________
____
____

Time 2 (write time you started __________)

a. ______________________________
____
____

b. ______________________________
____
____

c. ______________________________
____
____

d. ______________________________
____
____

Time 3 (write time you started __________)

a. ______________________________
____
____

b. ____
____
____

c. ____
____
____

d. ____
____
____

Check which of the following indicates what you got out of this practice exercise.

a. Completely useless _____
b. Somewhat useless _____
c. So-so _____
d. Somewhat useful _____
e. Extremely useful _____

Explain how you feel about this practice exercise and what you got out of it.

____
____
____
____
____

Concluding Follow-Up Form for Family Dimensions

Name ______________________ Sex _____Date ______

The purpose of this concluding follow-up form is to review whether this practice exercise was helpful to you.

1. Check the answer that best fits how you feel about this practice exercise.

   a. I did not like working on this practice exercise at all. I wish I never saw it. _____
   b. I did not like this practice exercise at all, but I am glad I got to work on it. _____
   c. I am delighted I got a chance to work on this practice exercise. _____
   d. I am not only delighted about this practice exercise, but I wish all families had a chance to work on it. _____

2. How helpful was it to work on this practice exercise? Please check the answer that applies to you.

   a. Not helpful at all _____
   b. Somewhat helpful _____
   c. Helpful _____
   d. Very helpful _____

3. Which practice exercise did you like best? Rank as No. 1 the one that you liked best, rank as No. 2 the one you liked next best, and so on, down to the one you did not like at all.

Dimensions	*Rank-order*	*Dimensions*	*Rank-order*
a. Description	________	f. Brainstorming	________
b. Evaluation	________	g. Play	________
c. Self-expression	________	h. Negotiation	________
d. Reflection	________	i. Role taking	________
e. Touching	________		

4. Which practice exercise was the most helpful to you? Sometimes what we like most is not necessarily the most helpful. Rank as No. 1 the most helpful, rank as No. 2 the next most helpful, and so on, down to the least helpful practice exercise (No. 9).

Dimensions	*Rank-order*	*Dimensions*	*Rank-order*
a. Description	________	f. Brainstorming	________
b. Evaluation	________	g. Play	________
c. Self-expression	________	h. Negotiation	________
d. Reflection	________	i. Role taking	________
e. Touching	________		

5. Why did you rank-order the practice exercises the way you did?

____

____

____

____

6. Feel free to write any comments that might improve this practice exercise.

____

____

____

____

Family Functioning

The purpose of this practice exercise is to help your family members learn from one another rather than to change anybody's feelings, opinions, or behaviors. After completing this practice exercise, get together by appointment to compare and contrast your answers with one another. See whether you can arrive at an agreement on what are the dimensions that are important to your family by adding individual rank-orders and finding those that are rank-ordered the highest by this family.

Practice Exercise 1. Definitions and Examples

Name______________________________ Sex ______Date ________

The purpose of this practice exercise is to learn how you see your family along a variety of dimensions.

1. Define each dimension of family functioning by using a dictionary or asking other family members, friends, or relatives. For each definition, give at least two examples of how that definition applies to your family.

Dimensions	*Definitions and Examples*
a. Cohesive	Example 1 ______________
______________	______________
______________	Example 2 ______________
______________	______________
b. Expressive	Example 1: ______________
______________	______________
______________	Example 2: ______________
______________	______________
c. Conflictual	Example 1: ______________
______________	______________
______________	Example 2: ______________
______________	______________
d. Intellectual-cultural	Example 1: ______________
______________	______________
______________	Example 2: ______________
______________	______________
e. Active-recreational	Example 1: ______________
______________	______________
______________	Example 2: ______________
______________	______________
f. Religious	Example 1: ______________
______________	______________
______________	Example 2: ______________
______________	______________
g. Organized	Example 1: ______________
______________	______________
______________	Example 2: ______________
______________	______________

h. Sociable

Example 1: ____________________

Example 2: ____________________

i. External control

Example 1 ____________________

Example 2 ____________________

j. Idealized

Example 1 ____________________

Example 2 ____________________

k. Disengaged

Example 1 ____________________

Example 2 ____________________

l. Democratic

Example 1 ____________________

Example 2 ____________________

m. Laissez-faire

Example 1 ____________________

Example 2 ____________________

n. Authoritarian

Example 1 ____________________

Example 2 ____________________

o. Enmeshed

Example 1 ____________________

Example 2 ____________________

3. Now that you have completed the definitions of these dimensions and given examples of how they apply to your family, rank-order these dimensions according to how they apply to your family. Rank as No. 1 the dimension that applies to your family the most, rank as No. 2 the dimension that applies second best, and so on, down to the last dimension that applies to your family very little or not at all.

Dimensions	*Rank-order*	*Dimensions*	*Rank-order*
a. Cohesive	________	i. External control	________
b. Expressive	________	j. Idealized	________
c. Conflictual	________	k. Disengaged	________
d. Intellectual-cultural	________	l. Democratic	________
e. Active-recreational	________	m. Laissez-faire	________
f. Religious	________	n. Authoritarian	________
g. Organized	________	o. Enmeshed	________
h. Sociable	________		

4. Write your reason for rank-ordering these dimensions the way you did.

____
____
____
____
____
____

Homework: During the coming week, and before your next family meeting, think about how you rank-ordered these dimensions the way you did. Write down your answer(s), and bring them to your family meeting to discuss with them.

Standard Practice Exercise for Family Functioning

Exercise No. _____Title of Dimension: ________________________

Name ______________________________Sex ______Date _______

The purpose of this practice exercise is to understand more about the dimension listed above.

1. How does this dimension get your family in trouble? Explain in detail.

____
____
____
____
____

2. How often does this dimension take place in your family?

a. Practically every day	_____	e. Once every 6 months	_____
b. Once a week	_____	f. Once a year	_____
c. A couple of times a month	_____	g. Once every few years	_____
d. Once a month	_____		

3. Please explain further:

____

____

____

____

____

4. How did this dimension come about? Do you remember when it started? Check which answer fits best:

   a. When I was a child (younger than 5 years of age) _____
   b. When I was in elementary school _____
   c. When I was in middle school _____
   d. When I was in high school _____
   e. After high school _____
   f. Any other time _____

5. Please explain further:

____

____

____

____

____

____

6. Give three specific examples of how this dimension gets your family in trouble

   Example 1

____

____

____

   Example 2

____

____

____

   Example 3

____

____

____

Homework: In the next few days, in order for you to learn more about yourself and your family ("Start it if you want to stop it!"), plan to repeat this behavior at preset times (for instance, at 8 a.m., 12 noon, 4 or 7 p.m.) on at least 3 days (on Monday, Wednesday, and Friday, or Tuesday, Thursday, and Saturday). Write down what happened in detail. For each time make sure to answer in writing the following four questions:

a. How did you start it?
b. What followed?
c. How did it end?
d. What did this behavior get you?

Time 1 (write the time you started __________)

a ______________________________
b ______________________________
c ______________________________
d ______________________________

Time 2 (write the time you started __________)

a ______________________________
b ______________________________
c ______________________________
d ______________________________

Time 3 (write the time you started__________)

a ______________________________
b ______________________________
c ______________________________
d ______________________________
____

Check which of the following shows what you got out of this practice exercise.

a. Completely useless _____
b. Somewhat useless _____
c. So-so _____
d. Somewhat useful _____
e. Extremely useful _____

Explain how you feel about this practice exercise and what you got out of it.

____
____
____
____

Concluding Feedback Form for Family Functioning

Name ______________________________ Sex _____ Date ______

The purpose of this concluding feedback form is to review whether this practice exercise was helpful to you.

1. Check the answer that best fits how you feel about this practice exercise:

   a. I did not like working on this practice exercise at all. I wish I never saw it. ____
   b. I did not like this practice exercise at all, but I am glad I got to work on it. ____
   c. I am delighted I got a chance to work on this practice exercise. ______
   d. I am not only delighted about this practice exercise but I wish all families had a chance to work on it. _____

2. How helpful was it to work on this practice exercise? Please check the answer that applies to you:

   a. Not helpful at all ____
   b. Somewhat helpful ____
   c. Helpful _____
   d. Very helpful _____

3. Which practice exercise did you like best? Rank as No. 1 the one that you liked best, rank as No. 2 the one you liked next best, and so on, down to the one you did not like at all.

Dimensions	*Rank-order*	*Dimensions*	*Rank-order*
a. Cohesive	_________	i. External control	_________
b. Expressive	_________	j. Idealized	_________
c. Conflictual	_________	k. Disengaged	_________
d. Intellectual-cultural	_________	l. Democratic	_________
e. Active-recreational	_________	m. Laissez-faire	_________
f. Religious	_________	n. Authoritarian	_________
g. Organized	_________	o. Enmeshed	_________
h. Sociable	_________		

4. Why did you rank-order order the practice exercises the way you just did?

____

____

____

____

5. Which practice exercise was the most helpful to you? Sometimes what we like most is not necessarily the most helpful. Rank as No. 1 the most helpful, rank as No. 2 the next most helpful, and so on, down to the least helpful.

Dimensions	*Rank-order*	*Dimensions*	*Rank-order*
a. Cohesive	________	i. External control	________
b. Expressive	________	j. Idealized	________
c. Conflictual	________	k. Disengaged	________
d. Intellectual-cultural	________	l. Democratic	________
e. Active-recreational	________	m. Laissez-faire	________
f. Religious	________	n. Authoritarian	________
g. Organized	________	o. Enmeshed	________
h. Sociable	________		

6. Explain why you arranged the practice exercises the way you did.

____

____

____

____

____

7. Feel free to write any comments that might improve this practice exercise.

____

____

____

____

____

Appendix A
Example of an Informed Consent Short Form[1]

I (We)____________________**(the undersigned) have been informed about the possible use of practice exercises**, either by themselves written at a distance (by mail, fax, or Internet), or as additions to other verbal, face-to-face professional approaches, such as prevention, psychotherapy, or rehabilitation. I (We) understand that this approach is still experimental and that it needs to be evaluated before being available to everybody. I am aware of the possible consequences that may be provoked by answering practice exercises at a distance. I agree to participate in this intervention with the full understanding that it may bring up painful memories in my past and that this approach, at least initially, may produce some upset in me, my partner, or my family.

I understand further that all information about me will be considered absolutely confidential because all of my writing will be between myself and the professional who is administering these written practice exercises. I can drop out from this type of intervention any time I want, and I can only disclose whatever I want at my discretion during the course of these practice exercises. If I were to become upset because of the nature of this approach, it will be up to me to deal with this upset in any way I deem satisfactory to me. First, I should discuss this upset with the professional who is administering this intervention. Second, I can discuss my upset with whomever I choose. I may keep it to myself or discuss it with friends, my clergy, or my physician.

I can answer and send my completed practice exercises through the Internet through whatever approach will guarantee absolute confidentiality. I do have the choice of using the Internet to communicate with the professional who is administering these homework practice exercise.

[1]This form is only an example. It can be changed to fit the setting and troublesome thoughts under which a practice exercise is administered.

L. L'Abate, *Sourcebook of Interactive Practice Exercises in Mental Health*, DOI 10.1007/978-1-4419-1354-8,

This professional, after proper evaluation, through either an interview or objective psychological tests, does have the option to inform me whether this approach will or will not be helpful to me. I will be informed of this option in writing.

I (We) undertake answering in writing practice exercises at a distance from a professional by my own free will and choice. I will not hold ______________________ ___________ responsible for any possible upset that may result from this intervention. Dr. (Mr. or Mrs.) ________________________is offering this intervention in good faith, using as many precautions as are humanly and professionally possible. I agree to complete in writing all practice exercises given to me until completion of an agreed-upon practice exercise and, if necessary, to be evaluated before administration and after completion of any practice exercise.

Signature of Participant(s) or Relative of Signature of Professional

*Patient*________________ Date_______ ___________________
Date________

One copy of this signed informed consent form should be kept by the patient and another copy by the professional.

Note: Do you presently use any antidepressant or mood-changing medication? If so, inform the mental health professional about this medication. Ask permission and consent from your attending physician to participate in this type of intervention. Make sure you obtain a written consent from your physician that indicates knowledge and consent for you to participate in programmed writing. Give a copy of the physician's consent to the professional. If necessary, have the mental health professional talk with your physician. In this case, you will need to give a written permission to this professional to talk with your physician.

Appendix B
General Standard Format

Practice Exercise No. ____Title of Behavior ________

Name ________________________________Sex________Date ______

The purpose of this practice exercise is to help you improve those behaviors (signs or troublesome thoughts) that were rated either 0, 1, 2, or 3 or that were rank-ordered from 1 to 6 in your first practice exercise. Usually you should not be working on more than four or five practice exercises.

1. Why does this behavior apply to you? Please explain in detail.

____
____
____
____
____

2. How often do you feel or are you aware of this behavior?
   a. Practically every day _______
   b. Once a week _______
   c. A couple of times a month _______
   d. Once a month _______
   e. Once every 6 months _______
   f. Once a year _______
   g. Once every few years _______

L. L'Abate, *Sourcebook of Interactive Practice Exercises in Mental Health*, DOI 10.1007/978-1-4419-1354-8,

3. Please explain further:

____
____
____
____
____

4. How did this behavior come about? Do you remember when you became aware of it? Check which answer fits best:
   a. When I was a child (younger than 5 years of age) _______
   b. When I was in elementary school _______
   c. When I was in middle school _______
   d. When I was in high school _______
   e. After high school _______
   f. Any other time _______

5. Please explain further:

____
____
____
____
____

6. Was this behavior acceptable or unacceptable? Why? Explain.

____
____
____
____
____

7. Give three specific examples of how this behavior affects you in the present.

   Example 1:

____
____
____
____
____

Example 2:

____

____

____

____

____

Example 3:

____

____

____

____

____

Homework: Next week, plan to write about this behavior at preset times (for instance, at 8 a.m., 12 noon, 4 or 7 p.m.) on at least 3 days (Monday, Wednesday, and Friday, or Tuesday, Thursday, and Saturday). If you can start thinking about it through writing, you might develop ways to make it stronger than it was in the past. Write down what happened in detail. For each time you start thinking about this behavior, make sure to answer in writing the following four questions:

a. How did you start thinking it?
b. What followed?
c. How did it end?
d. What did this behavior get you?

Time 1 (write the time you started__________)

a. ____

____

____

b. ____

____

____

c. ____

____

____

d. ____

____

____

Time 2 (write the time you started__________)

a. ____
____
____

b. ____
____
____

c. ____
____
____

d. ____
____
____

Time 3 (write the time you started__________)

a. ____
____
____

b. ____
____
____

c. ____
____
____

d. ____
____
____

Check which of the following indicates how you feel about this practice exercise:

a. Completely useless _______
b. Somewhat useless _______
c. So-so _______
d. Somewhat useful _______
e. Extremely useful _______

Explain in greater detail how you feel about this practice exercise and what you got out of it.

____
____
____
____

Appendix C
General Feedback Form for Practice Exercises

Name _____________________________ Sex ________ Date _______

Practice exercise _____________________ Practice Exercise No. ________

The purpose of this feedback form is to learn how this practice exercise affected you.

Now that you have completed this practice exercise, please respond to the following questions concerning it.

1. How useful did you find this task for understanding the practice exercise topic?
   a. Very useful _______
   b. Quite useful _______
   c. Somewhat useful _______
   d. Slightly useful _______
   e. Not useful at all _______

2. How important is the skill or attitude addressed by this practice exercise?
   a. Very important _______
   b. Quite important _______
   c. Somewhat important _______
   d. Slightly important _______
   e. Not important at all _______

3. Put into your own words what you got out of doing this practice exercise.

4. How could this practice exercise be improved or changed?

L. L'Abate, *Sourcebook of Interactive Practice Exercises in Mental Health*, DOI 10.1007/978-1-4419-1354-8,

Appendix D
General Concluding Feedback Form

Name ____________________________________ Sex ____ Date ____

The purpose of this form is to review whether this practice exercise was helpful to you or not.

1. Check the answer that best fits how you feel about this practice exercise:
   a. I did not like working on this practice exercise at all. I wish I never saw it. _______
   b. I did not like this practice exercise at all, but I am glad I got to work on it. _______
   c. I am delighted I got a chance to work on this practice exercise. _______
   d. I am not only delighted about working on this practice exercise, but I wish all people with anxiety had a chance to work on it. _______

2. How helpful was it to work on this practice exercise?
   a. Not helpful at all _______
   b. Somewhat helpful _______
   c. Helpful _______
   d. Very helpful _______

3. Can you explain why you liked or disliked this practice exercise?

____

____

____

____

____

L. L'Abate, *Sourcebook of Interactive Practice Exercises in Mental Health*, DOI 10.1007/978-1-4419-1354-8,

4. Which practice exercise did you like best?

5. Which practice exercise did you dislike the most?

6. If you had a choice, what kind of practice exercise would you like to work on?

7. Feel free to write any comments or suggestions that might improve this practice exercise.

Appendix E
Control/Comparison Practice Exercise

The goal of this practice exercise is to learn as much as possible about yourself. You can help by answering all the questions that will be asked in various practice exercises, to be completed at least once a week, writing for at least 20 minute for each practice exercise.

First Practice Exercise

Name ____________________________________ Sex ____ Date ____

In this practice exercise, help us to know as much as possible about your clothes, shirts, pants, jackets, coats, etc. Try to list them as you remember them from your past to the present. You can list all the clothes since you were a child to today. Try to describe each piece of clothing with as many details as possible, as if you were writing for someone who does not know and would like to know that particular piece of clothing.

1. Clothes in elementary school
   a. Every day
   b. Sunday meeting clothes and special occasions

2. Clothes in middle school
   a. Every day
   b. Sunday meeting clothes and special occasions

3. Clothes in high school or after middle school
   a. Every day
   b. Sunday meeting clothes and special occasions

L. L'Abate, *Sourcebook of Interactive Practice Exercises in Mental Health*, DOI 10.1007/978-1-4419-1354-8,

4. Clothes after high school or professional school
   a. Every day
   b. Sunday meeting clothes and special occasions

5. Clothes in college or after high school, when you started to work
   a. Every day
   b. Sunday meeting clothes and special occasions

Second Practice Exercise

Name ____ Sex ____ Date ____

In this practice exercise, help us to know all that there is to know about the furniture in your home. Try to list it all since as far back as you can remember in the past to the present. Try to write about each piece in as much detail as possible. List and write in detail about all the furniture in your home:

Your bedroom
Your parents' bedroom
Bedrooms of brothers and sisters
Bedroom of others
Kitchen
Dining room
Family room
Another room

Third Practice Exercise

Name ____ Sex ____ Date ____

Can you give us an idea of your home? Try to list all the houses (apartments) you have lived in since you can remember from the past to the present. If you can, write in detail each house (apartment) you have lived in since childhood:

List and write in detail:
The house or apartment where you live now
The house or apartment where you lived before than the present one
House or apartment of relatives (grandparents, uncles, aunts, in-laws, cousins, brothers, sisters)
A neighbor's house or apartment

Fourth Practice Exercise

Name ______________________________ Sex ____ Date ____

Write about your neighborhood in as much detail as possible, including streets, shops, industries, at least within four blocks of your house.

List and write in detail:
Roads
Churches
Shops
Schools
Gardens
Industries
Clinics or hospitals

Fifth Practice Exercise

Name ______________________________ Sex ____ Date ____

In this practice exercise, help us to know everything there is to know about your trips and vacations since your childhood to the present. Try to give years, destinations, length, and whatever else you can remember about your trips and vacation. List and write in detail about all your trips and vacations since you can remember to the present.

Sixth Practice Exercise

Name ______________________________ Sex ____ Date ____

List and write in detail about all the school or neighborhood friends you have had since you can remember. Tell in great detail all about friends as individuals and what kind of relationship you established with them.

Friends of the first order with whom you could talk freely about anything and everything

Friends of the second order with whom you were limited in talking about intimate matters

Family friends who you did not see very often and could not talk with about everything

Neighborhood friends who you were playmates with but not exactly close friends

Seventh Practice Exercise

Name ______________________________ Sex ____ Date ____

List all the states of the union with their capitals and important cities. Try to write in detail about the geography of each state, location, nature, and other details you know.

Eighth Practice Exercise

Name ______________________________ Sex ____ Date ____

List and tell about all the toys or transportation vehicles you used since childhood, starting with a tricycle, bicycle, etc., to the latest means of transportation you have used in the present.

The professional helper can choose among these practice exercises in any way or order that seems appropriate to a particular patient.

References

Aman, M. G., & Singh, N. N. (undated). *Aberrant behavior checklist (ABC): Residential and community version*. East Aurora, NY: Slosson.

American Psychiatric Association (1994). *Diagnostic and statistical manual of mental disorders* (4th ed.). Washington, DC: American Psychiatric Association Press.

Anthony, J. L., Lonigan, C. J., & Hecht, S. A. (1999). Dimensionality of posttraumatic stress disorder troublesome thoughts in children exposed to disaster: Results from confirmatory factor analysis. *Journal of Abnormal Psychology, 108*, 326–336.

Averill, J. R. (1997). The emotions: An integrative approach. In R. Hogan, J. Johnson, & S. Briggs (Eds.), *Sourcebook of personality psychology* (pp. 513–541). San Diego, CA: Academic.

Bearson, D. J., & Zimiles, H. (Eds.). (1986). *Thought and emotion: Developmental perspectives*. Hillsdale, NJ: Erlbaum.

Beltman, B. D., & Nair, J. (Eds.). (2004). *Self-awareness deficits in psychiatric participants: Neurobiology, assessment, and treatment*. New York: Norton.

Ben-Porath, Y. S. (1997). Use of personality assessment instruments in empirically guided treatment planning. *Psychological Assessment, 9*, 361–367.

Bergin, A. E., & Garfield, S. L. (Eds.). (1994) *Sourcebook of psychotherapy and behavior change*. New York: Wiley.

Blatt, S. J., Quinlan, D. M., Chevron, E. S., McDonald, C., & Zuroff, D. (1982). Dependency and criticism: Psychological dimensions of depression. *Journal of Consulting and Clinical Psychology, 50*, 113–124.

Bloom, B. L. (1985). A factor analysis of self-report measures of family functioning. *Family Process, 24*, 225–239.

Bloom, B. L. (1992). Computer-assisted psychological interventions: A review and commentary. *Clinical Psychology Review, 12*, 169–197.

Bodin, A. M. (1996). Relationship conflict – verbal and physical: Conceptualizing an inventory for assessing process and content. In F. W. Kaslow (Ed.), *Sourcebook of relational diagnosis and dysfunctional family patterns* (pp. 371–393). New York: Wiley.

Bodine, R. J., & Crawford, D. K. (1999). *Developing emotional intelligence: A guide to behavior management and conflict resolution in schools*. Champaign, IL: Research.

Bohart, A. C., & Tallman, K. (1999). *How participants make therapy work: The process of active self-healing*. Washington, DC: American Psychological Association.

Bonanno, G. A., & Keltner, D. (1997). Facial expression of emotion and the course of conjugal bereavement. *Journal of Abnormal Psychology, 106*, 126–137.

Brown, L., Black, D., & Downs, J. (1984). *School social skills (S3)*. East Aurora, NY: Slosson.

Brown, L., & Hammill, D. D. (1978). *Behavior rating profile (BRP-2)*. East Aurora, NY: Slosson.

Brown-Stanbridge, M. D. (1989). A paradigm for construction of family therapy tasks. *Family Process, 28*, 471–489.

Butcher, J. (1998). *Psychological treatment planning inventory: Test manual and interpretative guide*. San Antonio, TX: Psychological Corporation.

Cacioppo, J. T., & Gardner, W. L. (1999). Emotion. *Annual Review of Psychology, 50*, 191–214.

Campbell, L., Campbell, B., & Dickinson, D. (1999). *Teaching and learning through multiple intelligence*. Boston: Allyn & Bacon.

Chorpita, B. F., Albano, A. M., & Barlow, D. H. (1998). The structure of negative emotions in a clinical sample of children and adolescents. *Journal of Abnormal Psychology, 107*, 74–85.

Clark, L. A. (1990). Toward a consensual set of concern clusters for assessment of personality disorders. In J. H. Butcher, & C. D. Spielberger (Eds.), *Advances in personality assessment* (pp. 243–266). Hillsdale, NJ: Erlbaum.

Corrigan, P. W., Mueser, K. T., Bond, G. R., Drake, R. E., & Solomon, P. (2007). *The principles and practice of psychiatric rehabilitation: An empirical approach*. New York: Guilford.

Corrigan, P. W., Wassel, A., & Rafacz, J. (2008). An evidence-based approach to psychiatric rehabilitation. In L. L'Abate (Ed.), *Toward a science of clinical psychology: Laboratory evaluations and interventions*. Hauppauge, NY: Nova Science.

Costa, P. T. Jr., & Widiger, T. A. (1994). *Personality disorders and the five-factor model of personality*. Washington, DC: American Psychological Association.

Coyne, J. C., Thompson, R., & Palmer, S. C. (2003). Marital characteristic quality, coping with conflict, marital complaints, and affection in couples with a depressed wife. *Journal of Family Psychology, 16*, 26–37.

Cusinato, M., & L'Abate, L. (Eds.). (in press). *Advances in relational competence theory: With special attention to alexithymia*. New York: Nova Science.

Davis, R. D., & Millon, T. (1999). Models of personality and its disorders. In T. Millon, T. H. Blaney, & R. D. Davis. (Eds.), *Oxford textbook of psychopathology* (pp. 485–522). New York: Oxford.

De Giacomo, P., L'Abate, L., Pennebaker, J. M., & Rumbaugh, D. M. (2010). *Amplifications and applications of Pennebaker's analogic to digital model in health promotion, prevention, and psychotherapy*. Published in *Clinical Psychology & Psychotherapy*, 17, 355–362.

Demetrio, D., & Borgonovi, C. (2007). Teaching to remember ourselves: The autobiographical methodology. In L. L'Abate (Ed.), *Low-cost approaches to promote physical and mental health: Theory, research, and practice* (pp. 251–270). New York: Springer.

Dobson, K. S., & Craig, K. D. (Eds.). (1998). *Empirically supported therapies: Best practice in professional psychology*, Thousand Oaks, CA: Sage.

Dozois, D. J. A., Dobson, K. S., & Ahnberg, J. L. (1998). A psychometric evaluation of the Beck Depression Inventory – II. *Psychological Assessment, 10*, 83–89.

Eckhardt, C. L., Barbour, K. A., & Davison, G. C. (1998). Articulated thoughts of marital violence and nonviolent men during anger arousal. *Journal of Consulting and Clinical Psychology, 66*, 259–269.

Eckhardt, C. I., & Deffenbacher, J. L. (1995) Diagnosis of anger disorders. In H. Kassinove (Ed.), *Anger disorders: Definition, diagnosis, and treatment* (pp. 27–47). Philadelphia: Taylor & Francis.

Esterling, B. A., L'Abate, L., Murray, E., & Pennebaker, J. M. (1999). Empirical foundations for writing in prevention and psychotherapy: Mental and physical outcomes. *Clinical Psychology Review, 19*, 79–96.

Feindler, E. L. (1995). Ideal treatment package for children and adolescents with anger disorders. In H. Kassinove (Ed.), *Anger disorders: Definition, diagnosis, and treatment* (pp. 173–195). Philadelphia: Taylor & Francis.

Ferrari, J. R., Johnson, J. L., & McCown, W. G. (1995). *Procrastination and task avoidance: Theory, research, and treatment*. New York: Plenum.

Foa, U., & Foa, E. (1974). *Societal structures of the mind*. Springfield, IL: Thomas.

Fogarty, R., & Bellanca, J. (1998). *Multiple intelligences: A collection*. Boston: Allyn & Bacon.

Forgays, D. G., Forgays, D. K., & Spielberger, C. D. (1997). Factor structure of the State-Trait Anger Expression Inventory. *Journal of Personality Assessment, 69*, 497–507.

Frey, D. H., & Raming, H. E. (1979). A taxonomy of counseling goals and methods. *Personnel and Guidance Journal, 57*, 26–33.

Gardner, H. (1999). *Intelligence reframed: Multiple intelligences for the 21st century*. New York: Basic.

Goldberg, L. E. (1999). The curious experiences survey: A revised version of the dissociative experiences scale: Factor structure, reliability, and relation to demographic and personality variables. *Psychological Assessment, 11*, 134–145.

Goldberg, L. R. (1992). The development of markers for the Big-Five factor structure. *Psychological Assessment, 4*, 26–42.

Gottman, J. M. (1994). *What predicts divorce? The relationship between marital processes and marital outcomes*. Hillsdale, NJ: Erlbaum.

Gottman, J. M., Fainsilber, L., & Hooven, C. (1997). *Meta-emotion: How families communicate emotionally*. Mahwah, NJ: Erlbaum.

Greene, R. L., & Anderson, E. R. (1999). Minnesota multiphasic personality inventory (MMPI-2). In M. M. Maruish (Ed.), *The use of psychological testing for treatment planning and outcomes assessment* (pp. 1023–1050). Mahwah, NJ: Erlbaum.

Grieger, R., & Grieger, I. Z. (Eds.). (1982). *Cognition and emotional disturbance*. New York: Human Sciences.

Hartlage, S., Arduino, K., & Alloy, L. B. (1998). Depressive personality characteristics: State dependent concomitants of depressive disorder and traits independent of current depression. *Journal of Abnormal Psychology, 107*, 349–354.

Harwood, T. M., L'Abate, L. (2010). *Self-help in mental health: A critical review*. New York: Springer-Science.

Hassebrauck, M., & Fehr, B. (2002). Dimensions of relationship characteristic quality. *Personal Relationships, 9*, 253–270.

Henley, A. R. (1987). *Phobias: The crippling fears*. New York: Avon Books.

Hersen, M., & Last, C. G. (Eds.). (1990). *Sourcebook of child and adult psychopathology: A longitudinal perspective*. New York: Pergamon.

Hubble, M. A., Duncan, B. L., & Miller, S. D. (Eds.) (1999). *The heart and soul of change: What works in psychotherapy*. Washington, DC: American Psychological Association.

Hurtug, J., Audy, J. R., & Cohen, Y. A. (1998). *The anatomy of loneliness*. New York: International Universities Press.

Joiner, T. E., Jr., Steer, R. A., Beck, A. T., Schmidt, N. D., Rudd, M. D., & Catanzaro, S. J. (1999). Physiological hyperarousal: Construct validity of a central aspect of the tripartite model of depression and anxiety. *Journal of Abnormal Psychology, 108*, 290–298.

Kacewicz, E., Slatcher, R. B., & Pennebaker, J. W. (2007). Expressive writing: An alternative to traditional methods. In L. L'Abate (Ed.), *Low-cost approaches to promote physical and mental health: Theory, research, and practice* (pp. 271–284). New York: Springer.

Katz, R., Katz, J., & Shaw, B. F. (1999). Beck depression inventory and helplessness scale. In M. M. Maruish (Ed.), *The use of psychological testing for treatment planning and outcomes assessment* (pp. 831–870). Mahwah, NJ: Erlbaum.

Kazantzis, N., Deane, F. P., Ronan, K. R., & L'Abate, L. (Eds.) (2005). *Using homework assignments in cognitive behavior therapy*. New York: Routledge.

Kazantzis, N., & L'Abate, L. (Eds.). (2005). *Sourcebook of homework assignments in psychotherapy: Theory, research, and prevention*. New York: Springer.

Kelly, E. J. (1990). *Differential test of conduct and emotional problems*. East Aurora, NY: Slosson.

Kelly, E. J., & Vitali, G. J. (1992). *Conduct problem/emotional problem interventions*. East Aurora, NY: Slosson.

Kennedy-Moore, E., & Watson, J. C. (1999). *Expressing emotion: Myths, realities, and therapeutic strategies*. New York: Guilford.

King, D. W., Leskin, G. A., King, L. A., & Weathers, F. W. (1998). Confirmatory factor analysis of the clinician-administered PTSD scale: Evidence for the dimensionality of posttraumatic stress disorder. *Psychological Assessment, 10*, 90–96.

Kochalka, J., & L'Abate, L. (1997). Linking evaluation with structured enrichment: The Family Profile Form. *American Journal of Family Therapy, 25*, 361–374.

Kosson, D. S., Steuerwald, B. L., Forth, A. E., & Kirkhart, K. J. (1997). A new method for assessing the interpersonal behavior of psychopathic individuals: Preliminary validation studies. *Psychological Assessment, 9*, 89–101.

L'Abate, L. (1977a). *Enrichment: Structured interventions with couples, families, and groups*. Washington, DC: University Press of America.

L'Abate, L. (1977b). Intimacy is sharing hurt feelings: A reply to David Mace. *Journal of Marriage and Family Counseling, 3*, 13–16.

L'Abate, L. (1984). Beyond paradox: Issues of control. *American Journal of Family Therapy, 12*, 12–20.

L'Abate, L. (1986). *Systematic family therapy*. New York: Brunner/Mazel.

L'Abate, L. (1990). *Building family competence: Primary and secondary prevention strategies*. Newbury Park, CA: Sage.

L'Abate, L. (1991). The use of writing in psychotherapy. *American Journal of Psychotherapy, 45*, 87–98.

L'Abate, L. (1992). *Programmed writing: A self-administered approach for interventions with individuals, couples and families*. Pacific Grove, CA: Brooks/Cole.

L'Abate, L. (1997a). Distance writing and computer-assisted training. In S. R. Saber (Ed.), *Managed mental health care: Major diagnostic and treatment approaches* (pp. 133–163). Bristol, PA: Brunner/Mazel.

L'Abate, L. (1997b). The paradox of change: Better them than us! In R. S. Sauber (Ed.), *Managed mental health care: Major diagnostic and treatment approaches* (pp. 40–66). Bristol, PA: Brunner/Mazel.

L'Abate, L. (1997c). *The self in the family: A classification of personality, criminality, and psychopathology*. New York: Wiley.

L'Abate, L. (1999). Taking the bull by the horns: Beyond talk in psychological interventions. *The Family Journal: Counseling and Therapy for Couples and Families, 7*, 206–220.

L'Abate, L. (Ed.). (2001). *Distance writing and computer-assisted interventions in psychiatry and mental health*. Westport, CT: Ablex.

L'Abate, L. (2002). *Beyond psychotherapy: Programmed writing and structured computer-assisted interventions*. Westport, CT: Ablex.

L'Abate, L. (2003). *Family Psychology III: Theory building, theory testing, and psychological interventions*. Lanham, MD: University Press of America.

L'Abate, L. (2004a). *A guide to self-help practice exercises for clinicians and researchers*. Binghamton, NY: Haworth.

L'Abate, L. (Ed.). (2004b). *Using practice exercises in mental health: Resources in prevention, psychotherapy, and rehabilitation for clinicians and researchers*. Binghamton, NY: Haworth.

L'Abate, L. (2005). *Personality in intimate relationships: Socialization and psycho-pathology*. New York: Springer.

L'Abate, L. (2006). Toward a relational theory for psychiatric classification. *American Journal of Family Therapy, 34*, 1–15.

L'Abate, L. (2007a). A completely preposterous proposal: The dictionary as an initial vehicle of change in the family. *The Family Psychologist, 23*, 39–42.

L'Abate, L. (Ed.). (2007b). *Low-cost approaches to promote physical and mental health: Theory, research, and practice*. New York: Springer.

L'Abate, L. (2007c). Section IV: Secondary writing approaches. In L. L'Abate (Ed.), *Low-cost approaches to promote physical and mental health: Theory, research, and practice* (pp. 219–226). New York: Springer.

L'Abate, L. (2007d). What I really believe about family therapy. *Journal of Family Psychotherapy, 18*, 31–44.

L'Abate, L. (2008b). Proposal for inclusion of distance writing in couples therapy. *Journal of Relationship and Couple Therapy, 7*, 337–362.

L'Abate, L. (2008c). *The role of hurt feelings in health promotion, prevention, and psychotherapy*. Manuscript in preparation.

L'Abate, L. (Ed.). (2008d). *Toward a science of clinical psychology: Laboratory evaluations and interventions*. Hauppauge, NY: Nova Science.

L'Abate, L. (2009a). *A theory-derived structured interview for intimate relationships. The Family Psychologist*, 25, 12–14.

L'Abate, L. (2009a). *Handbook of play across the life cycle: Fun from infancy to old age*. Westport, CT: Greenwood.

L'Abate, L. (2009b). Hurt feelings: The last taboo for researchers and clinicians? In A. L. Vangelisti (Ed.), *Feeling hurt in close relationships* (pp. 479–498). New York: Cambridge University Press.

L'Abate, L. (2009c). The drama triangle: An attempt to resource a neglected pathogenic model in family therapy theory and practice. *American Journal of Family Therapy, 37*, 1–110.

L'Abate, L. Boyce, J., Fraizer, I., & Russ, D. A. (1992). Programmed writing: Research in progress. *Comprehensive Mental Health Care, 2*, 45–62.

L'Abate, L., & Cusinato, M. (2007). Linking theory with practice: Theory-derived interventions in prevention and family therapy. *The Family Journal: Counseling and Psychotherapy with Couples and Families, 15*, 318–327.

L'Abate, L., Cusinato, M., Maino, E., Colesso, W., & Scilletta, C. (2010). *Relational competence theory: Research and mental health applications*. New York: Springer-Science.

L'Abate, L., & De Giacomo, P. (2003). *Intimate relationships and how to improve them: Integrating theoretical models with preventive and psychotherapeutic approaches*. Westport, CT: Praeger.

L'Abate, L., Frey, J., & Holly, J. (1979). Intimacy is sharing hurt feelings: Comparison of three conflict resolution methods. *Journal of Marriage and Family Therapy, 5*, 35–41.

L'Abate, L., & Goldstein D. (2007). Practice exercises to promote mental health and life-long learning. In L. L'Abate (Ed.), *Low-cost approaches to promote physical and mental health: Theory, research, and practice* (pp. 285–302). New York: Springer.

L'Abate, L., & Harrison, M. G. (1992). Treating codependency. In L. L'Abate, J. E. Farrar, & D. A. Serritella (Eds.), *Sourcebook of differential treatments for addictions* (pp. 286–306). Boston: Allyn & Bacon.

L'Abate, L., & Sweeney, L. G. (Eds.). (in press). *Research on writing approaches in mental health*. Online Journal of Writting Research Amsterdam.

L'Abate, L., L'Abate, B. L., & Maino, E. (2005). A review of 25 years of part-time professional practice: Sourcebooks and length of psychotherapy. *American Journal of Family Therapy, 33*, 19–31.

L'Abate, L., Hevitt, D., & McMahan, O. (2007). An overview of paradoxical counseling and its consequence with biblical writings. *The Journal of Pastoral care & counseling, 61*, 231–242.

L'Abate, L., & Weinstein, S. E. (1987). *Structured enrichment programs for couples and families*. New York: Brunner/Mazel.

L'Abate, L. (in press-a). *Hurt Feelings: Theory, research, and applications in intimate relationships*. New York: Cambridge University Press.

L'Abate, L. (in press-b). Psychotherapy consists of homework assignments: A radical conoclastic conviction. In H. Rosenthal (Ed.), *Favorite counseling and therapy homework techniques: Classic Anniversary Edition*. New York: Routledge.

Lahey, B. B., Frick, P. J., Loeber, R., Tannenbaum, D. A., et al. (1990). *Oppositional conduct disorder: A meta-analysis review*. Unpublished manuscript. University of Georgia, Athens.

Lambert, M. J., & Whipple, J. L. (2008). Measuring and improving psychotherapy outcome: Laboratory methods in routine clinical practice. In L. L'Abate (Ed.), *Toward a science of clinical psychology: Laboratory evaluations and interventions*. Hauppauge, NY: Nova Science.

Lepore, S. J., & Smyth, J. M. (Eds.). (2002). *The writing cure: How expressive writing promotes health and emotional well-being*. Washington, DC: American Psychological Association.

Levine, M., & Calvanio, R. (2007). The recording of personal information as an intervention and as electronic health support. In L. L'Abate (Ed.), *Low-cost approaches to promote physical and mental health: Theory, research, and practice* (pp. 227–250). New York: Springer.

Levinson, H. N. (1986). *Phobia free*. New York: Evans.

Livesley, W. J., Jackson, D. N., & Schroeder, M. L. (1989). A study of the factorial structure of personality pathology. *Journal of Personality Disorders, 3*, 292–306.

Lorr, M., Youniss, R. P., & Stefic, E. C. (1991). An inventory of social skills. *Journal of Personality Assessment, 57*, 506–520.

Lynam, D. R. (1997). Pursuing the psychopath: Capturing the fledging psychopath in a nomological net. *Journal of Abnormal Psychology, 106*, 425–438.

Mascolo, M. F., & Griffin, S. (Ed.). (1998). *What develops in emotional development?* New York: Plenum.

Mash, L. J., & Barkley, R. A. (1996). *Child psychopathology*. New York: Guilford.

Mayer, J. D., & Salovey, P. (1995). Emotional intelligence and the construction and regulation of feelings. *Applied and Preventive Psychology, 4*, 197–208.

McCrae, R. R. (1994). A reformulation of Axis II: Personality and personality-related problems. In P. T. Costa & T. A. Widiger (Eds.), *Personality disorders and the five-factor model of personality* (pp. 303–309). Washington, DC: American Psychological Association.

McMahan, O., & Arias, J. (2004). Sourcebooks and psychotherapy with incarcerated felons: Replication in progress. In L. L'Abate (Ed.), *Using Sourcebooks in mental heath: Resources in prevention, psychotherapy, and rehabilitation for clinicians and researchers* (pp. 205–213). Binghamton, NY: Haworth.

McMahan, O., & L'Abate, L. (2001). Marital adjustment and programmed distance writing with seminarian couples. In L. L'Abate (Ed.), *Distance writing and computer-assisted interventions in psychiatry and mental health* (pp. 136–156). Westport, CT: Ablex.

Moras, K., Di Nardo, P. A., & Barlow, D. H. (1992). Distinguishing anxiety and depression: Reexamination of the reconstructed Hamilton scales. *Psychological Assessment, 4*, 224–227.

Morey, L. C. (1999). Personality assessment inventory. In M. E. Maruish (Ed.), *The use of psychological testing for treatment planning and outcome assessment* (pp. 1083–1122). Hillsdale, NJ: Erlbaum.

Morey, L. C., & Henry, W. (1994). Personality assessment inventory. In M. E. Maruish (Ed.), *The use of psychological testing for treatment planning and outcome assessment* (pp.185–216). Hillsdale, NJ: Erlbaum.

Mrazek, P. J., & Haggerty, R. J. (Eds.). (1994). *Reducing risks for mental disorders: Frontiers for preventive intervention research*. Washington, DC: National Academy Press.

Muller, K. L., Rego, S. A., & Sanderson, W. C. (2008). Manualized treatments in Psychotherapy. In L. L'Abate (Ed.), Toward a science of clinical psychology: Laboratory evaluations and interventions (pp. 149–160). Hauppage, NY: Nova Science Publishers.

Nathan, P. E., & Gorman, J. M. (Eds.). (1998). *A guide to treatments that work*. New York: Oxford University Press.

Newcomer, P. L., Barenbaum, E. M., & Bryant, B. R. (1994). *Depression and anxiety in youth scale*. Austin, TX: Pro-Ed.

Norcross, J. C. (2006). Integrating self-help into psychotherapy: 16 practical suggestions. *Professional Psychology: Research and Practice, 37*, 683–693.

Omer, H. (1985). Fulfillment of therapeutic tasks as a precondition for acceptance in therapy. *American Journal of Psychotherapy, 56*, 496–501.

Pennebaker, J. W., & Chung, C. K. (2008). Expressive writing, emotional upheavals, and health. In H. Friedman, & B. Silver (Eds.), *Handbook of health psychology* (pp. 263–284). New York: Oxford University Press.

Peplau, I. A., & Perlman, D. (Eds.). (1982). *Loneliness: A Sourcebook of current theory, research, and therapy*. New York: Wiley.

Perry, J. N., & Butcher, J. N. (1999). Butcher treatment planning inventory (BTPI): An objective guide to treatment planning. In M. E. Maruish (Ed.), *The use of psycho-logical testing for treatment planning and outcomes assessment* (pp. 1157–1171). Mahwah, NJ: Erlbaum.

Peterson, C., & Seligman, M. E. P. (2004). *Character strengths and virtues: A Sourcebook of classification*. New York: Oxford University Press.

Pinker, S. (2007). *The stuff of thought: Language as a window into human nature*. New York: Viking.

Pulier, M., Mount, T. G., McMenamin, J. P., & Maheu, M. M. (2007). Computers and the Internet. In L. L'Abate (Ed.), *Low-cost approaches to promote physical and mental health: Theory, research, and practice* (pp. 303–319). New York: Springer.

Reed, J. M., McMahan, O., & L'Abate, L. (2001). Sourcebooks and psychotherapy with incarcerated felons. In L. L'Abate (Ed.), *Distance writing and computer-assisted intervention in psychiatry and mental health* (pp. 157–167). Westport, CT: Ablex.

Root, L. M., & McCullough, M. E. (2007). Low-cost interventions for promoting forgiveness. In L. L'Abate (Ed.), *Low-cost approaches to promote physical and mental health: Theory, research, and practice* (pp. 415–434). New York: Springer.

Roth, A., & Fonagy, P. (1996). *What works for whom? A critical review of psychotherapy research.* New York: Guilford.

Sanford, K. (2003). Problem-solving conversations in marriage: Does it matter what topics couples discuss? *Personal Relationships, 10,* 97–112.

Schachner, D. A., & Shaver, P. R. (2004). Attachment dimensions and sexual motives. *Personal Relationships, 11,* 179–195.

Sifneos, P. E. (1973). The prevalence of "alexithymic" characteristics in psychosomatic participants. *Psychotherapy and Psychosomatic Research, 22,* 255–262.

Smyth, J. M., & L'Abate, L. (2001). A meta-analytic evaluation of Sourcebook effectiveness in physical and mental health. In L. L'Abate (Ed.), *Distance writing and computer-assisted interventions in psychiatry and mental heath* (pp. 77–90). Westport, CT: Ablex.

Snyder, C. R., & Ingram, R. E. (Ed.). (2000). *Sourcebook of psychological change: Psychotherapy processes & practice for the 21st century.* New York: Wiley.

Snyder, D. K. (1981). *Manual for marital satisfaction inventory.* Los Angeles, CA: Western Psychological Services.

Snyder, D. K., & Aikman, G. G. (1999). Marital satisfaction inventory – revisited. In M. E. Maruish (Ed.), *The use of psychological testing for treatment planning and outcome assessment* (pp. 1173–1219). Hillsdale, NJ: Erlbaum.

Spielberger, C. D., Reheiser, E. R., & Sydeman, S. J. (1995). Measuring the experience, expression, and control of anger.. In H. Kassinove (Ed.), *Anger disorders: Definition, diagnosis, and treatment* (pp. 49–67). Philadelphia: Taylor & Francis.

Sternberg, R. J. (1996). *Successful intelligence.* New York: Simon & Schuster.

Sternberg, R. J., & Kaufman, J. C. (1998). Human abilities. *Annual Review of Psychology, 49,* 479–502.

Taylor, S, Koch, K., Koch, W. J., Crockett, D. J., & Passey, G. (1998). The structure of posttraumatic stress troublesome thoughts. *Journal of Abnormal Psychology, 107,* 154–160.

Vangelisti, A. L. (Ed.). (2009). *Feeling hurt in close relationships.* New York: Cambridge University Press.

Vangelisti, A. L., & Beck, G. (2007). Intimacy and fear of intimacy. In L. L'Abate (Ed.), *Low-cost approaches to promote physical and mental health: Theory, research, and practice* (pp. 395–414). New York: Springer.

Vetter, H. (1970). *Language behavior and psychopathology.* Chicago, IL: Rand-McNally.

Weeks, G. R., & L'Abate, L. (1982). *Paradoxical psychotherapy: Theory and practice with individual couples, and families.* New York: Brunner/Mazel.

Weston, H. E., Boxer, P., & Heatherington, L. (1998). Children's attributions about family arguments: Implications for family therapy. *Family Process, 17,* 35–49.

Index

L. L'Abate, *Sourcebook of Interactive Practice Exercises in Mental Health*, DOI 10.1007/978-1-4419-1354-8,